James
Pathology

Tumors of the Bones and Joints

AFIP Atlas of Tumor Pathology

ARP PRESS

Silver Spring, Maryland

Editorial Director: Kelley A. Squazzo
Production Editor: Dian S. Thomas
Editorial/Scanning Assistant: Mirlinda Q. Caton
Copyeditor: Audrey Kahn
Scanning Technician: Kenneth Stringfellow

Available from the American Registry of Pathology
Armed Forces Institute of Pathology
Washington, DC 20306-6000
www.afip.org
ISBN 1-881041-93-X

AFIP ATLAS OF TUMOR PATHOLOGY

Fourth Series
Fascicle 2

TUMORS OF THE BONES AND JOINTS

by

K. KRISHNAN UNNI, MBBS
Consultant, Division of Anatomic Pathology, Mayo Clinic
Professor of Pathology and Orthopedic Surgery
Mayo Clinic College of Medicine
Rochester, Minnesota

CARRIE Y. INWARDS, MD
Consultant, Division of Anatomic Pathology, Mayo Clinic
Associate Professor of Pathology and Orthopedic Surgery
Mayo Clinic College of Medicine
Rochester, Minnesota

JULIA A. BRIDGE, MD
Professor of Pathology and Clinical Cytogenetics
Departments of Pathology, Pediatrics, and Orthopedic Surgery
University of Nebraska Medical Center
Omaha, Nebraska

LARS-GUNNAR KINDBLOM, MD, PhD
Department of Pathology
Göteborg University
Göteborg, Sweden

LESTER E. WOLD, MD
Consultant, Division of Anatomic Pathology, Mayo Clinic
Professor of Pathology
Mayo Clinic College of Medicine
Rochester, Minnesota

Published by the
American Registry of Pathology
Washington, DC
in collaboration with the
Armed Forces Institute of Pathology
Washington, DC
2005

AFIP ATLAS OF TUMOR PATHOLOGY

EDITORS' NOTE

The Atlas of Tumor Pathology has a long and distinguished history. It was first conceived at a Cancer Research Meeting held in St. Louis in September 1947 as an attempt to standardize the nomenclature of neoplastic diseases. The first series was sponsored by the National Academy of Sciences-National Research Council. The organization of this Sisyphean effort was entrusted to the Subcommittee on Oncology of the Committee on Pathology, and Dr. Arthur Purdy Stout was the first editor-in-chief. Many of the illustrations were provided by the Medical Illustration Service of the Armed Forces Institute of Pathology (AFIP), the type was set by the Government Printing Office, and the final printing was done at the Armed Forces Institute of Pathology (hence the colloquial appellation "AFIP Fascicles"). The American Registry of Pathology (ARP) purchased the Fascicles from the Government Printing Office and sold them virtually at cost. Over a period of 20 years, approximately 15,000 copies each of nearly 40 Fascicles were produced. The worldwide impact of these publications over the years has largely surpassed the original goal. They quickly became among the most influential publications on tumor pathology, primarily because of their overall high quality but also because their low cost made them easily accessible the world over to pathologists and other students of oncology.

Upon completion of the first series, the National Academy of Sciences-National Research Council handed further pursuit of the project over to the newly created Universities Associated for Research and Education in Pathology (UAREP). A second series was started, generously supported by grants from the AFIP, the National Cancer Institute, and the American Cancer Society. Dr. Harlan I. Firminger became the editor-in-chief and was succeeded by Dr. William H. Hartmann. The second series' Fascicles were produced as bound volumes instead of loose leaflets. They featured a more comprehensive coverage of the subjects, to the extent that the Fascicles could no longer be regarded as "atlases" but rather as monographs describing and illustrating in detail the tumors and tumor-like conditions of the various organs and systems.

Once the second series was completed, with a success that matched that of the first, ARP, UAREP, and AFIP decided to embark on a third series. Dr. Juan Rosai was appointed as editor-in-chief, and Dr. Leslie H. Sobin became associate editor. A distinguished Editorial Advisory Board was also convened, and these outstanding pathologists and educators played a major role in the success of this series, the first publication of which appeared in 1991 and the last (number 32) in 2003.

The same organizational framework will apply to the current fourth series, but with UAREP no longer in existence, ARP will play the major role. New features will include a hardbound cover, illustrations almost exclusively in color, and an accompanying electronic version of each Fascicle. There will also be increased emphasis (wherever appropriate) on the cytopathologic (intraoperative, exfoliative, and/or fine needle aspiration) and molecular features that are important in diagnosis and prognosis. What will not change from the three previous series, however, is the goal of providing the practicing pathologist with thorough, concise, and up-to-date information on the nomenclature and classification; epidemiologic, clinical, and pathogenetic features; and, most importantly, guidance in the diagnosis of the tumors and tumorlike lesions of all major organ systems and body sites.

As in the third series, a continuous attempt will be made to correlate, whenever possible, the nomenclature used in the Fascicles with that proposed by the World Health Organization's Classification of Tumors, as well as to ensure a consistency of style throughout. Close cooperation between the various authors and their respective liaisons from the Editorial Board will continue to be emphasized in order to minimize unnecessary repetition and discrepancies in the text and illustrations.

Particular thanks are due to the members of the Editorial Advisory Board, the reviewers (at least two for each Fascicle), the editorial and production staff, and—first and foremost—the individual Fascicle authors for their ongoing efforts to ensure that this series is a worthy successor to the previous three.

Steven G. Silverberg, MD
Leslie H. Sobin, MD

ACKNOWLEDGEMENTS

The authors gratefully acknowledge the assistance of many people without whose help this book would not have been possible.

Innumerable pathologists, radiologists, and orthopedic surgeons provided material through our consultation practice at Mayo Clinic. There are too many to be acknowledged individually, however, we have attempted to do so in the illustrations. The source of a few illustrations could not be identified. For this, we appologize.

Debbie Balzum originally typed the entire manuscript.

Dr. O. E. Millhouse, Margery Lovejoy, Kenna Atherton, and Roberta Schwartz from the Section of Scientific Publications at Mayo Clinic edited, formatted, and proofread the manuscript.

Many radiologists from the Department of Radiology at Mayo Clinic helped with the text, illustrations, and legends, especially Drs. J. Beabout, R. Swee, K. Cooper, M. Sundaram, D. Wenger, M. Adkins, M. Collins, P. Rouleau, and K. Amrami.

Dr. Andrew Rosenberg of the Department of Pathology at the Massachusetts General Hospital kindly provided the photomicrographs of epithelioid hemangioma.

Dr. Jorge Albores-Saavedra, who originally approached us about writing the Fascicle, helped and encouraged us.

Members of the Division of Media Support Services at Mayo Clinic did much of the work in obtaining old negatives and printing and reproducing innumerable illustrations.

Drs. Alberto Ayala and Leonard Kahn reviewed the manuscript and offered many helpful suggestions.

K. Krishnan Unni, MBBS
Carrie Y. Inwards, MD
Julia A. Bridge, MD
Lars-Gunnar Kindblom, MD, PhD
Lestor E. Wold, MD

Permission to use copyrighted illustrations has been granted by:

American Association for Cancer Research
Cancer Res 1993;53:16–8. For figure 5-102.
Clin Cancer Res 2002;8:782–7. For figure 5-103.

American Society for Investigative Pathology and Association for Molecular Pathology
J Mol Diagn 2001;3:16–21. For figures 12-14 and 12-15.

Edward Arnold Publishers
Malignant Lymphoma 2000. For Table 8-4.

Elsevier, Inc.
Cancer Genet Cytogenet 2001;124:127–31. For figure 5-13.
Hum Pathol 2000:31:306–11. For figure 4-66.

Humana Press, Inc.
Expression Profiling of Human Tumors: Diagnostic and Research Applications 2003. For figure 2-6.

John Wiley & Sons, Inc.
Genes Chromosomes Cancer 1999;26:237–46. For figure 4-85.
Genes Chromosomes Cancer 2002;33:133–40. For figure 5-125.

Journal of Bone and Joint Surgery, Inc.
J Bone Joint Surg Am 1998;80:11–7. For figure 4-87.

Lippincott Williams & Wilkins
Lab Invest 2000;80:1925–34. For figure 4-12.
Mod Pathol 1997;10:832–8. For figure 4-86.

Mayo Foundation
Dahlin's Bone Tumors: General Aspects and Data on 11,087 Cases, 5th ed., 1996. For figures 4-6, 4-36, 4-56, 4-88, 4-97, 4-98, 4-115, 8-2, 8-3, 10-26, 10-31, 10-32, 11-5, 11-8, 11-10, 12-2, 13-5, 14-23, 14-27, 14-58, 14-88, and 14-128.

Springer-Verlag
Skeletal Radiol 2000;29:63–74. For figure 10-4.

University of Chicago Press
Am J Hum Genet 1997;60:80–6. For figure 4-11.

TUMORS OF THE BONES AND JOINTS

1 INTRODUCTION

STRUCTURE OF NORMAL BONE

The skeleton serves several important functions, for which its structure is ideally suited. First, it performs a mechanical function by supporting the body and providing attachment sites for muscles and tendons that provide motion. Second, it protects vital organs and houses the bone marrow. Third, it serves as a reservoir for various minerals, especially calcium, and has a role in meeting the immediate needs of the organism for calcium (3).

Bones are divided into two main types: the flat bones of the axial skeleton (skull, scapula, clavicle, vertebra, jaw, and pelvis) and the tubular bones of the appendicular skeleton (9). Both types consist of cortical (or compact) bone and cancellous (or spongy) bone.

In a typical long bone such as the femur, the diaphysis, or shaft, is composed of cortical bone surrounding a voluminous marrow, or medullary, cavity (fig. 1-1). The epiphyses at the ends of long bones consist mostly of cancellous bone and a thin peripheral rim of cortical bone. In an immature skeleton, the epiphyses are separated from the diaphysis by the epiphyseal cartilage plates. The broad part of the long bone between the epiphyseal plate and the tubular diaphysis is termed the metaphysis. The epiphyseal cartilage and the metaphyseal portion form the growth apparatus.

The cortex of the bone consists of compact osseous tissue and the medullary cavity contains cancellous bone. Cancellous bone is made up of plates and bars that form an interconnecting network (fig. 1-2). These plates and bars are composed of varying numbers of contiguous thin layers (lamellae). The bony trabeculae are arranged along the lines of maximal pressure or tension.

The haversian system, or osteon, is the basic structural unit of cortical bone (fig. 1-3). It consists of a central haversian canal, which contains blood vessels, and lamellae of bone arranged concentrically around the central canal. The haversian canals form an anastomosing system of canals arranged along the long axis of the bone; thus, in cross section, bones appear as round openings surrounded by rings of bone. The lamellae have a large number of lacunae, which contain osteocytes and connect with one another through a series of canaliculi. The haversian canals are connected to the external surface of bone

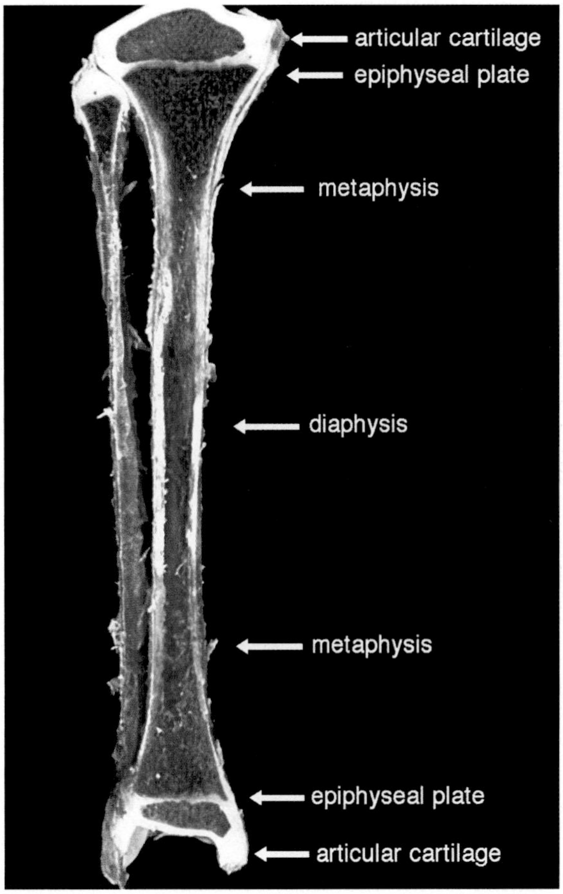

Figure 1-1

LONG BONE

The normal tibia and fibula of a 7-year-old boy illustrate the anatomy of a long bone.

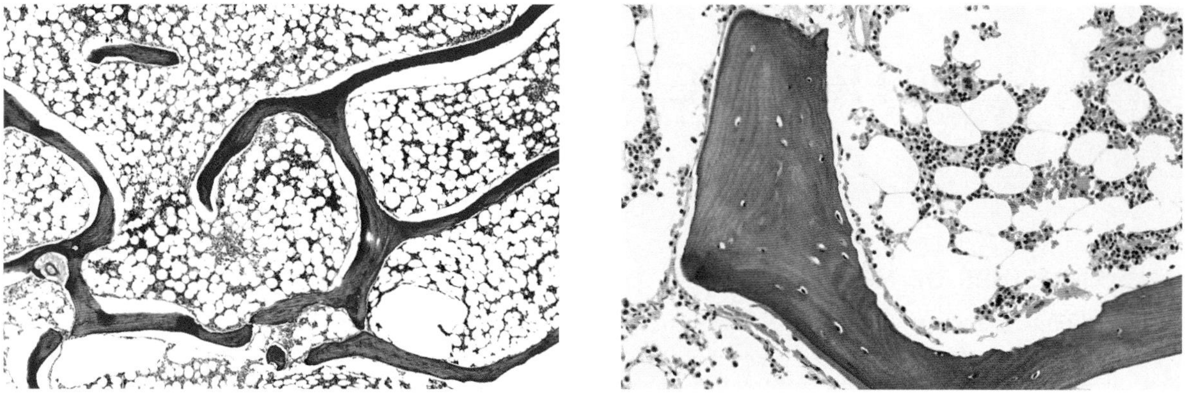

Figure 1-2

CANCELLOUS BONE

Left: An interconnecting network is created by plates and bars of lamellar bone.
Right: Higher-power view shows cancellous trabeculae surrounded by the marrow cavity containing fat and hematopoietic elements.

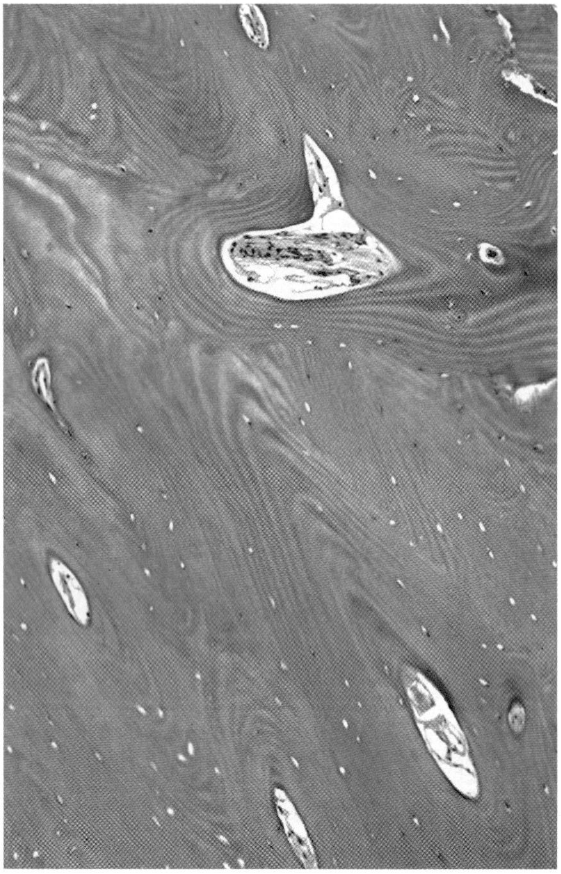

Figure 1-3

CORTICAL BONE

Dense compact cortical bone with haversian canals is surrounded by concentric lamellar bone.

and the marrow cavity through the canals of Volkmann.

Bone is covered by a connective tissue layer, the periosteum, except where it is in contact with the articular cartilage. The attachment between bone and periosteum is tight where bundles of collagen (Sharpey fibers) from the periosteum penetrate cortical bone. Large blood vessels and nerves enter the bone at these points. The periosteum has two layers: an outer layer composed of dense connective tissue and an inner cambium layer composed of loosely arranged collagen and elastic fibers and a few spindle cells. The inner aspect of the cortex is separated from the marrow space by a thin layer of connective tissue called the endosteum.

DEVELOPMENT OF BONE

Bone develops either from preexisting cartilage (endochondral ossification) or in membranous connective tissue (intramembranous ossification).

Intramembranous Ossification

The first signs of bone development are thin bars of a dense intercellular substance. The cells that remain in this meshwork are large, assume a polyhedral shape, and become osteoblasts. The cells are surrounded by a dense interstitial substance that undergoes calcification and becomes bone.

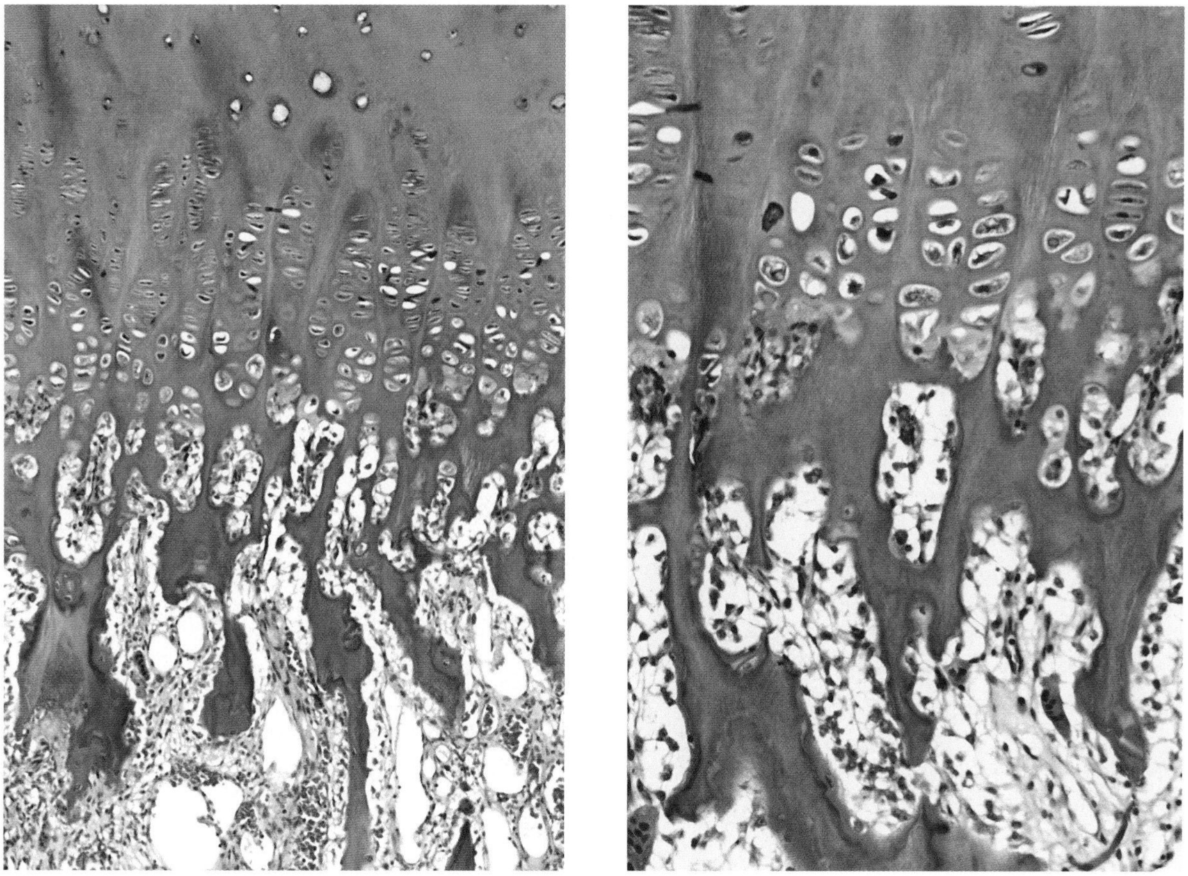

Figure 1-4

ENDOCHONDRAL OSSIFICATION

Left: Low-power appearance of an epiphyseal plate, with bone formation seen in the lower portion of the panel.
Right: Columns of cartilage cells in the zone of provisional calcification just before osteoid production.

Endochondral Ossification

Endochondral ossification is the mechanism by which long tubular bones grow in length, and is also is the process in fracture callus. The chondrocytes of the epiphyseal plate are arranged in columns, and near the metaphyseal end, they undergo hypertrophy and vacuolization of the cytoplasm and eventually become calcified (fig. 1-4). Loops of blood vessels and connective tissue invade the hypertrophic cartilage cells, which are then removed. The connective tissue cells are transformed into osteoblasts. Between the cartilage cells and osteoblasts, connective tissue becomes calcified, giving rise to columns of bone. With the cessation of longitudinal growth of bone, the epiphyseal plate disappears.

CLASSIFICATION OF BONE TUMORS

The classification of bone tumors is based on either the cytologic features of the tumor cells or the matrix produced by them (11,15). The classification system that follows is a slight modification of these two schemes. Malignant tumors rarely arise from benign ones, although it is convenient to divide tumors into benign and malignant counterparts (Table 1-1). Neoplasm simulators are discussed in chapter 14.

INCIDENCE OF BONE TUMORS

Primary tumors of bone are extremely rare, and no reliable statistics are available for the whole group. In the SEER (Surveillance, Epidemiology, and End Results) program, during 1973 to 1987, only 0.2 percent of all cancers were bone

Table 1-1

CLASSIFICATION OF BONE TUMORS[a]

Histologic Type	Total No.	Class %	Benign Tumor	Benign No. of Cases	Malignant Tumor	Malignant No. of Cases
Hematopoietic	1,788	18.8			Myeloma	986
					Lymphoma	802
Chondrogenic	2,914	30.6	Osteochondroma	946	Chondrosarcoma	1,023
			Chondroma	469	Secondary chondrosarcoma	128
			Chondroblastoma	138	Dedifferentiated chondrosarcoma	130
			Chondromyxoid fibroma	48	Mesenchymal chondrosarcoma	32
Osteogenic	2,480	26.0	Osteoid osteoma	369	Osteosarcoma	1,941
			Osteoblastoma	97	Parosteal osteosarcoma	73
Unknown	1,281	13.4	Giant cell tumor	627	Ewing's sarcoma	578
					Malignancy in giant cell tumor	36
					Adamantinoma	40
Histiocytic	99	1.0	Fibrous histiocytoma	9	Malignant fibrous histiocytoma	90
Fibrogenic	285	3.0			Desmoplastic fibroma	14
					Fibrosarcoma	271
Notochordal	411	4.3			Chordoma	411
Vascular	244	2.6	Hemangioma	131	Hemangioendothelioma	98
					Hemangiopericytoma	15
Lipogenic	10	0.1	Lipoma	8	Liposarcoma	2
Neurogenic	18	0.2	Neurilemmoma	18		
Total	9,530	100.0	Total	2,860	Total	6,670

[a]The number of cases in the Mayo Clinic files.

sarcomas (7). It has been estimated that 93,000 new cases of lung cancer and 88,000 cases of breast cancer occur annually in the United States, compared with only 1,500 cases of sarcoma of bone. Myeloma is the most common primary bone tumor, although one may argue that myelomas are tumors of bone marrow; most of them are diagnosed by biopsy of the bone marrow. In the SEER program, 35 percent of all sarcomas were osteosarcoma (however, myelomas and lymphomas were not included in that study). Chondrosarcoma and Ewing's sarcoma are the next most common types. There is a bimodal distribution, with osteosarcoma and Ewing's sarcoma occurring in the first and second decades of life and chondrosarcoma and myeloma in the older age groups.

METHODS OF BIOPSY

Diagnostic material from a bone tumor may be obtained in one of three ways: open biopsy, needle biopsy, or fine-needle aspiration (FNA).

Open Biopsy

Open biopsy is still the most common method for diagnosing bone tumors. It has the great advantage of obtaining the maximal amount of tissue. It is important to plan the biopsy so that the tract could be removed at the time of definitive surgical procedure. It is preferable for the surgeon who would perform the surgical procedure to perform the biopsy. An ill-conceived biopsy may preclude a limb salvage procedure (12). The biopsy should be planned with consultation among the radiologist, pathologist, and orthopedic surgeon.

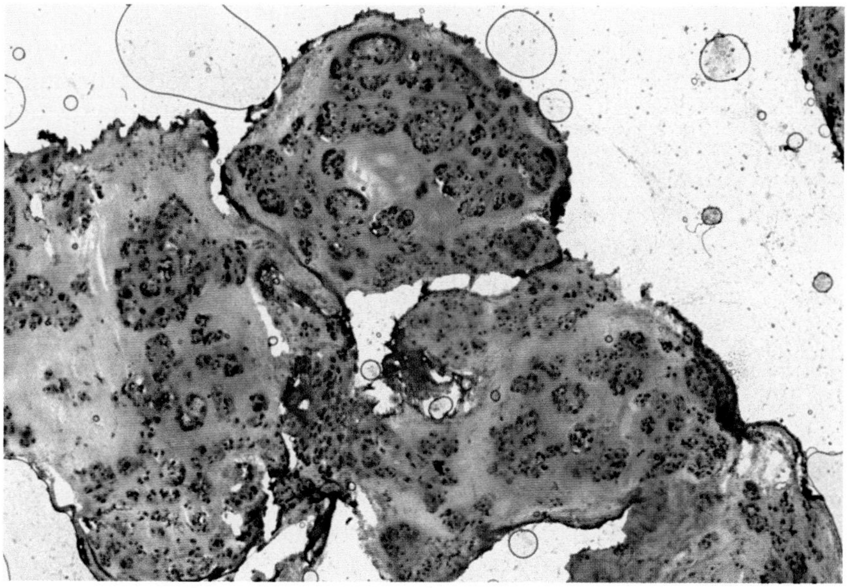

Figure 1-5

FROZEN SECTION

A hematoxylin and eosin–stained frozen section of synovial chondromatosis shows the characteristic clustering pattern of the chondrocytes.

It is important to examine the biopsy specimen before the wound is closed. Frozen sections are convenient for confirming that diagnostic material has been obtained.

Role of Frozen Sections in Diagnosis of Bone Tumors. The common misconception is that bone tumors are too hard (literally and figuratively) for frozen section diagnosis. However, if a few simple rules are followed, frozen sections can be made successfully. As with any diagnostic method (such as paraffin-embedded tissue and FNA), it is important to have good communication between the pathologist and the clinicians involved in caring for the patient. It is convenient to have the frozen section laboratory close to the surgical suites. Most bone tumors have soft material that can be used for frozen sections. The biopsy sample should be examined before the material is immersed in formalin or decalcification solution. The soft material should be separated from the bony fragments before the sample is processed. It is important to do this whether the material is used for frozen section or paraffin embedding procedures. Almost without exception, bone tumors can be processed without decalcification, and microscopic sections should be available within 24 hours.

Frozen sections can be made with either a cryostat or freezing microtome. Hematoxylin and eosin (H&E) or toluidine blue is used to stain the specimen (fig. 1-5). The nuclear details are excellent with the toluidine blue stain.

Frozen sections have several advantages over other diagnostic techniques. Perhaps the most important reason for making frozen sections is to check the adequacy of the specimen. If diagnostic tissue is received, part of it can be reserved for special studies such as microbiologic cultures, cytogenetics, and flow cytometry. Margins can be checked on frozen sections. It is not possible to check all the margins on large tumors, but those that are closest, such as the bone marrow margin, can be examined. In benign and low-grade malignant lesions, a definitive diagnosis can be made and immediate treatment instituted. With experience, a diagnosis can be based on frozen section specimens just as well as it can with paraffin sections.

Needle Biopsy

Percutaneous needle biopsy is an effective and safe technique (17) for obtaining diagnostic material from bone lesions, especially from metastatic carcinoma (2,13). Various needles have been used. The advantage over FNA is that a larger amount of tissue is obtained with a needle biopsy. Imprint cytologic preparations can also be made from the tissue.

Fine-Needle Aspiration Biopsy

The technique of FNA biopsy was pioneered eight decades ago by Ewing, Coley, Martin, and Ellis at Memorial Sloan-Kettering Cancer Center in New York City. Despite the accumulation of extensive experience with FNA worldwide, particularly in Scandinavia, many centers have not adopted it as a standard part of the diagnostic work-up of bone lesions.

The interpretation of FNA specimens of bone has problems similar to those of a histologic diagnosis based on open biopsy. However, the scarcity of morphologic material, the loss of certain architectural features, and the introduction of artifacts unique to FNA probably account for some of the reluctance of many centers to incorporate it into their routine diagnostic repertoire. Moreover, the accurate interpretation of FNA specimens of bone lesions requires a high degree of expertise within the specialty area, but this expertise is sparse because of the relative rarity of bone tumors, their wide morphologic spectrum, and diagnostic pitfalls. FNA findings must be interpreted in the context of the clinical and radiographic findings. Hence, FNA of bone lesions should be performed at medical centers that have experience and expertise in the diagnosis and treatment of musculoskeletal tumors. If FNA is performed in this setting, it is useful in most cases for determining whether a bone lesion is primary or metastatic, benign or malignant, and a low-grade or high-grade neoplasm. In many cases, a specific diagnosis can be suggested. The technique is particularly useful for rapidly distinguishing among primary bone tumor, metastasis, myeloma, and lymphoma. The technical aspects of performing FNA on bone lesions has been described in detail elsewhere (4,10,16,19,20).

Palpable lesions that have cortical thinning or breakthrough are easily aspirated, in most instances, with a 0.7- to 0.9-mm needle (20–22 gauge). Nonpalpable lesions with an intact cortex require a cutting needle or Tru-cut instrument as a leader for the needle; these biopsies usually are performed under the guidance of computerized tomography (CT) or other imaging techniques. Several aspirations are ideal to ensure that representative material has been obtained. May-Grünwald-Giemsa and H&E stains are preferable to the Papanicolaou stain for bone lesions because they enhance the matrix component of the lesion, which is critical in evaluating the lesion. Aspirates may be useful for performing routine histochemical stains, immunohistochemistry, DNA ploidy studies, fluorescence in situ hybridization studies, and the polymerase chain reaction as well as for tissue culture and karyotyping (provided the number of cells is adequate for the latter two studies). Also, aspirated material can be used for traditional light and electron microscopic studies.

HANDLING OF SPECIMENS

A special laboratory is not needed to handle gross specimens of bone lesions. At Mayo Clinic, the gross specimen is examined in the frozen section laboratory, which is adjacent to the surgical suites. The gross specimen may take the following forms.

Incisional Biopsy. It is important for the surgeon to take the biopsy specimen from the soft regions of the lesion. In instances of osteosarcoma, this usually involves the soft tissue extension. It rarely is necessary to take a biopsy specimen from the intraosseous component, which is usually more heavily mineralized.

Excisional Biopsy. In the case of bone tumors, excisional biopsy specimens usually are removed by curettage. If the specimen contains fragments of bone, the fragments should be separated from the tumor before the specimen is sectioned. No hard and fast rules exist for how many sections should be taken from any tumor. Areas that grossly appear to be different should be sampled.

Resection. Most patients who have high-grade sarcomas have preoperative chemotherapy, and the bone containing the tumor is resected. The specimen consists of the segment of bone with the surrounding soft tissue. An ellipse of skin containing the biopsy tract is also usually removed.

There are two ways to handle these specimens. First, the dissection can be performed immediately. All the soft tissue is dissected away, leaving the tumor with the involved bone. It is best to slice the bone open along the longitudinal axis, through the middle of the marrow cavity. The bone can be opened with either a band saw or butcher's meat saw (fig. 1-6). If the latter is used, the specimen has to be held in a vise. The cut surface should be washed with a brush (e.g., surgical scrub brush) under running water. This removes the bone dust from the specimen, thus reducing artifact. The surgeon usually sends a separate sample of bone marrow from the bony margin or margins. These can be checked by frozen section evaluation. It is not possible to

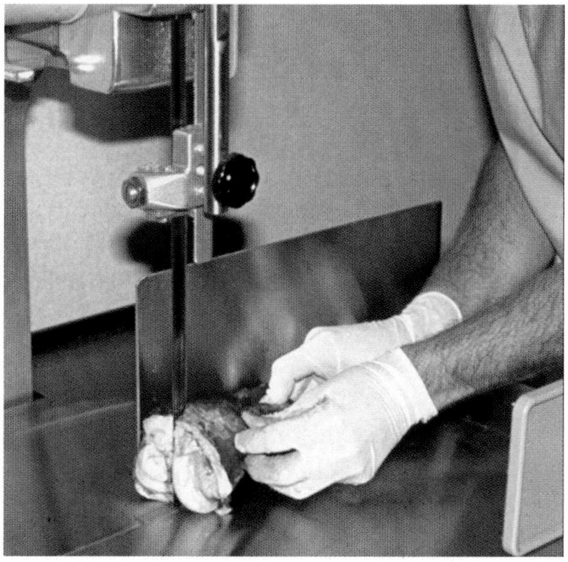

Figure 1-6

BAND SAW

A band saw is used to cut longitudinally through a resected femur.

use frozen sections to check all the radial margins of a large tumor. However, if the surgeon is concerned about a specific margin, such as the neurovascular bundle, it can be checked separately. This technique has several advantages: the margins can be checked grossly immediately; if necessary, tissue can be saved for special studies, such as cytogenetics; and gross photographs appear more natural when the tissue is not frozen.

The second method for handling resection specimens is to freeze the entire specimen until it becomes hard enough that it can be sliced open in its entirety. This has the advantage of keeping the gross contours of the tumor intact, including the relationships with other structures. However, it has the disadvantage of delay.

Decalcification

Several techniques are available for decalcifying bone specimens. Whatever method is used, it is important to saw the bone into thin slices to hasten decalcification. Thick cortical bone rarely needs to be decalcified for diagnostic purposes. Decalcifying it will only delay in making the sections. The slice should be washed to remove bone dust.

A practical method is to use a solution of 20 percent formic acid and 10 percent formalin, which is made by mixing 400 ml of formic acid in 1,600 ml of 10 percent formalin. The specimen should be checked frequently with a pair of forceps to avoid overdecalcification. Specimens without cortical bone are ready for sectioning within 24 hours. Other specialized decalcification solutions, such as ethylenediaminetetraacetic acid (EDTA), are available but not necessary for routine work. The addition of caustic acids has no advantage.

Assessment of Chemotherapy Effect

Most patients with high-grade sarcomas, especially osteosarcoma, are treated routinely with neoadjuvant chemotherapy before surgical removal of the neoplasm. Several studies (1,14) have shown a correlation between the effect of chemotherapy and survival. Hence, it is necessary to evaluate the extent of necrosis after chemotherapy. The gross specimen is dissected as described above, and the bone is cut along its longitudinal axis. One thin slice of the entire bone with tumor is obtained. This slice is put in a clear plastic bag and "photographed" on a photocopier. The photocopy image can be used as a template. The entire slice is decalcified. Decalcification may take several days because of cortical bone. When the bone is soft enough, it is cut into several smaller blocks, which should be numbered sequentially. These numbers are marked on the photocopy so that the location of each block can be identified. The number of blocks depends on the size of the tumor.

The effect of chemotherapy can take several forms. 1) The tumor is replaced with new bone formation. The marrow spaces, where the tumor was present, are filled with new bone. Malignant cells may or may not be present in the sclerotic bone; this is the feature that determines whether the tumor is viable. One problem is that osteoblastic osteosarcomas can have the same pattern, and it is impossible to decide whether the sclerotic bone is a result of chemotherapy. 2) The ghost outlines of the original neoplasm with infarct-like necrosis are present. 3) The part of the bone marrow containing the tumor is replaced with a proliferation of loosely arranged vessels and spindle cells. Frequently, there are collections of hemosiderin-containing histiocytes. It usually is possible to discern where the tumor was and where normal marrow is present.

The areas of viable tumor are identified with the microscope. Areas with viable tumor can be mapped on the photocopy image of the gross specimen and the amount of persistent tumor calculated. It is not always possible to be certain about the viability of some areas of the tumor. In spite of this problem, many studies have shown (1,14) that evaluation of response to chemotherapy is prognostically important. As recent studies have shown (1,14), it is only necessary to establish whether 95 percent or more of the tumor is viable. It has also been suggested that any residual viable tumor is important prognostically and, hence, it is only necessary to decide whether 99 percent or more of the tumor is necrotic.

GRADING OF BONE TUMORS

Grading is an attempt to predict the biologic behavior of a tumor on the basis of its histologic appearance. Many techniques of molecular biology are used to predict prognosis when a malignancy is diagnosed. Microscopic grading, however, is the basic attempt to describe the malignancy of a tumor. Interest has resurged in the histologic grading of tumors, and grading systems have proliferated which are unique to organs and even to specific tumors of an organ.

The grading system used at Mayo Clinic is based on the technique first described by Broders (5) while studying squamous cell carcinoma of the lip. He described four grades, depending on the "differentiation" of the tumor cells. Tumor cells were considered "differentiated" or "undifferentiated" on the basis of how similar or dissimilar their appearance was to that of normal precursor cells. This concept was similar to "anaplasia" described by Von Hansemann (18). The four grades were described as follows: grade 1, 0 to 25 percent of the cells are undifferentiated; grade 2, 25 to 50 percent of the cells are undifferentiated; grade 3, 50 to 75 percent of the cells are undifferentiated; and grade 4, 75 to 100 percent of the cells are undifferentiated. Broders showed a correlation between histologic grade of the tumor and survival of the patient.

Originally, Broders described this grading system for squamous cell carcinoma, but he later applied it to other epithelial malignancies. There is no logical reason why the principles cannot be applied to grading sarcomas.

Sarcomas of bone are graded predominantly on the basis of two features: cytologic atypia (anaplasia) and cellularity. Mitotic figures usually are more common in high-grade tumors, as is necrosis. Most sarcomas are diagnosed with a small biopsy sample; hence, necrosis and mitotic figures are hard to evaluate, but cytologic atypia is not. Grading requires that tumors show histologic variability. For example, one of the distinguishing features of Ewing's sarcoma is the uniformity of the cells in a tumor and between different tumors. Thus, Ewing's sarcoma cannot be graded. Studies have shown that histologic grading is not useful for chordoma, adamantinoma, or myeloma. It is helpful to grade chondrosarcomas, malignant vascular tumors, and spindle cell sarcomas of all kinds.

Grading is subjective, but this deficiency is not unique to the system described by Broders. The same caveat applies to reproducibility. Nevertheless, the results of each grading system have been shown to correlate with prognosis.

STAGING OF BONE TUMORS

Although a radiologic staging system for benign bone tumors has been proposed (and may be helpful in planning surgical management) (6), this section considers only the staging of sarcomas. The system that is used almost universally by musculoskeletal oncologists is that of Enneking et al. (8), which takes into account the histologic grade and anatomic extent of the neoplasm. Tumors are considered to occur in anatomic compartments. A sarcoma confined to the bone is intracompartmental; it is extracompartmental if it extends into soft tissues.

Sarcomas are graded as high-grade (grades 3 and 4) and low-grade (grades 1 and 2) tumors. The histologic grade and the anatomic description of the tumor are combined to define the stage: stage 1A—low-grade, intracompartmental; stage 1B—low-grade, extracompartmental; stage 2A—high-grade, intracompartmental; stage 2B—high-grade, extracompartmental; and stage 3—distant metastasis regardless of other factors.

This staging system also includes a description of surgical margins: 1) radical—the entire compartment involved by the tumor is removed; 2) wide—the tumor is removed with surrounding normal tissue, and the "reactive zone" (composed of the fibrovascular

Table 1-2

TNM CLINICAL CLASSIFICATION

T Primary Tumor			
TX	Primary tumor cannot be assessed		
T0	No evidence of primary tumor		
T1	Tumor 5 cm or less in greatest dimension	T1a	Superficial tumor
		T1b	Deep tumor
T2	Tumor more than 5 cm in greatest dimension	T2a	Superficial tumor
		T2b	Deep tumor

N Regional Lymph Nodes	NX	Regional lymph nodes cannot be assessed
	N0	No regional lymph node metastasis
	N1	Regional lymph node metastasis
M Distant Metastasis	MX	Distant metastasis cannot be assessed
	M0	No distant metastasis
	M1	Distant metastasis
G Histopathologic Grade	GX	Grade cannot be assessed
	G1	Well differentiated
	G2	Moderately differentiated
	G3	Poorly differentiated
	G4	Undifferentiated

Stage Grouping

Stage IA	Low-grade, small, superficial, deep	G1, T1a-b	N0	M0
Stage IB	Low-grade, large, superficial	G1-2, T2a	N0	M0
Stage IIA	Low-grade, large, deep	G1-2, T2b	N0	M0
Stage IIB	High-grade, small, superficial, deep	G3-4, T1a-b	N0	M0
Stage IIC	High-grade, large, superficial	G3-4, T2a	N0	M0
Stage III	High-grade, large, deep	G3-4, T2b	N0	M0
Stage IV	Any metastasis	Any G, any T	N1	M0
		Any G, any T	N0	M1

pseudocapsule) is removed intact; 3) marginal—the tumor is removed entirely, but the incision goes through the reactive zone; and 4) intralesional—the tumor is not removed intact, and margins are involved.

The TNM classification is given in Table 1-2.

REFERENCES

1. Ayala AG, Murray JA, Erling MA, Raymond AK. Osteoid-osteoma: intraoperative tetracycline-fluorescence demonstration of the nidus. J Bone Joint Surg Am 1986;68:747–51.
2. Ayala AG, Raymond AK, Ro JY, Carrasco CH, Fanning CV, Murray JA. Needle biopsy of primary bone lesions. M.D. Anderson experience. Pathol Annu 1989;24:219–51.
3. Bloom W, Fawcctt DW. A tcxtbook of histology, 8th ed. Philadelphia: WB Saunders; 1962:153–86.
4. Bommer KK, Ramzy I, Mody D. Fine-needle aspiration biopsy in the diagnosis and management of bone lesions: a study of 450 cases. Cancer 1997;81:148–56.
5. Broders AC. Squamous cell epithelioma of the lip. A study of 537 cases. JAMA 1920;74:656–64.
6. Campanacci M. Bone and soft tissue tumors: clinical features, imaging, pathology and treatment, 2nd ed. Padova, Italy: Piccin Nuova Libraria; 1999:1131.
7. Dorfman HD, Czerniak B. Bone cancers. Cancer 1995;75(Suppl):203–10.
8. Enneking WF, Spanier SS, Goodman MA. A system for the surgical staging of musculoskeletal sarcoma. Clin Orthop 1980:106–20.

9. Fechner RE, Mills SE. Tumors of the bones and joints. Atlas of Tumor Pathology, 3rd Series, Fascicle 8. Washington, DC: Armed Forces Institute of Pathology; 1993:1–16.
10. Kreicbergs A, Bauer HC, Brosjo O, Lindholm J, Skoog L, Soderlund V. Cytological diagnosis of bone tumours. J Bone Joint Surg Br 1996;78:258–63.
11. Lichtenstein L. Classification of primary tumors of bone. Cancer 1951;4:335–41.
12. Mankin HJ, Lange TA, Spanier SS. The hazards of biopsy in patients with malignant primary bone and soft-tissue tumors. J Bone Joint Surg Am 1982;64:1121–7.
13. Murphy WA, Destouet JM, Gilula LA. Percutaneous skeletal biopsy 1981: a procedure for radiologists—results, review, and recommendations. Radiology 1981;139:545–9.
14. Onikul E, Fletcher BD, Parham DM, Chen G. Accuracy of MR imaging for estimating intraosseous extent of osteosarcoma. AJR Am J Roentgenol 1996;167:1211–5.
15. Schajowicz F, Sissons HA, Sobin LH. The World Health Organization's histologic classification of bone tumors. A commentary on the second edition. Cancer 1995;75:1208–14.
16. Snyder RE, Coley BL. Further studies on the diagnosis of bone tumors by aspiration biopsy. Surg Gynecol Obstet 1945;80:517–22.
17. Stoker DJ, Cobb JP, Pringle JA. Needle biopsy of musculoskeletal lesions. A review of 208 procedures. J Bone Joint Surg Br 1991;73:498–500.
18. Von Hansemann HD. Cited by Broders AC. The microscopic grading of cancer. In: Pack GT, Livingston EM, eds. Treatment of cancer and allied diseases: by one hundred and forty-seven international authors, vol. 1. New York: Paul B. Hoeber; 1940:19–41.
19. Willems JS. Aspiration biopsy cytology of soft tissue tumors. In: Linsk JA, Franzén S, eds. Clinical aspiration cytology. Philadelphia: JP Lippincott; 1983:219–347.
20. Willen H. Fine needle aspiration in the diagnosis of bone tumors. Acta Orthop Scand Suppl 1997;273:47–53.

2 GENETICS OF BONE TUMORS

INTRODUCTION

The pathogenesis of cancer is a multistep process stemming from somatic mutations that impair the regulation of normal cell development, cell proliferation, and other fundamental cellular activities. The elucidation of this process has been challenging because the genetic events are unique for different tumor categories. Enormous progress has been achieved, however, with the advancement of cytogenetic and molecular genetic techniques. As a result, relevant oncogenes and tumor suppressor genes have been identified and localized. Further new gene constructs and their protein products resulting from translocations during sarcomagenesis have been determined. The identification of tumor-specific genetic markers for bone tumors such as Ewing's sarcoma has added a new dimension to the formulation of a diagnosis and the resolution of cellular origin. Many of the genetic markers have proved to have prognostic value, and studies are under way to determine their potential applications as specific therapeutic targets.

BASIC PRINCIPLES OF CANCER CYTOGENETICS

Cancer cytogenetics dawned in 1956 when Tjio and Levan (63) published what eventually proved to be the correct number of human chromosomes. In 1960, the first consistent karyotypic abnormality in a human neoplastic disorder, the Philadelphia (Ph) chromosome in chronic myelogenous leukemia, was discovered (41). The discovery of other tumor-associated chromosomal abnormalities, however, was slow because examination of different malignancies, such as commonly occurring carcinomas, revealed numerous anomalies of a seemingly random and chaotic nature. Moreover, human chromosomes could be distinguished only by their gross morphologic features of overall size and centromere location.

Propitiously, the situation changed dramatically in 1970 with the advent of chromosomal banding techniques (10). This completely revolutionized cytogenetic analysis. With this major breakthrough, each chromosome could be identified precisely by its unique alternating light and dark staining pattern. With banding analysis, an increasing number of cytogenetically aberrant benign and malignant neoplasms (including primary bone tumors) have been reported; over 45,000 karyotypically abnormal cases have been documented in an extraordinary database compiled by Mitelman et al. in 2004 (39).

CYTOGENETIC ANALYSIS

Specimen Requirements

For cytogenetic analysis tissue must be fresh (not frozen or fixed in formalin) because living, dividing cells are required. A sample of bone tumor submitted for cytogenetic analysis should be representative of the neoplastic process and preferably be part of the specimen submitted for pathologic study. Ideally, 1 to 2 cm^3 (approximately 0.5 to 1.0 g) of a fresh sample is provided for analysis (41,59). Also, small biopsy specimens or fine-needle aspirates (less than 500 mg) can be analyzed successfully, but prolonged culture may be needed to produce enough cells for examination (10). Necrotic tissue and nonneoplastic tissue should be dissected from the sample. The tumor tissue should be transported to the laboratory in sterile culture media or buffer solution (such as Hank's buffered salt solution) as soon as possible after surgical removal. Specimens sent over long distances (requiring 24 to 48 hours for delivery) to cytogenetic laboratories can be transported at room temperature or refrigerated (not frozen) in sterile isotonic saline or, preferably, culture media containing serum.

Cell Culture and Chromosome Banding

Generally, successful cytogenetic analysis of a primary bone tumor is more difficult to achieve than analysis of a soft tissue tumor.

Difficulties encountered with bone tumors include low cell density and the release of cells from the bone matrix. The basic process of cell culturing is the same for all bone lesions. Briefly, sterile tumor tissue is minced mechanically with scissors or a scalpel and enzymatically disaggregated by incubation in collagenase (33). The resulting single cells and small cell clusters are washed, diluted in culture medium, and allocated to tissue culture flasks, chamber slides, or coverslips. Standard culture media preparations such as RPMI 1640 supplemented with fetal bovine serum are used most commonly. To minimize contamination, a low concentration of antibiotics and antimycotics is added to the media (36,52).

The tissue cultures are incubated at 37°C with 5 percent CO_2 and inspected daily under an inverted microscope for growth. When an optimal number of mitoses is observed, the proliferating cells are arrested in mid-division with the addition of colchicine to block the assembly of the mitotic spindle. The time that a bone tumor may be cultured to attain satisfactory karyotypic findings varies depending on the histopathologic type, grade of tumor, tumor cellularity, and size of specimen submitted for analysis. A short-term culture usually results in a sufficient number of mitoses in 10 days or less. Lengthy culture times should be avoided because undesired overgrowth by normal fibroblasts is more likely to occur.

An alternative to tissue culture is direct harvest. With this technique, endemic dividing cells are arrested after a 1- to 12-hour incubation period in colchicine and culture medium. This method is useful for obtaining fast or preliminary results but is limited by the in vivo mitotic index (15). Thus, direct harvest is most useful for high-grade tumors. Also, for best success, it is imperative that the laboratory receive the tissue sample within 1 hour after biopsy.

Chromosomes, as they appear in a metaphase spread, consist of tightly coiled DNA and protein. A karyotype is the somatic chromosomal complement of an individual or species. For humans, the normal karyotype consists of 46 chromosomes aligned in a standard sequence according to size, centromere location, and banding pattern. A karyotype can be produced by photographing a metaphase spread under a microscope, manually cutting out the chromosomes from the photograph, and arranging and pasting them in order. Automated or computerized systems have been developed to facilitate analysis by eliminating the need for photography and manual preparation (6,52).

The karyotype is one of the basic tools of cytogeneticists. Certain properties of the chromosomes are identified to assist in distinguishing each pair. The primary constriction of a chromosome, the centromere, divides the chromosome into a short (upper) arm and a long (lower) arm, designated p (petit) and q, respectively. G-banding is the most common form of banding because of the relative ease of performing the technique, the reliability of the results, and the permanence of the preparations. G-bands can be visualized with Giemsa or Wright stain by pretreating the slide with trypsin or phosphate buffer, respectively. The number of alternating light and dark bands detectable with G-banding in the haploid genome varies with the level of chromosomal contraction in each metaphase cell, but it is in the range of 350 to 550 bands per haploid set. One band represents approximately 5 to 10 x 10^6 base pairs (bp) of DNA. A relationship exists between the different types of bands and gene density, base composition, and replication time; however, the functional basis for the interdependence of these features of chromosome structure and behavior is not known.

Nomenclature

An international system for designating bands in human chromosomes was introduced at a 1971 conference in Paris (44). In this system, the short and long arms are divided into several regions, each defined as an area of chromosome lying between two adjacent landmarks. Landmarks are consistent and distinct morphologic features important for identifying chromosomes. (Strictly, landmarks, like bands, are features of staining rather than morphologic features.) Regions are numbered consecutively from the centromere to the telomere (distal end of a chromosome) on each arm; within each region, the individual bands are numbered in the same direction. Thus, the complete designation of a band consists of the chromosome number, a letter to indicate the short or long

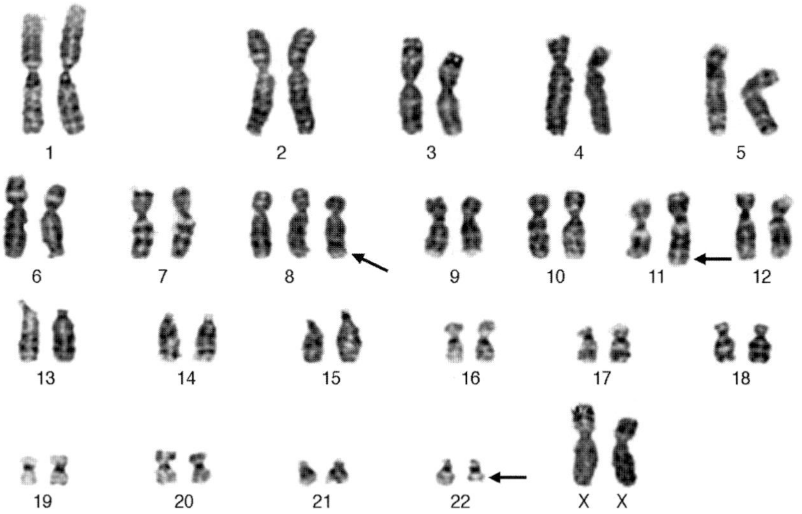

Figure 2-1

NOMENCLATURE USED TO DESIGNATE ABNORMALITIES IN A REPRESENTATIVE G-BANDED KARYOTYPE OF EWING'S SARCOMA: 47,XX,+8,t(11;22)(q24;q12)

Arrows show the presence of an extra copy of chromosome 8 and the translocation occurring between chromosomes 11 and 22.

arm, a number for the region, and a number for the band and subband; for example, Xp11.2 refers to the short arm of chromosome X, region 1, band 1, subband 2.

The two major types of chromosomal abnormalities are numerical and structural. Numerical abnormalities manifest as changes in complete sets of chromosomes (i.e., triploid [3N] or tetraploid [4N] complements) or in the number of individual chromosomes (i.e., loss of a single chromosome [monosomy] or gain of a single chromosome [trisomy]). Structural abnormalities of chromosomes result from chromosomal breakage and rejoining of the broken ends to form new combinations. A frequently observed structural abnormality is translocation. In a reciprocal translocation, chromosomal material is exchanged between two or more nonhomologous chromosomes. An example of the shorthand system used to describe numerical and structural aberrations is 47,XX,+8,t(11;22)(q24;q12), in which 47 indicates the total chromosome number, XX indicates the sex constitution, and +8 indicates an extra copy, trisomy, of chromosome 8 (fig. 2-1). The "t" is an abbreviation for translocation and in this example specifies an exchange of chromosomal material between the long arms of chromosomes 11 and 22 at bands q24 and q12, respectively. The 11;22 translocation is a characteristic rearrangement in Ewing's sarcoma, and trisomy 8 is a frequent secondary anomaly in this neoplasm. Aspects of the nomenclature and symbols likely to be encountered in most articles that discuss cancer cytogenetics are presented in Table 2-1. For more information, the International System for Human Cytogenetic Nomenclature (38) should be consulted.

MOLECULAR CYTOGENETICS

A revolutionary tool in the analysis and characterization of chromosomes and chromosomal abnormalities is the technique of in situ hybridization. Hybridization refers to the binding or annealing of complementary DNA or RNA sequences that serve as probes. With this approach, specific nucleic acid sequences can be detected in morphologically preserved chromosomes, cells, or tissue sections.

Molecular cytogenetic assays typically are performed with chromosome-specific probes labeled with fluorescent dyes such as fluorescein and rhodamine, and detected with fluorescence microscopy (fluorescence in situ hybridization [FISH]). Alternatively, hybridization signals can be detected with peroxidase or alkaline phosphatase, but these approaches are generally less sensitive.

Specimen

Traditional cytogenetic analysis depends on the success of tumor growth in culture and the production of quality metaphase preparations. A major advantage of FISH is that specific DNA target sequences can be detected in the nuclei of nondividing (i.e., interphase) cells. Thus, this technique can be performed on fresh or aged

Table 2-1

ABBREVIATIONS AND DEFINITIONS USED IN CYTOGENETICS

Abbreviation	Term
del	Deletion, or loss, of a chromosome segment Example: del(8)(q24) = deletion of band 24 located on the long arm of chromosome 8
der	Structurally abnormal chromosome created by the rearrangement of two or more chromosomes or more than one rearrangement in the same chromosome Example: der(22)t(11;22)(q24;q12) = replacement of one normal chromosome 22 by an unbalanced translocation product involving chromosomes 11 and 22
dup	Duplication, a replicated or duplicated chromosome segment next to itself; if in the same orientation = direct duplication (dir dup); if inverted = inverted duplication (inv dup) Example: dup(12)(q13q15) = direct duplication of the segment between bands 12q13 and 12q15
i	Isochromosome, a symmetric chromosome composed of duplicated long or short arms formed after misdivision of the centromere in a transverse plane Example: i(3)(p10), duplication of the short arm of chromosome 3 with loss of the long arm
ins	Insertion, a chromosomal segment from one chromosome is inserted into a nonhomologous chromosome; similar to a duplication, an insertion can be direct or inverted Example: dir ins(10;12)(q22;q13q14) = a direct insertion of the chromosomal segment of the long arm of chromosome 12(q13-14) into chromosome 10 at q22
inv	Inversion, a segment of a chromosome is reversed 180 degrees; a paracentric inversion does not involve the centromere in the inversion, a pericentric inversion does (a break in each chromosomal arm is necessary) Example: inv(12)(p12q13) is a pericentric inversion involving the centromere of chromosome 12
p	Short arm of a chromosome (from French "petit")
q	Long arm of a chromosome (letter following "p")
t	Translocation, an exchange of chromosomal material between two or more nonhomologous chromosomes (may be balanced or unbalanced); a robertsonian translocation involves acrocentric chromosomes with fusion at the centromere and loss of the short arms and satellites Example: t(11;22)(q24;q12) denotes a reciprocal translocation involving breaks at band q24 on the long arm of chromosome 11 and at band q12 on the long arm of chromosome 22, with exchange of the segments distal to those breakpoints
+	Added chromosome (+7) or chromosomal segment (7q+)
–	Lost (deleted) chromosome (–9) or chromosomal segment (9q–)

samples (such as blood smears, touch imprint cytologic preparations, or cytospin preparations), paraffin-embedded tissue sections, and disaggregated cells retrieved from fresh, frozen, or paraffin-embedded material. Importantly, this procedure can provide results (such as identification of a tumor-specific translocation or loss of a tumor suppressor gene locus) when the tissue is insufficient or unsatisfactory for cytogenetic analysis, when conventional cytogenetic analysis has failed to yield results, or when cryptic rearrangements are present.

Blood smears, touch imprint cytologic preparations, and cytospin preparations are air dried and subsequently fixed in methanol:glacial acetic acid (3:1) for 5 minutes. To visualize an anomaly within a specific region of a tumor or within a specific cell type, a 4- to 6-µm–thick paraffin-embedded tissue section is used. Analysis of thin sections, however, is limited because portions of most nuclei are lost during sectioning, and this may lead to false-positive results in the evaluation of chromosomal deletions or losses. For the most accurate assessment of subtle

Table 2-2

CHROMOSOMAL PROBES COMMONLY USED TO EXAMINE BONE TUMORS

Probe	Composition	Use
α-satellite	Organized tandem repeats of unique 171-bp[a] sequences present in as many as 5,000 copies at the (peri)centromeric region of each chromosome	Determining aneuploidy
Locus-specific	Collections of one or a few cloned unique or single copy DNA sequences May be cloned into large-insert vectors such as phage, cosmids, BACs, or YACs to provide the most preferable target size	Detecting numerical aberrations, particularly gene amplification or deletion Defining or detecting structural rearrangements, such as translocations
Whole chromosome ("paint probes")	A mixture of sequences that bind to entire length of a particular chromosome	Analyzing complex cytogenetic rearrangements in metaphase preparations

[a]bp = base pairs; BAC = bacterial artificial chromosome; YAC = yeast artificial chromosome.

aneuploidy changes, the preferred approach is to obtain whole or intact nuclei by disaggregating and releasing cells from a much thicker (50 to 60 μm) section. FISH is a same day or overnight procedure, depending on the probes used or the type of specimen analyzed (or both).

Probes

Chromosomal probes (complementary DNA sequences) frequently used to examine bone tumors can be divided into three categories: 1) chromosome-specific (peri)centromeric probes; 2) sequence- or loci-specific probes such as translocation breakpoint flanking or breakpoint spanning cosmid, bacterial, and yeast artificial chromosome probes; and 3) whole chromosome "painting" probes that bind to sequences along the length of a specific chromosome (Table 2-2). Probe detection or labeling with fluorescent molecules with different excitation and emission characteristics allows simultaneous analysis of several different probes (50).

Technical Variations

Conventional karyotyping is limited by its inability to detect cryptic translocations or to identify marker chromosomes accurately. With recently developed universal chromosome painting techniques, all chromosomes can be analyzed simultaneously. Two similar approaches have been developed: spectral karyotype analysis (SKY) (57) and multifluor fluorescence in situ hybridization (M-FISH) (60). Both techniques are based on the principle that the differential display of colored fluorescent chromosome-specific paints provides a complete analysis of the human chromosomal complement. With the use of combinations of 23 different colored paints as a "cocktail probe," subtle differences in fluorochrome labeling profiles after hybridization with the cocktail probe allow the computer to assign a unique color to each chromosome pair. Thus, abnormal chromosomes in the karyotype of a tumor can be identified by the pattern of color distribution along the axis of the chromosome, so that rearrangements between different chromosomes lead to a distinct transition from one color to another at the position of the breakpoint, greatly facilitating the identification of subtle or cryptic rearrangements (64). This technique is suited particularly to solid tumors in which the complexity of the karyotypes often masks the presence of recurrent chromosomal aberrations (fig. 2-2).

Comparative genomic hybridization (CGH), another valuable molecular cytogenetic technique, provides an overview of DNA sequence copy number changes (including losses or deletions and gains or amplifications) in a tumor specimen and maps these changes on normal chromosomes in a single hybridization (22,59). CGH is particularly useful for analysis of DNA sequence copy number changes in bone tumors such as osteosarcoma, in which high-quality metaphase preparations are often difficult to make and complex karyotypes with numerous markers, double minutes, and homogeneously

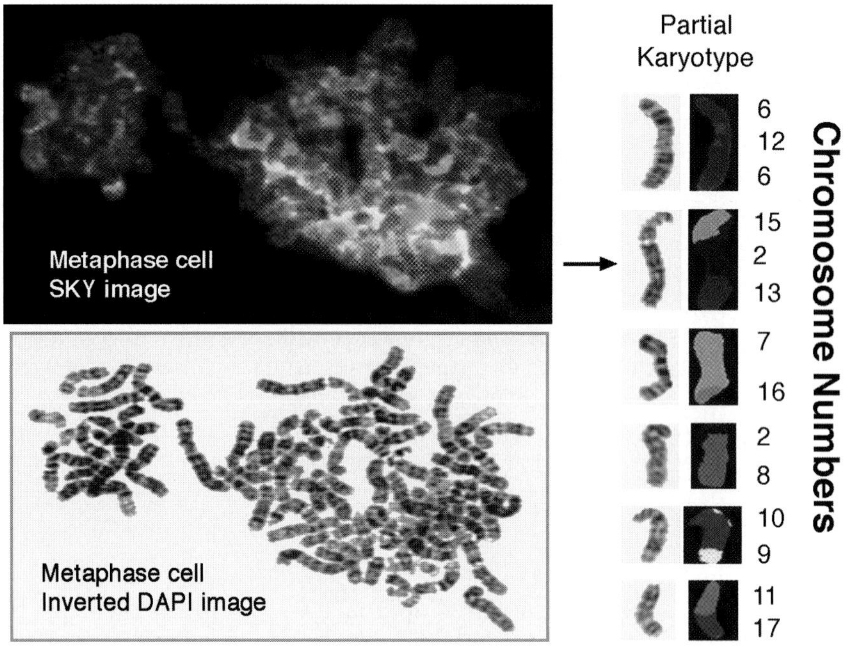

Figure 2-2

PARTIAL SPECTRAL KARYOTYPIC IMAGE OF ALVEOLAR RHABDOMYOSARCOMA CELL LINE

The numerous complex aberrations in the inverted DAPI (4,6-diamino-2-phenylindole) and spectral karyotypic (SKY)-imaged metaphase cell illustrated on the left include a three-way translocation variant (arrow on right) of the t(2;13)(q35;q14), characteristic of alveolar rhabdomyosarcoma. Recognition of many of these anomalies would be difficult without adjunctive SKY studies.

stained chromosomal regions are common (see below). CGH does not require previous knowledge of the aberrations in the test sample studied, and it can be performed with total genomic tumor DNA from fresh, frozen, or paraffin-embedded material.

The development of SKY, M-FISH, and CGH has permitted genome-wide screening to be performed with molecular techniques (17). These techniques, powerful adjuncts to FISH and classic banding methods, markedly improve the sensitivity and accuracy of karyotypic analysis. In turn, the information gained with these techniques can be used to guide positional cloning studies aimed at identifying neoplasia-associated genes.

MOLECULAR BIOLOGY

Recent advances in molecular technology have made possible the identification of mutations at the level of a single nucleotide and the isolation and characterization of individual genes from as little as a single tumor cell. Two broad classes of genes have been identified to contribute to carcinogenesis: oncogenes (62) and tumor suppressor genes (32).

Oncogenes

Proto-oncogenes are cellular genes that regulate normal cell division and differentiation. Recombination with a viral genome or a somatic mutational event may convert a proto-oncogene to an oncogene, which is a gene that induces uncontrolled cell proliferation (i.e., cancer-causing gene) (4). Numerous oncogenes have been identified through the study of tumorigenic retroviruses in animal systems. Retroviruses are RNA viruses that use the enzyme reverse transcriptase to transcribe their viral genome into DNA. They integrate into the genome of a host cell and replicate in unison with the genes of the host chromosome. If the virus carries an oncogene, the cell becomes transformed into a cancer cell. The first oncogenic virus to be described, the Rous sarcoma virus (*src*) (51), was identified in 1911 as a filterable agent capable of transferring sarcomas among chickens. Since then, more than 100 different viral oncogenes have been distinguished.

Although the identification of retroviral oncogenes has contributed significantly to understanding the control processes of cell proliferation, only a few human cancers have been shown to be caused by viruses, and most of these are due to DNA viruses (human papillomaviruses, adenoviruses, and herpesviruses). In contrast to RNA viruses, which promote tumor development by harboring or generating oncogenic alleles, many DNA tumor viruses encode proteins that inactivate or inhibit the activities of tumor suppressor protein products (29).

Most proto-oncogenes are included in one of the following categories: growth factors, cell surface receptors, transcription factors, or signal transmission proteins. The mutations that create oncogenes are dominant mutations; that is, only one gene allele needs to be mutated to produce an effect. When normal cellular proto-oncogenes are altered by somatic mutational events, such as point mutations, deletions, gene rearrangements, or amplification, expression of these genes may result in loss of growth control and, eventually, neoplastic transformation. Some oncogenes result from mutations that alter the regulatory region of the proto-oncogene, whereas others result from mutations in the structural (protein-encoding) portion.

Oncogene Detection

Two techniques have been particularly fruitful in identifying oncogenes in human tumors: DNA transformation and positional cloning. In transformation experiments, the introduction of DNA extracted from neoplastic cells into normal growth-regulated recipient cells or nontumorigenic immortalized cells (such as the murine fibroblastic NIH 3T3 cell line) results in neoplastic transformation of the morphologically normal cells when a transferred oncogene is expressed (43,61). Identification of the *ras* family of guanosine triphosphate (GTP)-binding proteins by this approach revealed that a single base change was sufficient to convert a gene member to a "transforming" oncogene, promoting uncontrolled growth. Activating point mutations for the *ras* gene family nonrandomly cluster in codons 12, 13, and 61 (5).

Translocations, or exchange of chromosomal material between two or more nonhomologous chromosomes, are encountered frequently as tumor-specific anomalies in hematologic malignancies (21) and mesenchymal neoplasms (7,14). These tumor-specific translocations serve as important signposts for molecular biologists conducting positional cloning studies of the genes at the translocation breakpoints.

Translocation events have two primary genetic consequences: 1) the juxtapositioning of inactive oncogenes within transcriptionally active chromosomal regions, such as those containing immunoglobulin or T-cell receptor genes, results in overexpression of an oncogene. For example, the t(14;18)(q32;q21) of follicular lymphoma results in the translocation of the *bcl2* oncogene (localized to 18q21) into the immunoglobulin heavy chain locus (localized to 14q32), resulting in overproduction of bcl2 messenger (m)RNA/encoded protein and loss of normal apoptosis (26); and 2) the fusion of two genes, one from each translocation partner, results in the formation of a chimeric gene. The fusion proteins encoded by these chimeric genes are not found in normal cells and are tumor specific. In sarcomas, the fusion genes most often code for aberrant transcription factors that result in inhibition of normal cellular differentiation, cell cycle activation, and loss of responsiveness to extracellular signals (Table 2-3) (2,48).

These highly specific gene rearrangements that occur from chromosomal translocations in bone and soft tissue tumors can be identified with reverse transcriptase polymerase chain reaction (RT-PCR) analysis (fig. 2-3). The PCR technique uses specific synthetic oligonucleotides to amplify a section of a gene in vitro. With the additional step of reverse transcription (mRNA into complementary [c]DNA), PCR can be carried out on RNA. Snap frozen tissue is preferred for RNA extraction and RT-PCR analysis, but this procedure can also be performed on archival (paraffin-embedded) material if the RNA is of sufficient quality.

RT-PCR analysis is remarkably sensitive. It may allow for the detection of abnormalities present in cells too few to be identified with traditional cytogenetic or FISH methods. It may be suitable for the detection or monitoring of minimal residual disease. Also, RT-PCR analysis is not dependent on successful cell culture and, similar to FISH, is rapid, with a short turnaround time. Compared with cytogenetic analysis, the greatest disadvantage of RT-PCR analysis is the inability to detect chromosomal anomalies other than those for which the test was designed. With conventional cytogenetic analysis, all major chromosomal abnormalities, including those not initially anticipated by the clinician or laboratorian, may be uncovered.

Gene Amplification

Amplification is another mechanism by which a proto-oncogene can function as an oncogene. Overproduction of a wild-type proto-oncogene

Table 2-3

CHARACTERISTIC AND VARIANT CHROMOSOMAL TRANSLOCATIONS AND ASSOCIATED FUSION GENES IN BONE AND SOFT TISSUE SARCOMAS

Neoplasm	Translocation	Fusion Gene(s)
Alveolar soft part sarcoma[a]	der(17)t(X;17)(p11.2;q25.3)	*ASPL/TFE3*
Alveolar rhabdomyosarcoma	t(2;13)(q35;q14) t(1;13)(p36;q14) t(X;2)(q13;q35) t(2;2)(q35;p23)	*PAX3/FKHR* *PAX7/FKHR* *PAX3/AFX* *PAX3/NCOA1*
Clear cell sarcoma	t(12;22)(q13;q12)	*EWS/ATF1*
Congenital fibrosarcoma[b]	t(12;15)(p13;q25)	*ETV6/NTRK3*
Epithelioid hemangioendothelioma	t(1;3)(p36;q25)	?
Ewing's sarcoma, pPNET[c]	t(11;22)(q24;q12) t(21;22)(q22;q12) t(7;22)(q22;q12) t(17;22)(q21;q12) t(2;22)(q33;q12) inv(22)(q12q12) t(16;21)(p11;q22)	*EWS/FLI1* *EWS/ERG* *EWS/ETV1* *EWS/EIAF* *EWS/FEV* *EWS/ZSG* *FUS/ERG*
Extraskeletal myxoid chondrosarcoma	t(9;22)(q22;q12) t(9;17)(q22;q11)	*EWS/NR4A3*[d] *RBP56*[e]*/NR4A3* *TCF12/NR4A3* *TFG/NR4A3*
Myxoid/round cell liposarcoma	t(12;16)(q13;p11) t(12;22)(q13;q12)	*TLS*[f]*/CHOP*[g] *EWS/CHOP*
Synovial sarcoma	t(X;18)(p11.2;q11.2) t(X;20)(p11.2;q13.3)	*SYT/SSX1* *SYT/SSX2* *SYT/SSX4* *SS18L1/SSX1*

[a]A balanced form of this translocation is seen also in a subset of pediatric renal neoplasms.
[b]This translocation is seen also in congenital mesoblastic nephromas.
[c]pPNET = peripheral primitive neuroectodermal tumor.
[d]Also referred to as *TEC, MINOR, CHN,* and *NOR-1.*
[e]Also referred to as *TAF2N.*
[f]Also referred to as *FUS.*
[g]Also referred to as *DDIT3.*

protein secondary to gene amplification has been described in various cancers, including bone tumors. In some cases, amplified DNA sequences are manifested karyotypically in the form of double minutes, homogeneously staining regions, or ring chromosomes. Double minutes are small chromatin bodies that replicate and segregate in the absence of centromeres, and homogeneously staining regions are segments of metaphase chromosomes that lack the cross-striational patterns revealed by chromosome banding (fig. 2-4). Ring chromosomes are formed when a break occurs on each arm of a chromosome, followed by fusion of the exposed ends to create a circular structure. In mitosis, ring chromosomes are often unstable, undergoing sister chromatid exchange and generating smaller or larger rings.

Neuroblastoma is a well-studied example of the relationship of double minutes, homogeneously staining regions, or both, and gene amplification. The presence of double minutes or homogeneously staining regions (or both) is associated with amplification of the N-*myc* gene

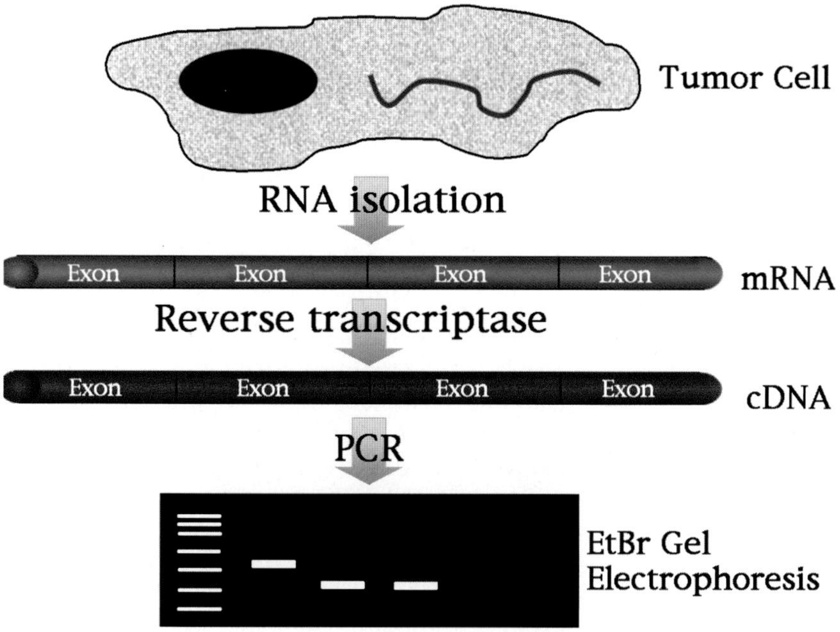

Figure 2-3

METHOD FOR THE REVERSE TRANSCRIPTASE POLYMERASE CHAIN REACTION

First, messenger RNA (mRNA) is isolated from tumor cells. This is followed by reverse transcription of the target mRNA into complementary DNA (cDNA) and polymerase chain reaction (PCR) amplification.

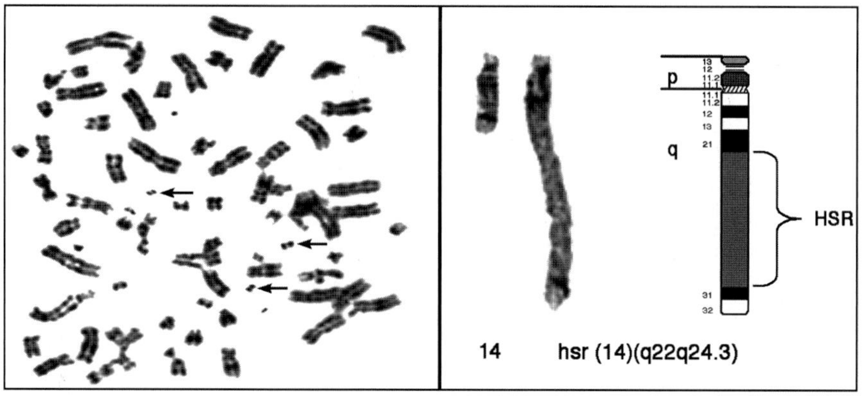

Figure 2-4

CYTOGENETIC MANIFESTATIONS OF GENE AMPLIFICATION

Left: Double minutes (arrows) are seen in a G-banded metaphase cell from a conventional osteosarcoma.

Right: Partial G-banded karyotype and schematic image of a homogeneously staining region on the long arm of chromosome 14 in a case of alveolar rhabdomyosarcoma.

(a member of the helix-loop-helix family of transcription factors) in neuroblastomas (58). Analysis for the presence of N-*myc* amplification is a routine step in the clinical work-up of a patient with neuroblastoma because this finding indicates a poor prognosis (independent of the clinical stage at the time of initial presentation) (8). Although the degree of N-*myc* amplification within neuroblastomas may range from a few to several hundred copies of N-*myc* per haploid genome, the level of amplification within a specific tumor is usually consistent (i.e., it does not change on serial biopsy studies) (9).

Amplification of sequences originating from the long arm of chromosome 12 (particularly 12q13-15) has been described in osteosarcomas and some soft tissue sarcomas (52). In this instance, more than one gene residing within this chromosomal region, such as *GLI, CHOP, SAS, CDK4,* and *HDM2*, may be amplified. The protein properties of these genes are summarized in Table 2-4. Notably, the size of the 12q region that is amplified may vary (even within the same histologic tumor subtype). Thus, it is necessary to examine the patterns of gene amplification and expression for many tumors of a histopathologic subtype to determine which gene or genes are consistently amplified (i.e., the target gene or genes). For example, parosteal osteosarcoma can be distinguished from conventional

Table 2-4

PROTEIN PROPERTIES OF 12q13-15 GENES

Gene	Protein Property
GLI	Transcription factor
CHOP	Transcription factor
SAS	Membrane protein
CDK4	Cyclin-dependent kinase
HDM2	p53 binding protein

osteosarcoma by the unique karyotypic finding of a supernumerary ring chromosome either as the sole anomaly or accompanied by a few other aberrations. The ring chromosomes are composed, at least in part, of chromosome 12 sequences, and amplification or coamplification and coexpression of *HDM2, CDK4*, and *SAS* have been detected in a high percentage of parosteal osteosarcomas and central low-grade osteosarcomas (18,40,49,68). These same genes also have been shown to be amplified in high-grade osteosarcomas, but in a much smaller subset. Amplification of a gene can readily be determined in tumor specimens with the Southern blot procedure, PCR, or FISH.

The phenomenon of multidrug resistance (i.e., patients are refractory to multiple structurally unrelated drugs to which they have never been exposed either in the absence of previous treatment [de novo resistance] or in response to previous treatment [acquired resistance]) is related to amplification or overexpression (or both) of the *MDR1* gene. This gene codes for a P-glycoprotein (p170), an energy-dependent drug efflux pump with multiple drug-binding sites (13). When P-glycoprotein is overexpressed, cytotoxic drugs are prevented from reaching the cellular sites of action because of enhanced drug efflux, ergo, resistance to antineoplastic agents.

Most of the mechanisms of drug resistance that have been described have been determined in cell culture and animal models. Many of these mechanisms also operate in human primary bone malignancies, but their relative importance in determining clinical drug resistance is still emerging (56). Immunohistochemistry and PCR are sensitive and specific methods for detecting P-glycoprotein and hold considerable promise for practical clinical application (12).

Tumor Suppressor Genes

Tumor suppressor genes normally regulate cell division. Thus, when one of these genes is mutated or deleted, there is loss of growth regulation. Tumor suppressor genes differ from proto-oncogenes in that both alleles of a tumor suppressor gene must be inactivated or lost to initiate cancer development (recessive mutations). Similar to proto-oncogenes, however, the normal functions of tumor suppressor genes are diverse, and the proteins encoded by these genes are found in many compartments of the cell.

Somatic cell hybrid studies and epidemiologic studies have provided strong evidence for the idea that, in some types of cancer, mutations must occur in both alleles of a gene to produce tumors in the host. Much of the current knowledge about tumor suppressor genes comes from extensive studies of retinoblastoma, a model for this class of genes. Knudson (25) first proposed that two distinct mutational events are necessary for the development of retinoblastoma (fig. 2-5); this was based on his observations of the age-specific differences in incidence between patients with hereditary retinoblastoma and those with sporadically occurring retinoblastoma. This "two-hit" kinetic model requires that a second somatic mutational event follow the primary mutation in germline cells of patients with the hereditary form of retinoblastoma or follow the primary somatic cell mutation that transpires in patients with sporadic retinoblastoma.

Peripheral blood or skin fibroblastic cytogenetic studies of patients with retinoblastoma provided the first clue to the chromosomal location of the retinoblastoma susceptibility gene (*RB*). Approximately 5 percent of patients with retinoblastoma exhibit a small interstitial deletion of the long arm of chromosome 13 at band q14 (16). Subsequently, the *RB* gene was cloned and found to be a relatively large gene, with 27 exons spanning nearly 200 kb of genomic DNA (31). Importantly, patients with germline mutations of *RB* are also at increased risk for the development of osteosarcomas, particularly in areas exposed to radiotherapy (e.g., the skull). In these patients, even sites remote

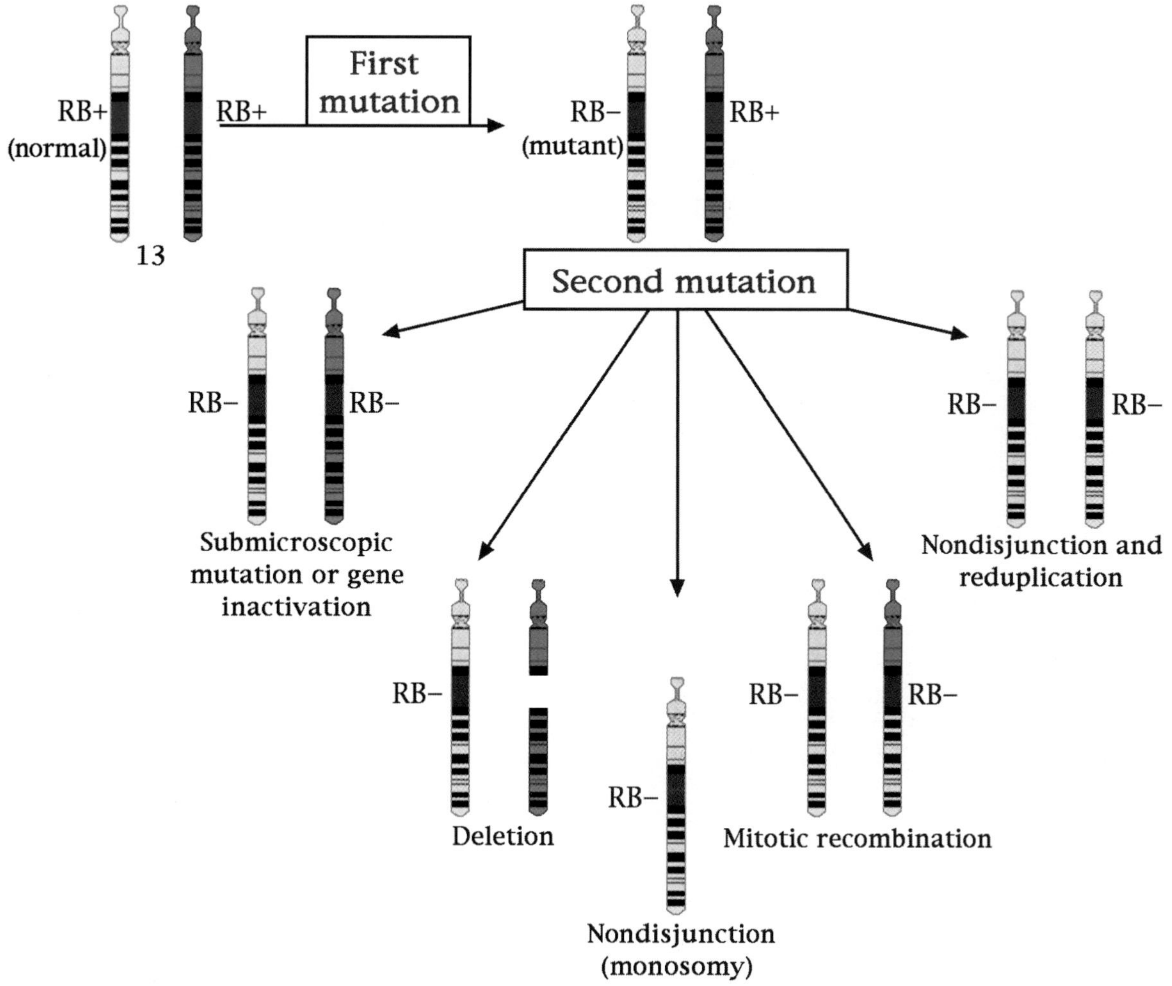

Figure 2-5

THE "TWO-HIT" TUMOR SUPPRESSOR GENE MODEL

This schematic representation of the model uses the retinoblastoma (*RB*) gene. Two normal chromosome 13 homologues are shown in the upper left corner. Two successive mutations are required to turn a normal cell into a tumor cell. The first mutation may be a germline mutation in a person with familial retinoblastoma or may be a somatic cell mutation in a person with sporadic retinoblastoma. Five examples are shown of ways in which the second mutational event may occur.

from radiotherapy are at increased risk for osteosarcoma, but the incidence is less than for sites within the field of radiation. The cloning of the *RB* gene has allowed the identification of specific inherited or somatic mutations in *RB*, resulting in a new era in the management of patients and families who have inherited cancer syndromes (20). The Li-Fraumeni syndrome and hereditary multiple exostoses (involving *TP53* and *EXT* tumor suppressor genes, respectively) are other examples of inherited cancer syndromes that have an important role in bone neoplasia.

DNA Mismatch Repair Gene Defects

DNA mismatch repair genes aid in correcting mispaired DNA bases. The repair of cellular DNA is an important mechanism for protecting the genome from the mutagenic effects of carcinogens. Loss of function of a DNA repair gene contributes to cancer by increasing the rate of mutations in other cellular genes, particularly proto-oncogenes and tumor suppressor genes (45). Germline mutations in DNA mismatch repair genes represent a basis for cancer

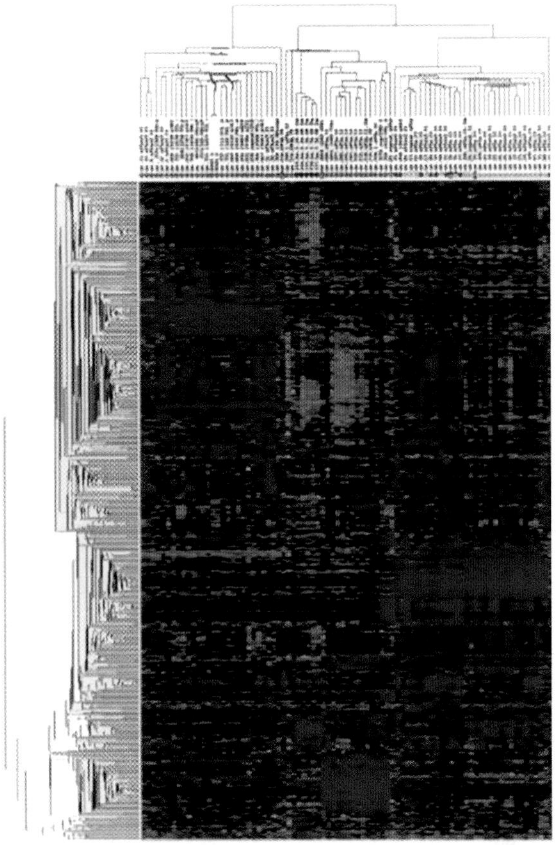

Figure 2-6

HIERARCHICAL CLUSTERING OF EXPRESSION MICROARRAY DATA

In this cluster diagram, columns represent tumor samples and rows indicate individual genes. Based solely on the gene-expression profiles, cluster analysis divided the tumors into three major groups, with osteosarcomas (blue) grouped on the left, neuroblastomas (black) and Ewing sarcomas (magenta) in the middle, and alveolar (green) and embryonal rhabdomyosarcomas (red) on the right. Relative gene expression is indicated by color ranges from very high (intense red) to very low (intense green). (Modified from fig. 3 from Schofield D, Wai D, Triche TJ. Expression profiling of bone tumors. In: Ladany M, Gerald WL, eds. Expression profiling of human tumors. Diagnostic and research applications. Totowa, NJ: Humana Press; 2003:359–91.)

predisposition. Some tumors caused by defects in mismatch repair behave differently from tumors due to other mutations (47). Studies of mismatch repair gene defects in bone tumors are evolving. Mismatch repair abnormalities can be diagnosed with microsatellite instability and antibody methods.

Microarray Technology

One of the most exciting advances in molecular biology in the last few years has been the development of microarray technology. Microarray approaches allow investigators to examine multiple (tens of thousands) genetic events concurrently in a single experiment. Microarray technology is providing insights into cancer that would be difficult, if not impossible, to obtain using a gene-by-gene approach (37). Importantly, this innovative technique is being widely used to investigate tumor classification, cancer progression, and chemotherapy resistance and sensitivity.

Microarray technology is based on the placement of multiple "probes" in orderly rows and columns on various substrates such as nylon, glass, or synthetic "chips." Although there are various options for producing microarrays, the advantages of using a glass substrate include: 1) an effective surface for probe immobilization; 2) a robust target-probe hybridization because glass can sustain high temperatures and is nonporous, allowing for minimal hybridization volumes and low background fluorescence; and 3) simultaneous hybridization of differentially fluorochrome-labeled probes in a single experiment, avoiding most of the complications of hybridization kinetics (11).

After the probe array has been prepared, the target of interest is hybridized to the array and the relative intensity of hybridization is correlated with the relative abundance of the corresponding target sequence. Depending on the substrate spotted on the microarray, changes occurring at the DNA, RNA, protein, or tissue level can be determined (19,34,46,53).

The greatest challenge of microarray analysis is analytical (i.e., data mining). Microarrays generate enormous amounts of data. Examining these datasets with scores of samples yields the deepest biologic insight; however, determining which types of datasets and analytical tools the computational scientists should use can be bewildering (3,27,28,30,35). Nevertheless, by applying mathematical tools for analyzing the gene expression patterns and grouping various tumor specimens that have similar patterns, it is possible to recognize two or more different classes of a tumor that previously appeared to be only a single clinicopathologic entity (28,35).

cDNA microarrays used for comprehensive RNA expression analysis have been applied to a small subset of bone tumors (1,23,24,42,54, 55,65–67). The resulting patterns of gene expression reflect the molecular basis of the sample phenotypes and are used for sample comparisons and classification (fig. 2-6). For example, a set of 96 genes was found to be capable of discriminating between four small round blue cell tumor types (neuroblastoma, Ewing's sarcoma, rhabdomyosarcoma, and Burkitt's lymphoma) in one expression-profiling study (23). Moreover, by using cDNA microarray analyses and appropriate antibodies on tissue microarrays, lineage-associated genes were demonstrated in specific tumor types, that is, prominent expression of neural proteins Ephrin B1 and NPYY1 in Ewing's sarcoma cases (66).

Methods have been described for isolating high-quality RNA from tumors with abundant extracellular matrix, such as chondrosarcoma (1). Other limitations applied to specimen samples include restricted quantity of the sample, RNA degradation associated with tumor necrosis, delay in handling, and cellular heterogeneity. Therefore, alternative sources of tumor and model systems, such as cell culture, xenografts, and animal models, are frequently used for investigative studies (55). For example, cells derived from osteosarcoma cell lines and normal human osteoblasts were used in a comparative cDNA microarray study to identify a consistent group of upregulated and downregulated genes (67). After RT-PCR confirmation, the authors concluded that the most significantly upregulated genes in the three osteosarcoma cell lines examined were heat shock protein 90β and polyadenylate-binding protein-like 1, whereas fibronectin 1 and thrombospondin 1 were among the group of genes that were downregulated. Genes possibly involved in the variable metastatic potential of individual osteosarcomas were identified in a murine osteosarcoma model in a separate cDNA microarray study (24). Although meaningful, valuable data can be obtained from both cell line and animal model studies, ultimate validation on human tumors is required (54,55).

Additional studies of bone sarcomas are needed to identify the large number of genes involved in the complex deregulation of cell homeostasis that occurs in these malignancies. Hopefully in the future, the likelihood of response to therapy for individual bone tumors will be predictable with this technology.

In conclusion, dramatic advances in cytogenetic and molecular biologic techniques have furthered our understanding of sarcomagenesis. Cytogenetic and molecular genetic assays have a direct, potentially decisive role in the examination of bone and soft tissue tumors, and many such assays are used routinely for diagnostic and prognostic purposes in molecular pathology laboratories. However, genetic analysis is not a replacement for histopathologic study, but rather it is a powerful adjunct to complement conventional microscopy and radiographic assessment in the formulation of an accurate diagnosis. By virtue of their exquisite sensitivity, molecular techniques appear superior to standard methods in the assessment of minimal residual disease or early relapse of disease. Future advancements in the clinical management of these malignancies will include the development of a new class of antineoplastic agents based on the underlying biologic events in bone and soft tissue sarcomas.

REFERENCES

1. Baelde HJ, Cleton-Jansen AM, van Beerendonk H, Namba M, Bovee NJ, Hogendoorn PC. High quality RNA isolation from tumours with low cellularity and high extracellular matrix component for cDNA microarrays: application to chondrosarcoma. J Clin Pathol 2001;54:778–82.
2. Barr FG. Translocations, cancer and the puzzle of specificity. Nat Genet 1998;19:121–4.
3. Bassett DE Jr, Eisen MB, Boguski MS. Gene expression informatics—it's all in your mind. Nat Genet 1999;21(Suppl):51–5.
4. Bishop JM. Viral oncogenes. Cell 1985;42:23–38.
5. Bos JL. The *ras* gene family and human carcinogenesis. Mutat Res 1988;195:255–71.
6. Bridge JA, Sandberg AA. Cytogenetics. In: Damjanov I, Linder J, eds. Anderson's pathology, vol. 1, 10th ed. St Louis: Mosby-Year Book, Inc; 1996:223–57.
7. Bridge JA, Sandberg AA. Cytogenetic and molecular genetic techniques as adjunctive approaches in the diagnosis of bone and soft tissue tumors. Skeletal Radiol 2000;29:249–58.
8. Brodeur GM, Azar C, Brother M, et al. Neuroblastoma. Effect of genetic factors on prognosis and treatment. Cancer 1992;70(Suppl):1685–94.
9. Brodeur GM, Hayes FA, Green AA, et al. Consistent N-myc copy number in simultaneous or consecutive neuroblastoma samples from sixty individual patients. Cancer Res 1987;47:4248–53.
10. Caspersson T, Zech L, Johansson C. Differential binding of alkylating fluorochromes in human chromosomes. Exp Cell Res 1970;60:315–9.
11. Cheung VG, Morley M, Aguilar F, Massimi A, Kucherlapati R, Childs G. Making and reading microarrays. Nat Genet 1999;21(Suppl):15–9.
12. Dalton WS. Overcoming the multidrug-resistant phenotype. In: DeVita VT Jr, Hellman S, Rosenberg SA, eds. Cancer: principles and practice of oncology, 4th ed. Philadelphia: JB Lippincott Company; 1993:2655–66.
13. Endicott JA, Ling V. The biochemistry of P-glycoprotein-mediated multidrug resistance. Annu Rev Biochem 1989;58:137–71.
14. Fletcher CD, Unni KK, Mertens F, eds. Pathology and genetics of tumours of soft tissue and bone. Lyon: IARC Press; 2002.
15. Fletcher JA, Kozakewich HP, Hoffer FA, et al. Diagnostic relevance of clonal cytogenetic aberrations in malignant soft-tissue tumors. N Engl J Med 1991;324:436–42.
16. Francke U. Retinoblastoma and chromosome 13. Birth Defects Orig Arctic Ser 1976;12:131–4.
17. Green GA, Schrock E, Veldman T, Heselmeyer-Haddad K, Padilla-Nash HM, Ried T. Evolving molecular cytogenetic technologies. In: Mark HF, ed. Medical cytogenetics. New York: Marcel Dekker, Inc.; 2000:579–92.
18. Gisselsson D, Palsson E, Hoglund M, et al. Differentially amplified chromosome 12 sequences in low- and high-grade osteosarcoma. Genes Chromosomes Cancer 2002;33:133–40.
19. Haab BB. Advances in protein microarray technology for protein expression and interaction profiling. Curr Opin Drug Discov Devel 2001;4:116–23.
20. Harbour JW. Overview of RB gene mutations in patients with retinoblastoma. Implications for clinical genetic screening. Ophthalmology 1998;105:1442–7.
21. Jaffe ES, Harris NL, Stein H, Vardiman JW, eds. Pathology and genetics of tumours of haematopoietic and lymphoid tissues. Lyon: IARC Press; 2001.
22. Kallioniemi A, Kallioniemi OP, Sudar D, et al. Comparative genomic hybridization for molecular cytogenetic analysis of solid tumors. Science 1992;258:818–21.
23. Khan J, Wei JS, Ringner M, et al. Classification and diagnostic prediction of cancers using gene expression profiling and artificial neural networks. Nat Med 2001;7:673–9.
24. Khanna C, Khan J, Nguyen P, et al. Metastasis-associated differences in gene expression in a murine model of osteosarcoma. Cancer Res 2001;61:3750–9.
25. Knudson AG Jr. Mutation and cancer: statistical study of retinoblastoma. Proc Natl Acad Sci U S A 1971;68:820–3.
26. Korsmeyer SJ. Bcl-2 initiates a new category of oncogenes: regulators of cell death. Blood 1992;80:879–86.
27. LaBaer J. Genomics, proteomics, and the new paradigm in biomedical research. Genet Med 2002;4(Suppl):2S–9.
28. Ladanyi M, Gerald WL. Present and potential impact of expression profiling studies of human tumors. In: Ladanyi M, Gerald WL, eds. Expression profiling of human tumors. Diagnostic and research applications. Totawa, NJ: Humana Press; 2003:3–7.
29. Lambert PF, Sugden B. Viruses and cancer. In: Abeloff M, Armitage J, Niederhuber J, Kastan M, McKenna W, eds. Clinical oncology, 3rd ed. New York: Elsevier; 2004:207–25.
30. Lander ES. Array of hope. Nat Genet 1999;21(Suppl):3–4.

31. Lee WH, Bookstein R, Hong F, Young LJ, Shew JY, Lee EY. Human retinoblastoma susceptibility gene: cloning, identification, and sequence. Science 1987;235:1394–9.
32. Levine AJ. The tumor suppressor genes. Annu Rev Biochem 1993;62:623–51.
33. Limon J, Dal Cin P, Sandberg AA. Application of long-term collagenase disaggregation for the cytogenetic analysis of human solid tumors. Cancer Genet Cytogenet 1986;23:305–13.
34. Lipshutz RJ, Fodor SP, Gingeras TR, Lockhart DJ. High density synthetic oligonucleotide arrays. Nat Genet 1999;21(Suppl):20–4.
35. Macgregor PF, Squire JA. Application of microarrays to the analysis of gene expression in cancer. Clin Chem 2002;48:1170–7.
36. Mandahl N. Methods in solid tumor cytogenetics. In: Rooney DE, Czepulkowski BH, eds. Human cytogenetics: a practical approach. Oxford: IRL Press; 1992:155.
37. Marx J. Medicine. DNA arrays reveal cancer in its many forms. Science 2000;289:1670–2.
38. Mitelman F, ed. ISCN 1995: an International System for Human Cytogenetic Nomenclature (1995): recommendations of the International Standing Committee on Human Cytogenetic Nomenclature, Memphis, Tennessee, USA, October 9-13, 1994. Basel: S Karger; 1995.
39. Mitelman F, Johansson B, Mertens F, eds. Mitelman database of chromosome aberrations in cancer (2004). Updated 5-26-04. Retrieved July 27, 2004, from the World Wide Web: http://cgap.nci.nih.gov/Chromosomes/Mitelman.
40. Noble-Topham SE, Burrow SR, Eppert K, et al. *SAS* is amplified predominantly in surface osteosarcoma. J Orthop Res 1996;14:700–5.
41. Nowell PC, Hungerford DA. A minute chromosome in human chronic granulocytic leukemia [Abstract]. Science 1960;132:1497.
42. Ochi K, Daigo Y, Katagiri T, et al. Prediction of response to neoadjuvant chemotherapy for osteosarcoma by gene-expression profiles. Int J Oncol 2004;24:647–55.
43. Parada LF, Tabin CJ, Shih C, Weinberg RA. Human EJ bladder carcinoma oncogene is homologue of Harvey sarcoma virus ras gene. Nature 1982;297:474–8.
44. Paris Conference (1971): standardization in human cytogenetics. Birth Defects Orig Arctic Ser 1972;8:1–46.
45. Peltomaki P. Role of DNA mismatch repair defects in the pathogenesis of human cancer. J Clin Oncol 2003;21:1174–9.
46. Pollack JR, Perou CM, Alizadeh AA, et al. Genome-wide analysis of DNA copy-number changes using cDNA microarrays. Nat Genet 1999;23:41–6.
47. Quirke P, Mapstone N. The new biology: histopathology. Lancet 1999;354(Suppl 1):SI26–31.
48. Rabbitts TH. Perspective: chromosomal translocations can affect genes controlling gene expression and differentiation—why are these functions targeted? J Pathol 1999;187:39–42.
49. Ragazzini P, Gamberi G, Benassi MS, et al. Analysis of *SAS* gene and CDK4 and MDM2 proteins in low-grade osteosarcoma. Cancer Detect Prev 1999;23:129–36.
50. Ried T, Baldini A, Rand TC, Ward DC. Simultaneous visualization of seven different DNA probes by in situ hybridization using combinatorial fluorescence and digital imaging microscopy. Proc Natl Acad Sci U S A 1992;89:1388–92.
51. Rous P. A sarcoma of the fowl transmissible by an agent separable from the tumor cells. J Exp Med 1911;13:397–411.
52. Sandberg AA, Bridge JA. The cytogenetics of bone and soft tissue tumors. Austin: R. G. Landes; 1994.
53. Schena M, Shalon D, Heller R, Chai A, Brown PO, Davis RW. Parallel human genome analysis: microarray-based expression monitoring of 1000 genes. Proc Natl Acad Sci U S A 1996;93:10614–9.
54. Schofield D, Triche TJ. cDNA microarray analysis of global gene expression in sarcomas. Curr Opin Oncol 2002;14:406–11.
55. Schofield D, Wai D, Triche TJ. Expression profiling of bone tumors. In: Ladanyi M, Gerald WL, eds. Expression profiling of human tumors. Diagnostic and research applications. Totawa, NJ: Humana Press; 2003:359–91.
56. Scholz RB, Christiansen H, Kabisch H, Winkler K. Molecular markers in the evaluation of bone neoplasms. In: Helliwell TR, ed. Pathology of bone and joint neoplasms. Philadelphia: WB Saunders; 1999:79–105.
57. Schrock E, du Manoir S, Veldman T, et al. Multicolor spectral karyotyping of human chromosomes. Science 1996;273:494–7.
58. Schwab M, Alitalo K, Klempnauer KH, et al. Amplified DNA with limited homology to myc cellular oncogene is shared by human neuroblastoma cell lines and a neuroblastoma tumour. Nature 1983;305:245–8.
59. Speicher MR, du Manoir S, Schrock E, et al. Molecular cytogenetic analysis of formalin-fixed, paraffin-embedded solid tumors by comparative genomic hybridization after universal DNA-amplification. Hum Mol Genet 1993;2:1907–14.
60. Speicher MR, Gwyn Ballard S, Ward DC. Karyotyping human chromosomes by combinatorial multi-fluor FISH. Nat Genet 1996;12:368–75.

61. Tabin CJ, Bradley SM, Bargmann CI, et al. Mechanism of activation of a human oncogene. Nature 1982;300:143–9.
62. Temin HM. The protovirus hypothesis: speculations on the significance of RNA-directed DNA synthesis for normal development and for carcinogenesis. J Natl Cancer Inst 1971;46:3–7.
63. Tjio JH, Levan A. The chromosome number of man. Hereditas 1956;42:1–6.
64. Veldman T, Vignon C, Schrock E, Rowley JD, Ried T. Hidden chromosome abnormalities in haematological malignancies detected by multicolour spectral karyotyping. Nat Genet 1997;15:406–10.
65. Wai DH, Schaefer KL, Schramm A, et al. Expression analysis of pediatric solid tumor cell lines using oligonucleotide microarrays. Int J Oncol 2002;20:441–51.
66. Wei J, Khan J, Welford S, et al. Elucidation of molecular targets of the EWS/FLI1 fusion gene found in Ewing's sarcoma using cDNA microarrays [Abstract]. Proc Am Assoc Cancer Res 2001;42:427.
67. Wolf M, El-Rifai W, Tarkkanen M, et al. Novel findings in gene expression detected in human osteosarcoma by cDNA microarray. Cancer Genet Cytogenet 2000;123:128–32.
68. Wunder JS, Eppert K, Burrow SR, et al. Co-amplification and overexpression of CDK4, SAS and MDM2 occurs frequently in human parosteal osteosarcomas. Oncogene 1999;18:783–8.

3 RADIOGRAPHIC APPEARANCE OF BONE TUMORS

Many advances, especially in computerized tomography (CT) and magnetic resonance imaging (MRI), have been made recently in skeletal radiology. However, plain radiographs remain the "gold standard" for the diagnosis of bone lesions. It was hoped that MRI would provide the information needed to make a histologic diagnosis, but this has not been realized.

Lodwick (5) has pointed out that a team approach is required to diagnose bone tumors. It is important for the team to consist of knowledgeable radiologists, pathologists, and orthopedic surgeons. Although pathologists and orthopedic surgeons need to have a working knowledge of the radiographic features of bone lesions, it is even more important that a knowledgeable radiologist review the films.

A systematic approach, outlined in this chapter, is needed when analyzing the various radiologic studies (5).

LOCATION

Radiographic studies usually are the first to identify a bone lesion. The bone involved and the location of the lesion within or on the bone provide important clues to the diagnosis.

Although most neoplasms can involve any skeletal site, some tumors have a predilection for certain bones. Adamantinoma almost exclusively involves the tibia and, less often, the fibula. The diagnosis of adamantinoma need hardly be considered for any other bone. A purely lytic destructive lesion that involves the distal radius (especially in a young woman) is almost certain to be a giant cell tumor (fig. 3-1). About 70 percent of all parosteal osteosarcomas involve the surface of the distal posterior femur.

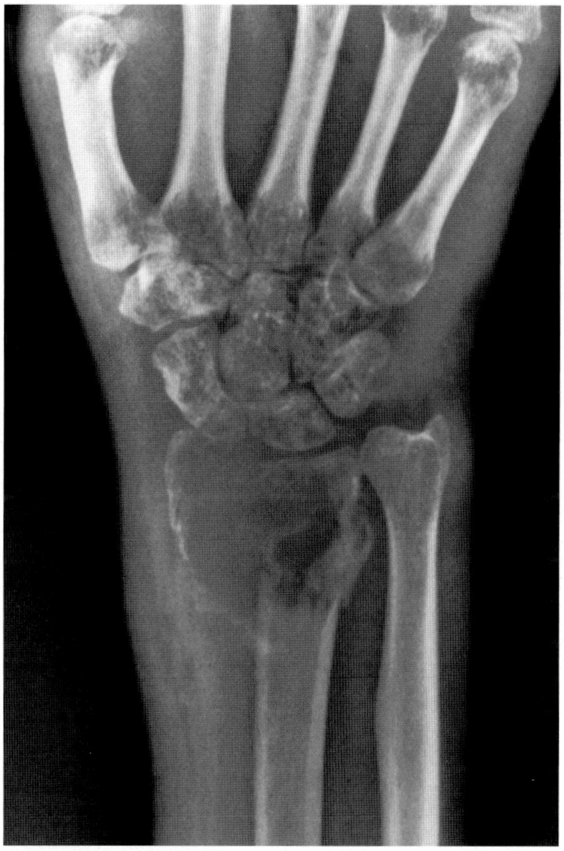

Figure 3-1

PURELY LYTIC LESION

A purely lytic lesion involving the distal radius suggests the diagnosis of giant cell tumor.

Equally important is the exact site of involvement of the bone. Most neoplasms and neoplasm-like lesions involve the metaphysis of long bones; a few involve almost exclusively the ends (epiphyses) of long bones. A lytic lesion that involves the epiphysis and extends across an open epiphyseal plate to involve the metaphysis is likely to be a chondroblastoma (fig. 3-2), whereas a purely lytic process that extends to the articular cartilage in an adult is likely to be a giant cell tumor. Although most bone tumors arise within the medullary cavity, some typically occur in the cortex and others are purely surface tumors. The main distinction between osteofibrous dysplasia and fibrous dysplasia is that the former is centered in the cortex. Adamantinoma is the only true neoplasm of bone with the propensity to involve the cortex.

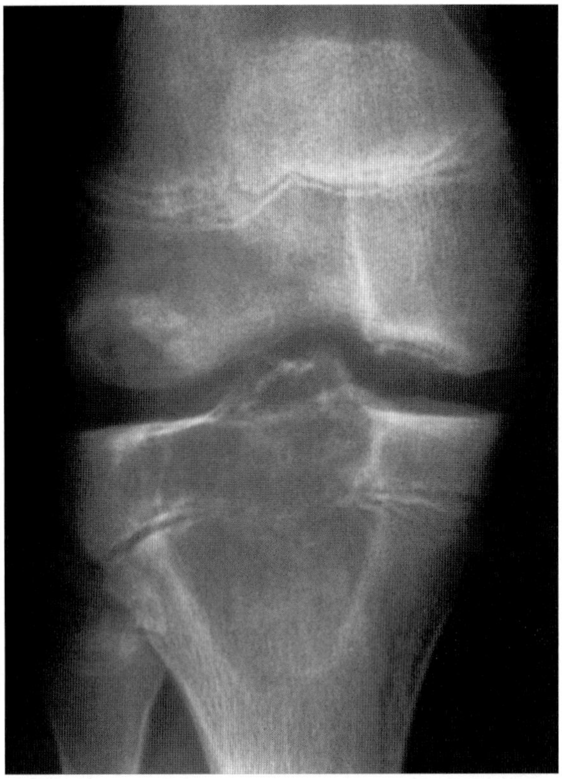

Figure 3-2

LYTIC LESION

A well-demarcated lesion involving the epiphysis and extending across an open epiphyseal plate is typical of chondroblastoma.

SIZE

Benign tumors tend to be relatively small, usually less than 6 cm in greatest dimension. Malignant tumors usually, but not invariably, are large. An osteosarcoma that is small and confined to bone is extremely unusual. A large cartilage tumor within the medullary cavity is more likely to be a chondrosarcoma than is a small lesion. Benign lesions such as aneurysmal bone cysts, however, can be extremely large (fig. 3-3).

INTERNAL MARGINS

The visualization of osteolysis depends on the structure of the bone, the degree of bone loss, and the amount of adjacent host bone available for contrast (6). Large amounts (30 to 50 percent) of trabecular bone must be destroyed before osteolysis is apparent on plain radiographs. The amount of host bone is important to consider. Older patients may have extensive permeative medullary lesions, especially in the shaft of a long bone, that are invisible on plain radiographs.

The growth of a bone tumor induces osteoblastic and osteoclastic activity, thus modifying bone structure. The patterns of bone destruction can be classified into three types (5): geographic, moth-eaten, and permeative. In the geographic pattern, the area of destruction is a well-circumscribed, single large defect in bone with a narrow zone of transition (the area between the lesion and normal bone) (fig. 3-4).

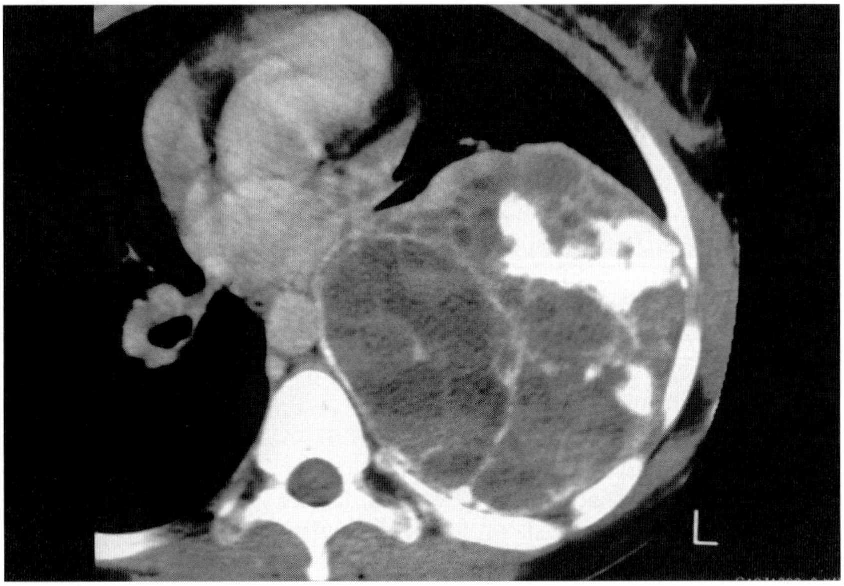

Figure 3-3

ANEURYSMAL BONE CYST

Fibrous dysplasia of rib associated with secondary aneurysmal bone cyst. Although large, the lesion is benign. (Courtesy of Dr. E.V. Perrin, Detroit, MI.)

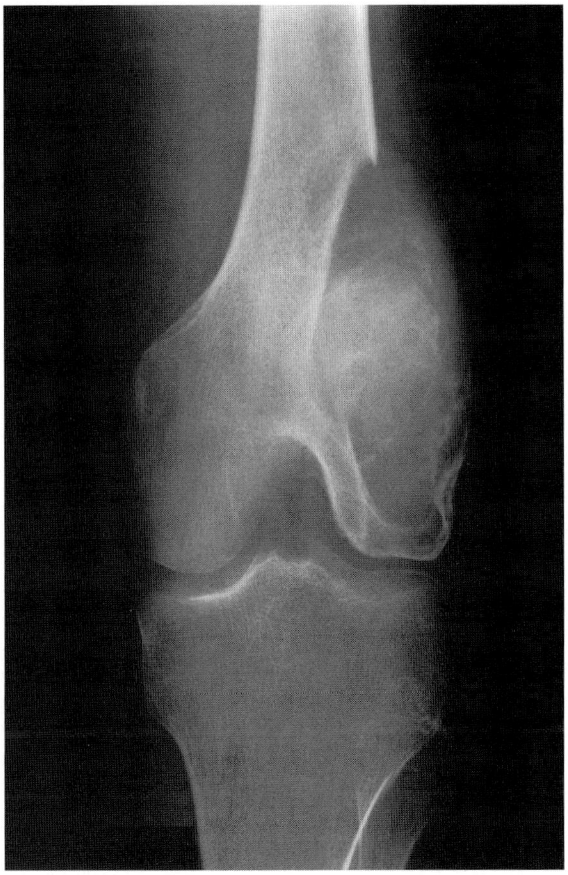

Figure 3-4

GEOGRAPHIC PATTERN OF DESTRUCTION

Giant cell tumor forms a large hole in the distal femur. This is typical of a geographic area of destruction.

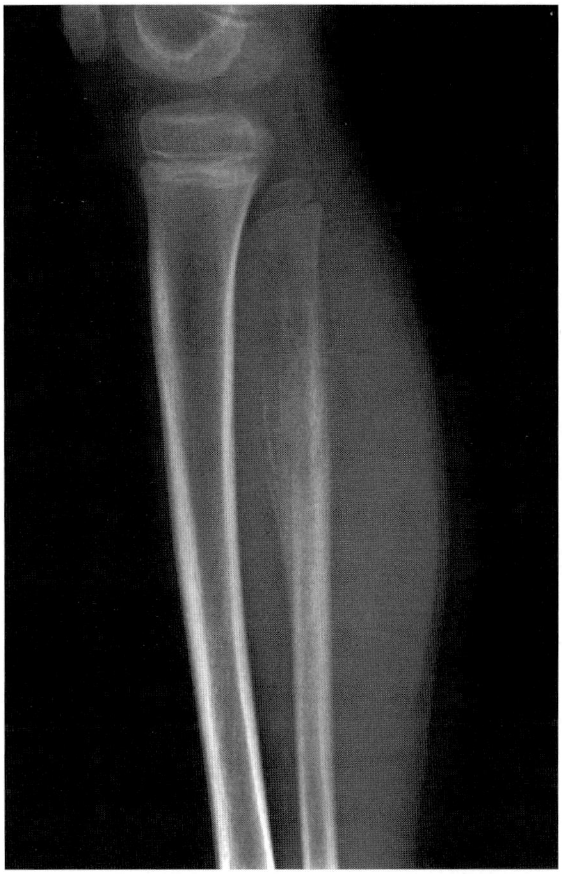

Figure 3-5

MOTH-EATEN PATTERN OF DESTRUCTION

Ewing's sarcoma involving the proximal fibula. The tumor is poorly demarcated and shows multiple small areas of destruction with intervening bone, giving rise to a moth-eaten appearance.

The lesion is usually, but not always, well demarcated. The geographic area may or may not be surrounded by sclerosis. This pattern is considered to be associated with a slow-growing process. With the moth-eaten pattern, the lesion consists of multiple scattered holes with cortical, cancellous, or both, bone types; these holes appear to arise separately and then coalesce. The moth-eaten pattern is associated with lesions that grow at a moderate rate (fig. 3-5). Permeative tumors have multiple, uniformly tiny lucencies that imperceptibly merge into normal bone (a wide zone of transition). These are the most rapidly growing tumors and include small cell malignancies (fig. 3-6).

MATRIX PATTERN

Some bone tumors produce matrix. The matrix frequently calcifies or ossifies, and this may be recognized by the radiologist. Calcification usually occurs in the form of calcium hydroxyapatite. However, other inorganic salts and a host of trace elements are also incorporated. Thus, "mineralization" is a more correct term than "calcification" (9). The pattern of mineralization helps to predict the type of matrix elaborated, but it generally does not aid in differentiating a benign process from a malignant one.

Osseous matrix results from the mineralization of the osteoid produced by neoplastic osteoblasts; it is the final step in the production of

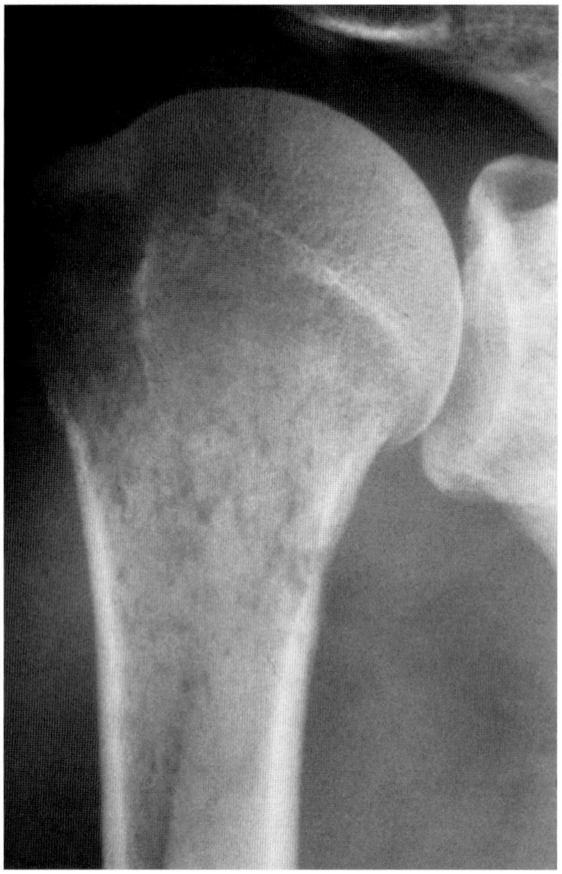

Figure 3-6

PERMEATIVE PATTERN OF DESTRUCTION

Malignant lymphoma of proximal humerus. The tumor is composed of minute areas of destruction that "fade" into normal bone.

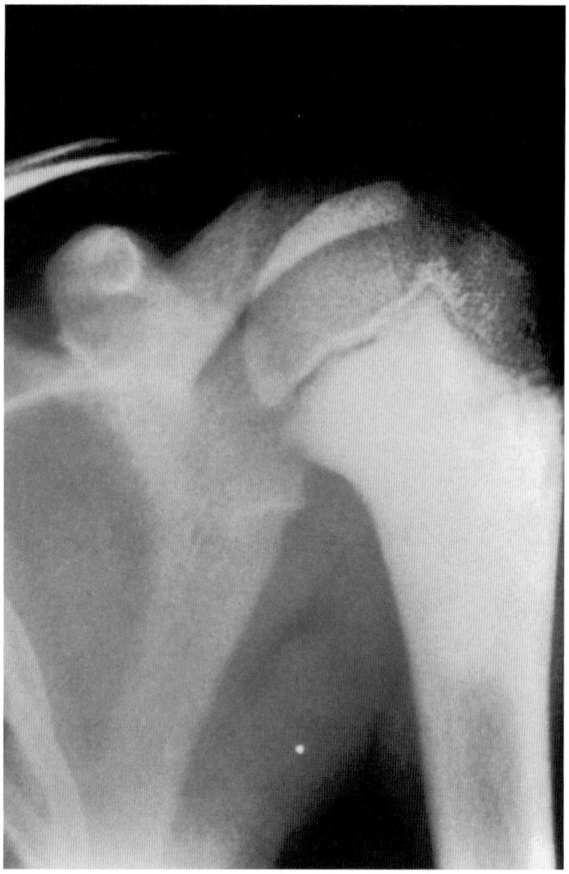

Figure 3-7

IVORY-LIKE DENSITY OF OSSEOUS MATRIX

Osteosarcoma of proximal humerus shows osteoid matrix, which is ivory-like.

a tumor. If the amount is sufficient, osseous matrix can be recognized on radiographs. The degree of density ranges from diffuse hazy (groundglass) to cloud-like and ivory-like (fig. 3-7).

Cartilage matrix may be stippled with small foci of calcification in the cartilage. The "stipples" may coalesce to form clumps of mineral (fig. 3-8). Arches and rings of calcification may form around lobules of cartilage to produce a ring-like pattern of mineralization.

PROLIFERATIVE BONE INDUCTION

Often, the response of a host to a tumor is the formation of bone by osteoblasts. This bone may be deposited on preexisting cancellous or cortical bone, or deposited in the soft tissues surrounding the bone as periosteal new bone.

Bone Formation within Bone. The patterns of reactive new bone formation can vary but be meaningful. For example, a slowly growing or static tumor within cancellous bone produces an organized type of response that results in sclerotic bone encapsulating the tumor (fig. 3-9). An aggressive tumor may evoke reactive new bone, but it is scattered or disorganized because some of it is destroyed by the tumor.

Periosteal New Bone Formation. Periosteal reactions have to be mineralized to be visible on radiographs. The pattern of periosteal reaction is related to the rate of growth of the underlying process and can be classified broadly into continuous and interrupted types (8). The earliest sign of involvement of the cortex is endosteal erosion. With progressive destruction of

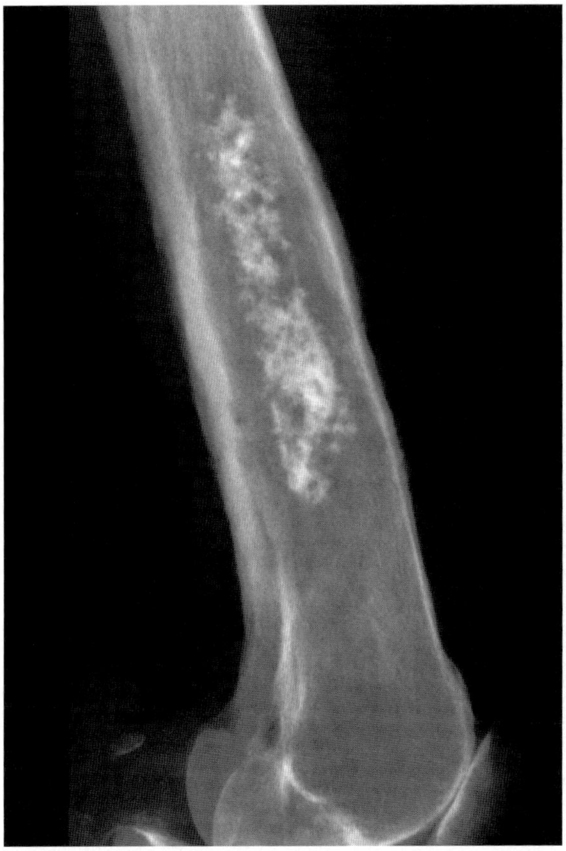

Figure 3-8

CARTILAGE MATRIX

Enchondroma of the distal femoral shaft shows typical cartilaginous calcification. The mineral is discrete and granular.

the cortex, new bone is laid down on the periosteal surface, producing the appearance of thickening of the cortex, expansion of the bone, or both. This appearance is typical of a chondrosarcoma. Continuous periosteal reactions may occur with a cortex that is either intact or destroyed. As indicated above, if periosteal new bone formation equals or exceeds the endosteal reaction, the bone appears thickened or expanded. If the rate of resorption of endosteal bone exceeds the rate of formation of appositional new bone, the cortex appears thinned and a bony shell eventually results. An intact bony shell suggests a benign but aggressive lesion such as an aneurysmal bone cyst.

A continuous periosteal reaction can form with partially or entirely intact cortex. The tumor may have permeated the cortex and invaded the periosteum. A solid continuous periosteal reaction consists of successive layers of periosteal new bone formation applied to the cortex in reaction to a slow-growing process such as eosinophilic granuloma, chronic osteomyelitis, or osteoid osteoma (fig. 3-10). A lamellated reaction is produced by concentric layers of periosteal new bone that produce an onionskin appearance. This appearance usually is associated with an aggressive process such as Ewing's sarcoma. It may be seen, however, in benign conditions such as osteomyelitis. A spiculated reaction consists of spicules of fine filamentous bone arranged perpendicularly to the underlying

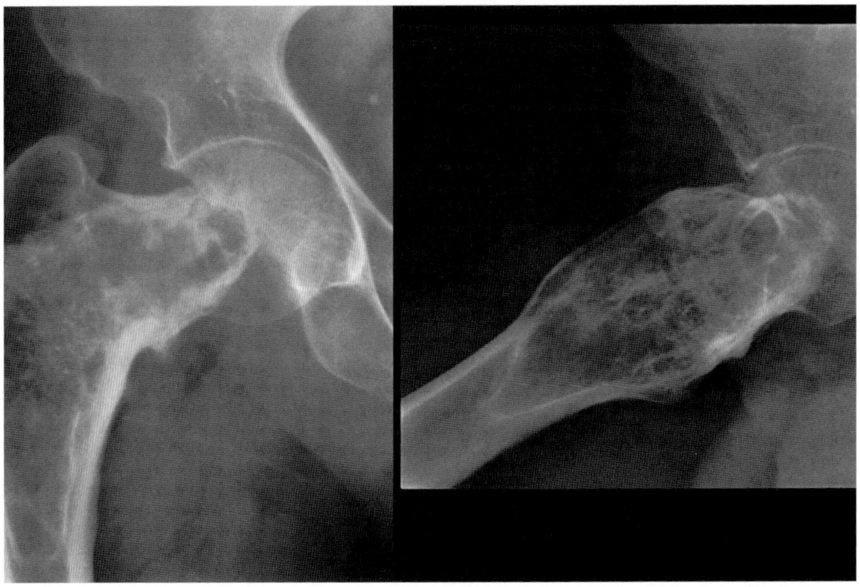

Figure 3-9

SCLEROTIC BONE ENCAPSULATING TUMOR

Fibrous dysplasia of proximal femur shows a well-demarcated area of lucency surrounded by a thick sclerotic "rind." The appearance virtually guarantees a benign lesion.

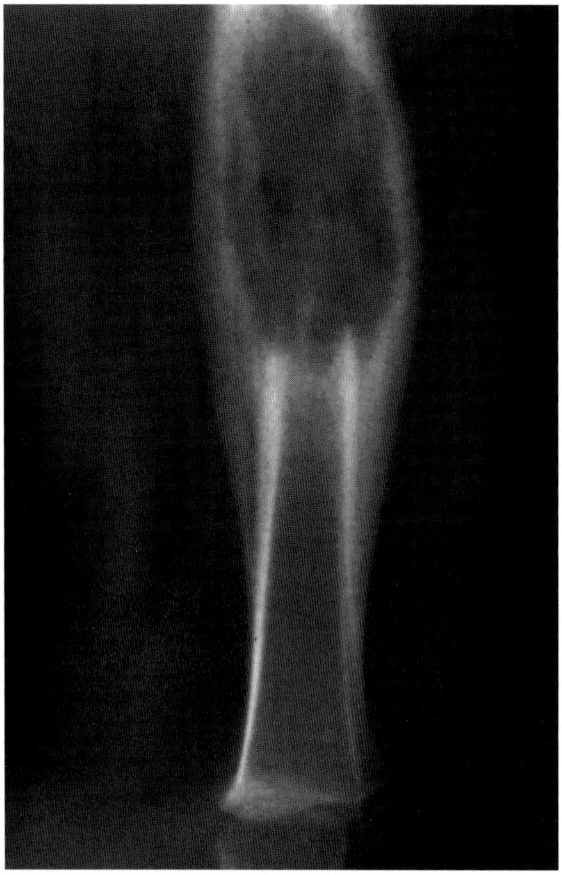

Figure 3-10

PERIOSTEAL NEW BONE

Thick, organized periosteal new bone suggests a benign lesion, such as this Langerhans' cell granulomatosis of the femur.

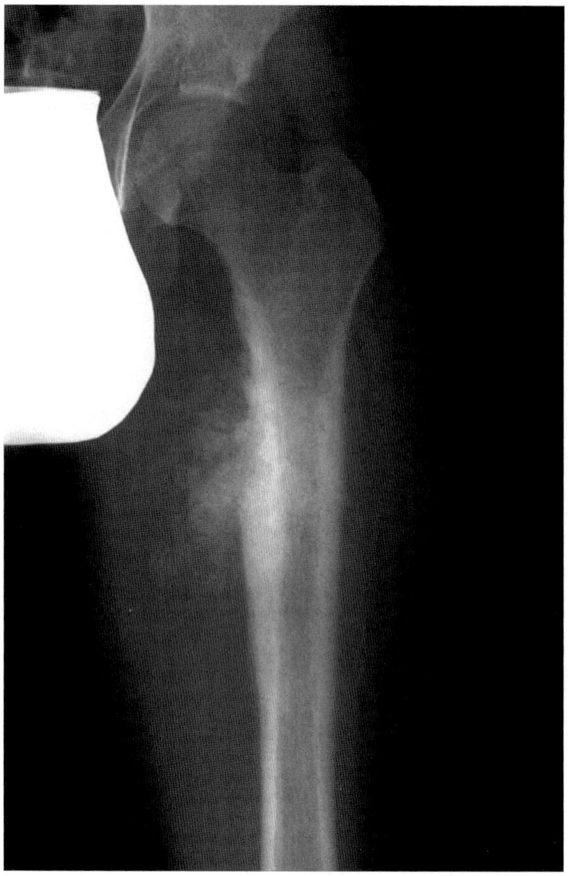

Figure 3-11

SPICULATED BONE

Spiculated bone in the periosteum, as in this sarcoma of the proximal femur, suggests an aggressive lesion. In this instance, the spiculated bone is part of the tumor.

bone. The spicules may be parallel ("hair-on-end") or disorganized ("sunburst"). This type of reaction usually is associated with a rapidly growing neoplasm. The spicules may be reactive (as in Ewing's sarcoma) or they may be evidence of matrix ossification by the tumor (as in osteosarcoma) (fig. 3-11).

INTERRUPTED PERIOSTEAL REACTION

As the term indicates, periosteal reactions may be incomplete in the middle (interrupted). If there is solid-appearing reactive bone on the two ends of the tumor, a buttress is formed (fig. 3-12). This usually means a benign, slow-growing process, for example, periosteal chondroma. If such a reaction is found only on one end, Codman's triangle (or angle) is formed (fig. 3-13). Codman's triangle usually is associated with a rapidly growing (but not necessarily malignant) tumor. Periosteal new bone formation is interrupted when the underlying process invades and destroys the periosteal new bone.

RADIONUCLIDE BONE IMAGING

Radionuclide scans depend on the propensity of the basic crystals of bone to absorb certain radioactive isotopes. After the radioactive agent has been injected into the vascular system, the patient is placed under a scintillation camera. The entire bone is scanned, and areas of abnormal accumulation of isotope are identified as hot spots. A bone scan is a sensitive and cost-effective way to identify skeletal lesions, especially in patients with metastatic carcinoma (2).

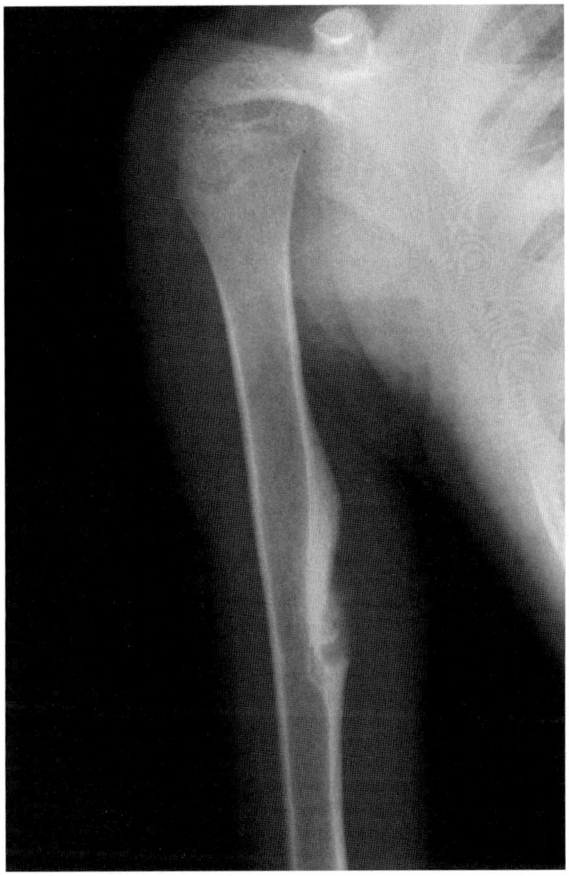

Figure 3-12

PERIOSTEAL REACTION

Reactive periosteal new bone formation forms a buttress on both ends of this periosteal chondroma.

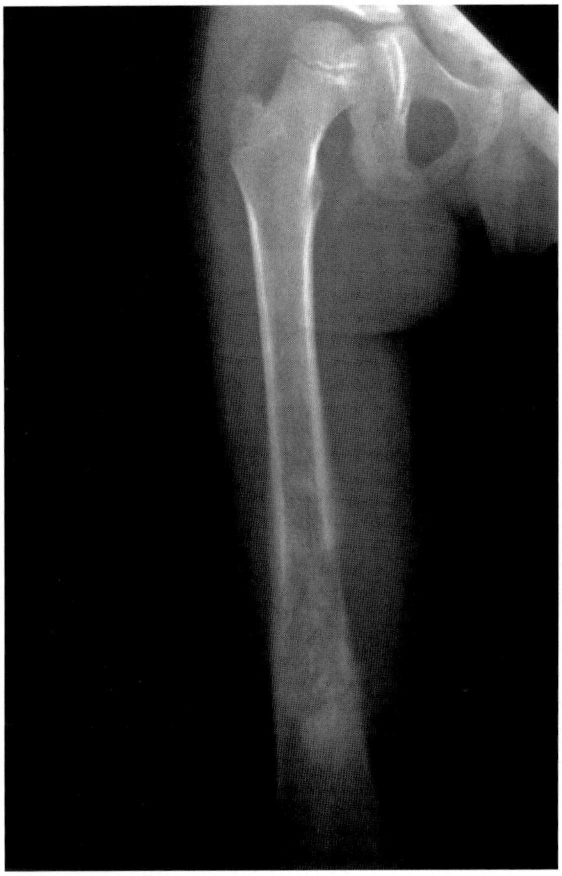

Figure 3-13

CODMAN'S TRIANGLE

Reactive new bone forms as the tumor grows through the cortex and lifts the periosteum. Codman's triangle is seen on the superior aspect of this osteosarcoma of the femur.

A bone scan is also useful for identifying multifocal disease as in malignant lymphoma and osteosarcoma. It is a sensitive method for identifying the nidus of osteoid osteoma (fig. 3-14), although CT is now considered better for this.

The disadvantage of bone scans is that they are nonspecific and merely identify increased bone formation, as in stress fractures.

COMPUTERIZED TOMOGRAMS

CT differs from plain radiography in that it uses a computer processing system instead of X-ray film to capture the image (1,4). A thin beam of X rays is passed through the patient, and a computer measures what passes through the tissues to the other side. The amount of X rays passing through the patient is determined by the attenuating properties of the tissues. The attenuation values are expressed in standard units called Hounsfield (H) units. The attenuation value for water is 0 and for air, -1,000 H. Bone has the highest value, +1,000 H. The CT numbers are assigned a range of gray shades, varying from black for air to white for bone. The display can be manipulated to highlight different units (windowing), such as bone or soft tissue. The CT scanner may be used to make a digital radiograph that can identify the area of interest. Although the computer collects data and formulates an axial image of the slices of variable thickness, from 0.3 cm to 1.5 cm, the data can be manipulated to project coronal and sagittal images.

CT images have several important advantages. The contrast resolution, which is far superior

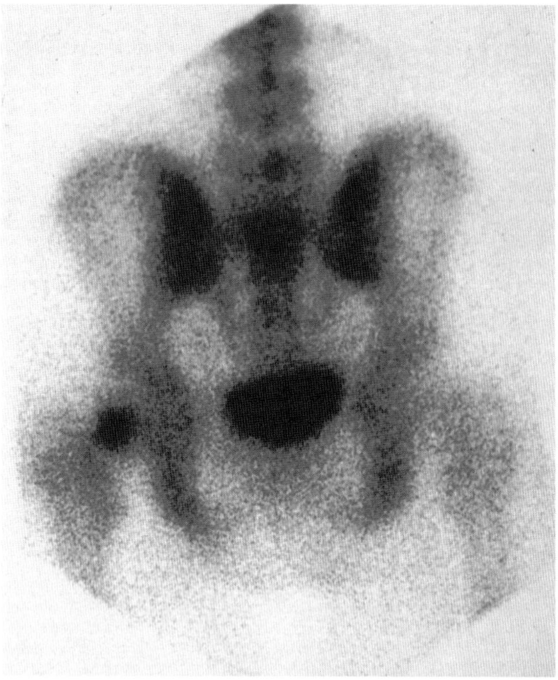

Figure 3-14

OSTEOID OSTEOMA

Osteoid osteoma of femoral neck presents as a "hot spot" on a bone scan.

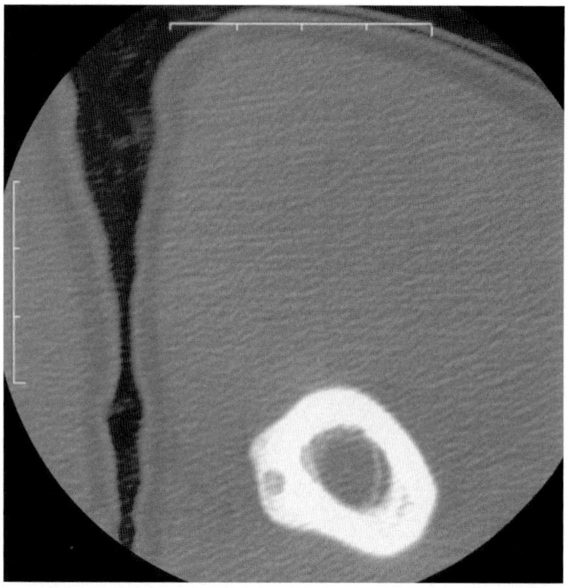

Figure 3-15

OSTEOID OSTEOMA

CT clearly identified the nidus of osteoid osteoma in the thickened femoral cortex.

to that of conventional radiographs, allows the extent of the tumor in bone and soft tissue to be defined for staging purposes. The axial orientation of the images is an advantage in regions of complex anatomy such as the pelvis, sacrum, and shoulder girdle, where overlying structures can obscure a lesion in plain radiographs. CT is very sensitive for identifying mineral that may not be seen with other methods. It is considered the best method for identifying the nidus of osteoid osteoma (fig. 3-15), and is useful for documenting the presence of fat, as in intraosseous lipoma. CT shows fluid-fluid levels, which is helpful in diagnosing aneurysmal bone cysts. It is sensitive in identifying metastatic deposits in the lung in patients with sarcomas. Finally, most needle biopsies of bone are performed under CT guidance; CT also is used for localization in radiofrequency ablation of osteoid osteoma.

The disadvantages of CT are that it is more expensive than plain radiography, metallic implants interfere with the images, and the patient has to remain motionless for long periods.

MAGNETIC RESONANCE IMAGING

MRI does not depend on radiation but on the reemission of absorbed radiofrequency while the patient is in a strong magnetic field. The image reflects the hydrogen intensity in tissue and the way mobile hydrogen protons respond to various sequences of radiofrequency stimulation. The response varies with the type of tissue (when the stimulation is discontinued, the protons return to their original alignment; this is called relaxation time). A bright (white) area of an image has high signal intensity and a dark (black) area has low signal intensity.

T_1 relaxation describes the absolute loss of energy, and T_2 relaxation describes the relative loss of energy due to the sum of wave phasing (Klein MJ, presented at the Radiological and Clinical Aspects of Bone Tumors meeting, University of Kyoto, Japan, October 2000). This differentiation is useful because different tissues display different signal intensities on T_1- and T_2-weighted images. Bone marrow fat is bright, and cortical bone is dark. Some tissues (edema, hematoma, tumor) have low intensity on T_1-weighted images but high intensity on T_2-weighted images (fig. 3-16). T_1 relaxation

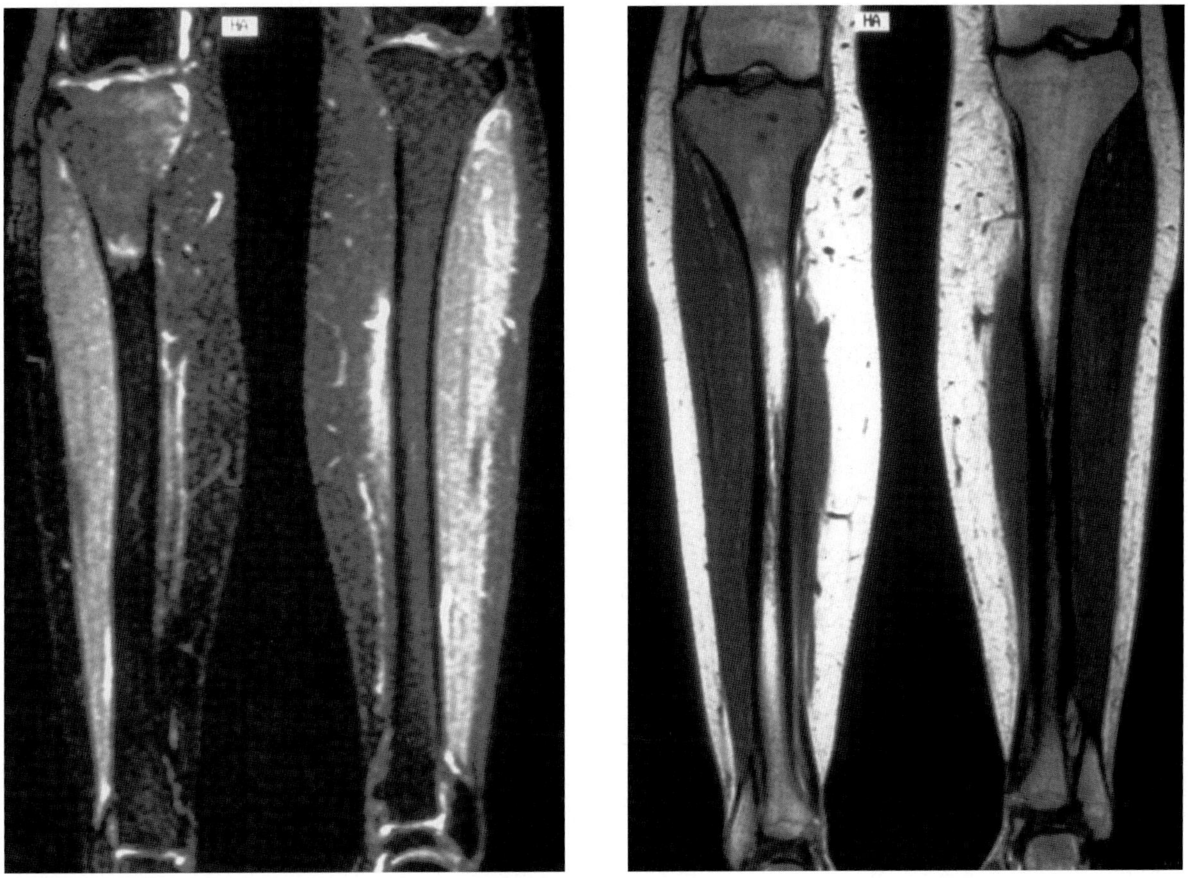

Figure 3-16

MAGNETIC RESONANCE IMAGE OF OSTEOSARCOMA OF TIBIA

The tumor is "dark" on T_1-weighted images (left) and "bright" on T_2-weighted images (right).

provides the best contrast between the low signal of tumor and the high signal of bone marrow and soft tissue fat. T_2 relaxation provides contrast between the high signal of tumor and low signal of cortical bone and skeletal muscle.

MRI has several advantages. The images have unsurpassed contrast resolution and, hence, accurately delineate the extent of the tumor both within the bone and outside it (7). The high sensitivity of MRI allows the detection of small lesions that may be missed on plain radiographs. This is especially true for lesions involving the bone marrow, such as myeloma and metastatic carcinoma. The patient is not exposed to ionizing radiation. The image can be displayed in multiple planes. Finally, dynamic MRI imaging appears to be sensitive for predicting response to chemotherapy (3).

The disadvantages of MRI are that it may be too sensitive and, hence, may exaggerate the size of the lesion, the appearance of tumors is nonspecific, it is not sensitive for identifying small amounts of mineral, it is an expensive and time-consuming method, and any metal in the patient (e.g., heart valves) may preclude using the technique.

REFERENCES

1. Andre M, Resnick D. Computed tomography. In: Resnick D, ed. Diagnosis of bone and joint disorders, vol. 1, 3rd ed. Philadelphia: WB Saunders; 1995:118–69.
2. Bassett LW, Gold RH, Webber MM. Radionuclide bone imaging. Radiol Clin North Am 1981;19: 675–702.
3. Fletcher BD, Hanna SL, Fairclough DL, Gronemeyer SA. Pediatric musculoskeletal tumors: use of dynamic, contrast-enhanced MR imaging to monitor response to chemotherapy. Radiology 1992;184:243–8.
4. Greenspan A, ed. Orthopedic radiology: a practical approach, 3rd ed. Philadelphia: Lippincott Williams & Wilkins; 2000:17–34.
5. Lodwick GS. A systematic approach to the roentgen diagnosis of bone tumors. In: Tumors of bone and soft tissue: a collection of papers presented at the Eighth Annual Clinical Conference of Cancer, 1963, at the University of Texas M.D. Anderson Hospital and Tumor Institute, Houston, Texas. Chicago: Year Book Medical Publishers; 1965:49–68.
6. Madewell JE, Ragsdale BD, Sweet DE. Radiologic and pathologic analysis of solitary bone lesions. Part I: internal margins. Radiol Clin North Am 1981;19:715–48.
7. McLeod RA, Berquist TH. Bone tumor imaging: contribution of CT and MRI. Contemp Issues Surg Pathol 1988;11:1–34.
8. Ragsdale BD, Madewell JE, Sweet DE. Radiologic and pathologic analysis of solitary bone lesions. Part II: periosteal reactions. Radiol Clin North Am 1981;19:749–83.
9. Sweet DE, Madewell JE, Ragsdale BD. Radiologic and pathologic analysis of solitary bone lesions. Part III: matrix patterns. Radiol Clin North Am 1981;19:785–814.

4 CARTILAGINOUS LESIONS

OSTEOCHONDROMA

Definition. Osteochondroma is a benign outgrowth of cortical and medullary bone, with a cartilaginous cap projecting from the surface of the involved bone (18). The term *exostosis* is sometimes used interchangeably with osteochondroma. However, exostosis is a more generic term that indicates an outgrowth of bone, as may be seen with an osteophyte in degenerative joint disease.

General Features. The prevalence of osteochondromas is unknown because many patients are asymptomatic and the tumor is never discovered. Until the year 2000, the surgical series at Mayo Clinic included 946 osteochondromas, which accounted for 33 percent of all benign bone tumors and 9.9 percent of all tumors. Of chondrogenic tumors, more than one third are osteochondromas (fig. 4-1).

Osteochondromas probably are not true neoplasms but rather growths of misplaced epiphyseal plates on the surface of bone. Osteochondromas have been reported to arise after radiotherapy in childhood: Libshitz and Cohen (31)

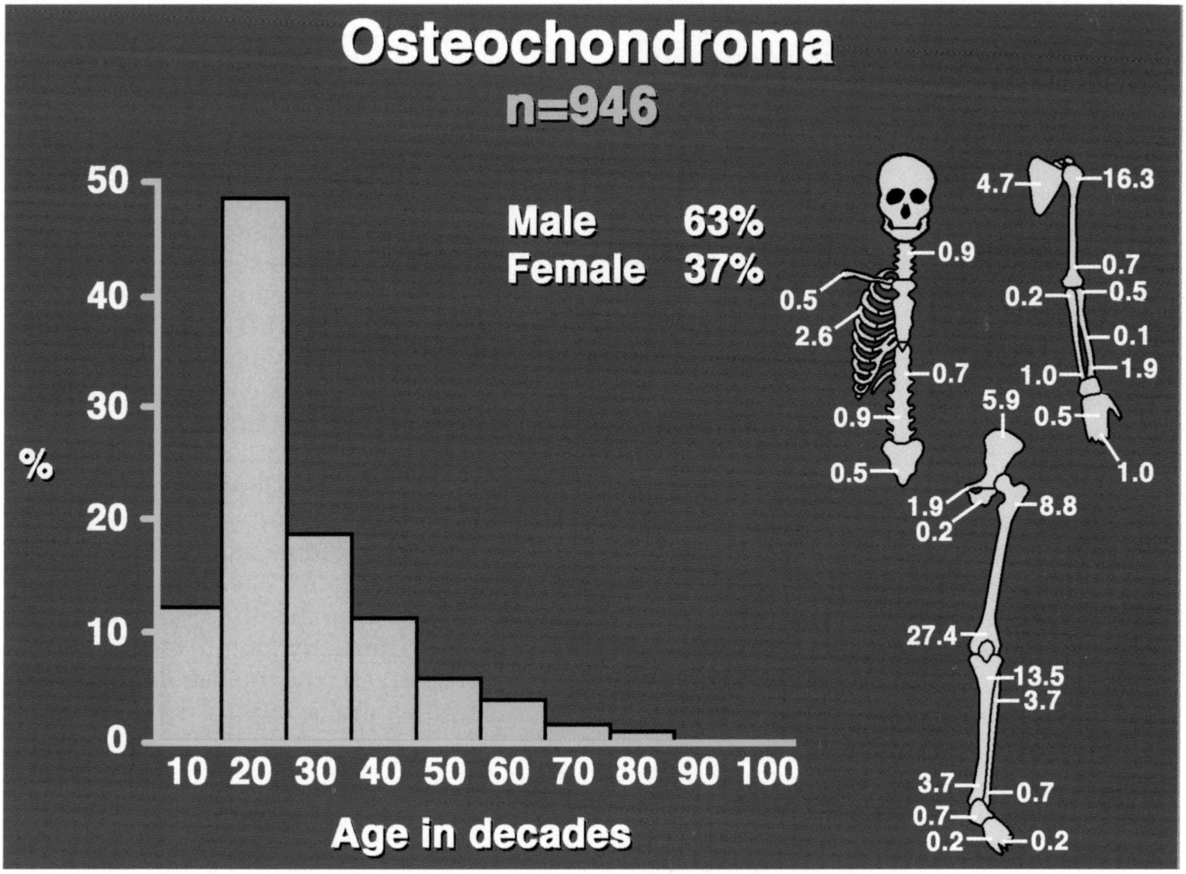

Figure 4-1

OSTEOCHONDROMA

The distribution of osteochondroma according to the age and sex of the patient and the site of the lesion.

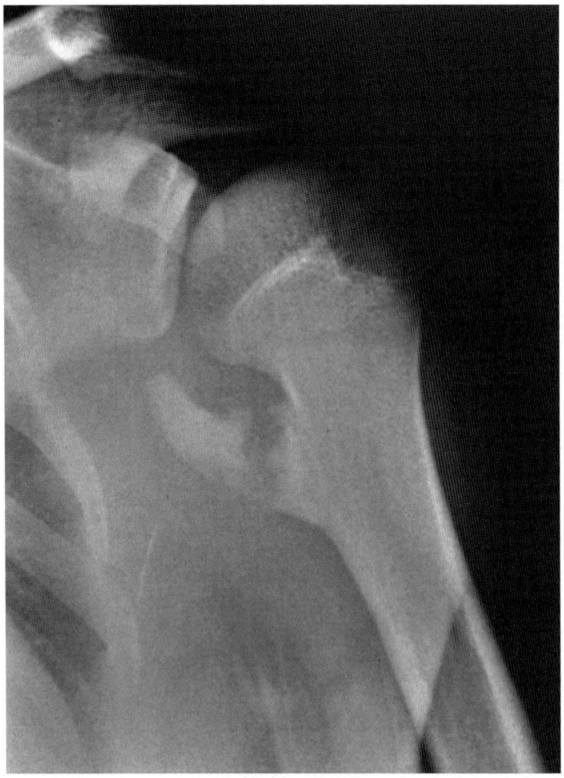

Figure 4-2

OSTEOCHONDROMA

Pathologic fracture of an osteochondroma involving the proximal humerus of a 15-year-old boy.

reported a 12 percent incidence of osteochondroma following radiotherapy for childhood malignancies. Of the 14 patients reported, 7 had multiple osteochondromas and 7 had solitary lesions. Any open epiphyseal plate is susceptible; the radiation dose has ranged from 1,000 to 6,000 rads, and the latent period can vary from 17 months to 16 years (24).

Clinical Features. Osteochondromas may present as a palpable mass or they may produce symptoms from pressure on nearby structures such as nerves. Occasionally, a fracture through the stalk of an osteochondroma produces pain (fig. 4-2). A bursa may overlie the cap of an osteochondroma and be large enough to form a palpable mass. Venous thrombosis and pseudoaneurysms of arteries may result from pressure from an osteochondroma. Although osteochondromas occur in any age group, about 60 percent of patients undergoing surgery are in the first two decades of life. There is a slight male predominance.

Sites. Osteochondromas may develop in any bone in which enchondral ossification occurs. The most frequently involved sites, in descending order, are the distal femur, proximal humerus, and proximal tibia. Osteochondromas may involve the pelvis or the spine; in the latter, the posterior elements are involved preferentially. It is rare for the small bones of the hands and feet to be involved in the absence of multiple osteochondromas. Osteochondromas usually do not occur in the skull or jawbones.

Radiographic Findings. The characteristic radiographic appearance is that of a projection, either pedunculated or sessile, from the surface of a bone, usually the metaphysis of a long bone (fig. 4-3). The cortex of the involved bone flares out into the cortex of the lesion. The medullary cavity of the osteochondroma is also continuous with the medulla of the involved bone. The outermost portion expands in a mushroom shape to form the cartilage cap. The cap may not be clearly visible on plain radiographs unless it is uniformly mineralized. Computerized tomography (CT) and magnetic resonance imaging (MRI) are better able to define the true thickness of the cartilage cap (28). Occasionally, especially in complex anatomic locations, plain radiographs may not be diagnostic because the relationship between the calcified density and the underlying bone is not obvious. CT can help delineate the relationship between the bone and the lesion.

The affected bone is often abnormally wide at the level of the osteochondroma, especially in cases of multiple lesions (fig. 4-4). A pedunculated osteochondroma typically points away from the nearest joint. The cartilage cap may be inconspicuous so that the lesion has the appearance of a thin bony spur (the so-called coathook deformity). If the osteochondroma is associated with a sizable bursa, a nonmineralized soft tissue mass may overlie the cap, raising suspicion of sarcomatous change. CT and MRI usually lead to the correct diagnosis by identifying the fluid-filled cyst (fig. 4-5).

Gross Findings. The gross features depend on the type of osteochondroma. *Sessile osteochondromas* have the appearance of a semicircle, with a thin regular cartilage cap covering the

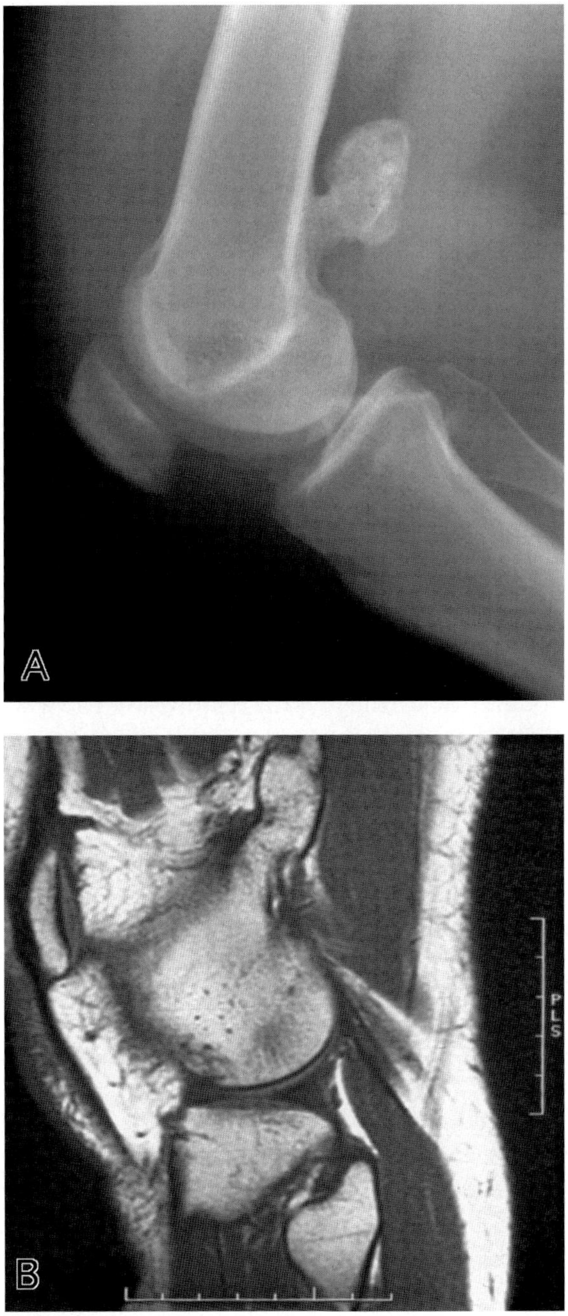

Figure 4-3

OSTEOCHONDROMA

A: A pedunculated osteochondroma characteristically points away from the nearest joint. The cortex is continuous with that of the underlying bone.

B: Magnetic resonance imaging (MRI) highlights continuous spongiosa between the underlying bone and osteochondroma. (Courtesy of Dr. N. Bramwell, Kalamazoo, MI.)

C: A sessile osteochondroma with a broad base projects from the distal femur.

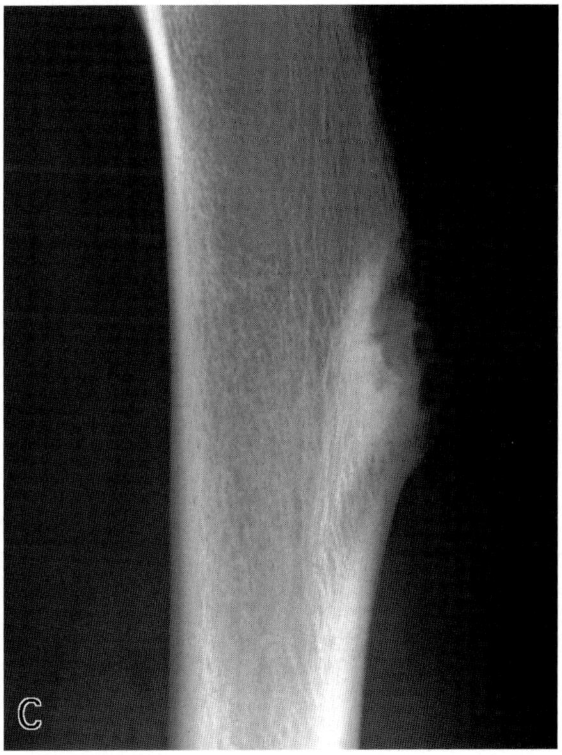

surface of the tumor. The surface is covered by a thin membrane that represents the periosteum lifted off the affected bone. Irregular lines of calcification demarcate the cartilage from the underlying cancellous bone. Fatty and hematopoietic bone marrow are present in the intertrabecular spaces, reflecting the status of the marrow in the involved bone.

Pedunculated osteochondromas resemble a mushroom with a bony stalk and a cartilage cap (fig. 4-6). The cap is smooth and usually no more than a few millimeters in thickness (fig. 4-7). It is important to slice the lesion perpendicularly to the stalk so that the true thickness of the cap can be appreciated. Although the cap may be somewhat bosselated, any irregular

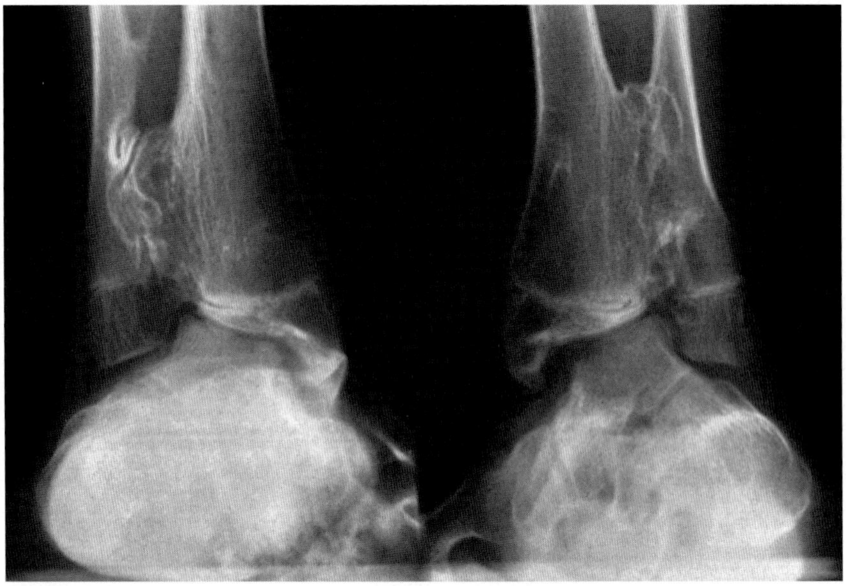

Figure 4-4

MULTIPLE OSTEOCHONDROMAS

Oblique views of the ankle show a large sessile tibial exostosis eroding into the fibula and forming a synostosis. A pedunculated fibula exostosis as well as abnormal bone modeling of the distal tibia are also present. (Courtesy of Dr. M. Costa, Sacramento, CA.)

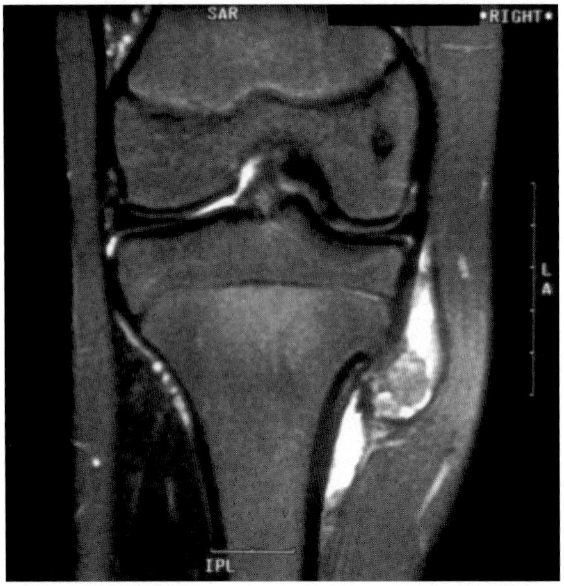

Figure 4-5

OSTEOCHONDROMA

Coronal T_2-weighted MRI shows an osteochondroma with a collection of bursal fluid proximal and distal to the tumor. (Courtesy of Dr. B. Sauli, Morristown, NJ.)

nodularity should make one consider the possibility of secondary chondrosarcoma.

It is not unusual to find a small inconspicuous bursa overlying the cap; rarely, the bursa becomes large and overshadows the osteochondroma giving rise to it. The bursa may contain nodules of cartilage with features of synovial chondromatosis (6).

Microscopic Findings. It is important to make a section through the cap and underlying bone for histopathologic examination. The outer aspect of the cap is covered with a thin pink membrane that represents the periosteum lifted off the underlying bone. A single slide should show both cartilage and bone; if not, chondrosarcoma should be suspected because the cartilage is so abundant. The cartilage cap is composed of chondrocytes in lacunae arranged in clusters, with an abundance of chondroid matrix between the clusters. Toward the base, the chondrocytes are arranged in columns, as in normal epiphyseal plates (fig. 4-8). Bony trabeculae arise from the cartilage plate (fig. 4-9). Fatty or hematopoietic bone marrow occurs between the bony trabeculae. Nodules of cartilage may be present within the bony trabeculae, a form of enchondral ossification (fig. 4-10).

Genetics and Other Special Techniques. Osteochondroma may occur as a sporadic solitary lesion or as multiple lesions. Multiple lesions characterize the autosomal dominant disorder, *hereditary multiple exostoses*, or the contiguous gene-deletion syndromes, *Langer-Giedion syndrome* and *DEFECT-11 (Potocki-Shaffer) syndrome* (3,25,33,38,40,42,49). Constitutional chromosomal deletions or structural rearrangements

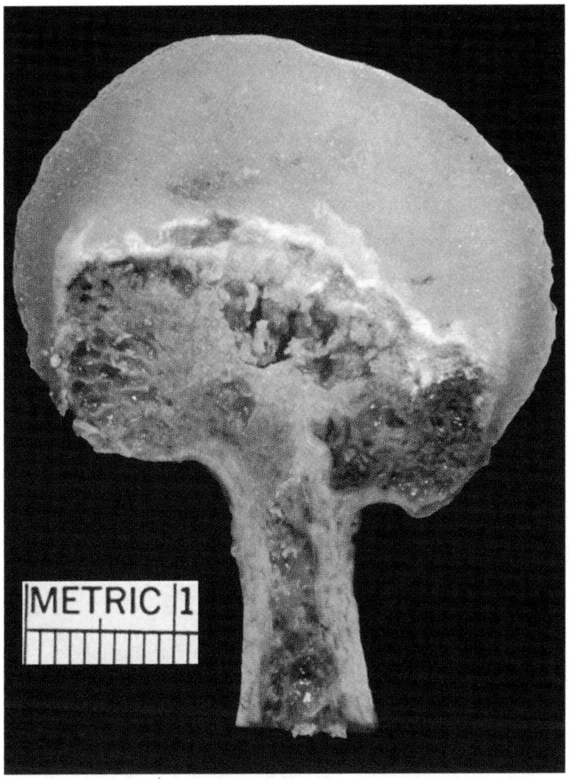

Figure 4-6

OSTEOCHONDROMA

The cartilage cap is somewhat thick but smooth. The chalky white areas are calcification. (Fig. 2-6 from Unni KK. Dahlin's bone tumors: general aspects and data on 11,087 cases, 5th ed. Philadelphia: Lippincott-Raven; 1996:15. By permission of Mayo Foundation.)

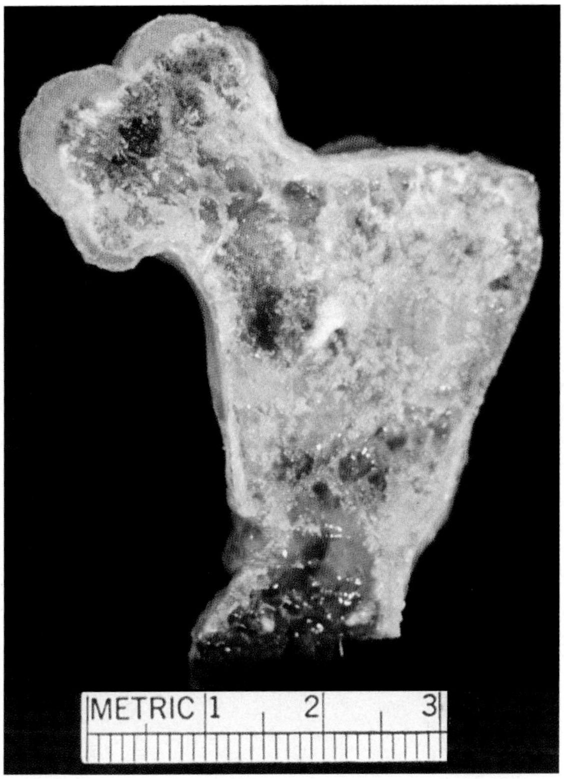

Figure 4-7

OSTEOCHONDROMA

A thin cartilage cap covers an osteochondroma arising from the femur of a 69-year-old man. Much of the osteochondroma is composed of a bony stalk.

of 8q24.1 are found in Langer-Giedion syndrome and of 11p11-12 in DEFECT-11 syndrome (3,25, 33,38,40,49). Langer-Giedion syndrome is characterized by multiple exostoses, dysmorphic facial features, mental retardation, and the loss of functional copies of both the *TRPS1* (trichorhinophalangeal syndrome type I) and *EXT1* (exostoses) genes (25,38). Patients with DEFECT-11 syndrome show interstitial deletions of chromosomal bands 11p11-12 (with loss of the *ALX4* [Aristaless-like 4] and *EXT2* genes), enlarged parietal foramina, multiple exostoses, craniofacial dysostosis, and mental retardation (3,40,49).

Hereditary multiple exostoses is genetically heterogeneous, with a prevalence of 1/50,000 (43). Three genetic loci for hereditary multiple exostoses have been identified: 8q24.1 (*EXT1*) (16), 11p11-12 (*EXT2*) (50), and 19p (*EXT3*) (30). Linkage studies have implicated the *EXT1* and *EXT2* genes in the majority of cases. The *EXT1* gene reportedly has shown linkage in 44 to 66 percent of families with hereditary multiple exostoses, whereas linkage for *EXT2* has been shown in approximately 27 percent (29,41). Preliminary studies suggest that these various chromosomal linkages may predispose to the location, percentage of involvement, and type (sessile or pedunculated) of osteochondromas, and the risk of malignant transformation, and thus explain the variable manifestations of the disease (13,20).

The *EXT1* gene has been cloned and sequenced, and the coding region is composed of 3.4 kb of complementary (c)DNA encoded in 11 exons (1). The *EXT2* gene has also been

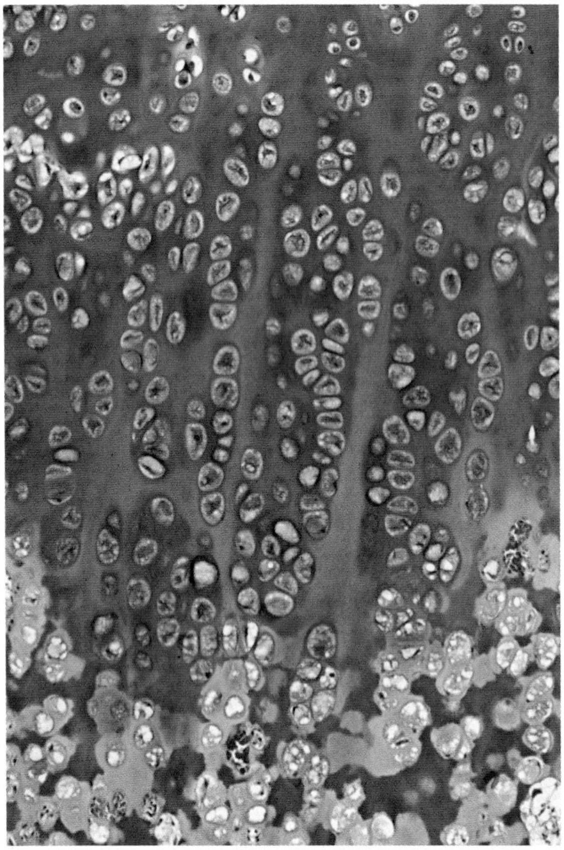

Figure 4-8

OSTEOCHONDROMA

Columns of maturing chondrocytes simulate the appearance of normal epiphyseal plate at the junction between the cartilage cap and stalk.

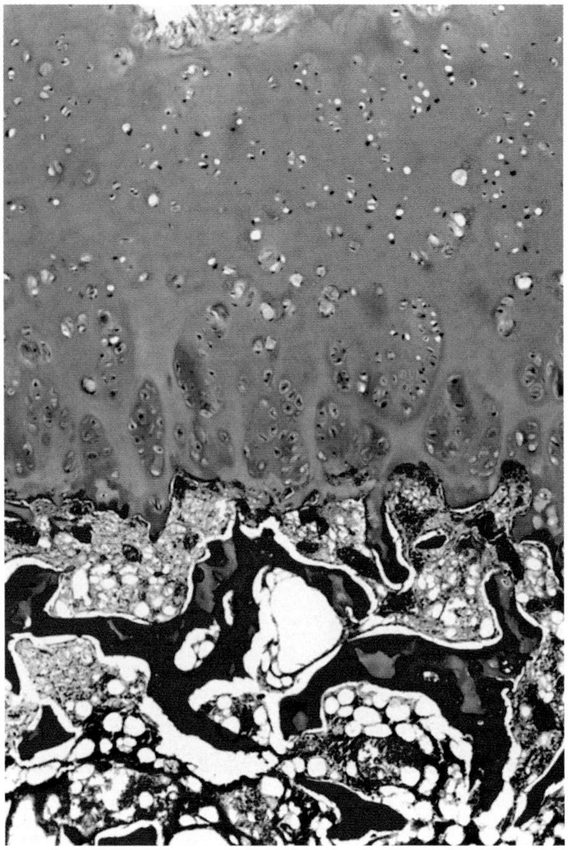

Figure 4-9

OSTEOCHONDROMA

A cartilage cap overlies cancellous bone of the stalk.

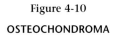

Figure 4-10

OSTEOCHONDROMA

Cancellous bone within the stalk contains islands of cartilage and is surrounded by fat and hematopoietic bone marrow.

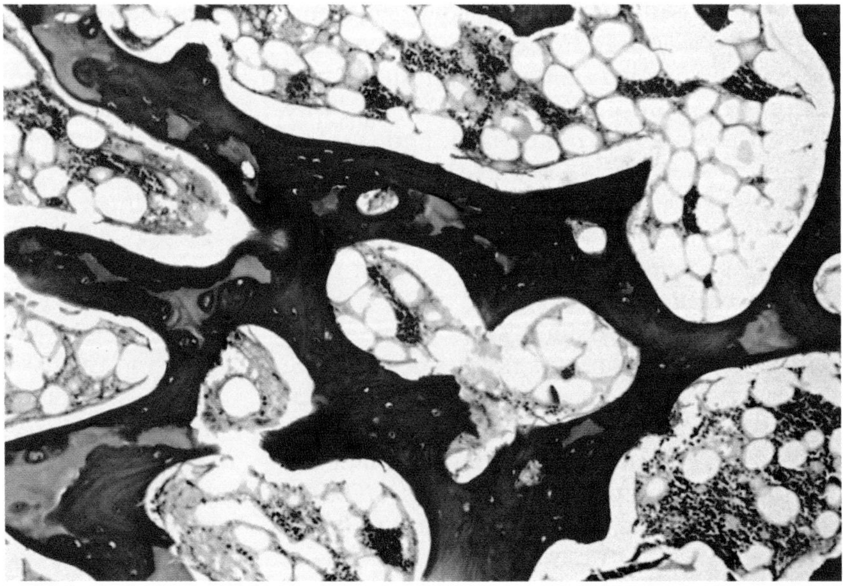

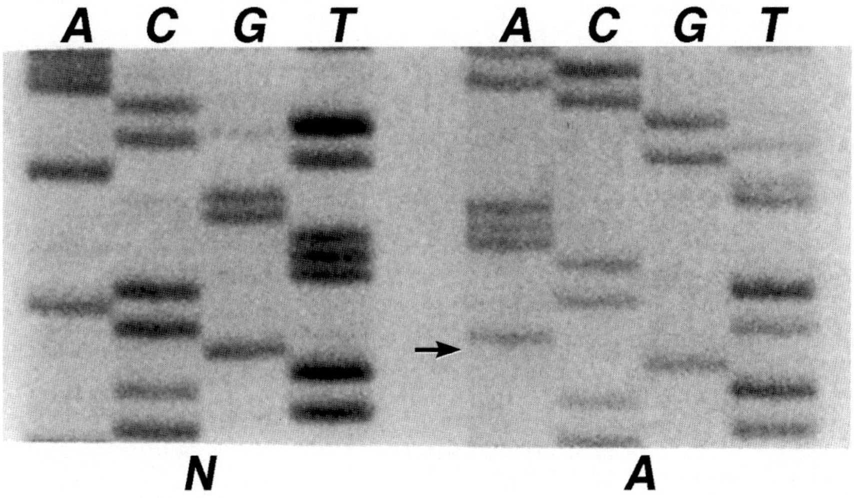

Figure 4-11

SOMATIC *EXT1* MUTATION IN A CHONDROSARCOMA

Normal constitutional DNA sequence, *N*, and chondrosarcoma demonstrating 8-bp deletion in exon 1 of the *EXT1* gene, *A*, both from a patient without a family history of hereditary multiple exostoses. This deletion resulted in a frameshift and premature stop codon at nucleotide 1213 of *EXT1*. (Fig. 4 from Hecht JT, Hogue D, Wang Y, et al. Hereditary multiple exostoses (EXT): mutational studies of familial EXT1 cases and EXT-associated malignancies. Am J Hum Genet 1997;60:80-6.)

identified and has an open reading frame encoding 718 amino acids with an overall homology of 30.9 percent with *EXT1* (52). *EXT3*, identified solely through linkage analysis, has not been isolated or characterized. Germline mutations of both *EXT1* and *EXT2* have been identified, and most result in truncated or nonfunctional proteins, supporting the hypothesis that *EXT1* and *EXT2* are tumor suppressor genes (1,52). Missense mutations of these two genes are less common (14, 51). A somatic mutation, an 8-bp deletion in exon 1 of *EXT1*, has been described in a patient with chondrosarcoma (fig. 4-11), and in an isolated sporadic osteochondroma, deletions involving both copies of the *EXT1* gene were detected (5,23).

The *EXT1* and *EXT2* genes encode for the type II transmembrane glycoproteins localized to the endoplasmic reticulum and required for heparan sulfate polymerization (32,36,44). Proteins EXT1 and EXT2 form a stable hetero-oligomeric complex in vivo that leads to the accumulation of both proteins in the Golgi apparatus; the complex possesses substantially higher glycosyltransferase activity than EXT1 or EXT2 alone, suggesting that the complex represents the biologically relevant form of the enzyme(s) (34). Heparan sulfate proteoglycans (HSPGs) participate in cell signaling pathways and consist of heparan sulfate glycosaminoglycans linked to a protein core (35). An *EXT1* drosophila homologue, *tout-velu (ttv),* has been identified and shown to have a role in HSPG biosynthesis in vivo (4,45,47).

The *ttv* gene is required for diffusion of Hedgehog, an important segment polarity protein and a homologue of the mammalian Indian Hedgehog (IHh) (4). During normal growth, IHh and parathyroid hormone-related peptide (PTHrP) are involved in the proliferation and differentiation of chondrocytes at the growth plate in an HSPG-dependent signaling pathway (2,9,17,48). Normal chondrocyte proliferation and differentiation are also dependent on another important HSPG-dependent pathway, the fibroblast growth factor (FGF) signaling pathway (17,22,48).

EXT gene inactivation results in altered heparan sulfate expression at the cell surface of chondrocytes and adversely affects IHh/PTHrP and FGF signaling. Inactivation of both copies of *EXT1* has been detected in hereditary osteochondromas (8). It has been hypothesized that IHh/PTHrP and FGF signaling defects have a role in the development of osteochondromas (fig. 4-12) (4,9,26,46). In one study, evaluation of the immunohistochemical expression of IHh/PTHrP and FGF signaling pathway members showed no immunoreactivity for PTHrP, FGF2, FGF receptor (R)1, bcl2, and $p21^{CIP1}$ in the majority of the 24 osteochondromas (hereditary and sporadic) analyzed, lending support to this hypothesis (9).

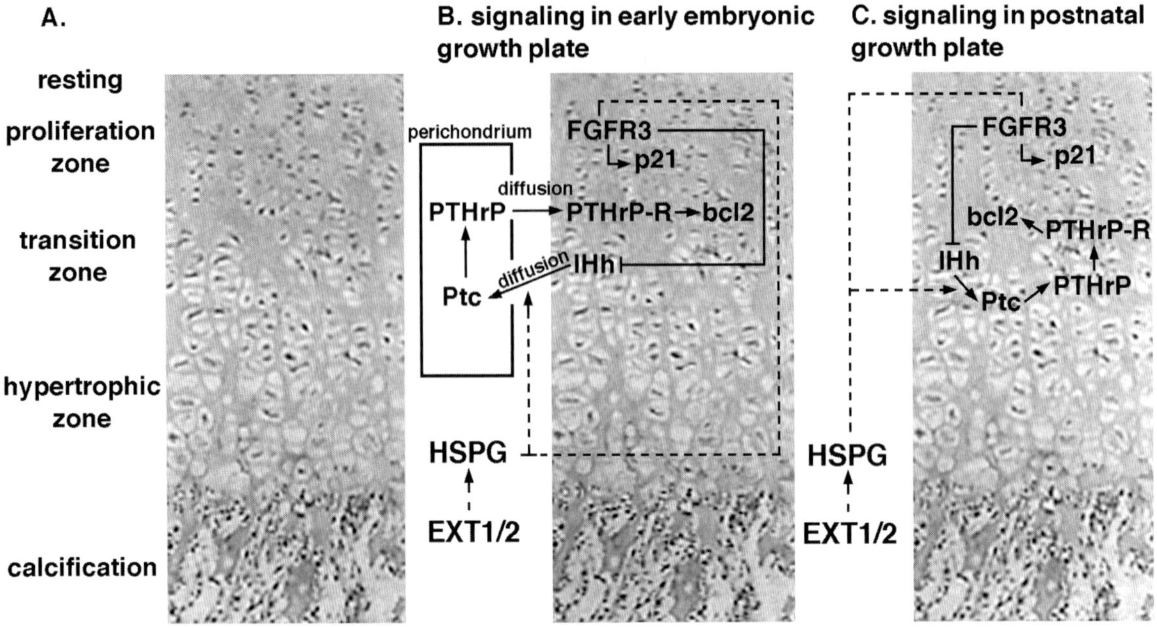

Figure 4-12

NORMAL POSTNATAL GROWTH PLATE

A: The normal postnatal growth plate is characterized by the orderly proliferation and maturation of chondrocytes in longitudinal columns, forming stratified zones of resting, proliferative, prehypertrophic/maturing, and hypertrophic cartilage. Ossification begins with invasion of calcified hypertrophic cartilage by capillaries, accompanied by apoptosis of terminal hypertrophic chondrocytes, resorption of cartilage matrix, and deposition of bone matrix by osteoblasts.

B: Growth signaling in the early embryonic growth plate is depicted. Chondrocytes in the transition zone secrete Indian hedgehog (IHh), which has to diffuse to the lateral perichondrium where its receptor, Ptc, is expressed. Binding induces upregulation of parathyroid hormone-related peptide (PTHrP) at the apical perichondrium, which then diffuses to its receptor localized at late proliferating chondrocytes. Via upregulation of bcl2, further differentiation of late proliferating chondrocytes is inhibited, resulting in fewer IHh-producing cells, which closes the feedback loop. Activation of fibroblast growth factor (FGF)R3, expressed at the proliferative zone by an as yet unknown ligand, inhibits chondrocyte proliferation via upregulation of $p21^{WAF1/CIP1}$ and represses IHh signaling.

C: Growth signaling in the postnatal growth plate. The IHh/PTHrP feedback loop is now confined to the growth plate. IHh binds to Ptc in the hypertrophic zone, stimulating PTHrP expression; PTHrP then binds its receptor in the hypertrophic zone, upregulating bcl2. (Fig. 1 from Bovée JV, van den Broek LJ, Cleton-Jansen AM, Hogendoorn PC. Up-regulation of PTHrP and Bcl-2 expression characterizes the progression of osteochondroma towards peripheral chondrosarcoma and is a late event in central chondrosarcoma. Lab Invest 2000;80:1925-34.)

Historically, the nature of osteochondroma (developmental aberration versus benign neoplasm) has been debated (39). The discovery of clonal chromosomal abnormalities in osteochondromas provided compelling evidence that they represent a true neoplasm (10,11,37). Clonal karyotypic abnormalities leading to loss or rearrangement of 8q24.1 or 11p11-12, the chromosomal loci of the *EXT1* and *EXT2* genes, have been detected as somatic aberrations in both sporadic and hereditary osteochondromas (fig. 4-13) (12). Fluorescence in situ hybridization (FISH) studies have confirmed the loss of the 8q24.1 locus in a subset of osteochondromas (19). The observation of clonal chromosomal loss of either 8q24.1 or 11p11-12 in sporadic osteochondromas suggests that, similar to hereditary multiple exostoses, sporadic exostoses are also genetically heterogeneous (12).

Malignant transformation of a sporadic osteochondroma is rare (less than 1 percent); however, it is a more frequent complication in patients with hereditary multiple exostoses (1.0 to 8.3 percent) (27). Peripheral chondrosarcomas are seen most commonly; osteosarcomas have also been reported. Loss of heterozygosity for *EXT1* has been observed in peripheral chondrosarcomas but not in central chondrosarcomas (7).

Differential Diagnosis. The differential diagnosis includes subungual exostosis, bizarre parosteal osteochondromatous proliferation, and secondary chondrosarcoma. Subungual exostosis involves the distal phalanx, usually of the big toe, and presents as a rapidly growing mass. Osteochondromas seldom occur in a subungual location. Radiographs show a lesion plastered onto the surface but without the cortical and medullary continuity typical of osteochondroma. Microscopically, cartilaginous nodules give rise to bone that has active osteoblastic proliferation and spindle cells between the trabeculae. The bone lacks the mature appearance seen in osteochondroma.

Bizarre parosteal osteochondromatous proliferation usually involves the surfaces of the small bones of the hand, although no bone of the skeleton is exempt. Radiographs show a heavily mineralized mass that is attached to the surface but not continuous with the medullary cavity. Microscopically, abundant cartilage is present, giving rise to irregular bony trabeculae. At the junction between the bone and cartilage, there is a deep blue to purple pattern of calcification, which is distinctive and never seen in osteochondroma.

When a malignancy arises in an osteochondroma, it is usually a chondrosarcoma (21). Radiographic, gross, and microscopic features have to be evaluated to differentiate osteochondroma from chondrosarcoma. A soft tissue mass with patchy mineralization suggests secondary chondrosarcoma. Grossly, a lobulated, thick (more than 2 cm) cartilage cap with myxoid change in the matrix that gives rise to liquefaction and cyst formation typifies secondary chondrosarcoma. Microscopically, the columnar arrangement of the chondrocytes typically present in osteochondroma is lost. The presence of nodules of cartilage separated from the main mass and embedded in soft tissue is diagnostic of chondrosarcoma.

Treatment and Prognosis. Surgical excision is indicated if the lesion causes symptoms. It is important to remove the entire cartilage cap to avoid recurrences. In the Mayo Clinic series, the recurrence rate was 2 percent; simple reexcision was curative in all instances. Chin et al. (15)

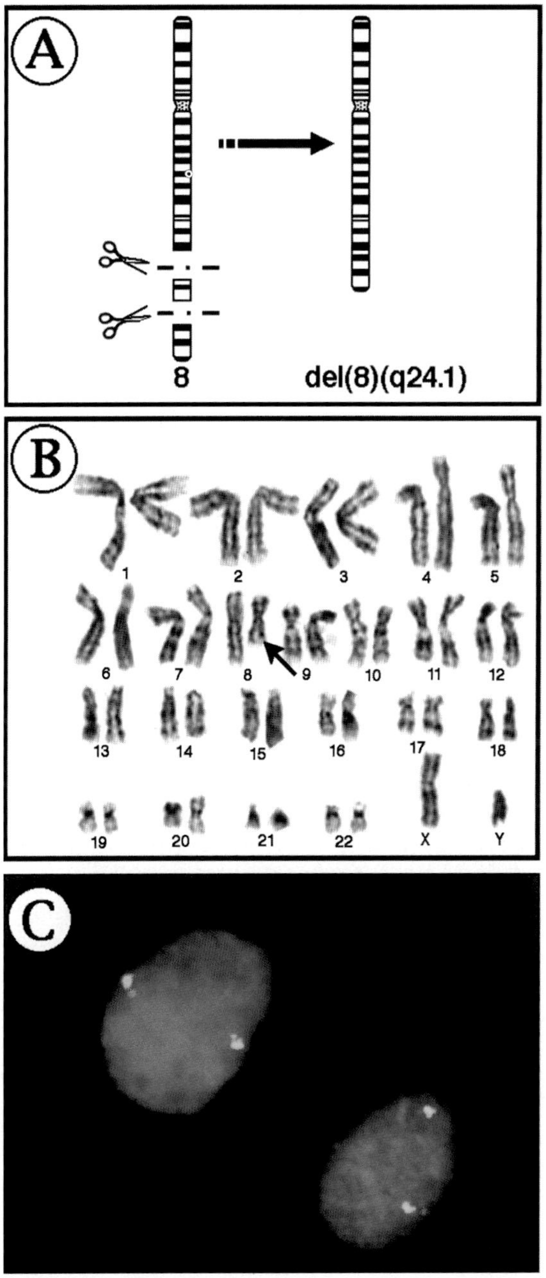

Figure 4-13

CHROMOSOME 8 CHANGES IN OSTEOCHONDROMA

A: Schematic of chromosome 8 illustrates loss of the *EXT1* gene locus at 8q24.1.

B: Loss of 8q, including 8q24.1, is observed in a sporadic osteochondroma (arrow).

C: Fluorescence in situ hybridization performed on a cytologic touch preparation of a sporadic osteochondroma, with a chromosome 8-specific centromeric probe in green and an 8q24 locus-specific probe (cosmid probe 59B5, courtesy of D. Wells, Houston, TX) in red, shows loss of one copy of the 8q24 locus (only one red signal).

described 23 patients with osteochondromas of the distal tibia and fibula; 4 had recurrences.

MULTIPLE HEREDITARY EXOSTOSES

Definition. This is a familial disorder in which patients present with multiple osteochondromas *(osteochondromatosis)*. The latter term is preferred, but multiple hereditary exostoses has been hallowed by tradition. Other terms used include *diaphyseal aclasis* and *hereditary deforming chondrodysplasia*.

General Features. Osteochondromatosis is inherited as an autosomally dominant condition, and about 65 percent of patients have similarly affected family members. It is the most common systematized anomaly of skeletal development (54).

Clinical Features. The clinical range of expression is quite variable (55). Patients may have few or innumerable osteochondromas. The condition is associated with other deformities such as ulnar deviation in the wrist, ankle valgus, or genu valgum (54).

Radiographic Findings. The radiographic findings are identical to those of solitary osteochondroma, except for the associated anomalies. Lack of tubulation of the long bones, especially noticeable in the proximal femur where the neck is as wide as the head, is nearly constant.

Gross Findings. The gross pathologic findings are similar to those of solitary osteochondroma.

Microscopic Findings. There are no distinctive microscopic features.

Genetics and Other Special Techniques. A description of the molecular alterations identified in multiple hereditary exostoses is included within the section on osteochondroma.

Differential Diagnosis. Chondrosarcoma arising in an osteochondroma has to be differentiated from osteochondroma. The criteria used are similar to those used with solitary lesions.

Treatment and Prognosis. Lesions that cause symptoms need to be excised surgically. The most serious complication is the development of chondrosarcoma. The true incidence of malignant change is unknown. In a study reported by Garrison et al. (53), the incidence of secondary chondrosarcoma in a series of surgically removed multiple osteochondromas was 27.3 percent. However, patients with clinically suspected chondrosarcoma are likely to be overrepresented in a surgical series. Peterson (54) suggested that the incidence of sarcomatous change is less than 1 percent. Schmale et al. (55) followed more than 46 kindreds with multiple exostoses. Of the 130 members affected, 1 developed chondrosarcoma (less than 1 percent). However, as the authors pointed out, more than half the patients were younger than 40 years and longer follow-up may yield more examples.

ENCHONDROMA

Definition. Enchondroma is a benign intramedullary neoplasm composed of hyaline cartilage. The term *chondroma* is sometimes used synonymously with enchondroma. However, chondroma is more inclusive, for example, it includes lesions of the periosteum and soft tissue.

General Features. The Mayo Clinic series includes 469 cases of enchondroma, constituting 16.3 percent of all benign tumors and 4.9 percent of all bone tumors (fig. 4-14). However, these values do not reflect the true incidence of enchondromas because patients are generally asymptomatic and biopsy is not performed.

Clinical Features. Enchondromas involving the small bones of the hands and feet are different in many respects from enchondromas involving large tubular bones (62). Lesions of the large tubular and flat bones do not cause symptoms. Frequently, these lesions are discovered as a positive focus on radionuclide bone scans usually performed to determine whether metastatic carcinoma is present in the skeleton. If a chondroid lesion of a large bone causes symptoms, the possibility of a chondrosarcoma should be considered. Patients with enchondromas of the small bones, however, frequently present with a pathologic fracture that produces pain (62). Enchondromas are found in all age groups, although patients in the second, third, and fourth decades of life predominate. There is a slight female predominance.

Radiographic Findings. Enchondromas produce a localized, central region of rarefaction. Any portion of the bone may be involved, but in long bones, the tumors tend to be metaphyseal. The amount of mineralization varies from slight to marked (fig. 4-15). Mineralization not visible on plain radiographs may be visualized on CT. The mineralization within the lesion tends to be uniform, and large areas

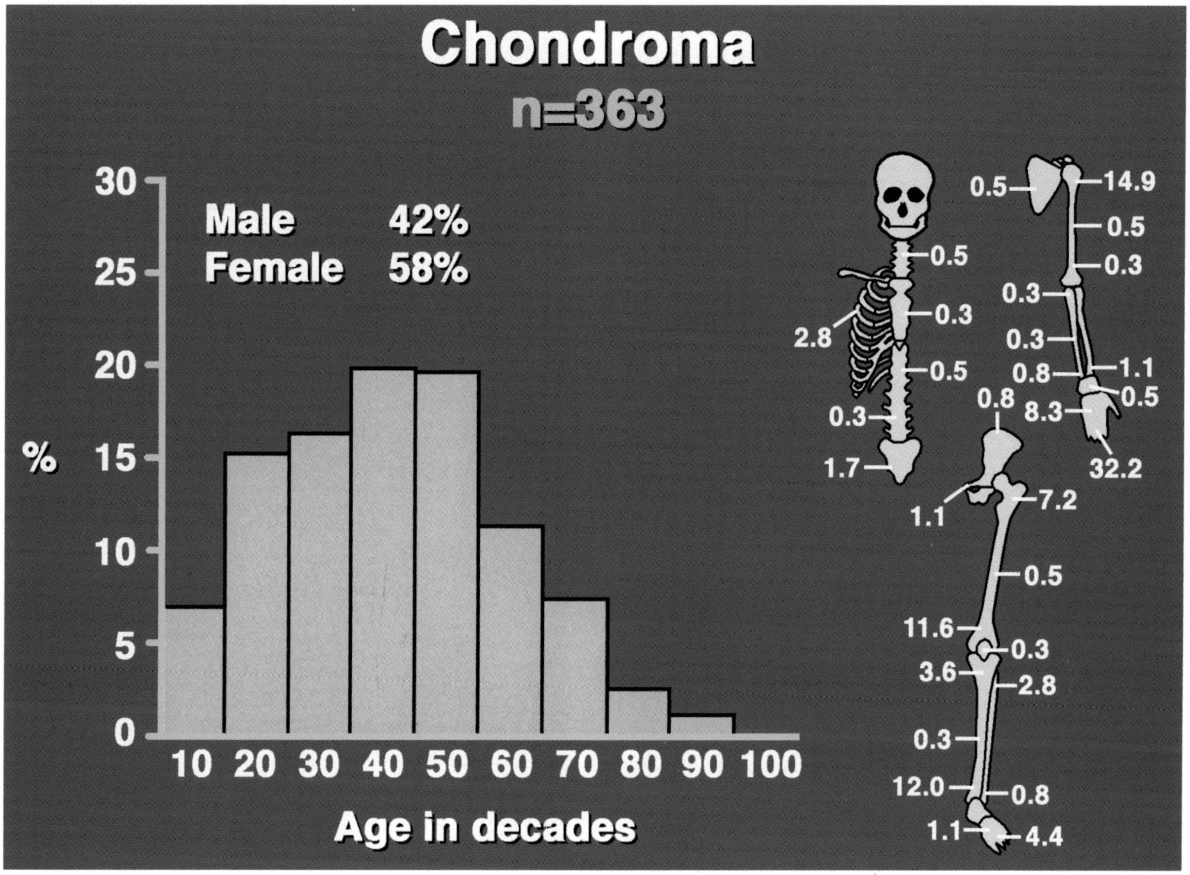

Figure 4-14

CHONDROMA

Distribution of chondroma according to the age and sex of the patient and the site of the lesion.

of lucency should arouse suspicion of chondrosarcoma. The calcification usually defines the extent of the sharply demarcated lesion. The mineralization varies from powder-like to dense aggregates. Ring-like calcification may be present within the lesion. The bony cortex overlying the enchondroma is not involved. We consider any scalloping of the overlying cortex to be a worrisome sign.

The radiographic features of small-bone enchondromas are somewhat different. They frequently involve the entire bone and show concentric thinning of the overlying cortex (fig. 4-16). Calcific foci are less common than in long-bone enchondromas. The uniform thinning of the cortex frequently gives rise to pathologic fractures.

CT and MRI do not show specific features. However, these modalities may help to better define the extent of the lesion and to document lack of involvement of the cortex. On MRI, enchondromas have a lobulated appearance (fig. 4-17).

Gross Findings. Enchondromas generally are curetted, and intact specimens are rare. The fragments of curetted enchondromas usually have lobulated, translucent, blue hyaline cartilage with variable amounts of calcification. Grossly, the matrix lacks the mucoid or myxoid quality frequently seen in chondrosarcomas.

If the resected lesion is intact, the lobulated architecture is seen to better advantage (fig. 4-18). Even in apparently solitary enchondromas, it is not unusual to find a multicentric growth pattern consisting of isolated nodules within the bone marrow cavities, separate from the main tumor.

Microscopic Findings. The histologic features vary considerably depending on the location of

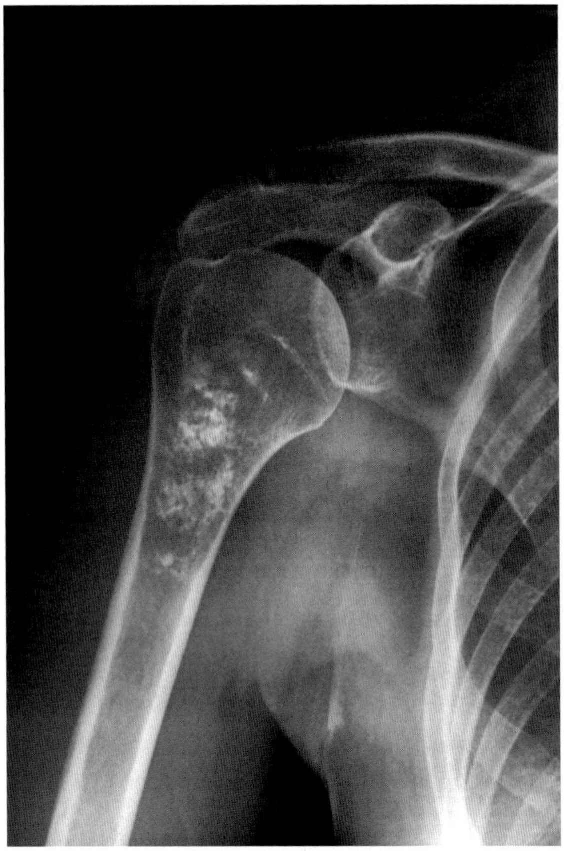

Figure 4-15

ENCHONDROMA

The proximal humerus contains a long segment of punctated and curvilinear calcifications without endosteal scalloping.

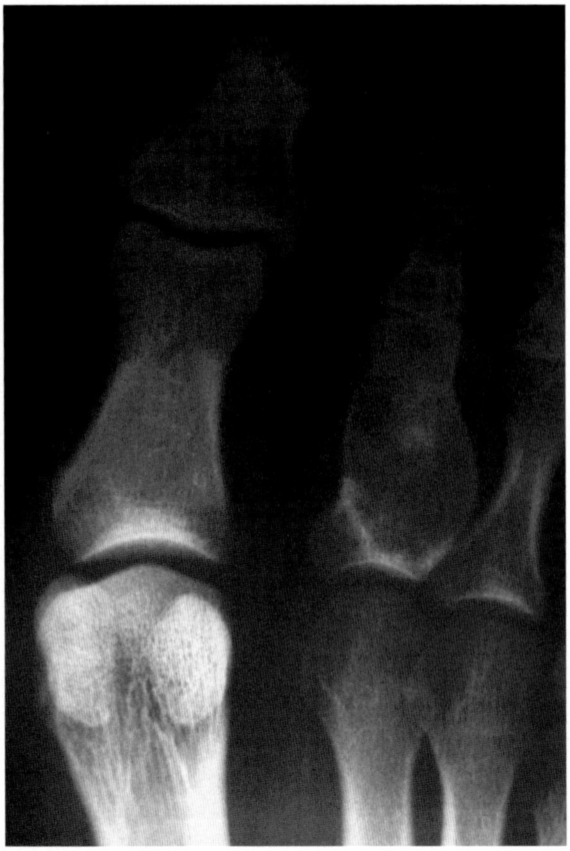

Figure 4-16

ENCHONDROMA

A lytic lesion with calcification arises in a proximal second phalanx. Despite the expansion and scalloping of the bone, this would be considered an enchondroma rather than chondrosarcoma because of the location of the lesion.

the lesion. Under low-power magnification, enchondromas of long and flat bones show a lobulated growth pattern (fig. 4-19). Frequently, these lobules of cartilage are encircled with a reactive rim of bone formation (fig. 4-20). Although the lesion may appear multicentric, with nodules of cartilage in the bone marrow separate from the main tumor, they do not show destructive permeation of surrounding tissue. The lobules of cartilage are relatively hypocellular, with clusters of chondrocytes separated by solid, blue-staining, hyaline cartilage matrix. Although some myxoid change in the matrix is manifested as fraying of the matrix and eventual loss may be seen focally (fig. 4-21), large areas of liquefactive myxoid change should not be present in enchondroma. The chondrocytes always lie within lacunae. Although any number of cells may be seen within a space, double-nucleated cells are rare. The chondrocytes are uniform and round, and the nuclei are dense. Calcification may be seen as a fine granular precipitate or as large chunks. Occasionally, calcification is the predominant feature of the lesion.

Enchondromas of the small bones of the hands and feet have distinct histologic features. Under low-power magnification, they are usually lobulated, and this lobulation may scallop the overlying cortex. However, the lesion is still well demarcated, without permeation. An enchondroma of a small bone is frequently hypercellular (fig. 4-22). The nuclei are large, and double-nucleated cells may be frequent (fig. 4-23). A moderate amount of myxoid change in the matrix is not

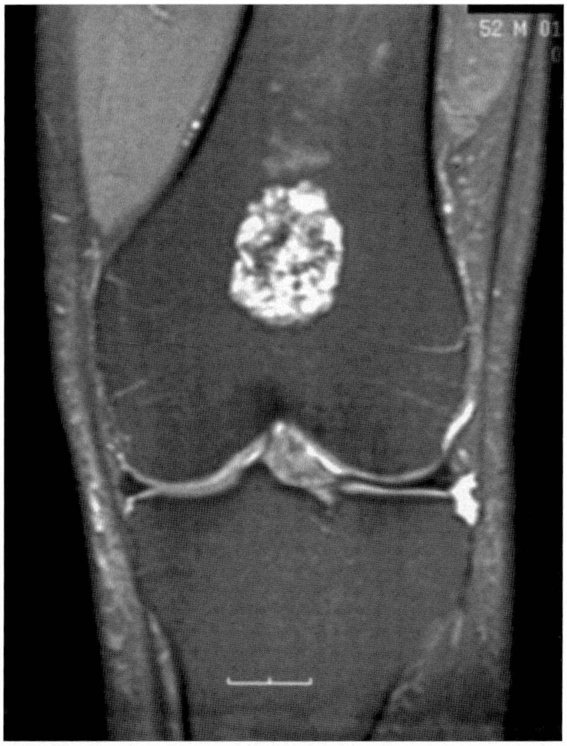

Figure 4-17

ENCHONDROMA

T_2-weighted coronal MRI of the knee shows a well-circumscribed high-signal lesion with several areas of low-signal intensity, consistent with an enchondroma. This is a frequent incidental finding considering the large number of MRI studies of the knee that are performed. The image, however, should always be correlated with a plain radiograph. (Courtesy of Dr. D. McClure, Denver, CO.)

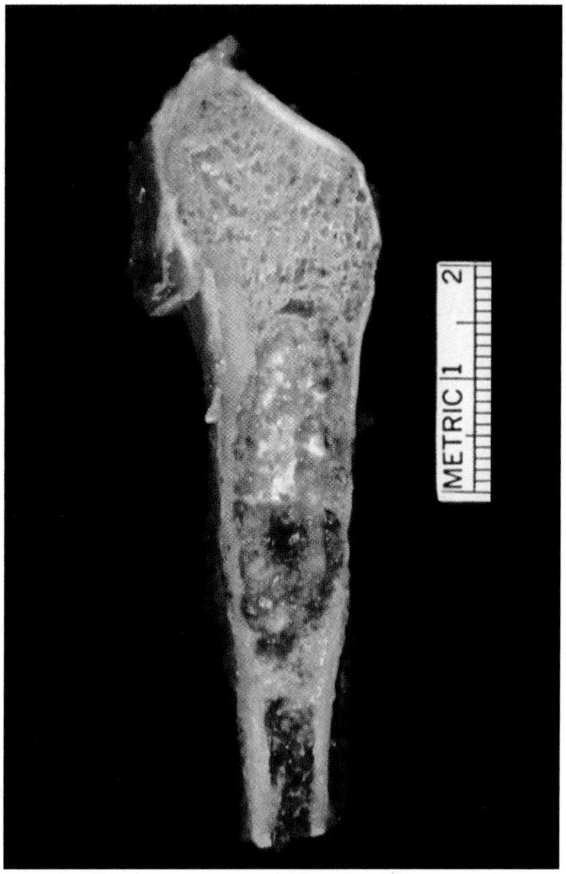

Figure 4-18

ENCHONDROMA

The lobulated tumor is gray-white, and the cortex is not violated.

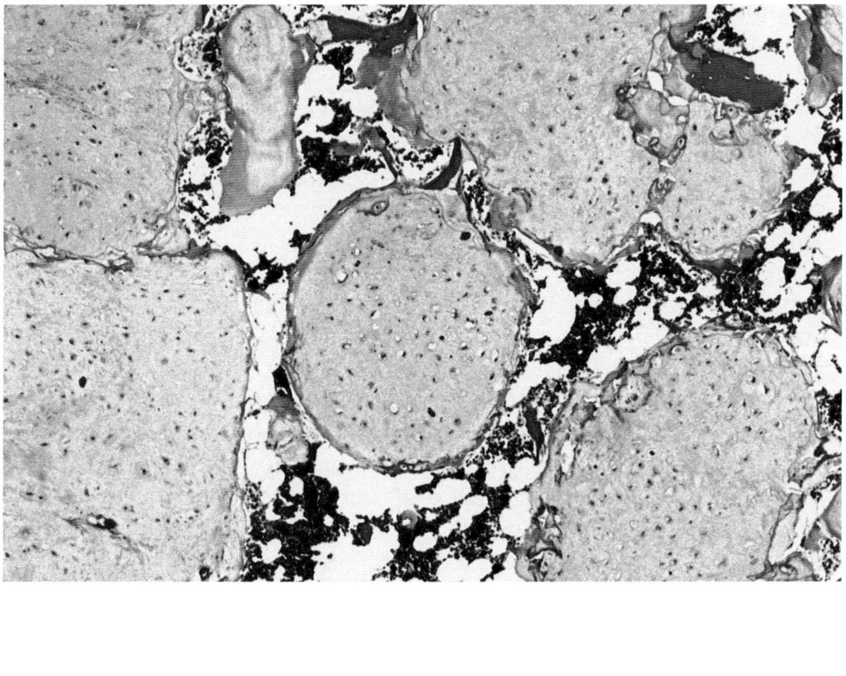

Figure 4-19

ENCHONDROMA

There is a lobular growth pattern with bone marrow elements between the lobules.

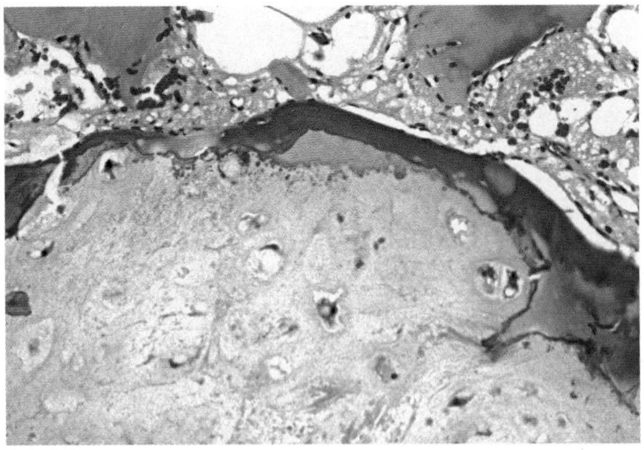

Figure 4-20

ENCHONDROMA

A thin rim of bone partially surrounds a lobule of the tumor.

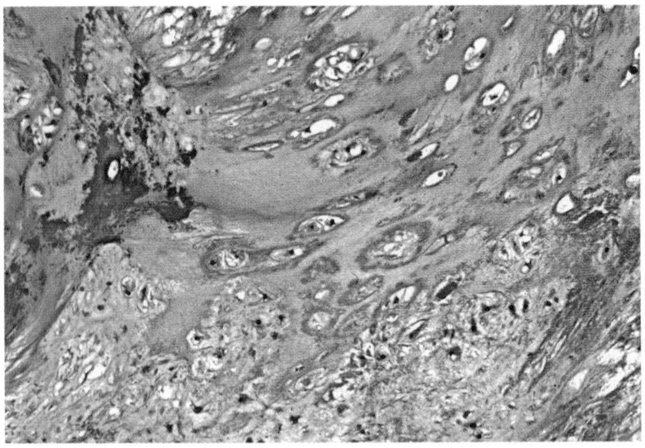

Figure 4-21

ENCHONDROMA

A purple-stained granular area of calcification is associated with degenerative changes.

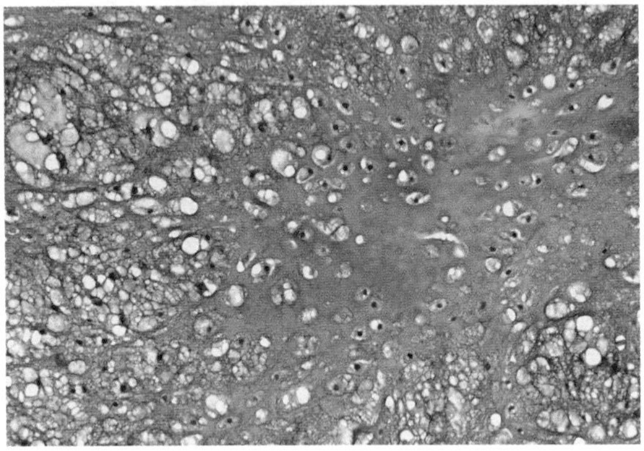

Figure 4-22

ENCHONDROMA OF A SMALL BONE

There is increased cellularity and focal myxoid change.

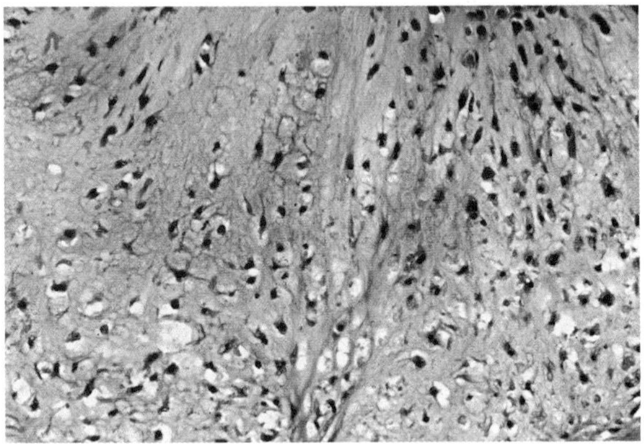

Figure 4-23

ENCHONDROMA OF A SMALL BONE

The tumor shows myxoid change and nuclear hyperchromasia.

unusual. In a larger bone, these histologic findings would be diagnostic of chondrosarcoma.

Frozen Sections. Frozen section evaluation can help determine a definite diagnosis of enchondroma. Toluidine blue staining is not appropriate for cartilage tumors because it stains the matrix metachromatically, making it difficult to identify nuclear details. Hence, hematoxylin and eosin (H&E) is a better stain. As with permanent sections, it is important to correlate the radiographic and clinical findings to arrive at the correct diagnosis.

Immunohistochemical Findings. As with other cartilaginous neoplasms, enchondromas stain for S-100 protein. However, no special stains help to differentiate enchondromas from chondrosarcomas.

Cytologic Findings. With the use of May-Grünwald-Giemsa stains, both osteochondroma and enchondroma are characterized by rather small, uniform chondrocytes embedded in an abundant, purple, fibrillary, myxoid to hyaline matrix (fig. 4-24). The degree of cellularity may vary from low to high in lesions such as digital enchondroma. In addition to hypercellularity, periosteal and soft tissue chondromas as well as synovial chondromatosis may show moderate cellular and nuclear pleomorphism that

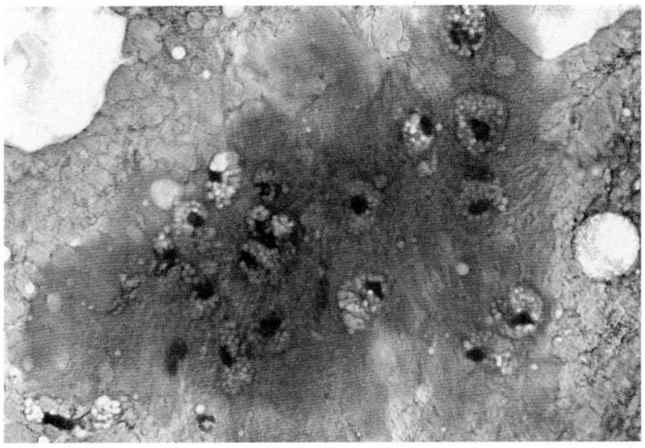

Figure 4-24

FINE-NEEDLE ASPIRATION BIOPSY OF ENCHONDROMA

Small, uniform chondrocytes with finely vacuolated cytoplasm are enclosed in an abundant, intensely stained, fibrillary, myxoid matrix (May-Grünwald-Giemsa stain).

could be misinterpreted as chondrosarcoma. Such cases emphasize the importance of clinical and radiographic correlation.

Genetics and Other Special Techniques. Diploid or near-diploid complements with simple structural abnormalities, particularly involving chromosomes 6 and 12, have been detected by conventional cytogenetic analysis in enchondromas (fig. 4-25) (56,57,59,61,63). Molecular studies have shown that the *HMGA2* gene (localized to 12q15) is a frequent target for chromosomal rearrangements in enchondromas and soft tissue chondromas, as well as chondrosarcomas, and that variable mechanisms are responsible for transcriptional activation (58).

A mutant PTH/PTHrP type I receptor (*PTHR1*) has been identified in enchondroma specimens from a subset of patients with enchondromatosis (Ollier's disease) (60). In one patient, the *PTHR1* mutation was germline, and in another, it could not be determined if it was a somatic mutation or if the patient was mosaic. The mutant PTH/PTHrP type I receptor constitutively activates Hedgehog signaling, and excessive Hedgehog signaling with overexpression of the transcription factor Gli2 is sufficient to cause formation of enchondroma-like lesions in mice.

Differential Diagnosis. Chondrosarcoma has to be differentiated from enchondroma. As indicated above, enchondromas of the small bones have histologic features that, out of context, may suggest the diagnosis of chondrosarcoma.

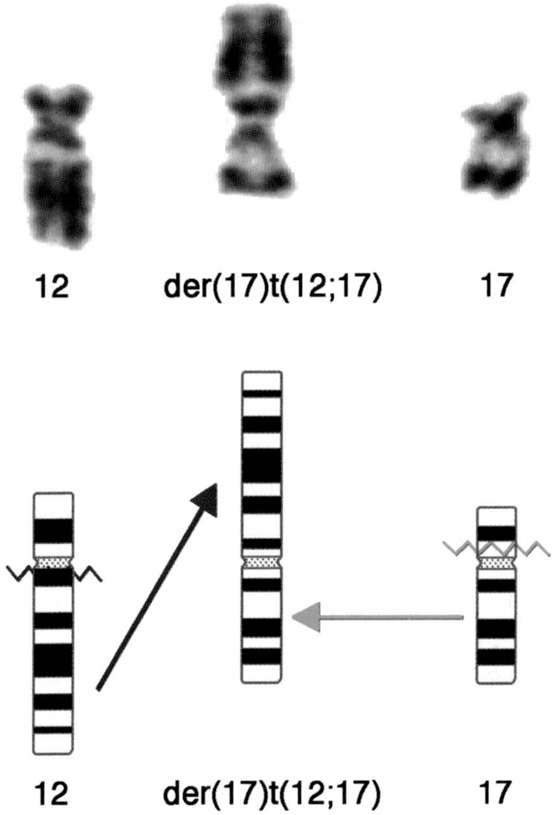

Figure 4-25

PARTIAL GTG-BANDED KARYOTYPE OF AN ENCHONDROMA

This partial karyotype and schema show an unbalanced rearrangement occurring between chromosomes 12 and 17 (arrows).

The radiographic features of chondrosarcomas of large bones are practically diagnostic. They tend to show expansion of the bone and thickening of the cortex. In comparison, enchondromas are well demarcated and do not invade the cortex. Increased cellularity, marked myxoid change of the matrix, and cytologic features of malignancy all support the diagnosis of chondrosarcoma. Perhaps the single best criterion to distinguish between the two is permeation. In enchondroma, it is common to see attenuated trabeculae surrounding lobules of cartilage. In chondrosarcoma, trabeculae of preexisting bone seem to be embedded within the advancing tumor.

Radiographic features are even more important in differentiating enchondroma of a small bone from chondrosarcoma. Enchondromas show thinning of the cortex but not permeation through the cortex into soft tissue. This is probably the single best criterion for differentiating an enchondroma from a chondrosarcoma in a small bone. Microscopically, if the sections include the cortex, the cartilage tumor may permeate through the interstices of the cortex into the soft tissue in a chondrosarcoma but not in an enchondroma.

Treatment and Prognosis. Enchondromas of the larger bones are frequently incidental findings. They need no treatment. The possibility that an enchondroma will undergo malignant change is so small that it does not justify surgical removal. Some patients with large-bone enchondromas may complain of pain. However, it is difficult to know if the pain is related to the enchondroma. If it is thought that the lesion is indeed symptomatic, simple curettage should be curative. Enchondromas of the small bones frequently cause symptoms and therefore require surgical removal. Simple curettage should be curative. Recurrence is extremely uncommon, and if the tumor does recur, the original diagnosis should be questioned.

MULTIPLE CHONDROMAS

Definition. Multiple chondromas are defined as a condition in which multiple cartilaginous nodules occur in the skeleton.

General Features. The presence of multiple chondromas, or *enchondromatosis*, generally is considered a congenital nonhereditary disorder. There are three main types of enchondromatosis: *Ollier's disease, Maffucci's syndrome,* and an unclearly defined type involving especially small bones of the hand. The most common type is Ollier's disease, which is characterized by multiple cartilaginous masses involving the entire skeleton, half of the body, or even one limb. Rare cases of Ollier's disease possibly involve a single bone. Maffucci's syndrome is characterized by chondroid nodules associated with soft tissue hemangiomas. Although Ollier's disease and Maffucci's syndrome appear to be identical both clinically and radiographically, their malignant potential is significantly different. The third type of enchondromatosis is not clearly defined but consists of multiple chondromas, involving especially the small bones of the hands. This last condition probably is related more to solitary enchondromas, whereas Ollier's disease and Maffucci's syndrome represent skeletal dysplasias.

Clinical Features. Patients present with multiple chondromas in the first few years of life (fig. 4-26). They may have skeletal deformities such as short stature or localized swellings, especially in the hands and feet (fig. 4-27). Pathologic fracture may be the presenting symptom.

Sites. Chondrodysplasias may involve any portion of the skeleton. As indicated above, there is a tendency to involve half of the skeleton to a greater extent, although some patients have involvement of the entire skeleton. True multiple chondromas usually involve the small bones of the hands and feet.

Radiographic Findings. The radiographs are usually diagnostic when the patient is young. As the skeleton matures, some of the specific features are lost. In the small bones of the hands, multiple chondromas appear as lytic defects involving multiple bones (fig. 4-28). In the long bones, chondromas appear as tumefactive masses, typically involving the metadiaphyseal region of long bones, which appear expanded. Both ends of the bone are involved, but the shaft generally is spared. The masses typically show longitudinal striations of mineralization that extend from the epiphyseal plate toward the diaphysis (fig. 4-29). These masses within the bone usually are associated with tumors of the periosteum (*periosteal chondromas*). This feature should not be mistaken for an invasive, destructive chondrosarcoma. In flat bones, the mineralization may appear to extend into the soft tissue and have a "hair-on-end" appearance. As the skeleton matures, this characteristic mineralization pattern is lost, although the bones appear expanded and deformed (fig. 4-30).

The radiographic findings in Maffucci's syndrome are identical to those of Ollier's disease. In the early stages, the soft tissue hemangiomas may not be obvious. However, they become apparent in later stages because of the presence of phleboliths, which are seen on radiographs as calcific nodules in the soft tissue (fig. 4-31).

Gross Findings. If an intact bone is removed, the ends will be seen to be expanded with large masses of cartilage containing longitudinal streaks of calcification. The cartilaginous masses

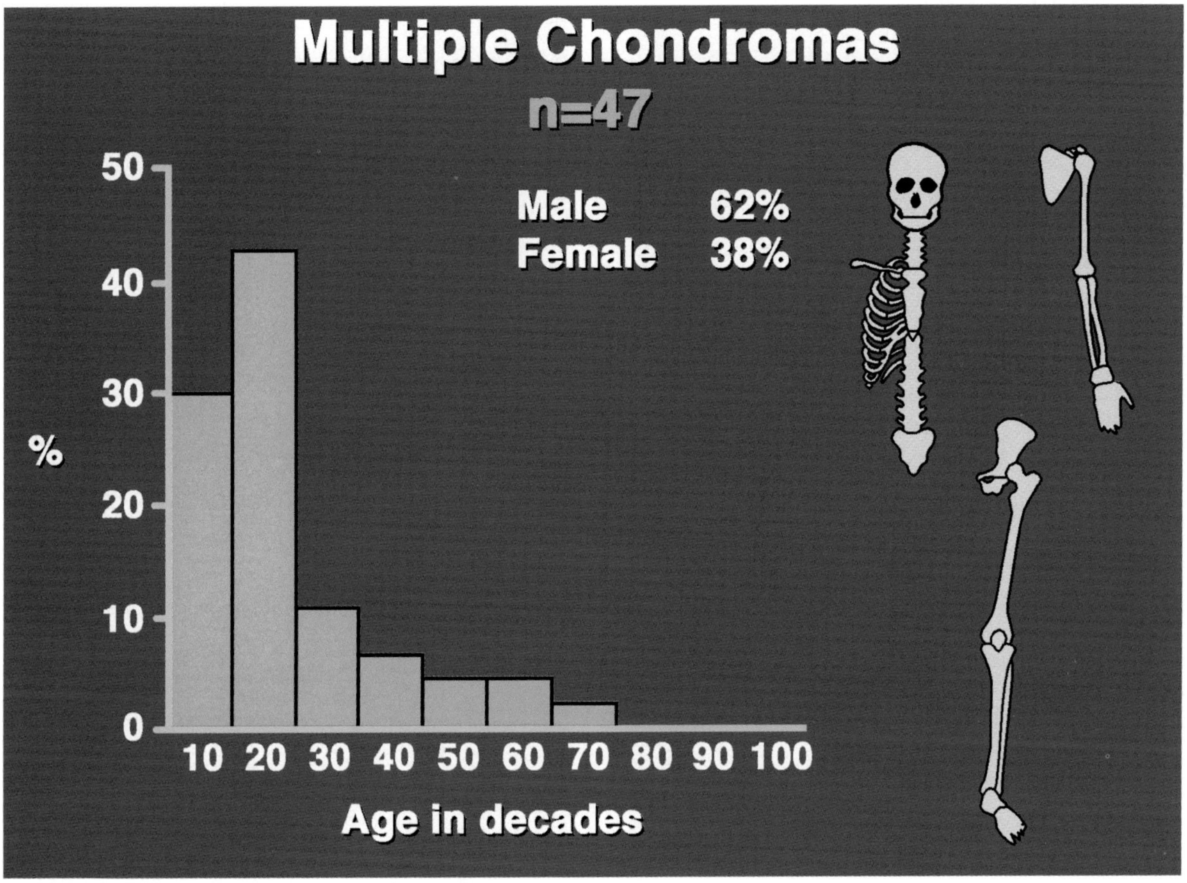

Figure 4-26

MULTIPLE CHONDROMAS

The distribution of multiple chondromas according to the age and sex of the patient.

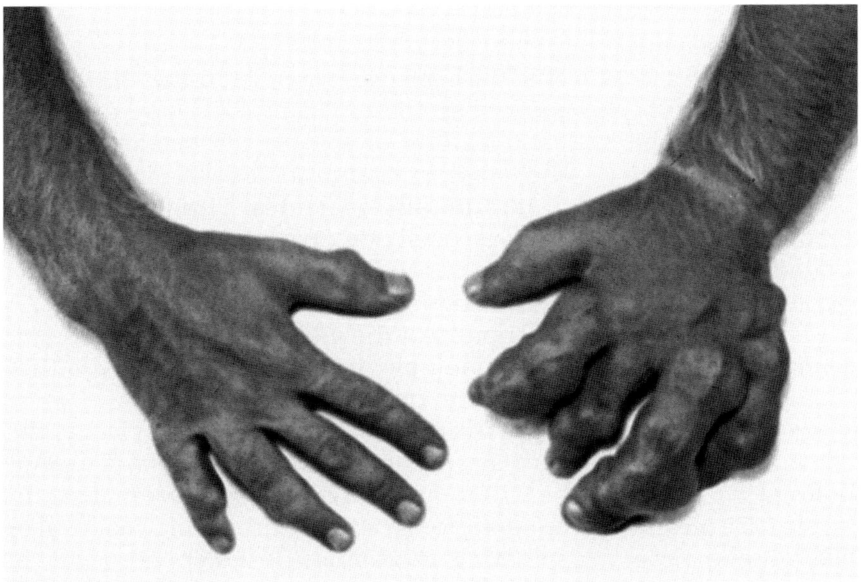

Figure 4-27

MULTIPLE CHONDROMAS IN OLLIER'S DISEASE

The left hand of this 27-year-old man with Ollier's disease contains multiple deforming chondromas.

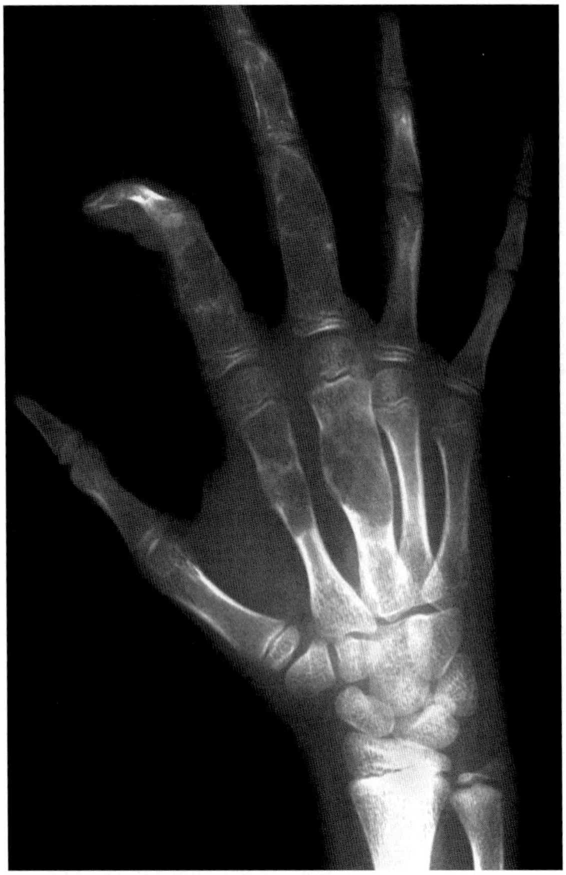

Figure 4-28

MULTIPLE CHONDROMAS

The tumors involve the bones of the second and third rays with sparing of the joint spaces. (Courtesy of Dr. Sidhu, Johnson City, NY.)

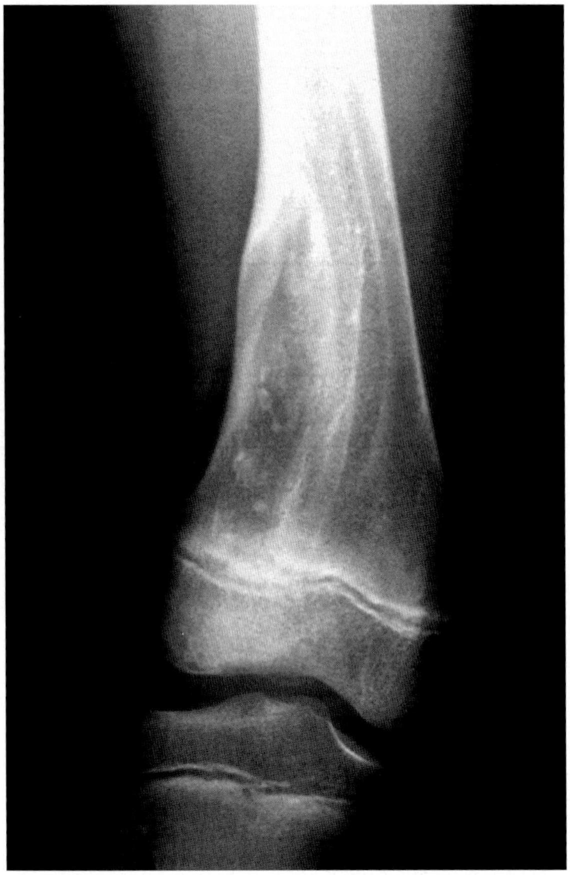

Figure 4-29

MULTIPLE CHONDROMAS

A plain radiograph shows the linear striations with interspersed calcification and abnormal bone modeling characteristic of Ollier's disease. (Courtesy of Dr. E. Marley, Las Vegas, NV.)

have a distinctly multinodular arrangement, with intervening normal bone marrow (fig. 4-32). Frequently, the cortex appears not to be present, and an expansile mass extends into the periosteum. However, the matrix is solid and is a characteristic light blue.

Microscopic Findings. Microscopically, the cartilage present in multiple chondromas tends to be hypercellular, the nuclei tend to be enlarged, and double-nucleated cells may be abundant. The nuclei still lie in lacunae but may be somewhat elongated (fig. 4-33, top). Because of the hypercellularity and nuclear enlargement, the pathologic process may be mistaken for a chondrosarcoma (fig. 4-33, bottom).

In Maffucci's syndrome, the cartilage present in bone is similar to that in Ollier's disease. However, the hemangiomas of soft tissues distinguish the former. These hemangiomas have the histologic features of spindle cell hemangioendotheliomas, at least in some cases (64).

Immunohistochemical Findings. As with cartilage of all other types, stains for S-100 protein are positive in chondrodysplasia.

Genetics and Other Special Techniques. A description of the molecular alterations identified in multiple chondromas is included within the section on enchondroma.

Differential Diagnosis. Histologically, the cartilage present in chondrodysplasia cannot be differentiated confidently from that of enchondroma, although the somewhat oval or spindling appearance of the chondrocytes in chondrodysplasia can be a clue. The two conditions have clearly different radiographic and clinical features.

Differentiating a chondrosarcoma from the cartilage of multiple chondromas (especially because of the worrisome histologic features of the latter) can be a challenge. If a patient with a known chondrodysplasia complains of new symptoms, such as a mass or pain, chondrosarcoma should be suspected. Although radiographs of chondrodysplasia can show periosteal masses (which may be mistaken for permeation), they do not have indistinct borders and unmineralized soft tissue masses. MRI may help identify such masses. The gross appearance of a secondary chondrosarcoma is distinctly different. The typical appearance of the benign cartilage is that of nodules of intact blue cartilage, whereas secondary chondrosarcoma has a distinct myxoid quality with liquefaction and cyst formation. This may be the most important criterion to differentiate chondrosarcoma from a preexisting cartilage precursor. Microscopically, the hallmarks of chondrosarcoma are marked myxoid change of the matrix and destructive permeation of medullary bone, with entrapment of preexisting bony trabeculae.

Treatment and Prognosis. Treatment consists of supportive surgical measures for the skeletal deformities and the occasional pathologic fracture. Rarely, the swelling and deformity require amputation.

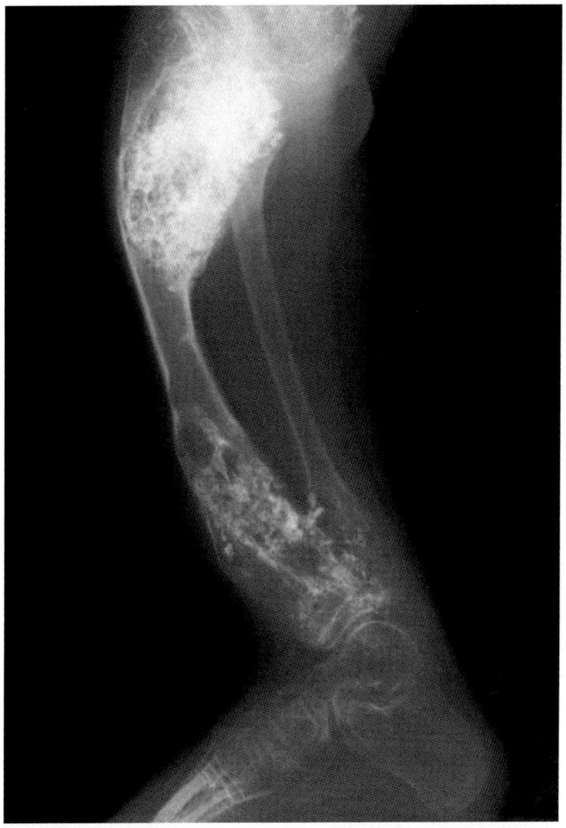

Figure 4-30

MULTIPLE CHONDROMAS

This patient with Ollier's disease eventually had an above-knee amputation because of marked deformity involving the right lower extremity. The radiograph shows abnormal modeling with heavy calcification proximally and distally.

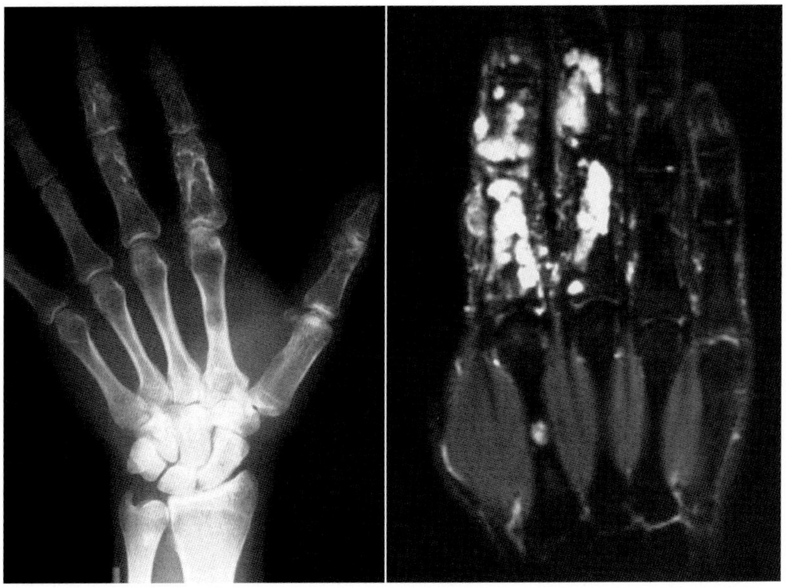

Figure 4-31

MAFFUCCI'S SYNDROME

Left: Multiple benign cartilage tumors involve the metacarpals and phalanges of the first to third digits. Soft tissue swelling and masses with calcified phleboliths are compatible with soft tissue hemangiomas.

Right: Coronal short tau inversion recovery image shows multiple high signal intensity lesions in phalanges of the second and third digits and second metacarpal, consistent with enchondromas. The small soft tissue mass in the second digit and serpiginous vessels in the second and third digits are compatible with hemangiomas.

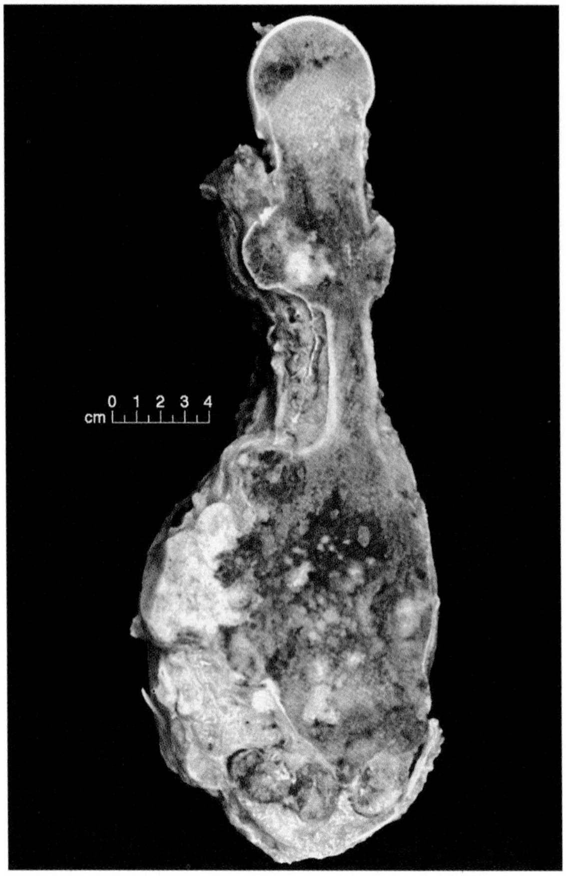

Figure 4-32

MULTIPLE CHONDROMAS

This femur is an autopsy specimen from a patient with Ollier's disease who died of an unrelated illness. There is massive involvement by multiple benign chondromas that form nodules of cartilage throughout the specimen.

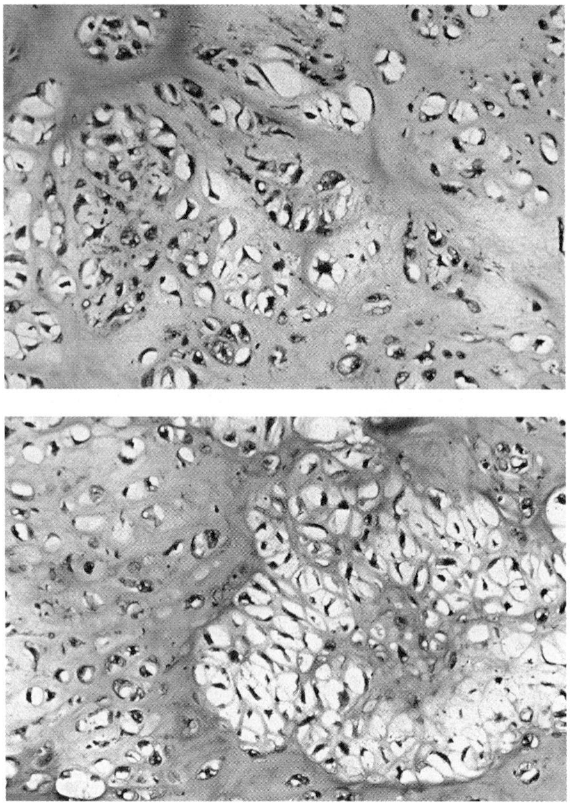

Figure 4-33

OLLIER'S DISEASE

Top: The tumor is hypercellular, with mild cytologic atypia.

Bottom: The nuclei within the lacunae are elongated.

It is difficult to evaluate the true incidence of chondrosarcoma arising from multiple chondromas. Dedifferentiated chondrosarcomas and osteosarcomas are also associated with multiple chondromas. In a Mayo Clinic series, approximately 25 percent of patients with Ollier's disease developed chondrosarcoma (66), as did almost 60 percent of those with Maffucci's syndrome (66,68). In a review of patients with Maffucci's syndrome, Lewis and Ketcham (65) reported a 15.2 percent incidence of chondrosarcoma. Schwartz et al. (67) followed 37 patients with Ollier's disease and 7 with Maffucci's syndrome; 4 of the patients with Ollier's disease and 4 with Maffucci's syndrome developed sarcoma. Three of the latter also developed visceral malignancies, which were fatal. No patient in this series died of chondrosarcoma. The authors estimated that malignancy develops in 25 percent of patients with Ollier's disease, whereas some sort of malignancy is inevitable in patients with Maffucci's syndrome.

PERIOSTEAL CHONDROMA

Definition. Periosteal chondroma is a benign hyaline cartilage tumor situated on the surface of bone.

General Features. As indicated above, it is not unusual to find surface lesions in patients with chondrodysplastic syndromes. They are not included in the statistics on periosteal chondroma. Soft tissue chondromas of the hands and feet may erode the underlying bone and simulate the appearance of periosteal chondroma.

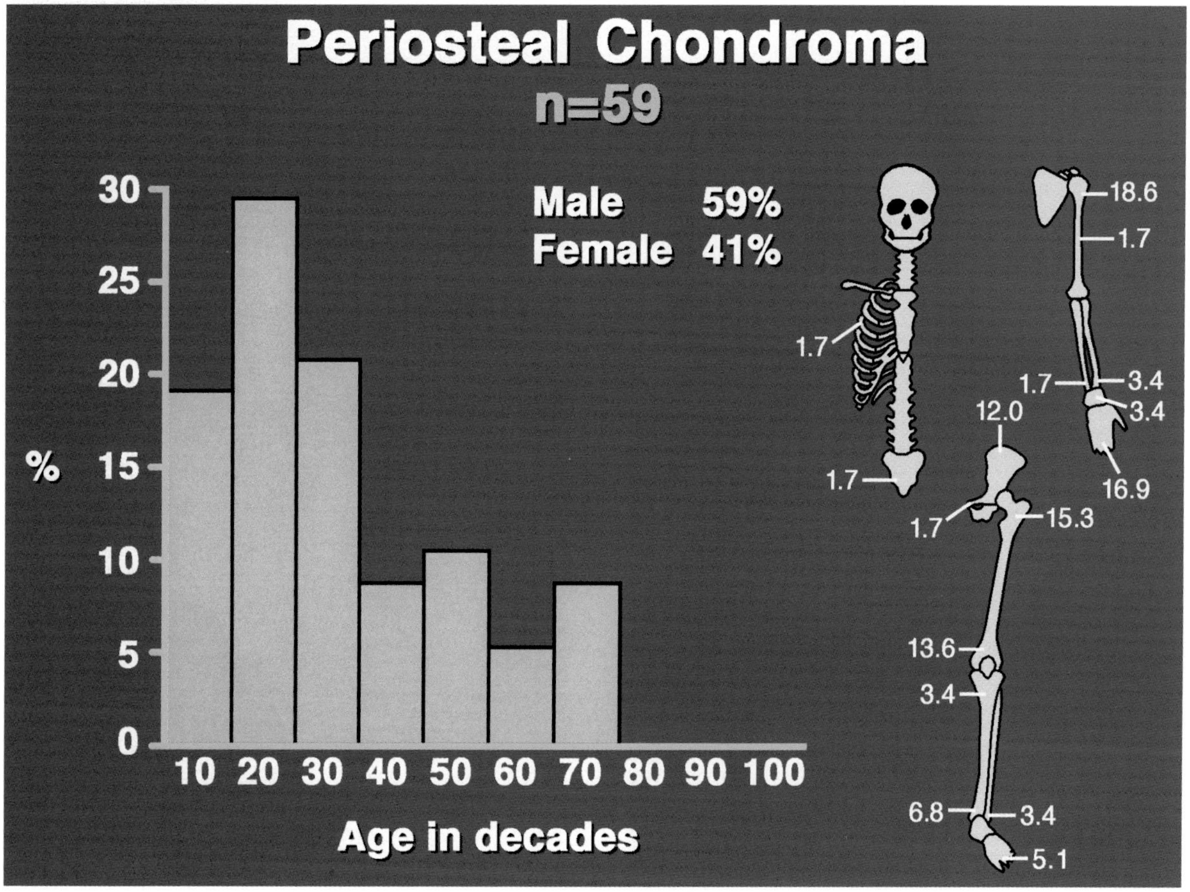

Figure 4-34

PERIOSTEAL CHONDROMA

The distribution of periosteal chondroma according to the age and sex of the patient and the site of the lesion.

Clinical Features. The Mayo Clinic files include 59 cases of periosteal chondroma, which account for less than 1 percent of bone neoplasms. Patients present with a swelling that may be slightly painful. Young adults are usually affected, and males outnumber females 3 to 2 (fig. 4-34).

Sites. Periosteal chondroma has a peculiar tendency to involve the proximal humerus and distal femur (74). The tumor is situated usually on the metaphysis.

Radiographic Findings. Periosteal chondroma presents as a well-demarcated lucency on the surface of bone (69,71). The lesion is situated in a saucer-shaped depression in the cortex and is demarcated from the underlying medullary cavity by a thin rim of sclerosis. Periosteal new bone formation is present as a buttress at both ends of the lesion (fig. 4-35). The lesion may be separated from the soft tissues by a thin line of new bone formation. CT and MRI are helpful in evaluating the size and character of the external surface of the tumor.

Gross Findings. Periosteal chondroma is a well-circumscribed, blue, lobulated mass (fig. 4-36). The outer surface may be covered by a fibrous capsule, which represents the periosteum of the involved bone. The matrix is solid, without a sticky myxoid quality. The most important feature is that the tumor is always small: periosteal chondromas rarely exceed 3 cm in greatest dimension. Any surface cartilage lesion larger than 5 cm should be suspected to be malignant.

Microscopic Findings. Periosteal chondroma is a well-circumscribed, lobulated, hyaline cartilage tumor that does not permeate the

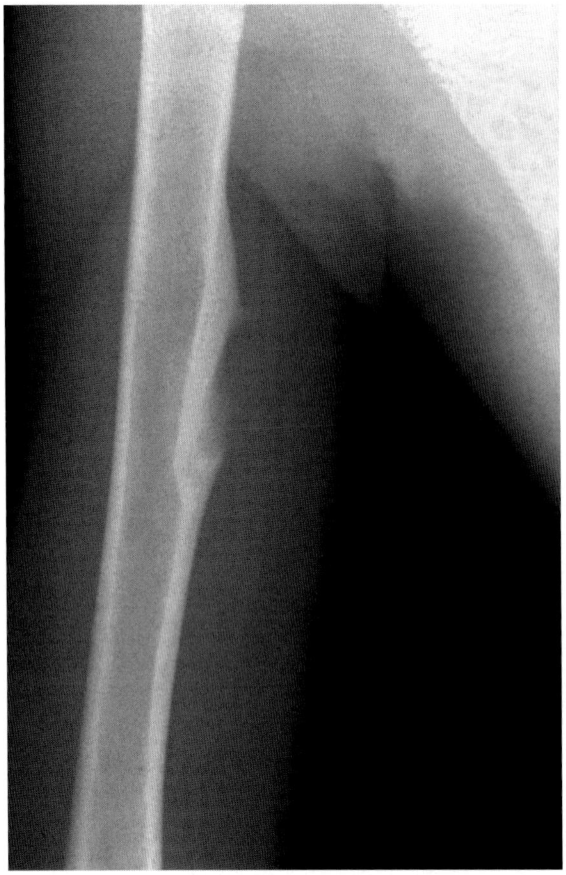

Figure 4-35

PERIOSTEAL CHONDROMA

Periosteal lesion with characteristic marginal beaking. (Courtesy of Dr. D. Carpentieri, Philadelphia, PA.)

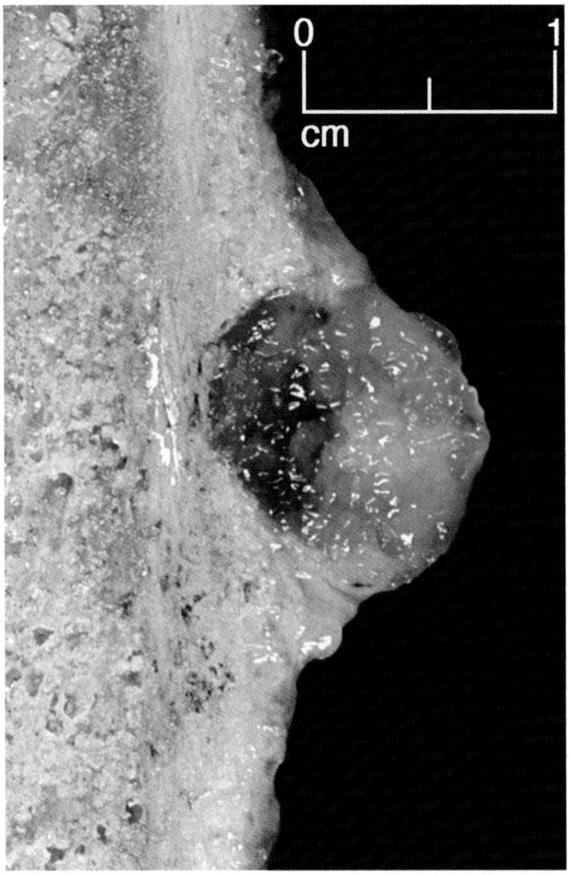

Figure 4-36

PERIOSTEAL CHONDROMA

The lesion, involving the cortex and extending into soft tissue, is small and well circumscribed. The medullary cavity is not involved. (Fig. 3-10 from Unni KK. Dahlin's bone tumors: general aspects and data on 11,087 cases, 5th ed. Philadelphia: Lippincott-Raven; 1996:31. By permission of Mayo Foundation.)

surrounding soft tissues. However, microscopic nodules of cartilage may be seen in the underlying bone marrow. These nodules are small and do not have a permeative growth pattern. The appearance suggests a dysplastic condition rather than a sarcoma. The chondrocytes frequently are enlarged and hyperchromatic (fig. 4-37). Double-nucleated cells are common, and moderate myxoid change may be seen in the matrix. Out of context, these features suggest the diagnosis of chondrosarcoma.

Immunohistochemical Findings. The S-100 protein stain is positive. Special stains do not help rule out sarcoma.

Genetics and Other Special Techniques. Clonal karyotypic abnormalities have been described in four cases of periosteal chondroma (70, 73,75). In one case, structural changes of the same band occurred on both chromosome 12 homologues, leading to speculation that a homozygous gene alteration, possibly an inactivating mutation of a tumor suppressor gene, was the salient DNA-level outcome (73). An abnormality of the long arm of chromosome 4 was detected in two cases (70).

Differential Diagnosis. Periosteal chondrosarcoma and periosteal osteosarcoma are the main differential diagnostic considerations. Periosteal chondrosarcomas are large (over 5 cm) masses with poorly defined margins and irregular

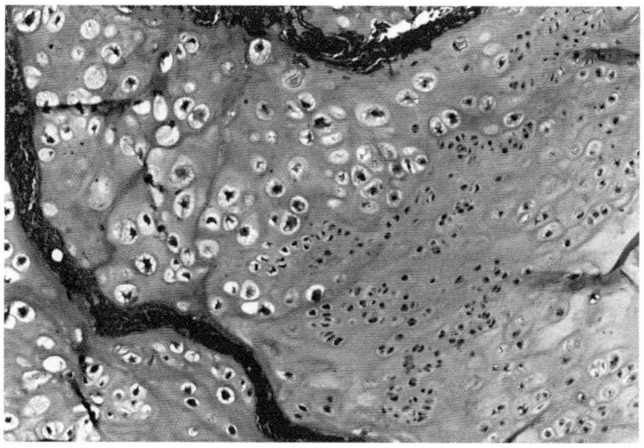

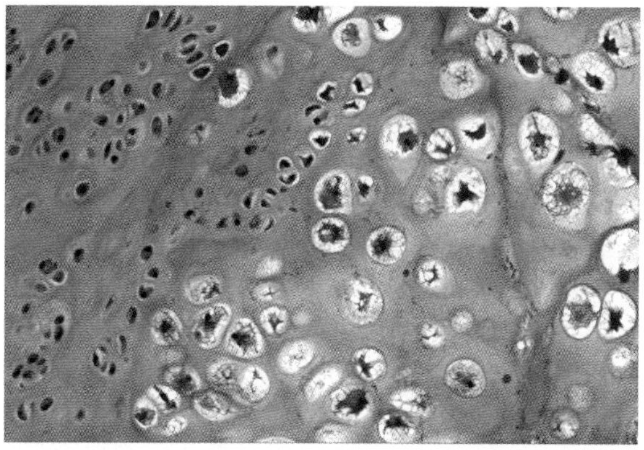

Figure 4-37

PERIOSTEAL CHONDROMA

Left: There is increased cellularity and variability in nuclear size and shape. The cells tend to cluster. Right: There is mild nuclear atypia with hyperchromasia.

mineralization. In contrast, periosteal chondromas are small (about 3 cm) and well circumscribed. Microscopically, chondrosarcomas permeate into soft tissue and chondromas do not.

Periosteal osteosarcomas also present as small lucencies on the cortex; however, they lack the buttress formation typical of periosteal chondromas and tend to fade into the soft tissues. Microscopically, both are predominantly chondroid. However, periosteal osteosarcomas have spindled nuclei at the periphery of the chondroid lobules and trabeculae of bone in the center, features not seen in periosteal chondromas.

Treatment and Prognosis. Periosteal chondroma is treated usually with surgical excision. Recurrences are extremely uncommon (72).

SOFT TISSUE CHONDROMA

Definition. Soft tissue chondroma is a benign lobulated lesion that is composed of hyaline cartilage and is located in the soft tissues.

General Features. Soft tissue chondromas share many features with synovial chondromatosis. Indeed, the histologic features are identical. They probably have the same derivation because the tendons and ligaments of the hands and feet have a synovial lining.

Clinical Features. Soft tissue chondromas present as lobulated, painless, soft tissue masses that may be present for years and have a slow growth. The lesion affects older adults, and there is a slight male predominance (78).

Sites. Most soft tissue chondromas involve the soft tissues of the hands or, less commonly, the feet; similar neoplasms are rarely seen elsewhere.

Radiographic Findings. Radiographs show a well-circumscribed soft tissue swelling with variable mineralization (fig. 4-38). The lesion may be densely mineralized and multinodular and erode the underlying bone.

Gross Findings. Soft tissue chondromas are lobulated, white to light blue masses with focal chalky calcification (fig. 4-39).

Microscopic Findings. Soft tissue chondromas have clusters of chondrocytes, with an abundance of solid chondroid matrix between the clusters (fig. 4-40). The chondrocytes generally have enlarged and hyperchromatic nuclei, features suggesting a chondrosarcoma out of context. Occasionally, a flattened layer of synovial cells surrounds the nodules of cartilage. Calcification varies from fine and powdery to coarser deposits (fig. 4-41). Occasionally, the mononuclear cells have oval nuclei with longitudinal grooves, simulating those seen in chondroblastoma (fig. 4-42) (77,83). About 10 to 15 percent of soft tissue chondromas have foci of epithelioid-appearing cells admixed with giant cells, suggesting the diagnosis of giant cell tumor of tendon sheath origin (79). Indeed, in some cases, the elements may be so mixed that it is difficult to decide whether to make a diagnosis of soft tissue chondroma or giant cell tumor of tendon sheath origin.

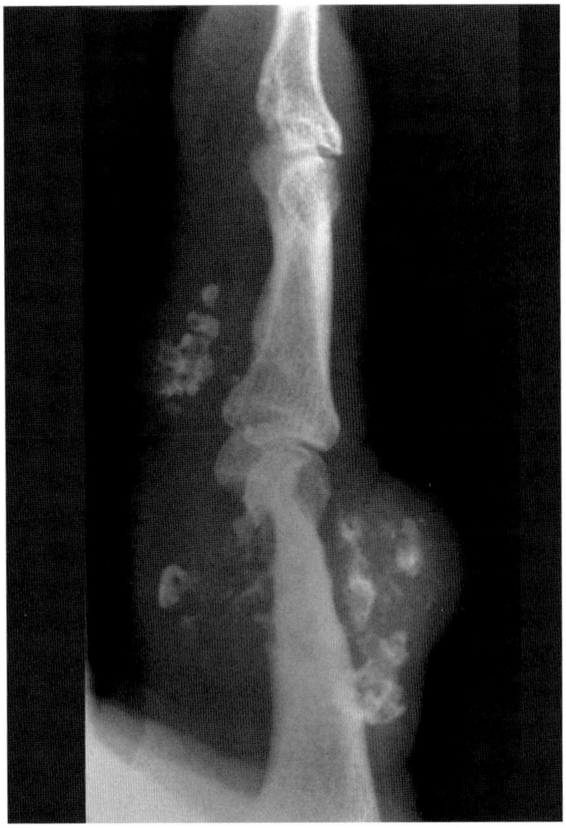

Figure 4-38

SOFT TISSUE CHONDROMA

Mineralized soft tissue masses surround the phalanges of a young man with secondary extrinsic cortical erosion of the proximal phalanx.

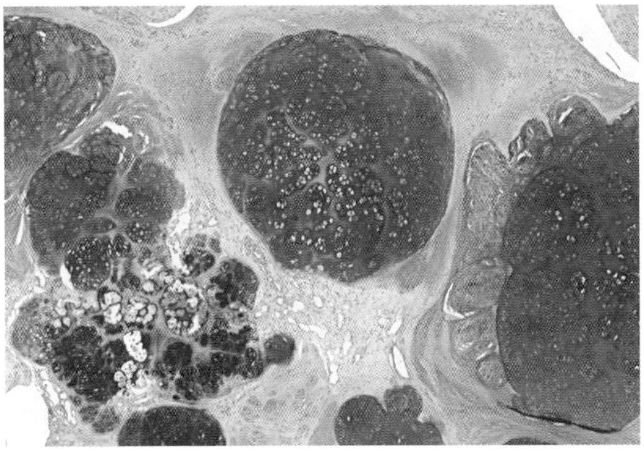

Figure 4-40

SOFT TISSUE CHONDROMA

There are multiple nodules of hyaline cartilage of various sizes. The clustering arrangement of the chondrocytes is typical of soft tissue chondromas and synovial chondromatosis.

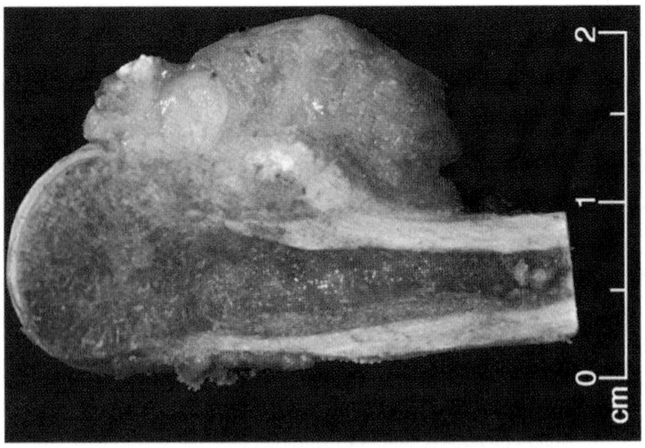

Figure 4-39

SOFT TISSUE CHONDROMA

A lobulated, gray-blue, cartilaginous soft tissue mass with focal calcifications adheres to the surface of the underlying bone.

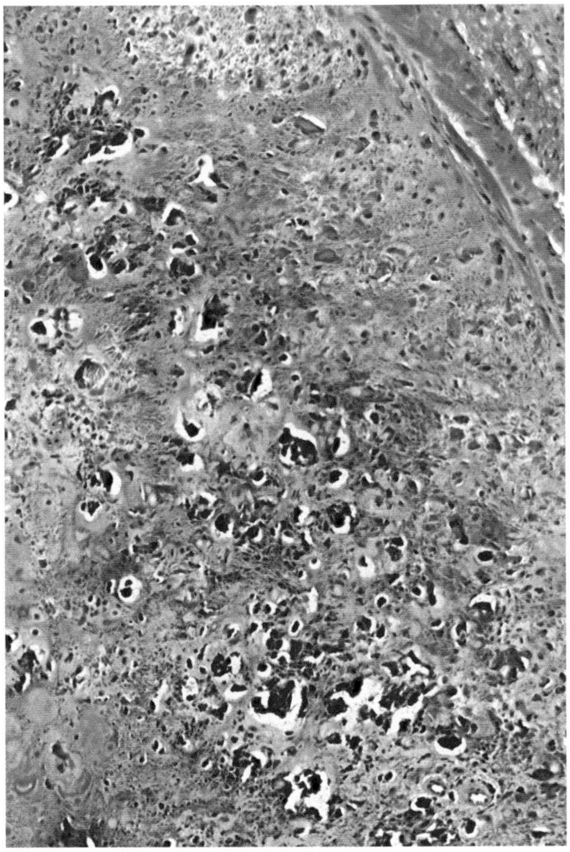

Figure 4-41

SOFT TISSUE CHONDROMA

Coarse and granular calcifications within a lobulated soft tissue chondroma.

Genetics and Other Special Techniques. Abnormalities of chromosomal region 12q14-15 and extra copies of chromosome 5 have been prominent in the few cases that have been characterized cytogenetically (76,80–82).

Differential Diagnosis. As indicated above, chondrosarcomas of pure hyaline cartilage rarely occur in soft tissues. The characteristic clustering arrangement of the chondrocytes is rarely seen in chondrosarcoma. If sheets of chondrocytes are present, a diagnosis of soft tissue chondroma is not tenable. The characteristic myxoid background, with a cording arrangement of cells typically seen in myxoid chondrosarcoma, is not a feature of soft tissue chondroma.

Treatment and Prognosis. Simple surgical excision is the treatment of choice. Recurrences are common, and the tumor may recur multiple times and produce multinodular masses. The development of chondrosarcoma is so rare that it is not a practical consideration.

CHONDROBLASTOMA

Definition. Chondroblastoma is a primary neoplasm of bone with a peculiar tendency to involve the ends of long bones. It has many histologic similarities to a giant cell tumor but, unlike the latter, has cartilaginous differentiation.

General Features. Chondroblastomas are rare, accounting for less than 2 percent of all bone tumors in the Latin American Bone Tumor Registry (101). The Mayo Clinic files contain 138 chondroblastomas, which account for more than 1.4 percent of bone tumors and almost 5 percent of benign tumors (fig. 4-43). The nature of the proliferating cell has been debated, but electron microscopic and immunohistochemical studies clearly suggest cartilaginous differentiation (94).

Clinical Features. Patients generally present with localized pain, usually mild and from a few weeks to a few years in duration. Patients may also note a swelling over the involved bone. A palpable mass and localized tenderness are the sole findings on physical examination. Patients range in age from 2 to 83 years (92), but most are in the second decade of life. There is a definite male predominance (92,96).

Sites. Approximately 60 percent of chondroblastomas involve the long tubular bones (96). The femur, usually the distal epiphysis, is the most common site. In some large series, the proximal humerus (102) or the proximal tibia (98) is the usual site. About one fourth of tumors involve the apophyses, either the greater trochanter of the femur or the tuberosity of the humerus. Tumors involving the ilium commonly arise from the region of the triradiate cartilage. In the skull, the temporal bone is the preferred site. In a large series of consultation cases reported by Kurt et al. (92), the most common site was the calcaneus and talus together.

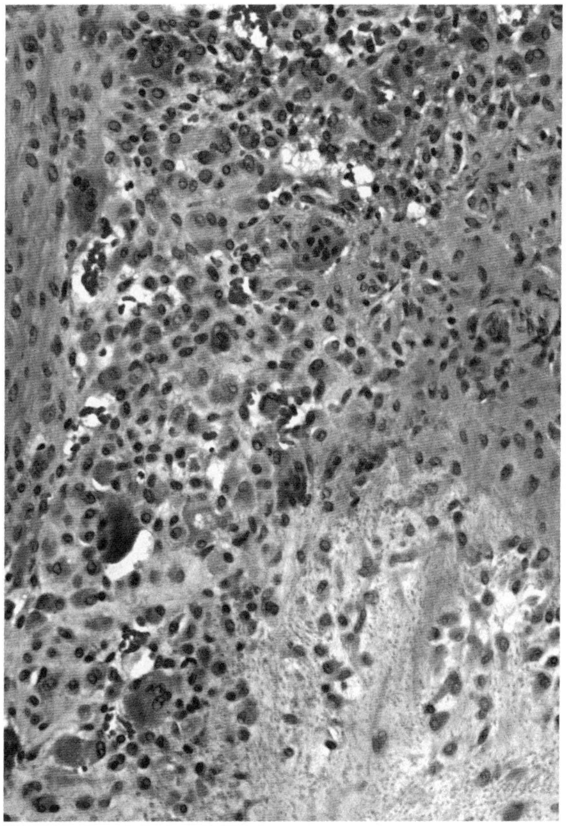

Figure 4-42

SOFT TISSUE CHONDROMA

A chondroblastoma-like soft tissue chondroma contains hypercellular areas with mononuclear cells and multinucleated giant cells.

Radiographic Findings. The typical radiographic feature is a lucent defect at the end of a long bone (fig. 4-44A). The majority of lesions involve the medulla, but a small percentage seem to arise in the cortex or, rarely, even on the surface of the bone. Although some chondroblastomas attain a considerable size, most are less than 5 cm in greatest dimension. Typically, they

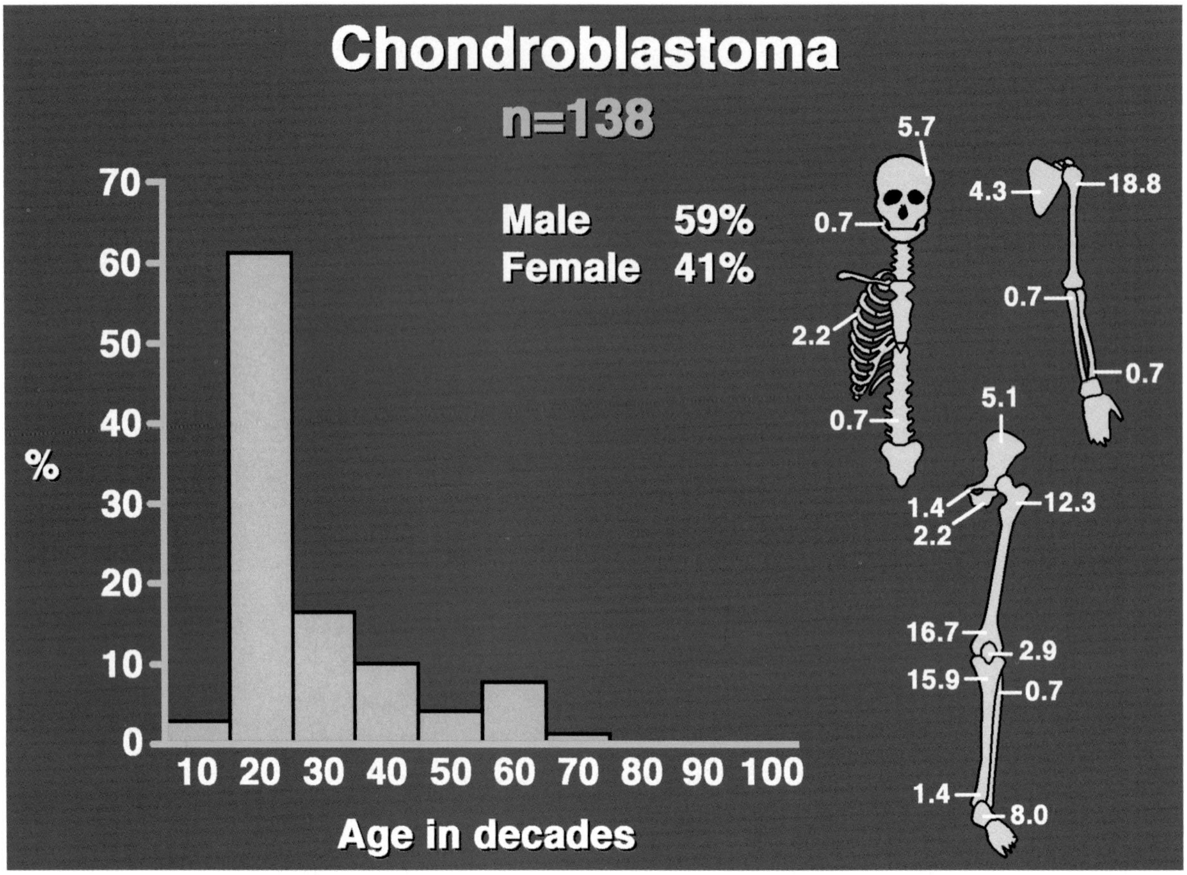

Figure 4-43

CHONDROBLASTOMA

The distribution of chondroblastoma according to the age and sex of the patient and the site of the lesion.

appear as a round or oval lucency located eccentrically or in the middle of the epiphysis. Although 40 percent of the lesions are confined to the epiphysis, slightly more than half extend to involve the metaphysis. A lucency that has an epicenter in the epiphysis and extends across an open epiphyseal plate to involve the metaphysis is typical of chondroblastoma. More than 50 percent of the tumors have a sclerotic rim. Calcification, seen rarely on plain radiographs, may be visible on CT (fig. 4-45). Periosteal new bone formation is found in about 10 percent of cases. The presence of a secondary aneurysmal bone cyst may suggest an aggressive neoplasm.

Chondroblastomas tend to be positive on radionuclide bone scans (89). The extent of the process, especially joint involvement, can be better defined with CT. MRI shows a thin lobulated rim, which is quite typical (97,106), and usually shows peritumoral edema, which may be alarming to the unwary (fig. 4-44B,C). Periosteal new bone formation is better defined with MRI.

Gross Findings. Chondroblastomas are usually treated with curettage. Fragments of soft pink to gray tumor tissue may show chalky white deposits of calcium (fig. 4-46). Areas of hemorrhage and small cystic spaces are common. Grossly visible cartilage is uncommon. If the lesion is resected, the tumor appears as a well-circumscribed lobulated neoplasm, often containing small cystic areas. Rarely, the lesion is predominantly cystic and the tumor is a mural nodule.

Microscopic Findings. Chondroblastomas consist of mononuclear cells and giant cells. The mononuclear cells have well-defined cytoplasmic boundaries and an oval-to-elongated

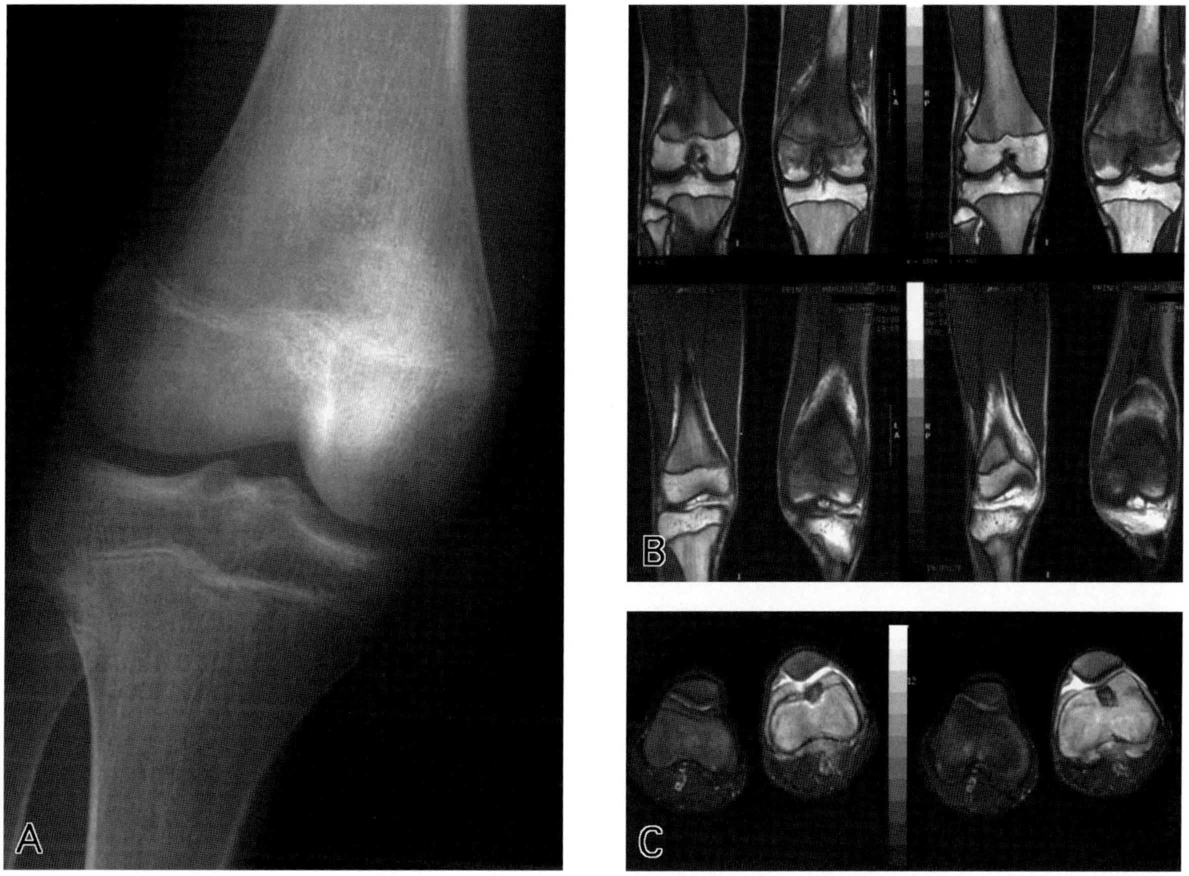

Figure 4-44

CHONDROBLASTOMA

A: A small epiphyseal lesion in the femur of a 16-year-old patient with open growth plates.

B: T_1-weighted coronal MRI shows an extensive abnormality suggesting a lesion much larger than that seen in the radiograph. This is caused by extensive edema, which in this sequence masks the lesion and could mislead the unwary.

C: T_2-weighted axial MRI shows the lesion to be of low signal intensity, corresponding in size to the radiographic abnormality, and surrounded by extensive edema.

nucleus with a characteristic longitudinal groove, producing a "coffee bean" appearance. The chromatin is distributed evenly, and nucleoli are not prominent. Although mitotic figures are nearly always present, they are not numerous (fig. 4-47). The number of multinucleated giant cells is quite variable. Some lesions have a larger number of giant cells similar to the pattern seen in giant cell tumor. The giant cells have a variable number of nuclei, from about 10 to 40. The nuclei are rounded and do not resemble those of mononuclear cells.

Although the nuclear characteristics of chondroblastoma cells are quite typical, matrix formation has to be identified to confirm the diagnosis. About 95 percent of the tumors form cartilage, which may be focal or abundant. The cartilage matrix stains pink rather than blue (fig. 4-48). About 35 percent of chondroblastomas contain calcification (fig. 4-49), which occurs in a lace-like arrangement between individual tumor cells, hence, the term "chicken wire" calcification. Rarely, the calcification occurs in lumps and may obscure the underlying neoplasm.

The mononuclear cells may have vesicular nuclei and abundant pink cytoplasm. Such epithelioid cells are found more commonly in chondroblastomas of the skull (fig. 4-50). The cells of some chondroblastomas contain brown granular pigment in the cytoplasm. This feature

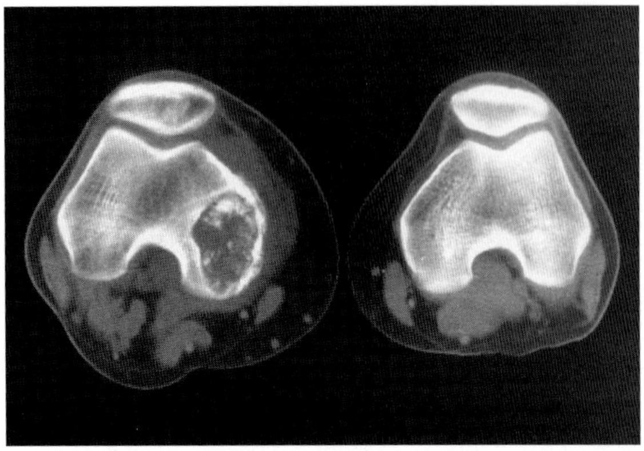

Figure 4-45

CHONDROBLASTOMA

Axial computerized tomography (CT) demonstrates an osteolytic lesion in a 19-year-old patient. The lesion is well demarcated and contains stippled calcification.

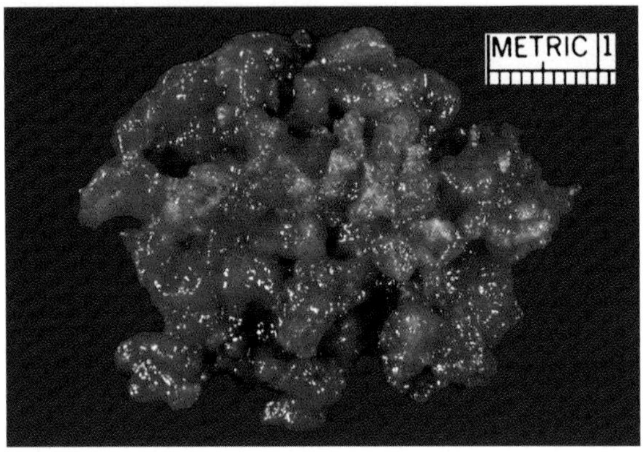

Figure 4-46

CHONDROBLASTOMA

This gray-brown lobulated tumor contains several pale yellow areas of calcification.

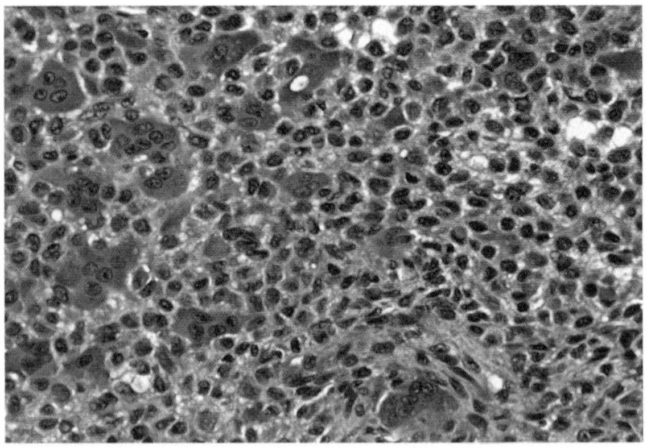

Figure 4-47

CHONDROBLASTOMA

Occasional mitotic figures are present in chondroblastoma.

is also more common in tumors of the skull. Rarely, tumors have mononuclear cells that are spindled and have a hemangiopericytomatous vascular pattern or have enlarged bizarre nuclei (fig. 4-51). The chondroid matrix usually undergoes ossification and a bone-forming neoplasm may be suggested. This pattern is more common in chondroblastomas that involve the talus and calcaneus.

A secondary aneurysmal bone cyst is found in more than one third of chondroblastomas (fig. 4-52), usually seen as microscopic cystic spaces within the tumor. Occasionally, however, the aneurysmal bone cyst pattern may dominate and the chondroblastoma consists of mural nodules.

Frozen Sections. Chondroblastoma can be diagnosed confidently on the basis of fresh frozen section analysis. The nuclear characteristics described above are well recognized in toluidine blue- or H&E-stained sections. The calcification is seen as crystalline rods between individual tumor cells.

Immunohistochemical Findings. The mononuclear cells in chondroblastomas stain for S-100 protein.

Cytologic Findings. The fine-needle aspiration appearance of chondroblastoma is typically cellular, with cell clusters and single, dispersed cells; these are uniform and round, with well-defined cytoplasm, variable cytoplasmic pseudoinclusions, and a single, uniform, grooved nucleus with one or more small nucleoli (fig. 4-53). Small osteoclasts are frequently encountered in addition to a variable amount of purple, fibrillary, myxoid matrix (86,87,90,91,105).

Genetics and Other Special Techniques. Clonal abnormalities have been described in six benign chondroblastomas and one aggressive chondroblastoma (84,95,103,104). The observation of recurrent structural anomalies involving chromosomes 5 and 8 suggests that these chromosomes may be preferentially involved (103). The *CORS-26* (collagenous repeat-containing sequence of 26-kDa protein) gene has been localized to the short arm of chromosome 5. CORS-26 mRNA has been shown to be

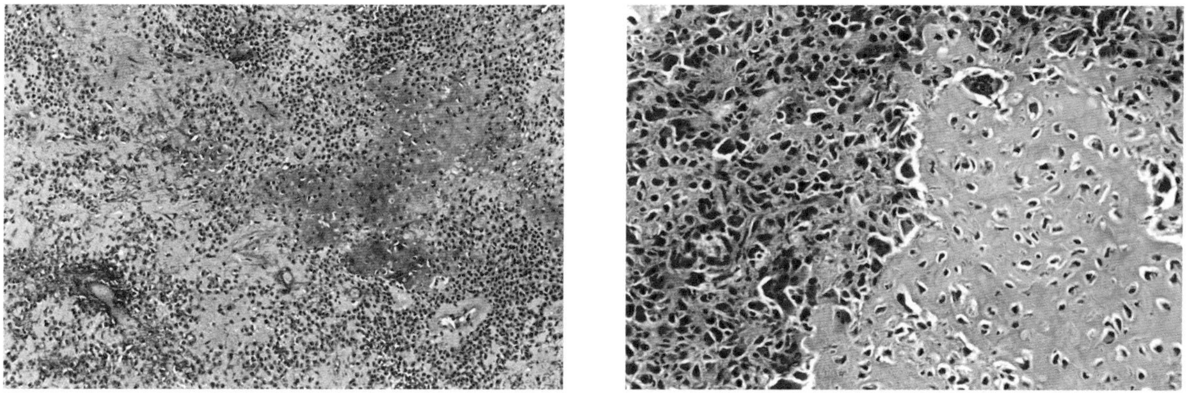

Figure 4-48

CHONDROBLASTOMA

Left: Typical low-power appearance with irregularly shaped pink to pale blue chondroid lobules, calcification, and sheets of mononuclear cells.

Right: Pink chondroid surrounded by mononuclear cells with scattered longitudinal grooves.

strongly expressed in chondroblastoma and may play a role in the pathogenesis of this neoplasm (100). Growth plate signaling molecules and a transmembrane molecule essential for regulating osteoclast formation and activity have also been shown to be expressed in chondroblastoma (88,99). These findings indicate that chondroblastoma may originate from a mesenchymal cell committed to chondrogenesis via active growth plate signaling pathways and this neoplasm may induce recruitment of osteoclast-like cells, resulting in osteolytic bone destruction, respectively.

Differential Diagnosis. The differential diagnosis includes giant cell tumor, chondromyxoid fibroma, and osteosarcoma. Both giant cell tumors and chondroblastomas occur at the ends of bones. On radiographs, chondroblastomas tend to be better demarcated than giant cell tumors. Giant cell tumors do not show reactive sclerosis at the periphery, as do chondroblastomas. The mononuclear cells in giant cell tumors lack the longitudinal groove in the nucleus so typical of the mononuclear cells in chondroblastomas. Also, chondroblastomas are characterized by chondroid matrix, calcification, or both, which is not a feature of giant cell tumors.

Chondromyxoid fibromas involve the metaphysis, whereas chondroblastomas involve the epiphysis. Chondromyxoid fibromas have a lobulated growth pattern, with a myxoid background. The mononuclear cells in chondromyxoid fibromas can be very similar to those in chondroblastomas, and in a biopsy sample, it may be impossible to distinguish the two except on the basis of location within the bone.

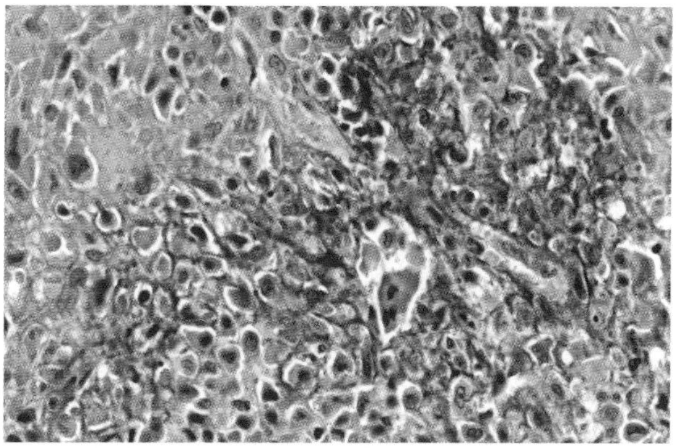

Figure 4-49

CHONDROBLASTOMA

There is lace-like calcification between the mononuclear tumor cells.

A rare type of osteosarcoma has cytologic features similar to those of chondroblastoma; however, in these osteosarcomas, the cells are arranged in a sheet-like pattern and permeate bony trabeculae.

Treatment and Prognosis. Curettage is the treatment of choice. Reported recurrence rates vary from 6 (101) to 15 percent (98,102). Most recurrences have been managed with recurettage

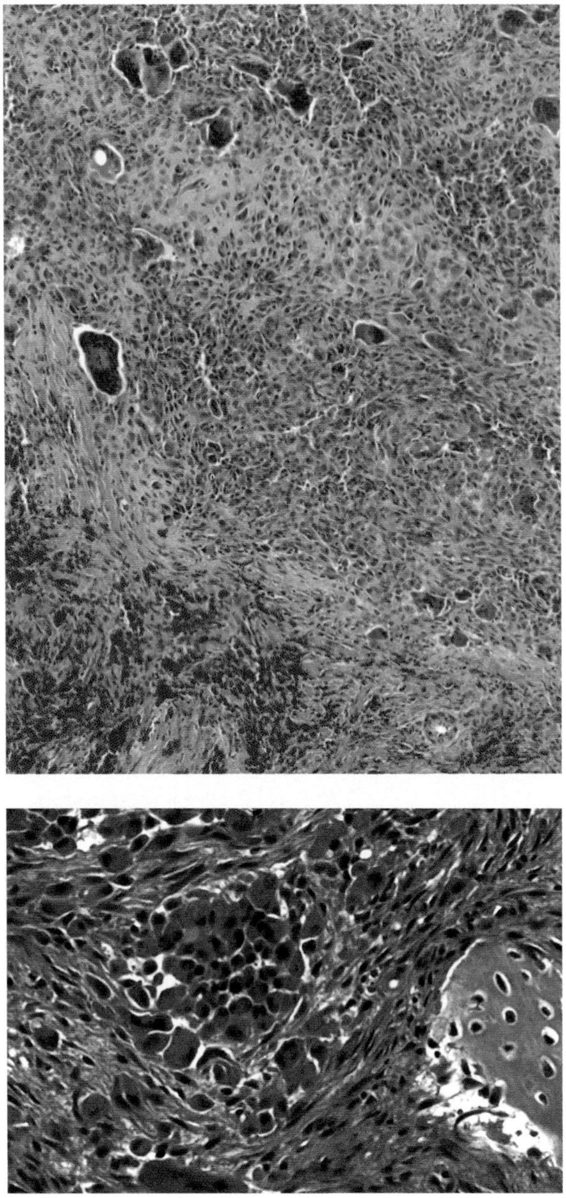

Figure 4-50

CHONDROBLASTOMA

Top: This chondroblastoma arising in a temporal bone contains areas of spindled mononuclear cells, hemosiderin deposition, and multinucleated giant cells. The lesion is histologically similar to giant cell reparative granuloma.

Bottom: Some of the mononuclear cells with abundant cytoplasm have an epithelioid appearance.

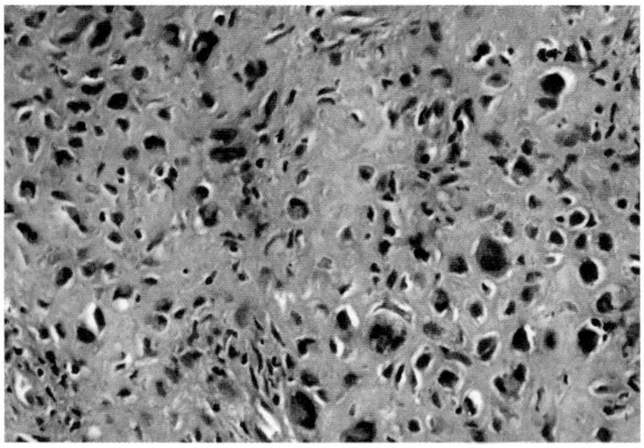

Figure 4-51

CHONDROBLASTOMA

This tumor contains atypical cells with enlarged, irregular, and hyperchromatic nuclei. However, there is no overall increase in the nuclear-cytoplasmic ratio.

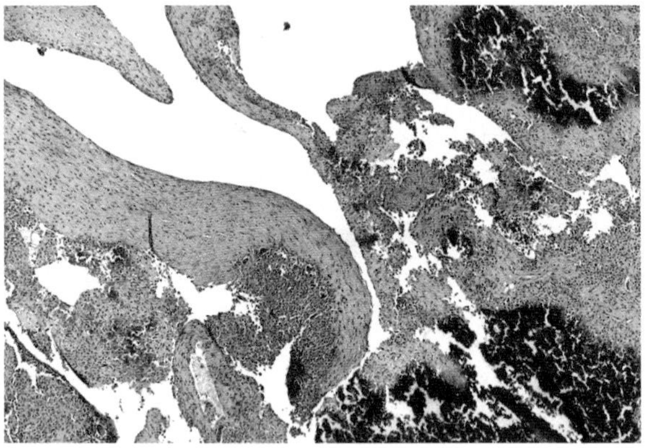

Figure 4-52

CHONDROBLASTOMA

Tumor with a secondary aneurysmal bone cyst.

(85). For lesions that recur aggressively, the term "aggressive chondroblastoma" has been used. However, this is more a clinical description than a pathologic entity. As with giant cell tumor, "benign" pulmonary metastases occur with chondroblastoma, although the rate is lower. Kurt et al. (92) reported a metastatic rate of less than 2 percent. Ramappa et al. (98) described 47 patients, of whom 2 developed metastases. One of these two patients died. Kyriakos et al. (93) described a patient who died of progressive metastatic chondroblastoma. Distant metastases are so rare that not enough information is available about the prognosis of such patients. Although there are well-documented examples of patients dying of metastatic chondroblastoma, these are exceptions. In most cases, a good outcome can be expected. There are

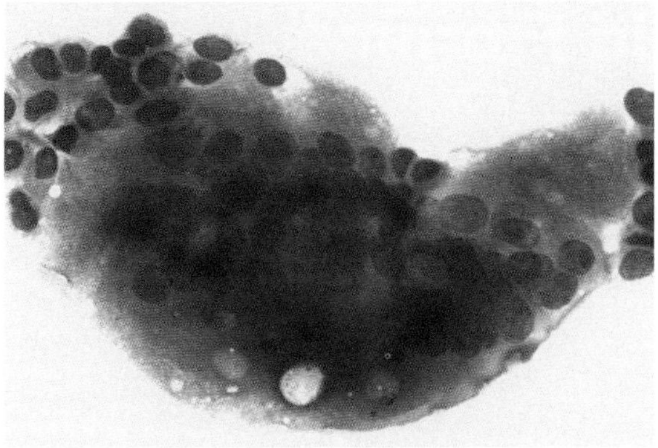

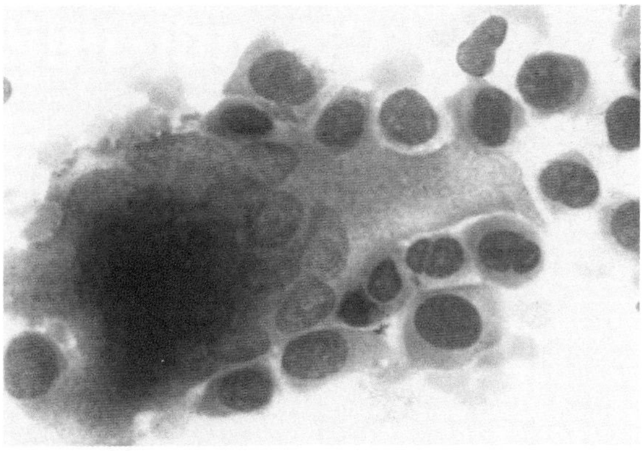

Figure 4-53

FINE-NEEDLE ASPIRATION BIOPSY OF CHONDROBLASTOMA

The tumor has uniform, round "chondroblastic" cells with well-defined cytoplasm and oval to round nuclei with evenly distributed chromatin next to multinucleated osteoclasts (May-Grünwald-Giemsa stain).

rare examples of malignant transformation but usually after radiotherapy.

CHONDROMYXOID FIBROMA

Definition. Chondromyxoid fibroma is a benign lobulated neoplasm composed of spindle- and stellate-shaped cells that are embedded in a myxoid matrix. Generally, it occurs in the metaphysis of a long bone and has a benign radiographic appearance.

General Features. The tumor was first described by Jaffe and Lichtenstein (111) in 1948, when they presented eight cases culled from a group of chondrosarcomas in their files. They realized that a small group of tumors previously classified as chondrosarcoma had a benign clinical evolution and unique histologic characteristics. Dahlin (107) pointed out the similarities between chondromyxoid fibroma and chondroblastoma. Most cases that have been reported in the literature as myxoma and fibromyxoma of bone probably are examples of chondromyxoid fibroma. Chondromyxoid fibroma is one of the rarest bone neoplasms, accounting for less than 0.5 percent of all tumors and 1.6 percent of all benign tumors in the Mayo Clinic files, which up to the year 2000 included 48 cases of chondromyxoid fibroma (fig. 4-54).

Clinical Features. Pain is the common presenting symptom, and it may be noted for a considerable time (121). Swelling is noted less commonly (114). Pathologic fracture is uncommon. Some reports have suggested a male predominance (120). Patients range in age from 3 to 87 years. The peak incidence is in the second and third decades of life.

Sites. Approximately 45 percent of the lesions occur in the long bones; the proximal tibia is the most common site. The iliac wing and ribs are also relatively common sites. Although more than one third of the lesions of the hands and feet involve the metatarsals, rarely are the metacarpals involved.

Radiographic Findings. The typical radiographic appearance is that of an eccentrically located, purely lucent, lobulated defect of the metaphysis of a long bone (fig. 4-55). It is unusual to identify mineral in the substance of the lesion, but when it is present, it occurs in clumps, suggesting cartilage. The rare chondromyxoid fibroma that occurs on the surface of a bone tends to become heavily mineralized (fig. 4-56) (115). The scalloped appearance of the margins is accentuated on MRI. The tumor may abut the epiphyseal plate and extend to involve the epiphysis or, less commonly, the diaphysis. In the large series reported by Wu et al. (120), the diaphysis alone was involved in 11 cases and the tumor was purely epiphyseal in only 1 case.

The cortex is thinned in most cases and expanded in almost as many cases. In about half of the cases, the cortex is absent, at least partly. Nearly always, the margin is sharply demarcated and about half of the tumors have a sclerotic rim. Periosteal new bone formation is rare.

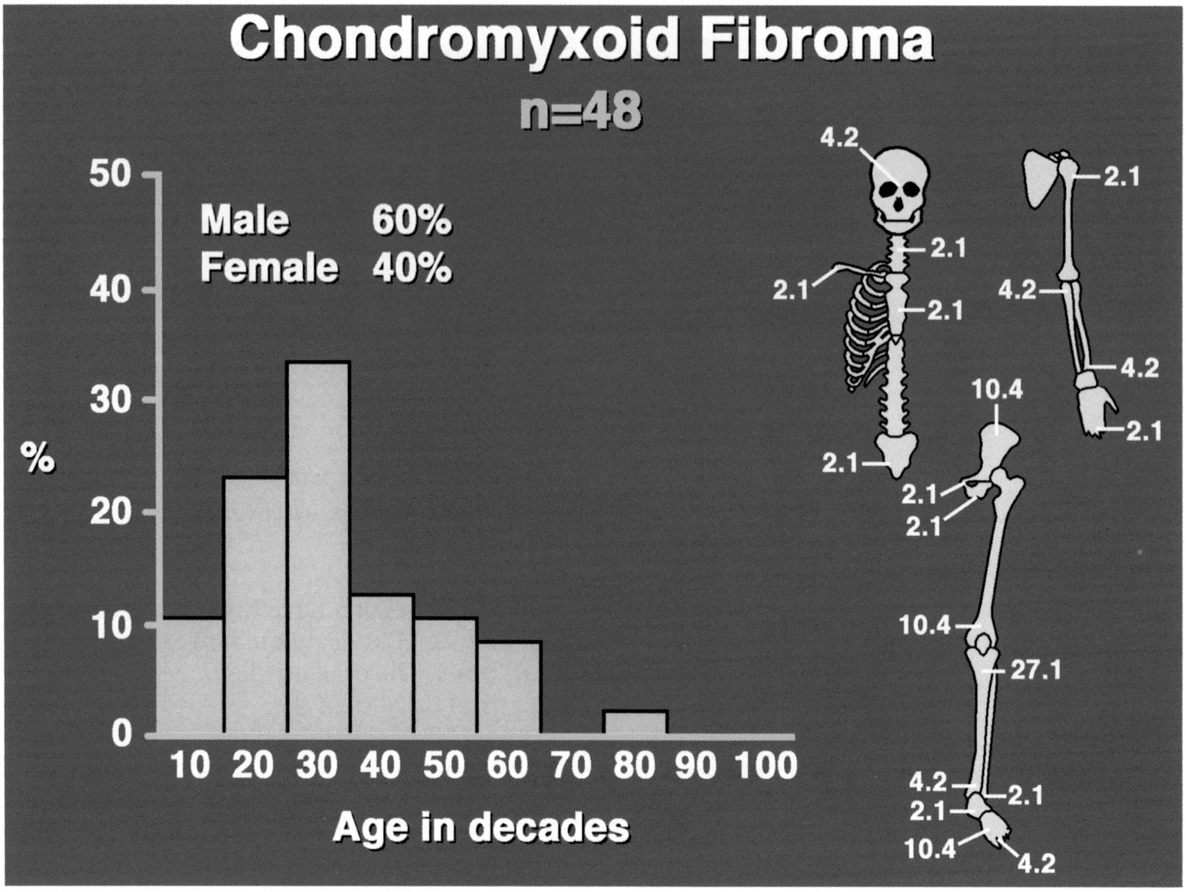

Figure 4-54

CHONDROMYXOID FIBROMA

The distribution of chondromyxoid fibroma according to the age and sex of the patient and the site of the lesion.

In the small bones, the tumor is located centrally and shows fusiform expansion of the bone. The epiphysis is involved more often in small bones than in long bones (fig. 4-57). In flat bones, especially the iliac crest, the lesion may become large and markedly scalloped, producing a bubbly appearance (fig. 4-58).

The radiographic features of chondromyxoid fibroma are nonspecific, but they almost invariably suggest a benign process.

Gross Findings. Because chondromyxoid fibromas are treated frequently with curettage, intact gross specimens are uncommon. Curetted fragments are blue-gray, with a chondroid "aura," although well-developed cartilage is not seen (fig. 4-59). The gross specimen usually has a semitranslucent appearance that suggests a myxoid process. If the lesion is removed intact, it is well circumscribed and lobulated, and tends to retract from the surrounding bone (fig. 4-60). Liquefactive myxoid change is not found.

Microscopic Findings. If one histologic feature characterizes chondromyxoid fibroma, it is a lobulated growth pattern, although this growth pattern is occasionally absent (120). If the lesion is removed intact and the sections contain bone, the edges of the tumor are rounded and retract from the surrounding bone.

The lobules may be large and obvious (macrolobular pattern) on low-power examination or less distinct and smaller (microlobular pattern) (fig. 4-61). The lobules consist of spindle and stellate cells embedded in a myxoid background (fig. 4-62). The cells frequently have abundant pink cytoplasm, producing an epithelioid appearance.

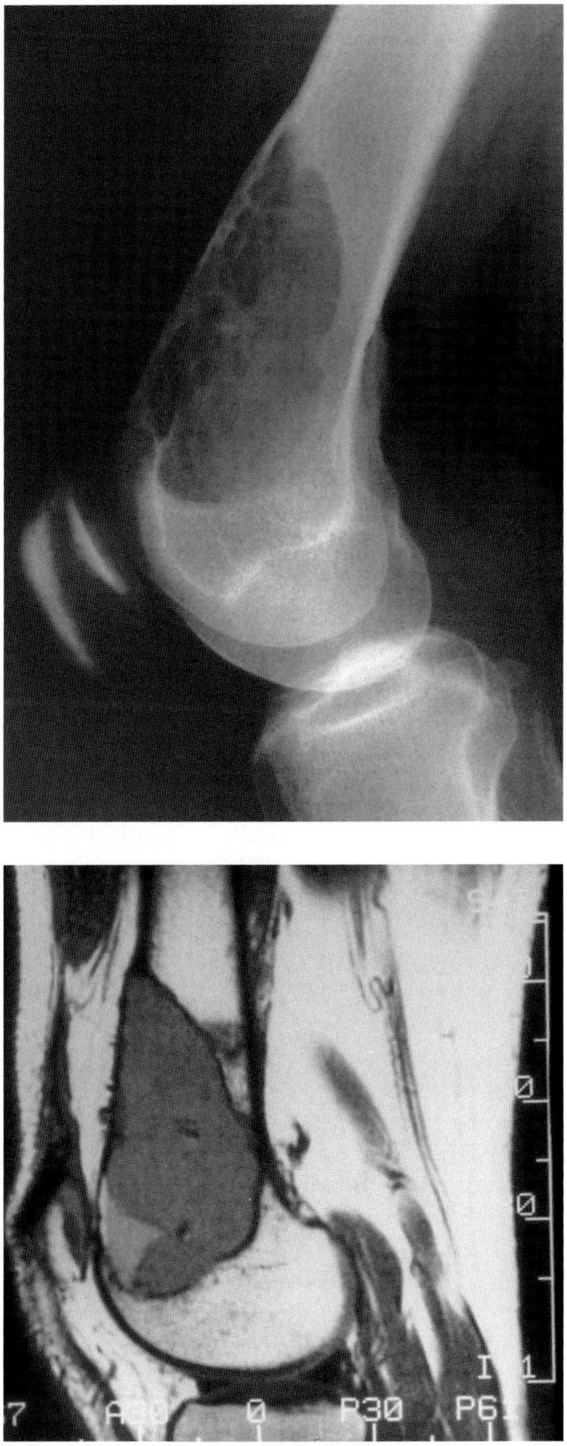

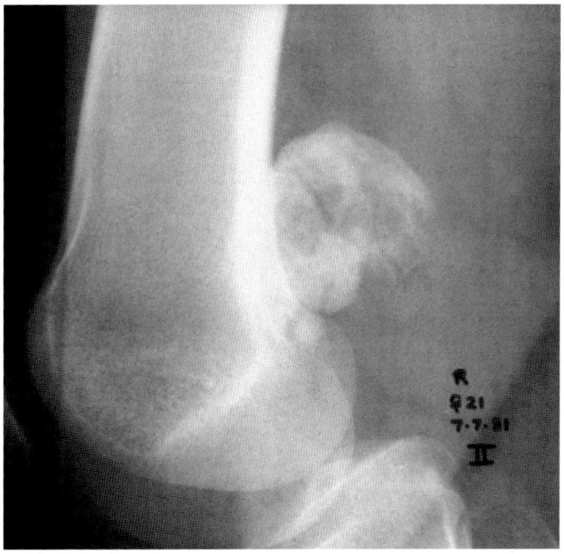

Figure 4-56

CHONDROMYXOID FIBROMA

The lesion in this 27-year-old man is heavily mineralized, not unusual for a surface lesion. (Fig. 5-10 from Unni KK. Dahlin's bone tumors: general aspects and data on 11,087 cases, 5th ed. Philadelphia: Lippincott-Raven; 1996:62. By permission of Mayo Foundation.)

Figure 4-55

CHONDROMYXOID FIBROMA

Top: A well-marginated, lytic, and trabeculated lesion arises in the supracondylar area of the distal femur.

Bottom: T_1-weighted MRI shows a lobulated lesion of intermediate signal intensity confined to bone.

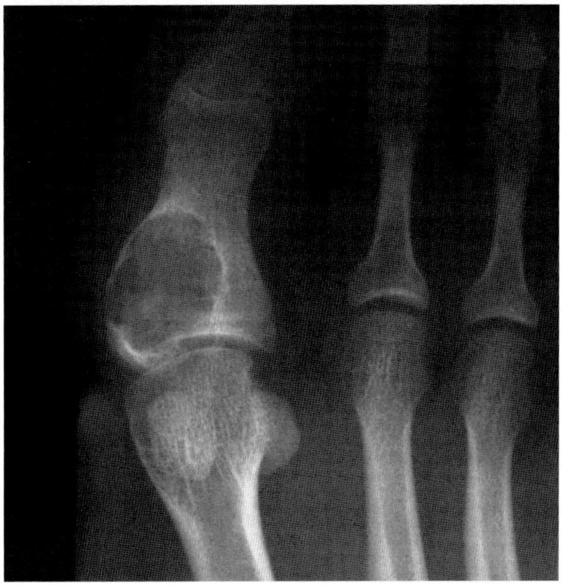

Figure 4-57

CHONDROMYXOID FIBROMA

An expansile lytic lesion is located eccentrically in the proximal phalanx of the great toe. The radiographic features are similar to those of enchondroma (see figure 4-16). (Courtesy of Dr. C. Clark, Cartersville, GA.)

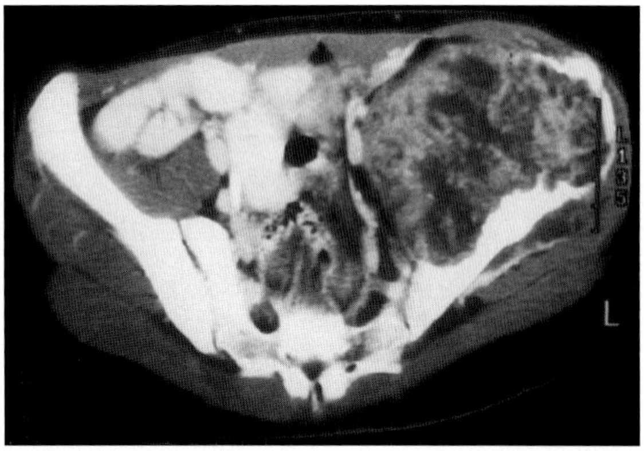

Figure 4-58

CHONDROMYXOID FIBROMA

CT shows a large, heterogeneous, and destructive mass arising from the left ilium. There is some evidence of scalloping peripherally. (Courtesy of Dr. K. Chang, Duarte, CA.)

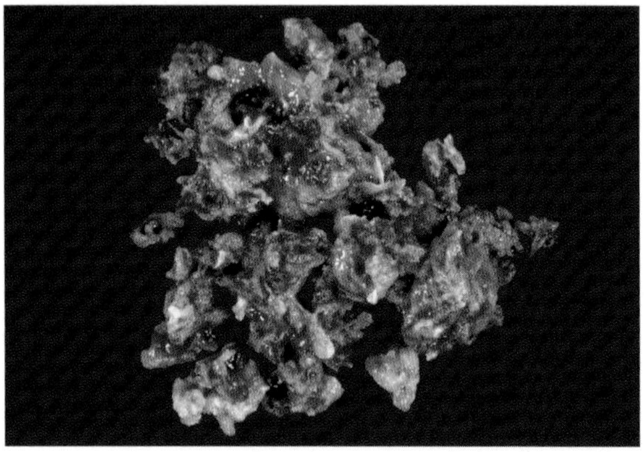

Figure 4-59

CHONDROMYXOID FIBROMA

Curetted fragment of a glistening, blue-gray tumor. There is no obvious evidence of cartilaginous tissue.

The center of the lobule is hypocellular, and the periphery has a condensation of nuclei. Frequently, the periphery contains a proliferation of polyhedral cells, suggesting a chondroblastoma. Clusters of benign giant cells occur at the edges of the lobules in about half of the cases.

The matrix uniformly stains light blue with the H&E stain; liquefactive myxoid change is rare and, if present, focal. Well-formed hyaline cartilage is present in less than 20 percent of cases (fig. 4-63). Calcification occurs in about one third, either as fine granules or denser and plaque-like (fig. 4-64). Surface lesions tend to become heavily calcified.

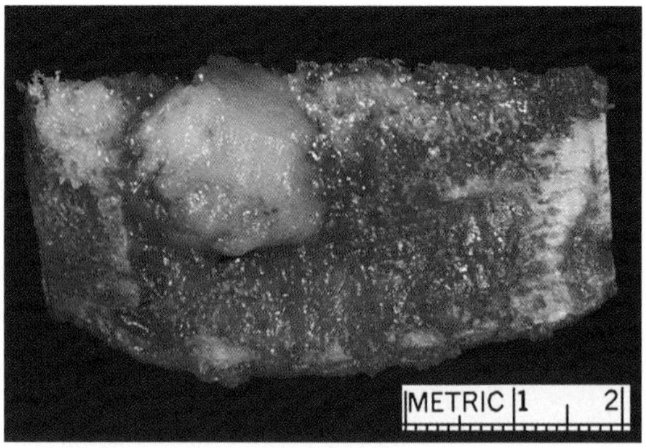

Figure 4-60

INTRACORTICAL CHONDROMYXOID FIBROMA

The tumor forms a well-circumscribed nodular mass within the cortical bone of the proximal tibia.

A secondary aneurysmal bone cyst is distinctly unusual. Bizarre cytologic features of the stellate cells are more common. The nuclei may become enlarged and hyperchromatic. The smudgy appearance of the nuclei, the abundance of the cytoplasm, and the lack of mitotic activity all help label these cells as "pseudomalignant" (fig. 4-65). Rarely, a chondromyxoid fibroma appears permeative, with entrapment of preexisting bony trabeculae. This feature is more common in lesions of flat bones.

Cytologic Findings. Few reports mention the appearance of chondromyxoid fibroma on fine-needle aspiration specimens. The cytologic differentiation of chondromyxoid fibroma from chondroblastoma and chondrosarcoma may be difficult at times (110,113).

Genetics and Other Special Techniques. Few cytogenetic studies of chondromyxoid fibroma are available; however, clonal abnormalities of chromosome 6 appear to be nonrandom (108,109,116,117,119). In particular, rearrangements of the long arm of chromosome 6 at bands q13 and q25 are recurrent in this neoplasm (fig. 4-66). Pronounced expression of hydrated proteoglycans (major constituent of the myxoid matrix) and focal expression of collagen type II (a marker of chondrocytic cell differentiation) as well as collagen types I, III, and VI are characteristic of the matrix composition and gene expression pattern in chondromyxoid fibroma (118).

Differential Diagnosis. Chondromyxoid fibroma may be mistaken for chondrosarcoma and

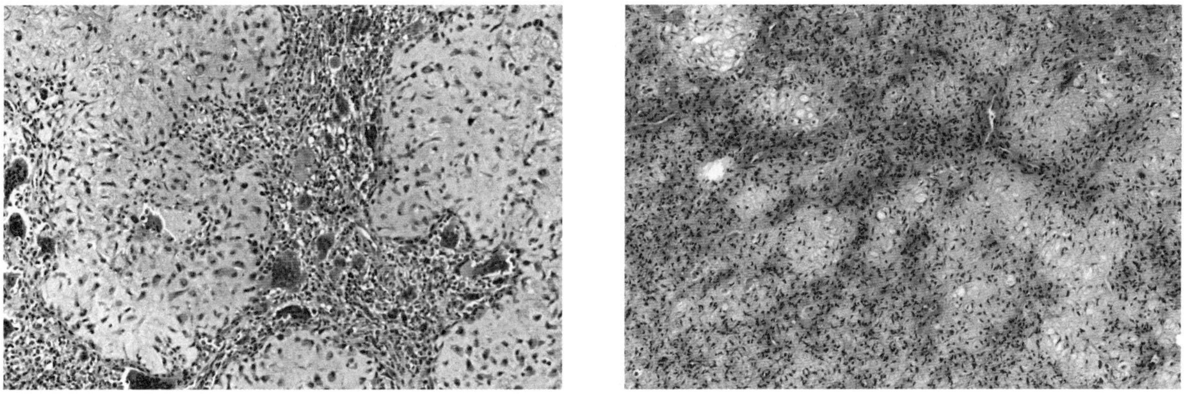

Figure 4-61

CHONDROMYXOID FIBROMA

Left: Macrolobular growth pattern with multinucleated giant cells at the periphery of the lobules.

Right: Microlobular growth pattern characterized by pale, less well-formed nodules containing stellate-shaped cells in a myxoid background.

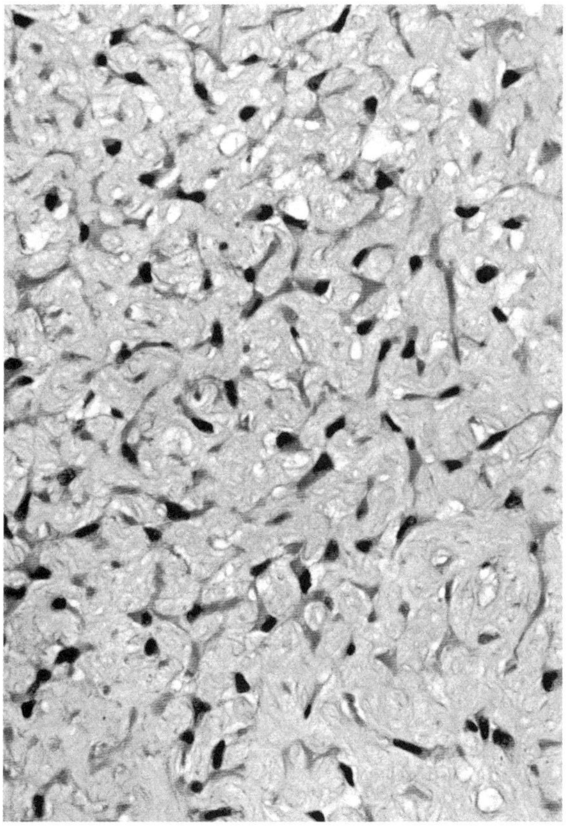

Figure 4-62

CHONDROMYXOID FIBROMA

Cells within the lobules of the tumor have small, oval to spindle-shaped nuclei with eosinophilic cytoplasmic extensions.

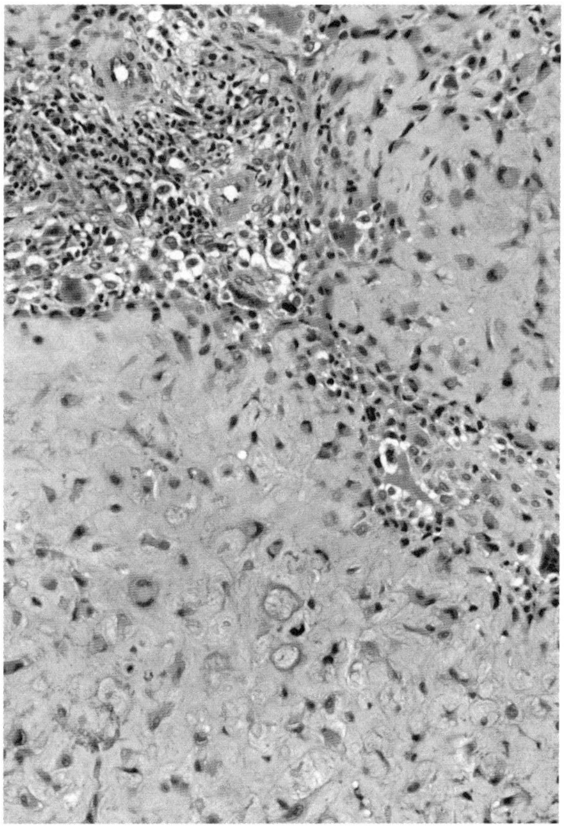

Figure 4-63

CHONDROMYXOID FIBROMA

Well-formed hyaline cartilage seen here is not commonly seen in chondromyxoid fibromas.

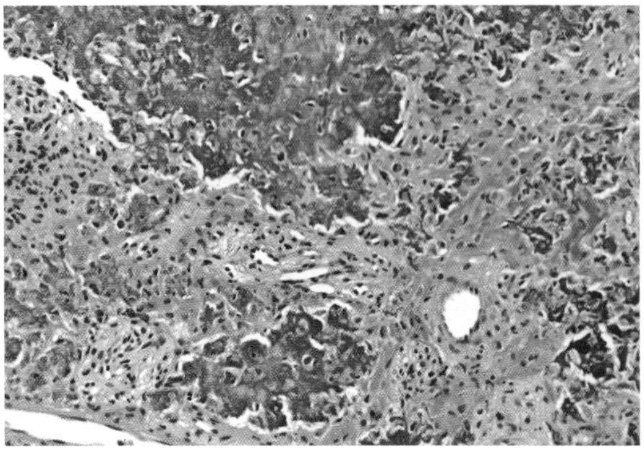

Figure 4-64

CHONDROMYXOID FIBROMA

Chunky, plaque-like calcification in a tumor located in the femoral metaphysis. The calcification is similar to what is commonly seen in surface lesions.

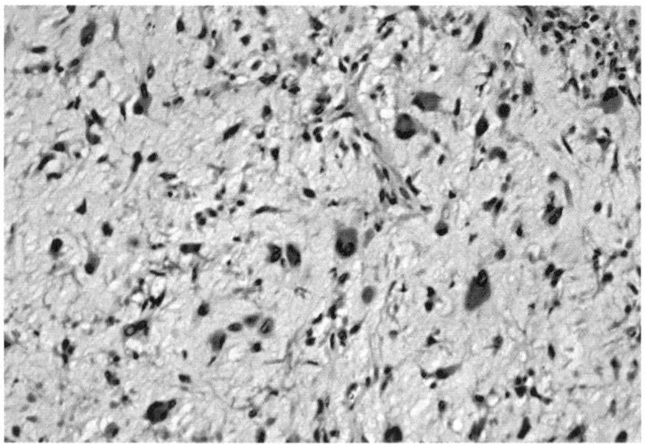

Figure 4-65

CHONDROMYXOID FIBROMA

The tumor occasionally contains atypical cells. The nuclei are enlarged and irregularly shaped, with smudgy chromatin and scattered vacuoles. Abundant eosinophilic cytoplasm surrounds the nuclei, giving some cells an epithelioid appearance.

Figure 4-66

KARYOTYPE OF CHONDROMYXOID FIBROMA

Right: Representative karyotype of a chondromyxoid fibroma exhibiting the following abnormal chromosomal complement: 46,XX,t(6;9) (q25;q22), t(7;12)(q32;q13) (arrows show breakpoints).

Below: Spectral karyotypic image of the case shown on the right illustrates the 6;9 and 7;12 translocations. (Figs. 3 and 4 from Safar A, Nelson M, Neff JR, et al. Recurrent anomalies of 6q25 in chondromyxoid fibroma. Hum Pathol 2000; 31:306–11.)

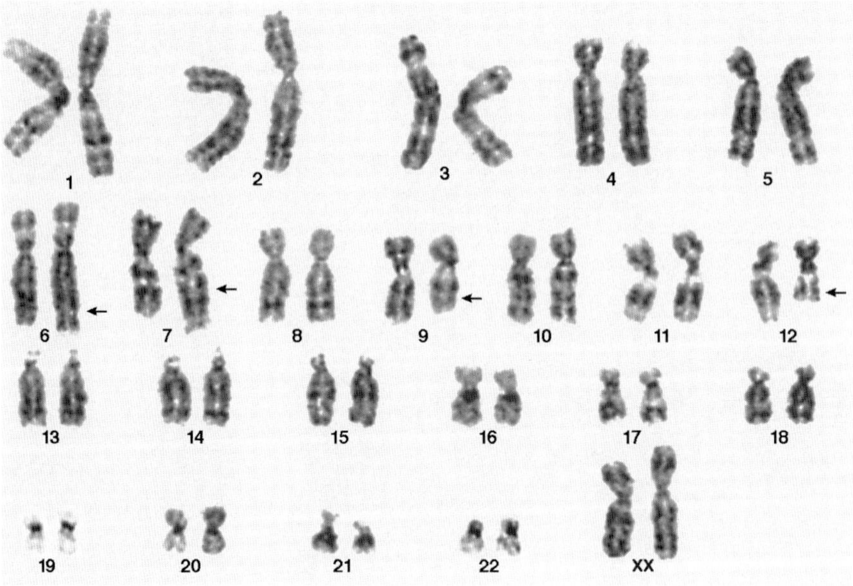

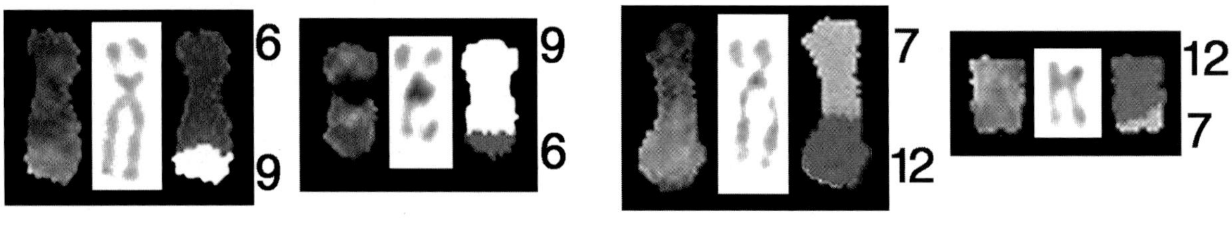

vice versa. A chondrosarcoma, which grows in a lobulated pattern with myxoid change, is usually a high-grade tumor and, hence, easily distinguished from chondromyxoid fibroma. In such instances, it is important to correlate the radiographic features, which are invariably benign in chondromyxoid fibroma. Although both chondromyxoid fibroma and chondrosarcoma appear lobulated, the distinct hypocellularity in the center of the lobule of chondromyxoid fibroma is not a feature of chondrosarcoma.

Treatment and Prognosis. Curettage or limited resection is the treatment of choice. About 20 percent of patients have recurrence, which may involve soft tissue (112). No examples of benign metastases are known. We are aware of one high-grade sarcoma that arose in association with a chondromyxoid fibroma. There also have been examples of postradiation sarcoma.

CHONDROSARCOMA

Definition. Chondrosarcoma is a malignant tumor composed entirely of a hyaline cartilage matrix and chondrocytes in lacunae. The matrix may become myxoid and the cells oval-shaped, floating in the matrix. Calcification and reactive bone formation may be present but not osteoid produced by tumor cells.

General Features. Chondrosarcoma is the third most common primary malignant neoplasm of bone, exceeded only by myeloma and osteosarcoma. The Mayo Clinic files include 1,023 cases of chondrosarcoma, which account for 10.7 percent of all tumors and 15.3 percent of malignant tumors (fig. 4-67).

Chondrosarcoma can be subclassified in many ways depending on the site, presence of a preexisting lesion, and histologic peculiarities. The common type is termed *conventional chondrosarcoma*. This type preferentially involves the pelvic and shoulder girdles of adults. Chondrosarcomas that arise de novo are called primary, and those that arise in relation to a preexisting lesion are called secondary; the latter are considered in a separate section. Chondrosarcomas also have been divided into central and peripheral (147). In our experience, central chondrosarcomas are more common and peripheral ones tend to be special types (secondary to osteochondroma and periosteal chondrosarcoma) and are discussed in separate sections. More than 86 percent of chondrosarcomas are considered primary. Chondrosarcomas in special and unusual sites such as small bones and histologic variants such as dedifferentiated, mesenchymal, and clear cell are considered separately.

Clinical Features. Males are affected more frequently than females; the reported ratio varies from 1.1 to 1 (168,212) to 2 to 1 (147). Chondrosarcoma is a disease of adulthood and old age. Of the cases in the Mayo Clinic files, the youngest patient was 3 years old and the oldest was 85. More than 60 percent of the patients are in the fourth through sixth decades of life. Young et al. (218) reported 47 patients younger than 17 years, but only 14 received treatment at Mayo Clinic. Huvos and Marcove (157) reported 79 patients younger than 21 years (this series included 5 patients with dedifferentiated, 1 with clear cell, and 20 with mesenchymal type chondrosarcoma). In both series, more than 25 percent of the chondrosarcomas were considered secondary.

Pain, occasionally the referred type, is the most common presenting symptom. A small percentage of chondrosarcomas are incidental findings on radiographs. The duration of symptoms varies from a few months to many years. A rapid increase in size and pain in a preexisting lesion suggests that the chondrosarcoma arises from a precursor, such as an osteochondroma. A small percentage of patients present with pathologic fracture. The physical examination may demonstrate a palpable mass, especially in the case of a peripheral chondrosarcoma.

Sites. More than two thirds of chondrosarcomas involve the pelvic and shoulder girdles and the upper ends of the femur and humerus. It is rare to find a chondrosarcoma distal to the wrist and ankle joints. Also, bones of the face and skull are rarely involved. Most cartilage tumors at the base of the skull are chondroid chordomas, and most cartilaginous tumors of the jawbones are chondroblastic osteosarcomas. Chondrosarcomas of the facial skeleton usually involve the nasal septum. Chondrosarcomas of the upper respiratory tract are unusual, locally aggressive tumors. Chondrosarcomas involving the synovium may arise from synovial chondromatosis or be primary tumors. Of the five chondrosarcomas of joints in the Mayo Clinic files, two involved the knee and one each the hip, ankle, and elbow.

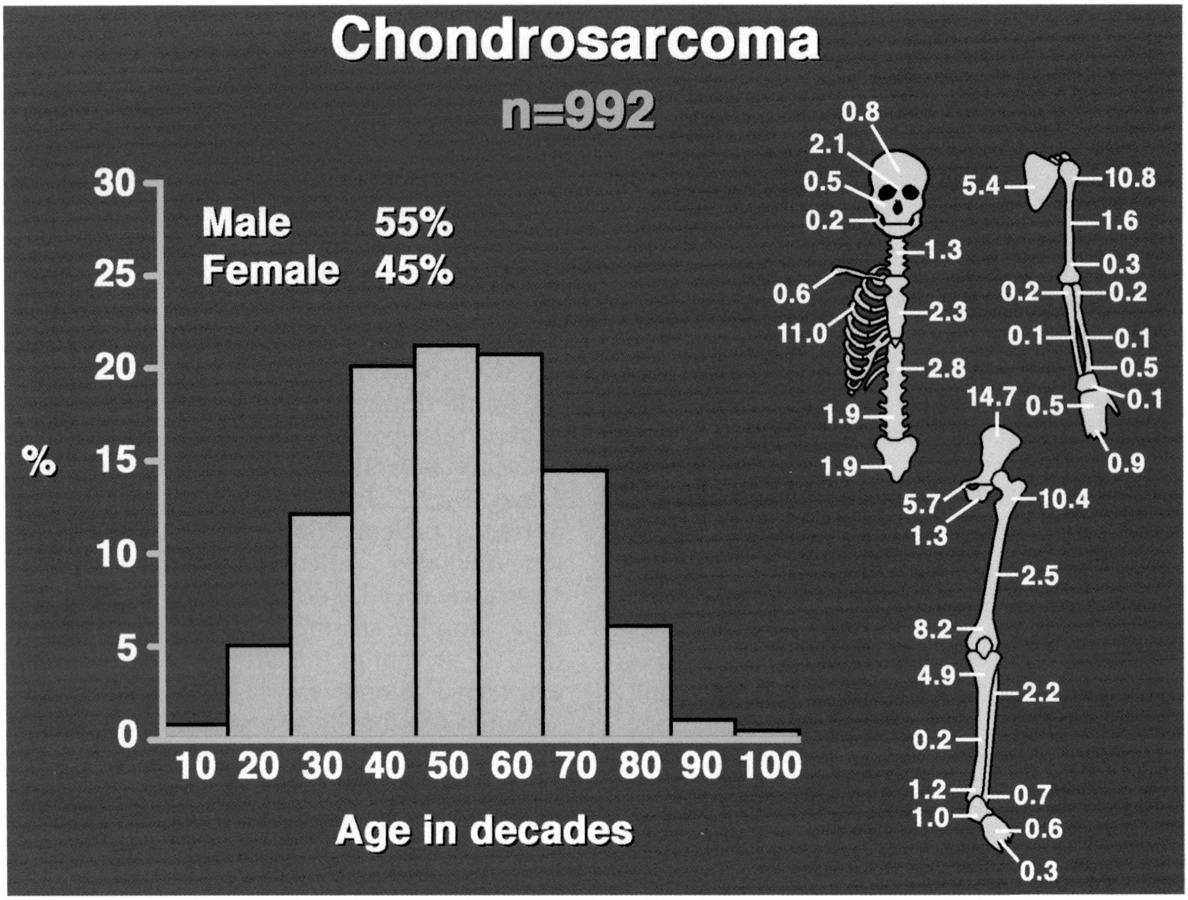

Figure 4-67

CHONDROSARCOMA

The distribution of chondrosarcoma according to the age and sex of the patient and the site of the lesion.

Radiographic Findings. Chondrosarcomas of long bones involve the diaphysis or metaphysis; epiphyseal chondrosarcomas are rare. In the ilium, they tend to arise near the acetabulum. This area is difficult to visualize on plain radiographs and tumors may be overlooked. Thus, chondrosarcomas are usually large when detected. In the study of Bjornsson et al. (128), the mean size of the tumors evaluated on radiographs was 9.5 cm. Smaller lesions are round or oval, and larger ones conform to the shape of the involved bone.

Although calcification is considered a hallmark of a tumor of the cartilage, mineral is seen on plain radiographs of only about 75 percent of chondrosarcomas. CT is more sensitive than plain radiographs for detecting calcification (fig. 4-68): about 40 percent of tumors show slight mineralization; heavy mineralization is uncommon. The mineral may be ring shaped, popcorn-like, or comma shaped (148). It has been suggested that the low-grade tumors are more heavily calcified than high-grade ones (145). An area of lucency in an otherwise uniformly mineralized cartilage tumor suggests chondrosarcoma or even dedifferentiation (fig. 4-69). Approximately 80 percent of chondrosarcomas are poorly marginated; less than 5 percent are sharply marginated. A sclerotic rim is almost never present.

The majority of chondrosarcomas involve the cortex, either by endosteal erosion or by frank destruction. About one third of the lesions widen or expand the bone, and about half thin the cortex; approximately one fifth combine expansion

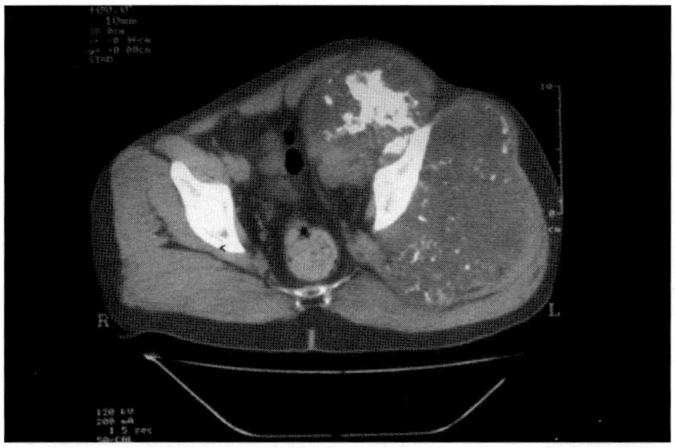

Figure 4-68

CHONDROSARCOMA

CT shows a large, partially calcified mass arising from the left pelvis. (Courtesy of Dr. D. Trinh, Alexandria, MN.)

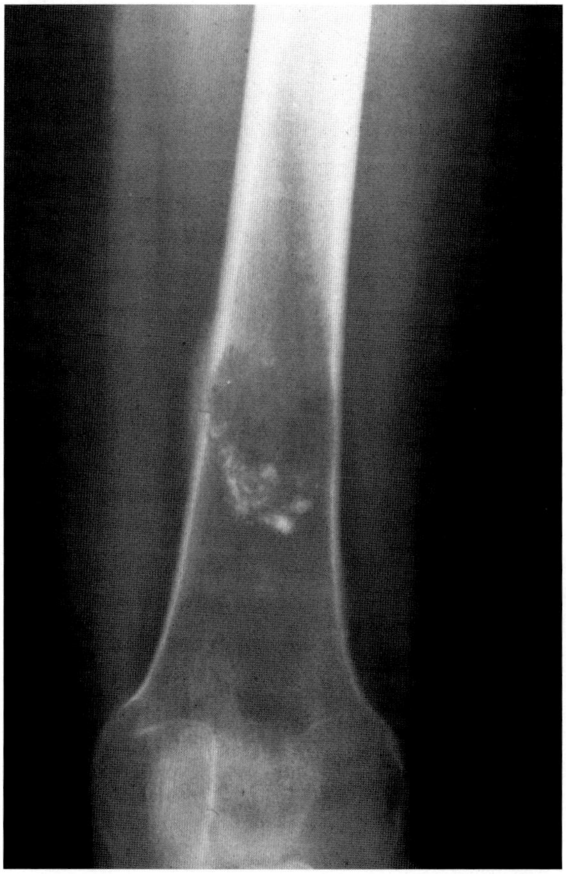

Figure 4-69

CHONDROSARCOMA

This radiograph shows an intramedullary tumor with an eccentric, nonuniform pattern of mineralization that is suggestive of chondrosarcoma. Endosteal scalloping and a periosteal reaction are also apparent.

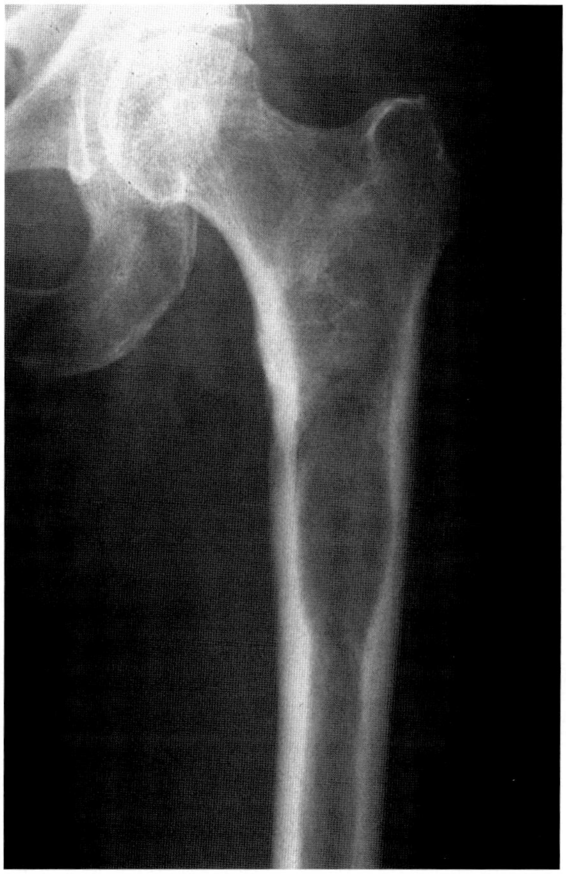

Figure 4-70

CHONDROSARCOMA

An osteolytic mass causes endosteal scalloping, which indicates a slow-growing lesion. (Courtesy of Dr. J. Koett, Riverside, CA.)

of bone and thickening of the cortex (fig. 4-70). This combination is practically diagnostic of chondrosarcoma. Periosteal new bone formation is rare and, when present, minimal. CT and MRI are better for delineating the extent of the neoplasm, especially soft tissue extension, than plain radiographs (fig. 4-71).

Gross Findings. Chondrosarcomas are lobulated, light blue or white masses (fig. 4-72). The matrix may be solid or have a sticky mucoid quality. When the myxoid change is pronounced, the matrix undergoes liquefaction and the tumor "runs" when it is cut. The cut surface of such a tumor is mucoid and contain cystic cavities full of liquid (fig. 4-73). This appearance is not seen in benign cartilage tumors. Calcification may be present as chalky white deposits.

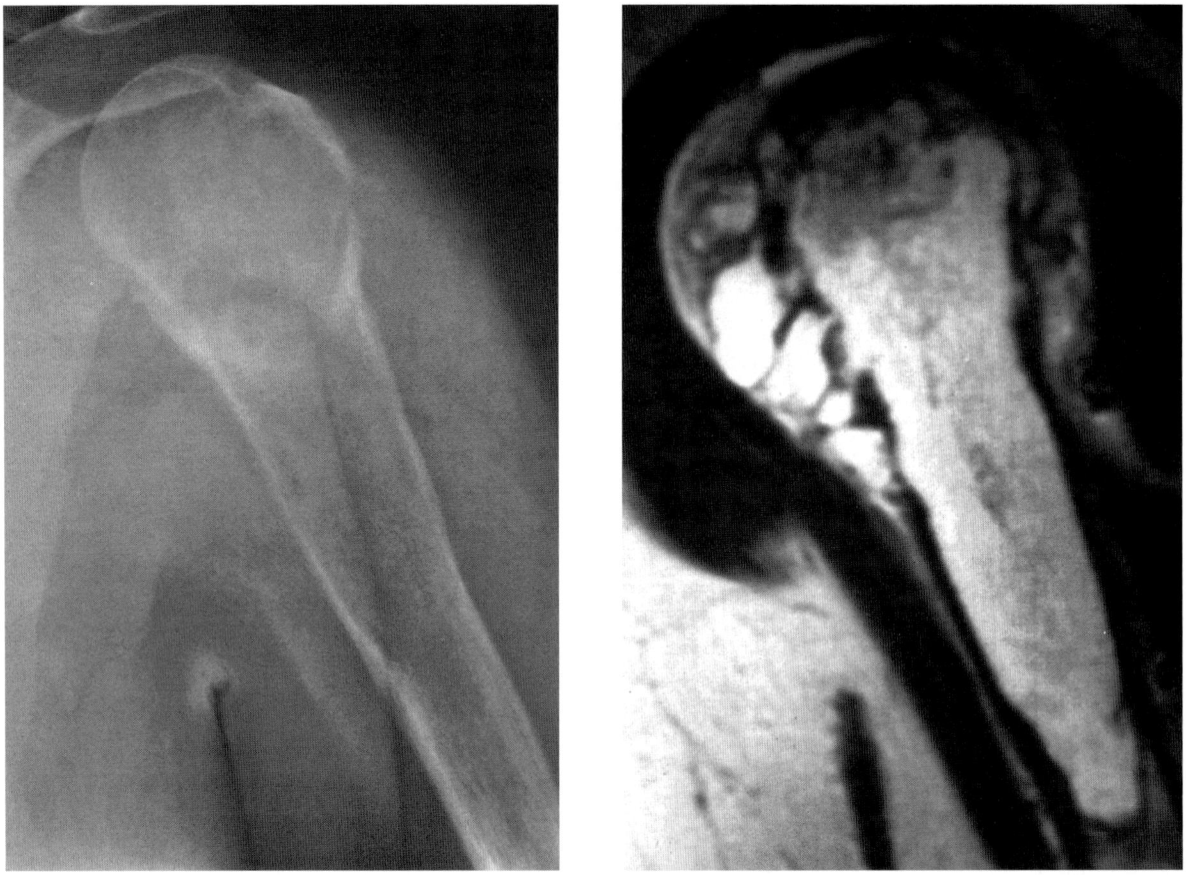

Figure 4-71

CHONDROSARCOMA

Left: An unmineralized osteolytic lesion in the proximal humerus has destroyed the medial cortex.
Right: T_2-weighted MRI shows the intramedullary extent and soft tissue extension beyond the medial cortex.

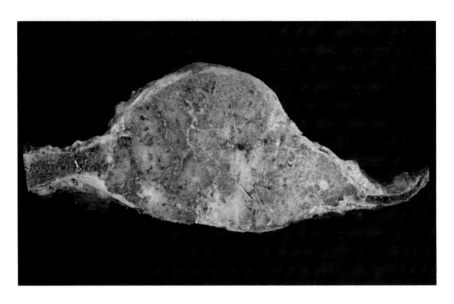

Figure 4-72

CHONDROSARCOMA

The tumor arose in the sternum. It has a characteristic gray-blue appearance, is lobulated, and has chalky white calcific deposits. Cartilage tumors at this site are almost always malignant.

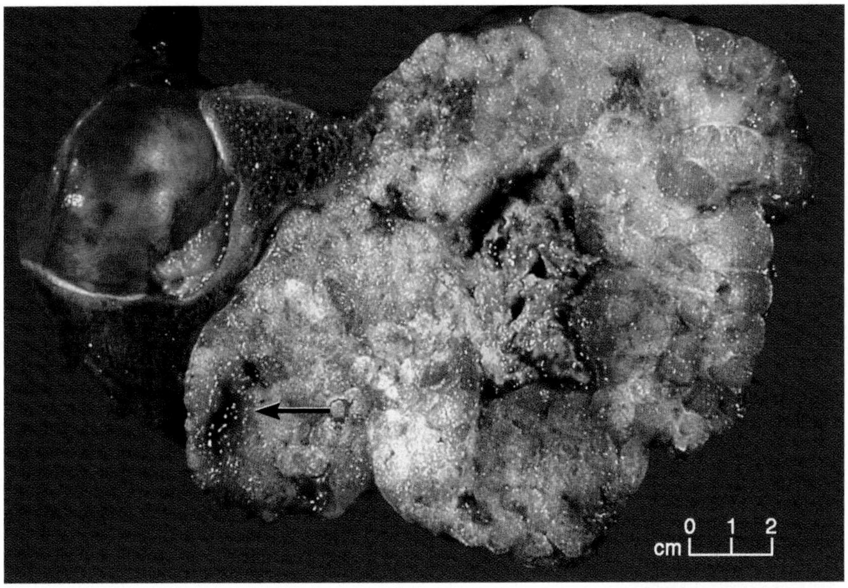

Figure 4-73

CHONDROSARCOMA

The tumor, in the right ilium, shows central cystic degeneration, with necrosis and areas of myxoid change peripherally (arrow).

If the lesion is resected intact, it will be seen to fill the bone marrow cavity, and the junction between the tumor and the marrow is distinct. If the specimen is dissected immediately, the margins can be checked grossly. Knowledgeable surgeons remove the tumor with an envelope of normal tissue; hence, the soft tissue margins are generally clear. However, if the surgeon is particularly concerned about one special site, it can be examined by frozen section. The bone will appear expanded (like an aneurysm), corresponding to the appearance on radiographs (fig. 4-74). A thickened cortex has semicircular defects on the endosteal aspect, a sign of endosteal erosion. Small or large cystic areas containing liquid material may be present. The tumor may have broken through the cortex to form a soft tissue mass, which is generally well circumscribed and pseudoencapsulated.

Microscopic Findings. Conventional chondrosarcomas have the essential hallmarks of all cartilage tumors: a blue chondroid matrix and neoplastic cells located within lacunae. The variation in the relative proportions of the matrix and cells (cellularity), the character of the matrix (whether myxoid or solid), the cytologic features of the chondrocytes, and the relationship of the tumor to the bone (whether permeative or not) help to diagnose and grade the chondrosarcoma.

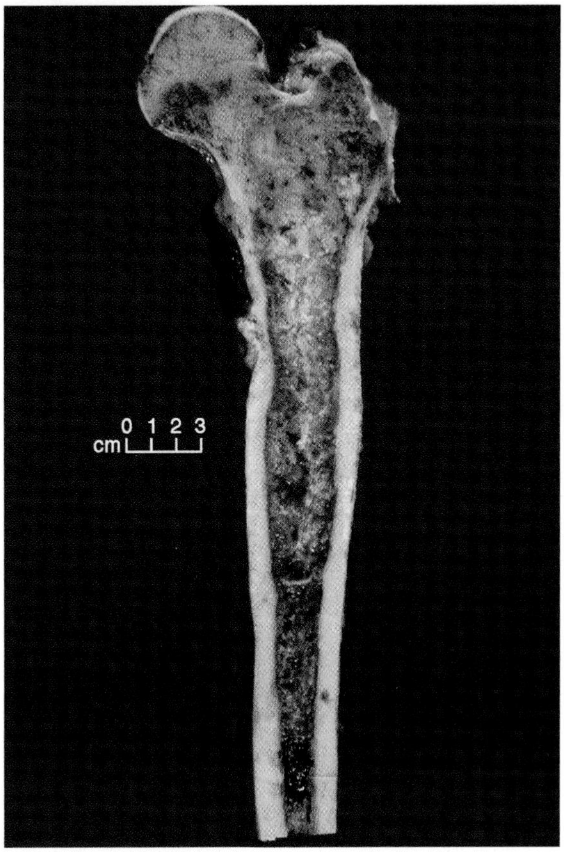

Figure 4-74

CHONDROSARCOMA

The tumor has thickened the cortex. The distal diaphyseal component glistens because of myxoid change in the matrix.

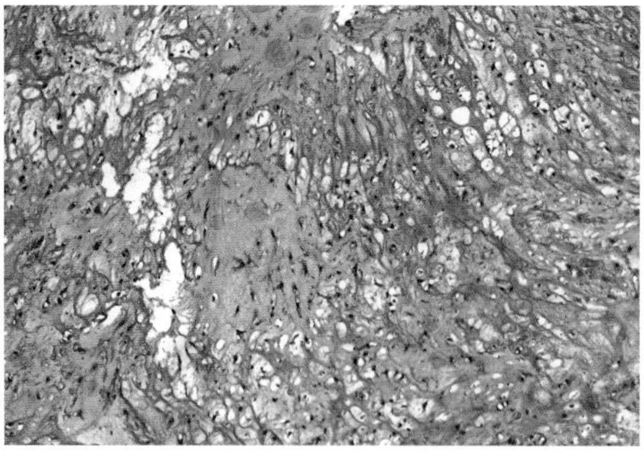

Figure 4-75

CHONDROSARCOMA

Degenerative myxoid change is seen in the matrix.

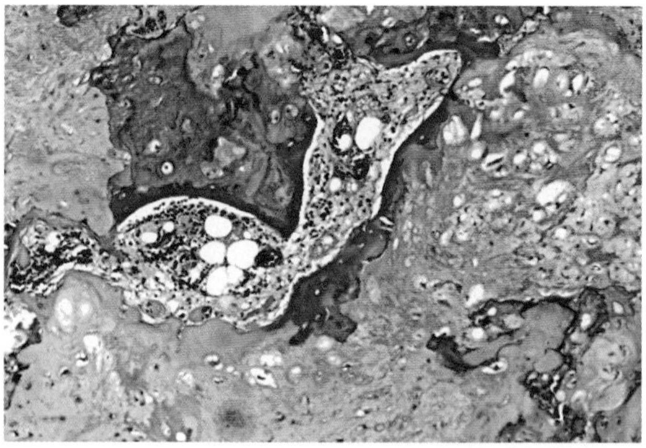

Figure 4-76

CHONDROSARCOMA

A shell of bone at the periphery of cartilaginous nodules, a feature of enchondroma, may also be seen in chondrosarcoma.

As do cartilage tumors generally, chondrosarcomas tend to grow in lobules of varying sizes, some of which coalesce. The chondrocytes are always located within lacunae, although some of the cells, especially at the edge of lobules, seem to lie outside lacunae in some high-grade tumors. The matrix may be solid or myxoid. The solid matrix has a pale blue, uniform, unbroken appearance. Myxoid change in the matrix is manifested as fraying of the matrix, a bubbly appearance, and occasionally, liquefaction, so that one may find only the matrix with a few cells floating in it. This liquefactive change is diagnostic of chondrosarcoma (fig. 4-75).

Calcification may be present as coarse or granular precipitates. Reactive bone formation, when present, is in the form of attenuated semicircles of bony trabeculae around lobules of cartilage (fig. 4-76).

If the tumor is resected and appropriate sections are made, the permeative and destructive qualities of the tumor are apparent. The cortex may show tumor abutting against cortical bone and producing concave impressions (scalloping). Nodules of tumor may permeate the interstices of the cortex.

Perhaps the most distinctive characteristic of chondrosarcoma is permeation of medullary bone (the chondrosarcoma permeation pattern, according to Mirra et al. [174]). The tumor fills the bone marrow cavity so that the trabecular bone becomes trapped within the advancing tumor. The tumor has to be present on either side of the trabecula and hug it to confirm permeation (fig. 4-77).

As indicated above, chondrocytes are located in lacunae; many cells may occupy one space. Lichtenstein and Jaffe (169) pointed out the importance of double-nucleated cells in the diagnosis of chondrosarcoma; more than one nucleus has to be identified in a cytoplasmic body. The chondrocytes are arranged in sheets, but in a small percentage of chondrosarcomas, the tumor cells are arranged in clusters, similar to the pattern seen in synovial chondromatosis. The nuclei are enlarged and more open than those in enchondroma. Mitotic figures are uncommon in chondrosarcoma and are not useful in diagnosis or grading (128).

Foci of necrosis may be identified by chondrocyte nuclei that do not stain with hematoxylin (fig. 4-78).

Grading. Many studies have shown the prognostic significance of histologic grading of chondrosarcomas (128,144,147,157,186). Although there are some differences in the criteria used by authors, the basic concepts of grading are similar. Chondrosarcomas are divided into only three grades, unlike spindle cell sarcomas, which are divided into four grades.

Grade 1 chondrosarcoma is differentiated from enchondroma with difficulty. The tumor is more cellular than an enchondroma, and the nuclei are slightly enlarged and irregular (fig. 4-79). Double-nucleated cells are present, and

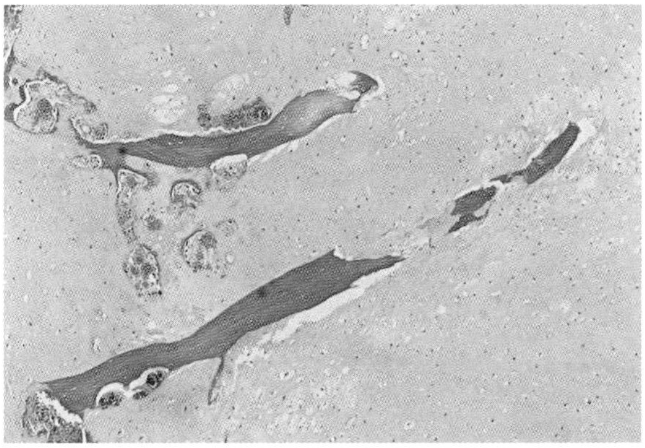

Figure 4-77

CHONDROSARCOMA

The tumor permeates between bony trabeculae, fills the bone marrow spaces, and is closely juxtaposed to preexisting bone.

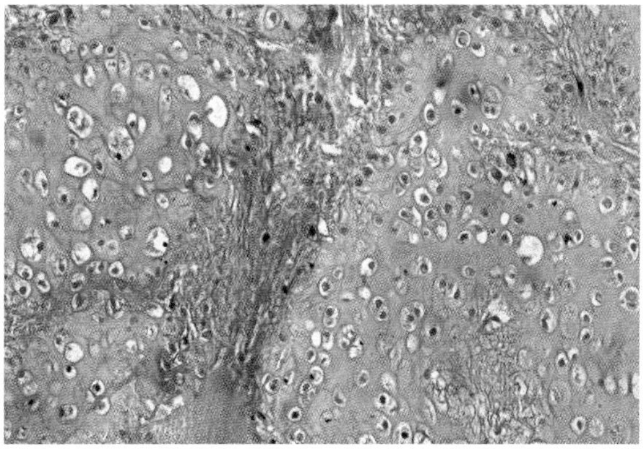

Figure 4-78

CHONDROSARCOMA

An area of necrosis, with only pale pink ghost cells left in lacunar spaces.

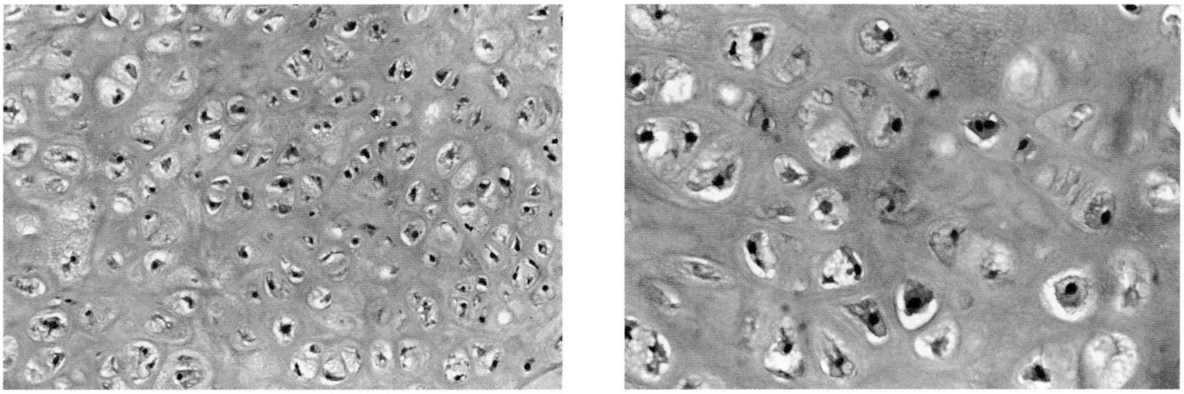

Figure 4-79

GRADE 1 CHONDROSARCOMA

Left: Low-power view shows increased cellularity compared with the number of cells typically seen in enchondroma. Right: High-power view shows some degree of cytologic atypia with nuclear enlargement and binucleation.

there are small foci of necrosis, which are characterized by lack of nuclear staining. Grade 2 chondrosarcoma is sufficiently different from enchondroma that the diagnosis can be made confidently without knowledge of other clinical features. The lesion is more cellular than grade 1 chondrosarcoma. The tumor usually is lobulated, and the periphery of the lobules has a condensation of nuclei, which are enlarged, irregular, and hyperchromatic. Double-nucleated cells and foci of necrosis are present (fig. 4-80). Grade 3 chondrosarcoma is very cellular, and the nuclei are enlarged and hyperchromatic and may become fusiform, especially at the periphery of the lobules (fig. 4-81). Sheets of spindle cells are not seen. Mitotic figures may be present, and necrosis may be prominent.

Grading is a subjective exercise; it is difficult to quantify "atypia" and "cellularity." Thus, there is some variability in the proportions of different grades of chondrosarcoma reported by different institutions. In the Mayo Clinic series, about half of the tumors are grade 1, more than 40 percent are grade 2, and between 5 and 10 percent are grade 3 (128,186). In contrast, the group from M.D. Anderson Hospital reported that 25 percent

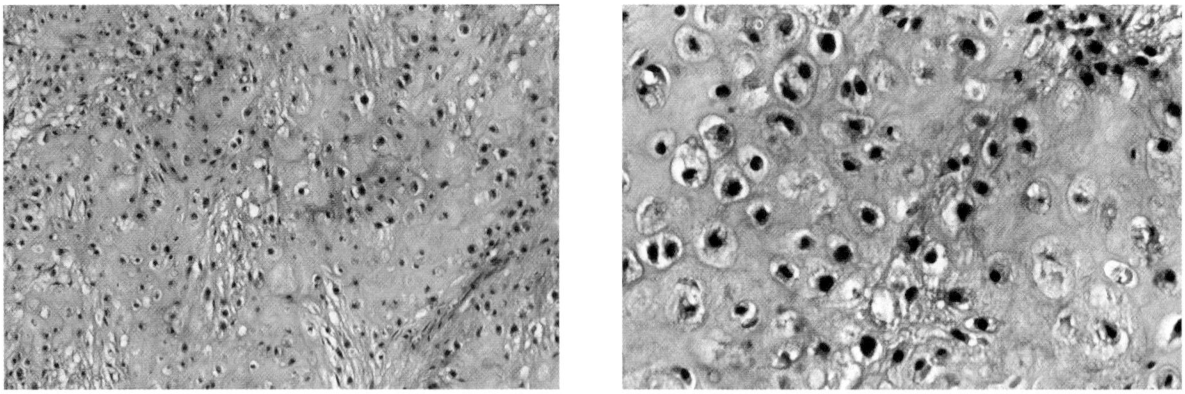

Figure 4-80

GRADE 2 CHONDROSARCOMA

Left: Low-power view shows that the tumor is more cellular than grade 1 tumors.
Right: High-power view shows many more enlarged, hyperchromatic nuclei than in grade 1 tumors.

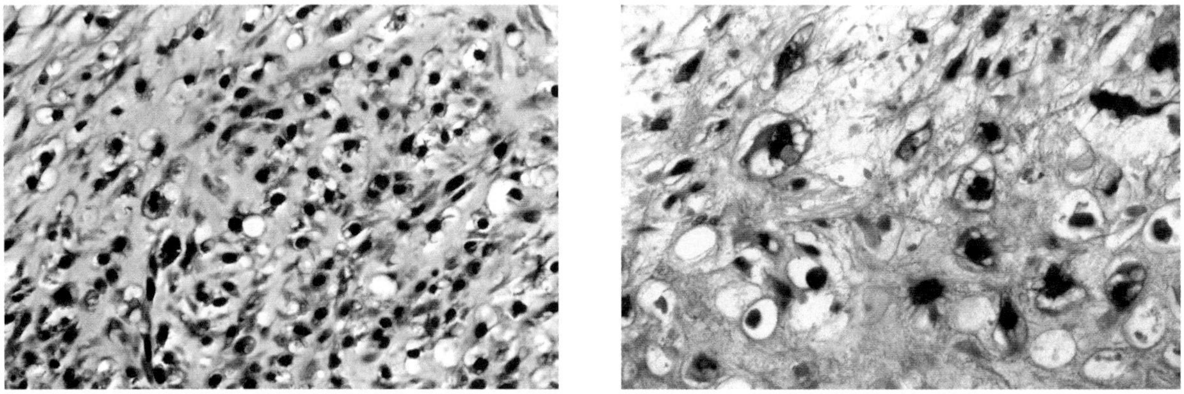

Figure 4-81

GRADE 3 CHONDROSARCOMA

Left: There is a marked increase in cellularity and areas where tumor cells begin to appear spindle shaped.
Right: Nuclear pleomorphism of chondrocytes.

of the tumors are grade 3 (144) and at the Istituto Orthopedico Rizzoli, 44 percent are grade 3 (147).

Cytologic Findings. The majority of low-grade, well-differentiated chondrosarcomas may be impossible to differentiate from benign cartilaginous lesions solely on the basis of fine-needle aspiration biopsy evaluation (fig. 4-82). The cellularity of the aspirate from some benign lesions overlaps with that of many well-differentiated chondrosarcomas, and the degree of atypia may also be similar. For practical purposes, however, confirmation of the chondroid nature of a tumor is usually sufficient because malignancy is best assessed with imaging studies, and decisions about treatment are based primarily on the clinical setting and radiographic features of the lesion (122,203,211,216).

In contrast, high-grade chondrosarcomas are readily identified with fine-needle aspiration biopsy (fig. 4-83). The main problem is differentiating chondrosarcoma from chondroblastic osteosarcoma and chordoma when the base of the skull and the spine are involved (216). Special studies, including alkaline phosphatase stain for osteosarcoma, cytokeratin and epithelial membrane antigen immunostains for chordoma, and electron microscopy, usually help the diagnosis when interpreted in the clinical context.

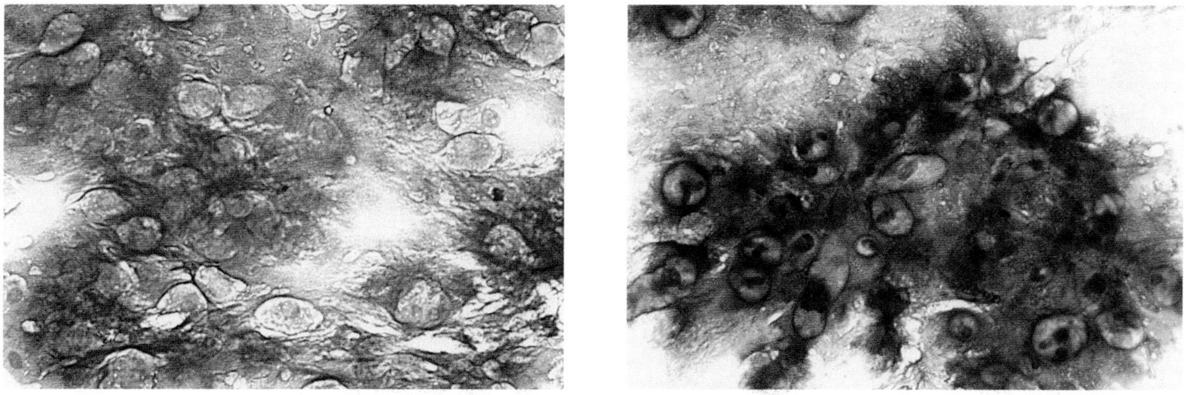

Figure 4-82

FINE-NEEDLE ASPIRATION BIOPSY OF CHONDROSARCOMA

Well-differentiated chondrosarcoma shows coherent clusters of tumor cells with chondrocytic features and moderate atypia enclosed in a prominent myxoid to hyaline matrix, partly forming lacunar structures (May-Grünwald-Giemsa stain).

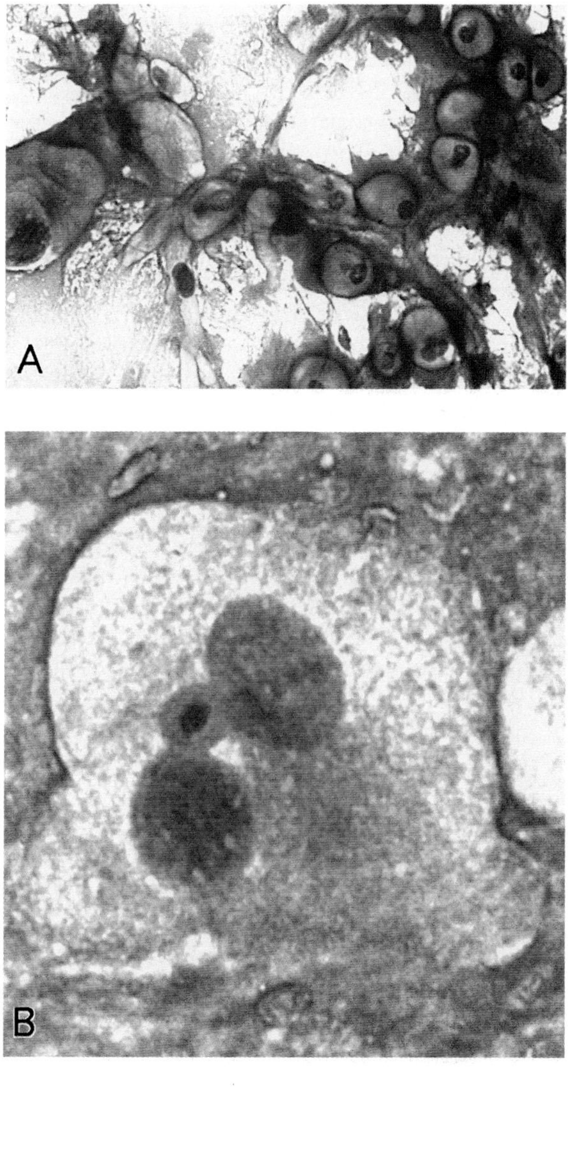

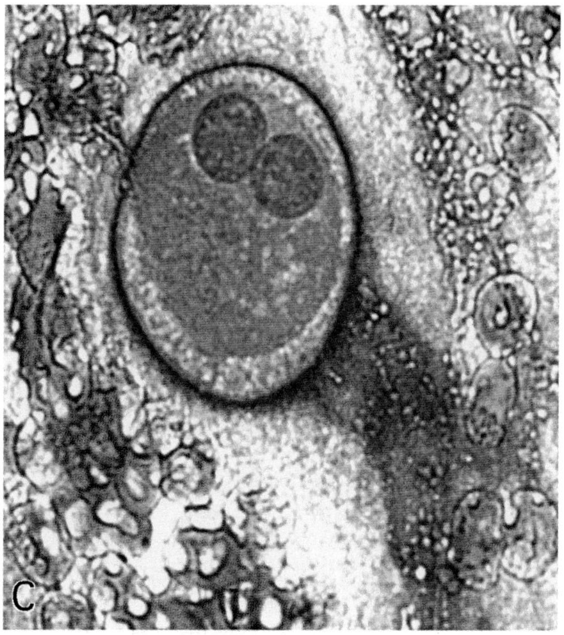

Figure 4-83

FINE-NEEDLE ASPIRATION BIOPSY
OF HIGH-GRADE CHONDROSARCOMA

A: The aspirate is similar to the aspirate in figure 4-82, although the cellular and nuclear atypia is more pronounced.

B,C: The occurrence of large, atypical, binucleated and multinucleated tumor cells with abundant cytoplasm and areas of clearing is reminiscent of the fine-needle aspirate appearance of chordoma. However, the distinct rim-like condensation of the surrounding myxoid matrix indicates that the cells lie within the lacunar spaces (May-Grünwald-Giemsa stain).

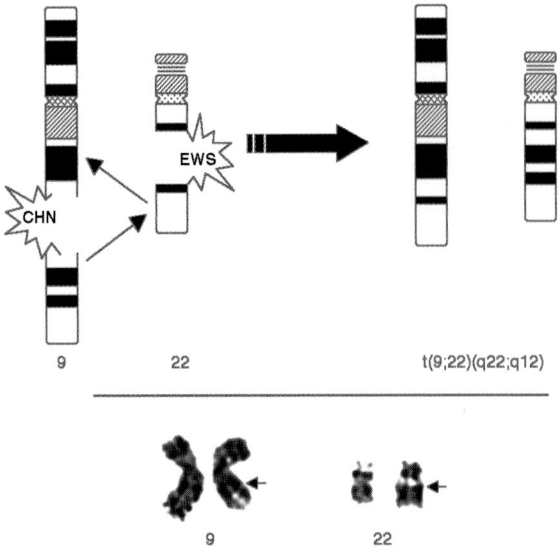

Figure 4-84

EXTRASKELETAL MYXOID CHONDROSARCOMA

Schematic (top) and partial karyotype (bottom) of the 9;22 translocation [t(9;22)(q22;q12)] and associated fusion of the *CHN* (also known as *NR4A3, TEC,* or *NOR1*) and *EWS* genes characteristic of extraskeletal myxoid chondrosarcoma.

Genetics and Other Special Techniques. The multiple forms of benign osteochondroma (autosomal dominant hereditary multiple exostoses) and enchondroma (nonhereditary Ollier's disease and nonhereditary Maffucci's syndrome) have a higher rate of malignant transformation than the corresponding solitary lesions. Malignant transformation of a solitary osteochondroma or enchondroma is rare (less than 1 percent), whereas in patients with hereditary multiple exostoses, Ollier's disease, or Maffucci's syndrome, malignant transformation is more frequent (1.0 to 8.3 percent and 15 to 30 percent, respectively) (162,171,205). Some patients with hereditary multiple exostoses or multiple enchondromatosis develop more than one chondrosarcoma, either synchronously or metachronously (129,135).

Tumor Cytogenetics. In addition to conventional chondrosarcoma, which comprises approximately 80 to 85 percent of cases, there are several less common clinicohistopathologic variants, including dedifferentiated (6 to 10 percent), myxoid (5 percent), mesenchymal (2 percent), juxtacortical (2 percent), and clear cell (2 percent) chondrosarcoma (141,204). Skeletal and extraskeletal myxoid chondrosarcomas cannot be distinguished on clinical or light microscopic grounds other than by their site of origin (143,156). Genetically and ultrastructurally, however, extraskeletal and skeletal myxoid chondrosarcoma represent two distinct entities in the chondrosarcoma family of tumors (124,134). Extraskeletal myxoid chondrosarcoma is characterized cytogenetically by a t(9;22)(q22;q12) which results in the fusion of the *NR4A3* (or *CHN, TEC,* or *NOR1*) gene at 9q22 with the *EWS* gene at 22q12 (fig. 4-84) or, less commonly, by variant t(9;17)(q22;q11.2), resulting in the fusion of the *NR4A3* gene with the *TAF2N* (*RBP56*) gene at 17q11.2 or variant t(9;15)(q22;q21), resulting in the fusion of the *NR4A3* gene with the *TCF12* gene at 15q21 or variant t(3;9)(q11-12;q22), resulting in the fusion of the *NR4A3* gene with the *TFG* gene at 3q11-12 (124,134,137,154,155,166, 182,200,202). Moreover, the der(16)t(1;16)(q21;q13), a secondary structural aberration common to other fusion gene–distinguished sarcomas such as Ewing's sarcoma and alveolar rhabdomyosarcoma, has been detected in extraskeletal myxoid chondrosarcoma but not in skeletal myxoid chondrosarcoma (139). Early cDNA microarray studies indicate that extraskeletal myxoid chondrosarcoma exhibits a tumor-specific gene expression profile that may be useful in distinguishing it from other mesenchymal neoplasms (201). A recurrent or specific genetic aberration has not been detected in skeletal myxoid chondrosarcoma.

The etiologic, diagnostic, and prognostic value of the cytogenetic analysis of benign and malignant cartilaginous lesions has been examined (133,172,191,207). Overall, the most frequent structural abnormalities involve 1cen-q21, 5q13, 6q13, 12q13, 15p11, and 17p13, and loss of material from 1p, 3, 4p, 6q, 9p, 10, 11, 13, 14, 17p, and 22 and gain of material from 1q, 2, 5, 7, 8, 12, 15, 19, 20, and 21 represent the most common imbalances. Of potential diagnostic relevance is the exclusive or near-exclusive aberrancy of chromosomes 1 and 7 in malignant cartilaginous neoplasms. Prognostically, there is a strong correlation between the presence of chromosomal abnormalities and increasing histologic grade ($P = 0.001$) (191). Similar relationships have been found with DNA flow cytometric studies (the proportion of aneuploid tumors increases with tumor grade) and Ki-67 expression studies (123,152,153,164,165,173,175,195,198). Furthermore, karyotypically complex aberrations appear most prominent in high-grade chondrosarcomas (133,150,181,187,206,207).

In one study, chromosomal aberrations of 6q13-21 were proposed to correlate with locally aggressive behavior in both benign and malignant cartilaginous neoplasms (192). In another study, gain of 8q24.1-qter was associated with a shorter overall survival period (167). Chromosomal abnormalities of 9p and extra copies of chromosome 22 are prominent in central chondrosarcoma when contrasted with peripheral chondrosarcoma (131).

Tumor Suppressor Genes. Growing evidence has shown the importance of tumor suppressor gene mutations in the development or progression (or both) of malignant neoplasms. The *TP53* gene, localized to 17p13, is a well-characterized tumor suppressor gene. Wild-type, but not mutant, p53 protein regulates the progression through the G_1 phase of the cell cycle into the S phase, activates the mechanisms for DNA repair if there is a replication error or mutation, and triggers apoptosis in tumor cells. An abnormal p53 protein, the product of a mutated *TP53* gene, is metabolically stable and accumulates in the nucleus; thus, it can be detected with immunohistochemistry. Overexpression, structural alterations (gene mutations and karyotypic rearrangements), or loss of heterozygosity of the *TP53* gene (or locus) has been observed in a small proportion of chondrosarcomas (130,138,140,177,180,199,208, 215,217). Altered patterns of p53 expression and *TP53* mutations have been detected primarily in high-grade, advanced tumors and their variants. Inactivation of the *TP53* gene appears to be a late occurrence in chondrosarcoma and may be associated with disease progression.

A key regulatory function of the *TP53* gene, the ability to arrest the cell cycle, occurs with proper activation of the retinoblastoma (RB) pathway. Studies for loss of heterozygosity (LOH) on 13q or *RB* gene mutations in chondrosarcomas are few (130,142,217). In one study, a significant association between local recurrence and LOH on 13q was seen in primary grade 1 and grade 2 chondrosarcomas (217). Cytogenetically, loss of 13q appears to be an independent prognostic factor for chondrosarcoma metastasis regardless of tumor size or grade (172).

Cyclin-dependent kinase (CDK) inhibitory molecules are capable of blocking protein (p)RB phosphorylation and methylation. Deletions of the $p16^{INK4a}$ (*CDKN2A*) gene or the $p15^{INK4b}$ (*MTS2*) gene, members of the CDK inhibitory molecule family, have been observed in a small subset of primary chondrosarcomas as well as in four chondrosarcoma cell lines (125,158). Moreover, genomic loss of the chromosomal locus for the $p16^{INK4a}$ and $p15^{INK4b}$ genes, 9p21, has also been detected, by comparative genomic hybridization analysis, as one of the more common regions of loss in chondrosarcoma (167) and is frequently rearranged cytogenetically, particularly in central chondrosarcomas (131). Loss of $p16^{INK4a}$ protein expression in central chondrosarcoma has been shown to correlate with increasing histologic grade (214).

Frequent LOH for polymorphic markers on chromosomal arm 10q in chondrosarcoma has also been observed (130,188). In one study, 12 of 18 (67 percent) chondrosarcomas analyzed exhibited LOH for at least one marker, and in most of these tumors, the region of loss spanned all or large portions of the chromosome (188). The critical region of LOH in these tumors was identified as a 7- to 12-cM interval in the proximal long arm of chromosome 10 bounded by markers D10S578 and D10S568. The tumor suppressor gene *PTEN* localized to 10q23 has been shown to be an unlikely candidate for this loss (170). LOH on chromosomal arm 10q has been observed in both peripheral and central chondrosarcomas and in early-stage lesions with no correlation with grade or prognosis (130,188).

To investigate potential genetic differences in peripheral and central chondrosarcomas, Bovée et al. (130–132) subjected a series of peripheral and central chondrosarcomas to cytogenetic, molecular cytogenetic, DNA flow cytometric, and LOH analyses. The authors concluded that peripheral chondrosarcomas exhibit a high percentage of LOH, with prominent involvement of the *TP53, RB*, and *EXT1* loci, in contrast to absence of LOH of these loci in most central chondrosarcomas (fig. 4-85). In addition, a subset of low-grade peripheral chondrosarcomas

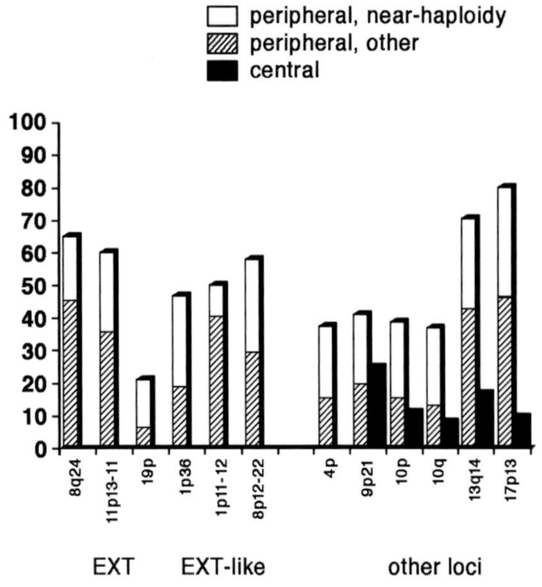

Figure 4-85

CENTRAL AND PERIPHERAL CHONDROSARCOMAS

Percentages of loss of heterozygosity (LOH) for several loci are depicted in this study of central and peripheral chondrosarcomas. Peripheral chondrosarcoma is subdivided into two groups: the upper part of the bar is formed by five tumors showing either near haploidy or polyploidization of near-haploid tumor clones. The lower part of the bar consists of all other peripheral chondrosarcomas (n = 14). Percentages were calculated as number of tumors showing LOH for at least one of the markers divided by the total number of informative cases. (Fig. 2 from Bovée JV, Cleton-Jansen AM, Kuipers-Dijkshoorn NJ, et al. Loss of heterozygosity and DNA ploidy point to a diverging genetic mechanism in the origin of peripheral and central chondrosarcoma. Genes Chromosomes Cancer 1999;26:237-46.)

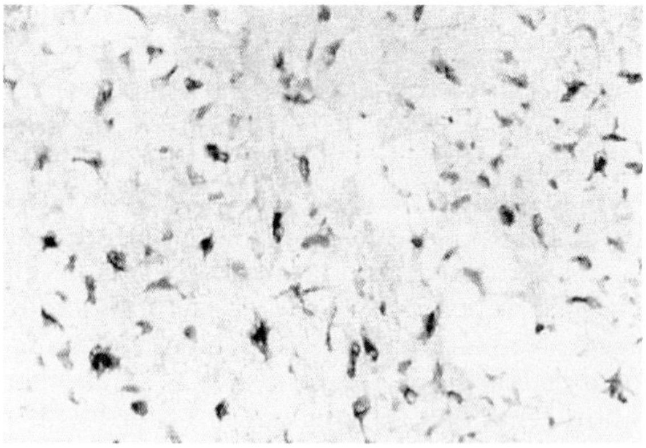

Figure 4-86

CHONDROSARCOMA OF THE PROXIMAL METAPHYSIS OF THE HUMERUS

c-MET expression is observed in the cytoplasm of more than half of all the observed tumor cells in this 75-year-old man (c-MET immunostain; original magnification, X66). (Fig. 2 from Naka T, Iwamoto Y, Shinohara N, Ushijima M, Chuman H, Tsuneyoshi M. Expression of c-met proto-oncogene product (c-MET) in benign and malignant bone tumors. Mod Pathol 1997;10:832-8.)

appears to be characterized by near haploidy, purportedly followed by polyploidization in high-grade peripheral chondrosarcoma (132).

Prognostic Markers and Other Genetic Markers. Proto-oncogenes are necessary for normal division and proliferation of cells. Structural alteration (mutation) or increased production (amplification) of a proto-oncogene may result in oncogenic activity (oncogene). The *abl* oncogenes are cellular homologues of the *v-abl* oncogene of the Abelson murine leukemia retrovirus. They encode nuclear and cytoplasmic protein tyrosine kinases that function in signal transduction, cell cycle-dependent and DNA damage-induced gene expression, and apoptosis inhibition. Intense expression of abl has been observed immunohistochemically in grades 1 and 2 chondrosarcomas, tumor grades in which there is negligible apoptosis and a low percentage of proliferating cells (178,179). Moderate to strong abl immunoreactivity has also been detected in immature fetal chondrocytes, suggesting that *abl* gene expression is associated with differentiation and apoptosis inhibition in fetal and neoplastic chondrocytes. Abl immunoreactivity is greatly reduced or absent in grade 3 chondrosarcoma.

Expression of the c-MET hepatocyte growth factor receptor, a transmembrane tyrosine kinase encoded by the *c-met* proto-oncogene, is associated with tumor progression in different human carcinomas (149,184). In studies of fetal vertebral tissue and benign and malignant bone and soft tissue tumors, c-MET expression was frequently detected in normal articular cartilage and in the cartilaginous tumors (fig. 4-86). The authors concluded that c-MET may have a role in the development of these neoplasms (176,194). Other genes, including *c-myc, n-myc, h-ras, c-fms, c-myb, c-fos, c-jun, HDM2, HER2/neu, CDK4, SAS, GADD153(CHOP), GLI,* and *A2MR,* have been examined in chondrosarcoma but have shown no or rare evidence of mutation or amplification (136,146,160,183,185).

Matrix metalloproteinases (MMPs) are zinc proteinases responsible for the degradation of

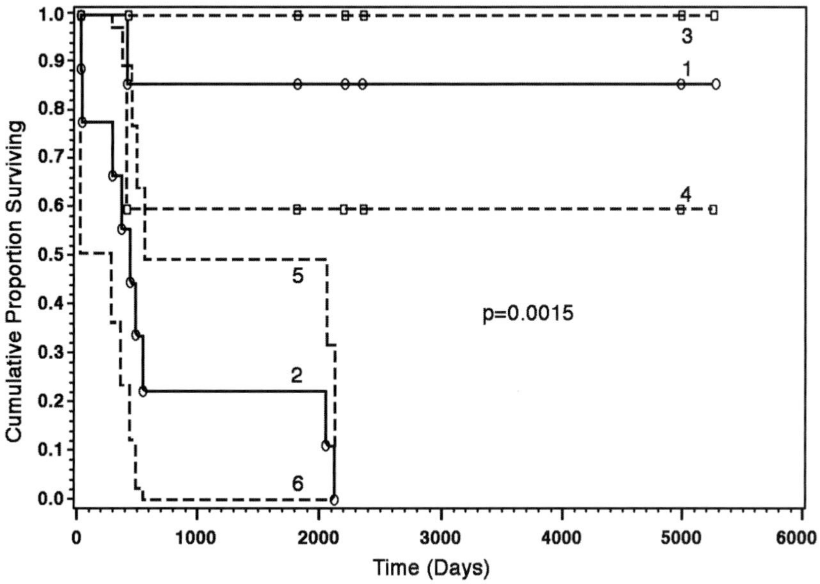

Figure 4-87

KAPLAN-MEIER CURVES OF DISEASE-FREE SURVIVAL FOR PATIENTS WITH CHONDROSARCOMA

Disease-free survival is significantly lower for patients whose tumors have a high ratio (> 0.8) of matrix metalloproteinase-1 to tissue inhibitor of metalloproteinase-1 (curve 2) than for those whose tumors have a low ratio (curve 1). Curves 3 and 4 and curves 5 and 6 represent the 95 percent confidence intervals for curves 1 and 2, respectively. (Fig. 3 from Berend KR, Toth AP, Harrelson JM, Layfield LJ, Hey LA, Scully SP. Association between ratio of matrix metalloproteinase-1 to tissue inhibitor of metalloproteinase-1 and local recurrence, metastasis, and survival in human chondrosarcoma. J Bone Joint Surg Am 1998;80:11-7.)

extracellular matrix macromolecules in pathophysiologic conditions such as embryonic development, angiogenesis, and tumor invasion. In studies of benign and malignant cartilaginous neoplasms, a pattern of increased expression of MMP-1, MMP-2, MMP-9, and MMP-13 and decreased expression of MMP-3 and MMP-8 have corresponded with a malignant phenotype (127,151,161,190,193,196,213). Moreover, observation of abundant aggrecan degradation products that result from cleavage in vivo at the MMP site, supports the concept that MMPs participate in the degradation of extracellular matrix in chondrosarcoma, thereby allowing neoplastic chondrocytes to escape local confinement, to migrate, and to invade neighboring and remote tissues (210). Similarly, high-grade but not low-grade chondrosarcomas express vascular endothelial growth factor (VEGF), a potent angiogenic factor (126). A high ratio of MMP-1 to TIMP-1 (tissue inhibitor of MMP-1) may correspond with a more aggressive clinical course and worse prognosis for patients with chondrosarcoma (fig. 4-87) (127,159).

Nephroblastoma overexpressed (NOV) protein and connective tissue growth factor (CTGF) are expressed in cartilage cells during fetal development. The *CTGF* and *NOV* genes are members of the CCN (Cyr61/Connective tissue growth factor/Nephroblastoma overexpressed) family. All CCN family members are thought to be involved in the control of cell proliferation and differentiation. Expression studies of CTGF, NOV, and other CCN family members in chondrosarcoma and enchondroma by semiquantitative reverse transcriptase polymerase chain reaction (RT-PCR), real-time PCR, Western blot, and immunohistochemical analysis have revealed a correlation between expression and tumor grade (197,219). The authors have suggested that the level of expression of CCN family members could be a useful adjunct in the determination of tumor grade and clinical course in patients with chondrosarcoma.

Malignant cartilaginous neoplasms demonstrate chemotherapeutic resistance through undetermined mechanisms. P-glycoprotein, the protein product of the multiple drug resistance gene

1 (*MDR1*), confers multidrug chemotherapeutic resistance in a variety of malignancies. MDR1 expression has been examined in benign and malignant chondromatous tumors by immunohistochemistry and in situ hybridization (189, 209). These studies have shown constitutive expression of P-glycoprotein in cartilaginous neoplasms, with greatest expression in high-grade chondrosarcomas. The findings may account for the resistance of some cartilage tumors to chemotherapeutic agents.

Differential Diagnosis. Chondrosarcoma has to be differentiated from enchondroma and chondroblastic osteosarcoma. The difficulty in distinguishing between enchondroma and low-grade chondrosarcoma is discussed above. Clinical (including site), radiographic, and histologic features have to be correlated to make the correct diagnosis. Indistinct margins and involvement of the cortex are the most important radiographic features, and abnormal cytologic features and a permeative growth pattern are the paramount histologic features.

Chondrosarcomas occur in older persons, whereas chondroblastic osteosarcomas affect children. In a child, a cartilage tumor that appears to be high grade is likely to be osteosarcoma. Sheets of spindle cells with the formation of lace-like osteoid characterize chondroblastic osteosarcoma.

Spread and Metastases. Chondrosarcomas usually are locally aggressive tumors that have limited potential for metastasis. When metastases occur, they are delayed and generally involve the lungs.

Staging. Grade 1 chondrosarcomas are considered stage 1, which can be divided into 1A and 1B, depending upon whether the tumor extends through the cortex or not. Grade 2 and grade 3 chondrosarcomas are stage 2 (also divided into 2A and 2B). It is rare for chondrosarcomas to have distant metastasis at presentation (stage 3).

Treatment and Prognosis. Because chondrosarcomas are locally aggressive tumors with limited potential for metastasis, treatment is surgical extirpation of the primary tumor. Systemic chemotherapy is not indicated. It is important to remove the tumor intact, with an envelope of normal tissue (wide resection).

Chondrosarcomas frequently recur after 5 and even 10 years; hence, 5-year survival is not considered a cure. In the group of patients reported by Pritchard et al. (186), the 5-year survival rate was 59 percent and 20-year survival rate was 35 percent. The location of the lesion, the grade of the tumor, and the adequacy of surgical removal all affect prognosis. Improvement in surgical technique has contributed to improved survival in the modern era (186). Pulmonary metastases, 14 percent in one series (128) and 28 percent in another (147), have been reported. Evans et al. (144) found no metastasis with grade 1 chondrosarcoma, a 10 percent rate with grade 2, and 71 percent with grade 3.

Chondrosarcoma of the Small Bones of the Hands and Feet

As indicated in the section on enchondroma, enchondromas of the small bones of the hands and feet have special characteristics, which in a larger bone would make the diagnosis of chondrosarcoma mandatory. Hence, the rules used to diagnose chondrosarcoma must also be different. Enchondroma of the small bones frequently produces pain associated with fracture; thus, this criterion is not used to differentiate enchondroma from chondrosarcoma. Radiographs show thinning of the cortex in an enchondroma. To confirm the diagnosis of chondrosarcoma, radiographs have to show the tumor extending through the cortex into soft tissues (fig. 4-88). Although enchondromas may be large and produce fusiform expansion of the bone, a thin cortex separates the tumor from soft tissues. In chondrosarcoma, the tumor permeates through the interstices of the cortex into soft tissues (fig. 4-89). Permeation of medullary bone is considered a sign of chondrosarcoma in a large bone. However, permeation with entrapment of bony trabeculae can be seen in tumors that are clearly benign on radiographs of small bones. Thus, to diagnose chondrosarcoma, the tumor must invade through the cortex (fig. 4-90).

Increased cellularity, cytologic atypia, and moderate myxoid change are frequently found in enchondroma. There is no clear answer to the question of how atypical an enchondroma can appear in a small bone. We believe that if the cytologic features suggest a grade 2 or grade 3 chondrosarcoma (fig. 4-91), a diagnosis of malignancy has to be made regardless of other features.

For patients with these rare chondrosarcomas, the prognosis is excellent. Distant metastases are

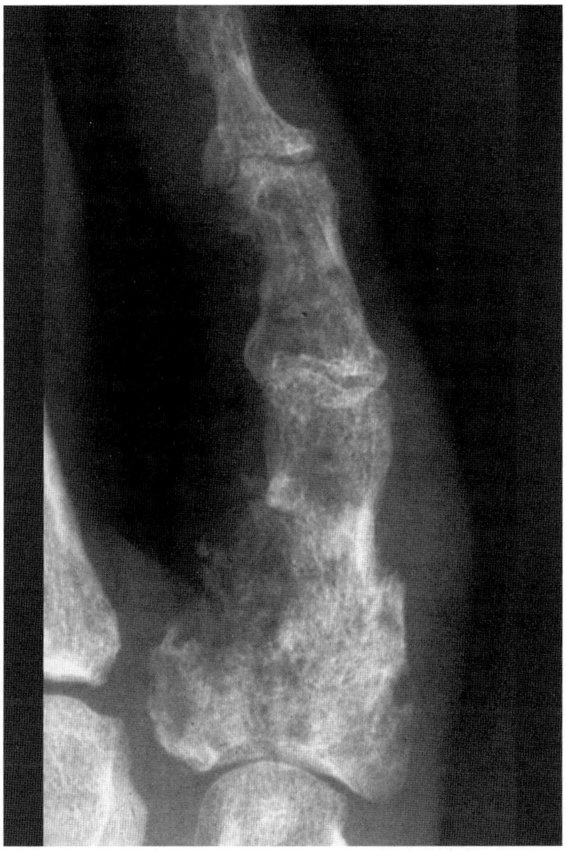

Figure 4-88

CHONDROSARCOMA OF SMALL BONE

The tumor, in a 52-year-old man, has destroyed the cortex and extended into the soft tissues. (Fig. 6-13 from Unni KK. Dahlin's bone tumors: general aspects and data on 11,087 cases, 5th ed. Philadelphia: Lippincott-Raven; 1996:81. By permission of Mayo Foundation.)

rare and occur mainly in tumors of the talus and calcaneus (223). It has been suggested that chondrosarcomas of the phalanges have an even more benign clinical evolution (220,222). Although rare, metastases occur, even from phalangeal chondrosarcomas (221); hence, we believe they have to be classified as malignant.

Periosteal Chondrosarcoma

Periosteal chondromas are extremely rare. They frequently have the cytologic features of malignancy. Thus, it is difficult to differentiate the rare periosteal chondrosarcoma (fig. 4-92) from its benign counterpart. Size is an important criterion: periosteal chondromas are small, usually less than 3 cm in greatest dimension;

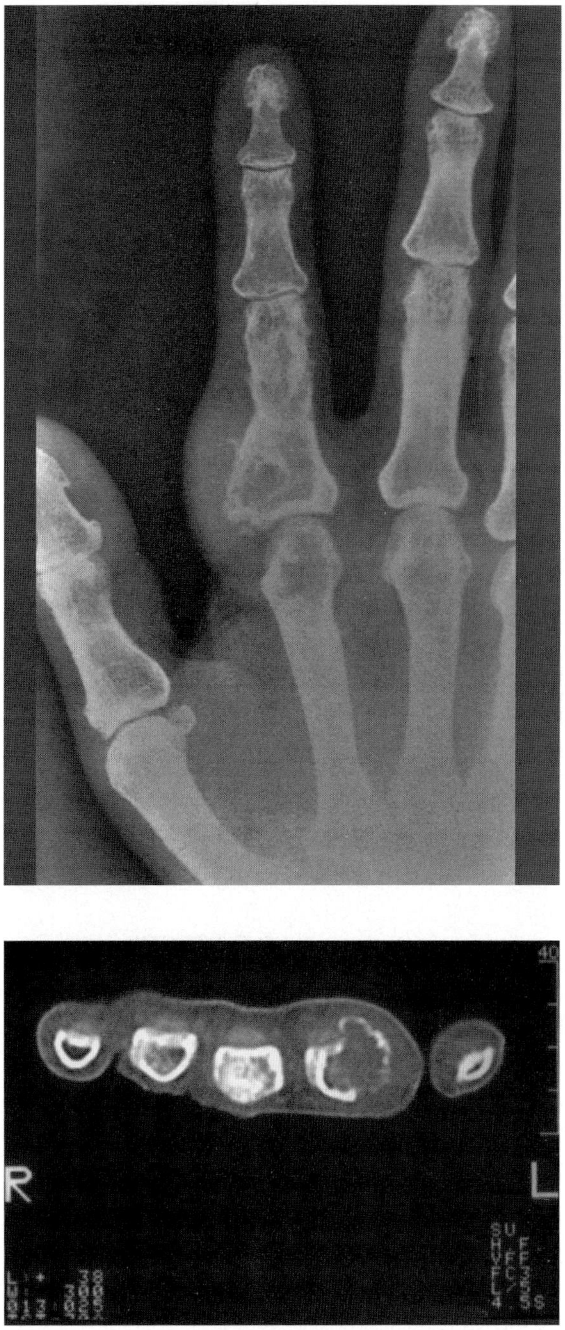

Figure 4-89

CHONDROSARCOMA OF SMALL BONE

Top: The plain radiograph shows an osteolytic lesion of the proximal phalanx of the index finger of a 74-year-old man, with cortical permeation and a partially mineralized soft tissue mass radially.

Bottom: CT of the index finger demonstrates cortical destruction and a soft tissue mass. Four years before this study, a radiograph of this finger was reported as "benign." (Courtesy of Dr. T. Matsuno, Asahikawa, Japan.)

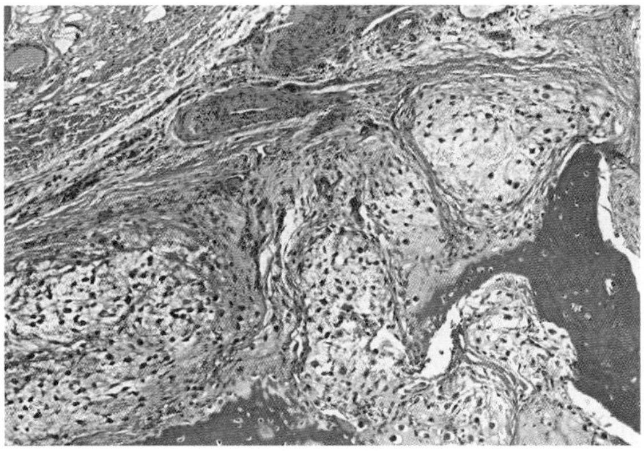

Figure 4-90

CHONDROSARCOMA OF SMALL BONE

Low-power view shows that the tumor has broken through the cortex and invaded the surrounding soft tissue.

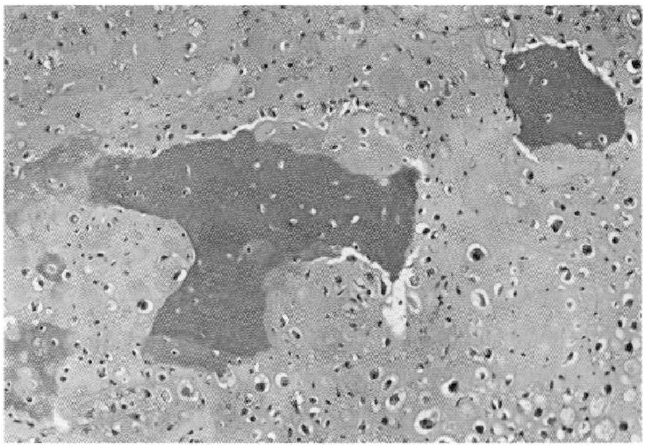

Figure 4-91

GRADE 2 CHONDROSARCOMA OF SMALL BONE

The tumor, involving the first metatarsal, has permeated through preexisting bone. The degree of cytologic atypia is more than would be seen in an enchondroma at this site.

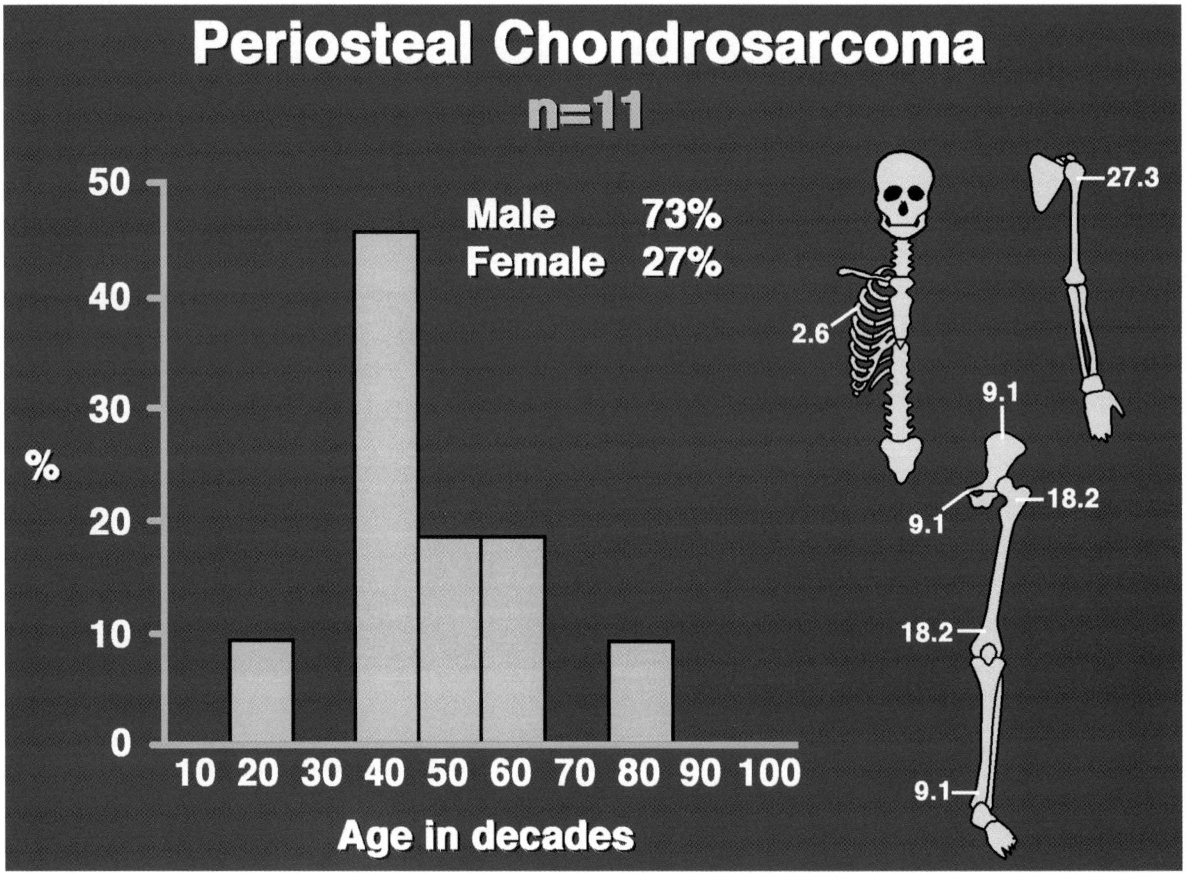

Figure 4-92

PERIOSTEAL CHONDROSARCOMA

The distribution of periosteal chondrosarcoma according to the age and sex of the patient and the site of the lesion.

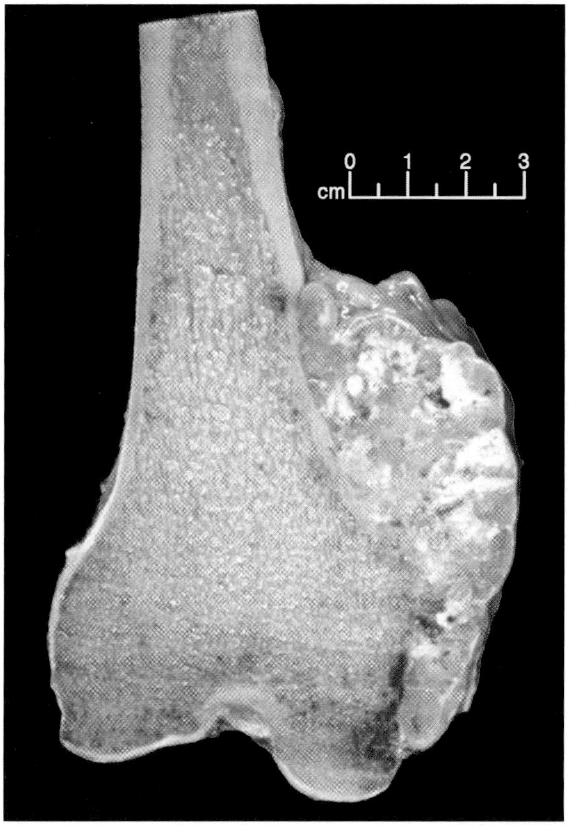

Figure 4-93

PERIOSTEAL CHONDROSARCOMA

Grossly, this gray-white cartilaginous tumor adheres to the surface of the distal femur with no intramedullary involvement. It is larger than a typical periosteal chondroma.

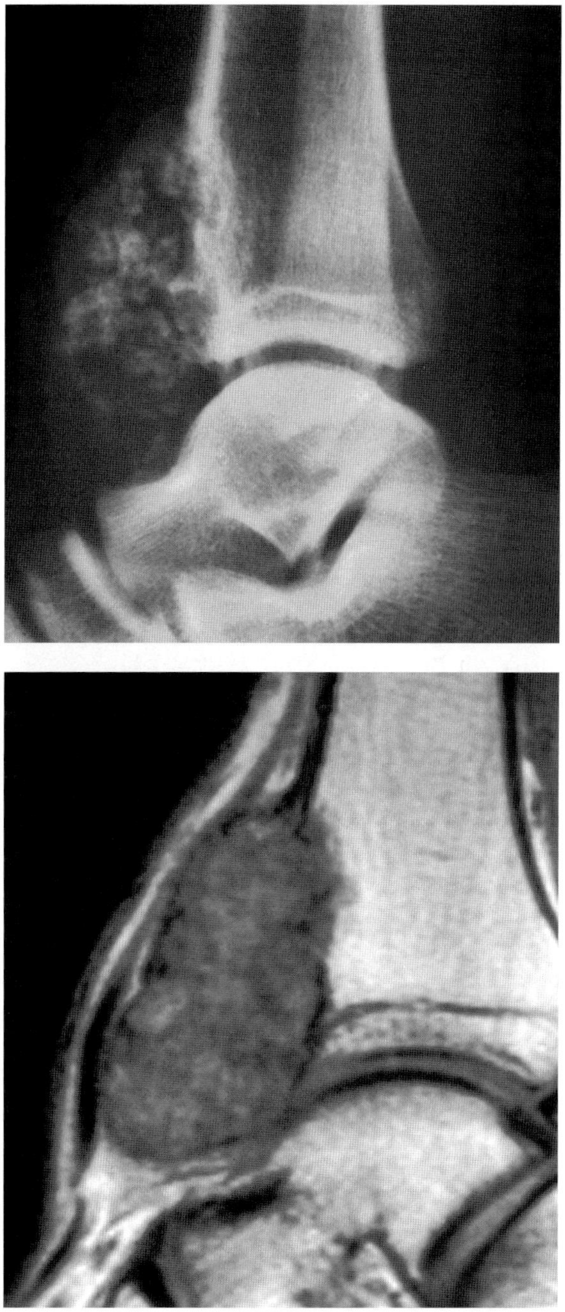

Figure 4-94

PERIOSTEAL CHONDROSARCOMA

Top: A plain radiograph shows a heavily and diffusely mineralized exophytic mass arising from the surface of the distal tibial metaphysis and epiphysis, with associated cortical destruction and adjacent medullary sclerosis.

Bottom: Sagittal T_1-weighted MRI shows a well-circumscribed heterogeneous mass with punctate foci of low signal intensity that correlate with the cartilaginous matrix. The image accurately delineates the size and extent of the soft tissue mass.

periosteal chondrosarcomas are usually more than 5 cm (fig. 4-93). Radiographs show clear demarcation of periosteal chondromas from the medullary cavity and soft tissues, whereas the margins of periosteal chondrosarcomas are indistinct (fig. 4-94, top). Histologically, permeation into the surrounding soft tissue is unequivocal evidence of malignancy (fig. 4-95).

Periosteal chondrosarcomas tend to behave in a locally aggressive fashion (224) but distant metastases do occur (225).

Secondary Chondrosarcoma

As with other sarcomas, chondrosarcomas usually arise without a known precursor lesion. However, in approximately 12 percent of the chondrosarcomas in the Mayo Clinic files, the tumor was secondary to a preexisting benign condition

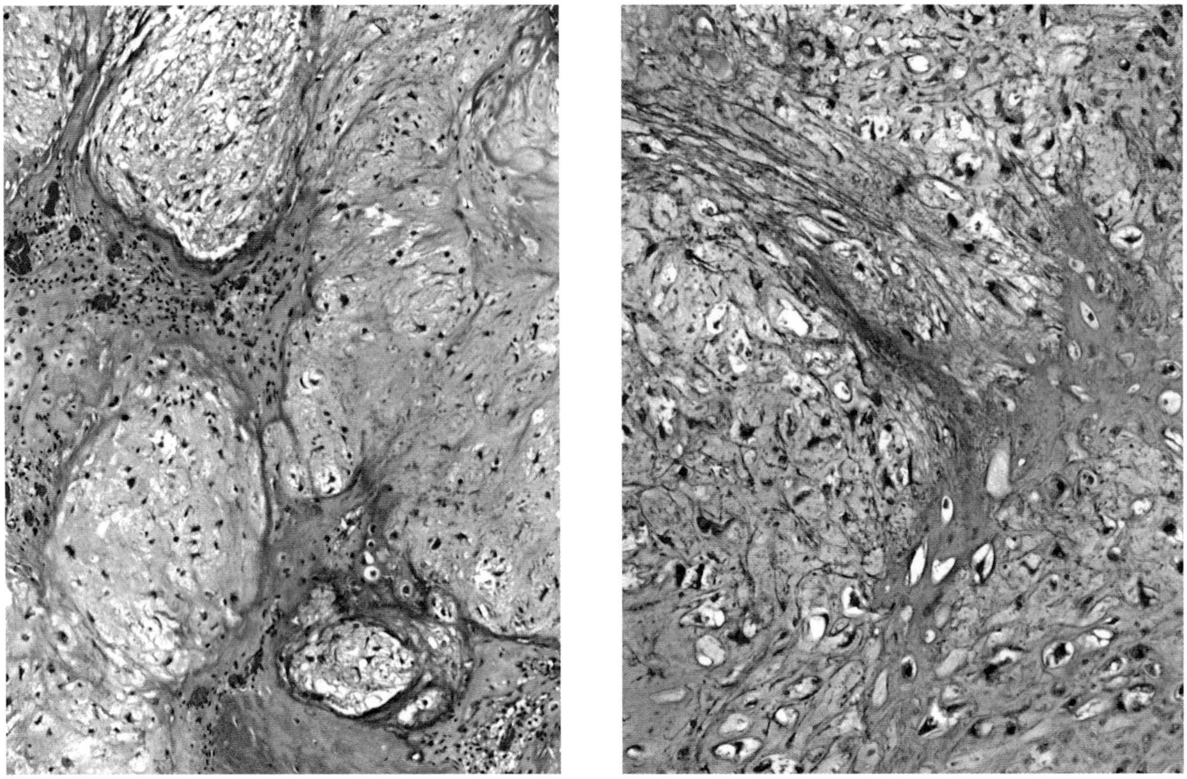

Figure 4-95

PERIOSTEAL CHONDROSARCOMA

Left: Low-power magnification shows lobules of the tumor permeating the surrounding soft tissue.

Right: High-power magnification shows extensive myxoid change in the matrix, which would not be seen in periosteal chondroma.

Table 4-1

THE NUMBER OF CASES OF CHONDROSARCOMA ARISING FROM BENIGN LESIONS IN 128 PATIENTS[a]

Benign Lesion	Number
Solitary osteochondroma	71
Multiple osteochondromatosis	41
Ollier's disease	10
Maffucci's syndrome	4
Multiple chondromas	2
Total	128

[a]In addition, there were two chondrosarcomas in fibrous dysplasia, four following radiotherapy, and five arising in synovial chondromatosis.

(fig. 4-96). It is difficult to document chondrosarcoma arising in a solitary enchondroma; there are, however, rare examples of chondrosarcoma associated with a well-documented preexisting enchondroma. These are so rare and difficult to document that they are not included in the statistics.

Patients with secondary chondrosarcoma tend to be a decade younger than those with primary chondrosarcoma. There is a slight male predominance. If a patient with a known benign lesion, such as an osteochondroma, complains of a sudden increase in swelling or pain, secondary chondrosarcoma should be suspected.

The Mayo Clinic files include 128 patients with secondary chondrosarcoma. The number of cases of chondrosarcoma arising from benign lesions is listed in Table 4-1.

The clinical, radiographic, and histologic features of these tumors are described with the benign lesions (figs. 4-97–4-101). Treatment is surgical. The prognosis is generally excellent, especially for patients whose chondrosarcomas arise from osteochondromas.

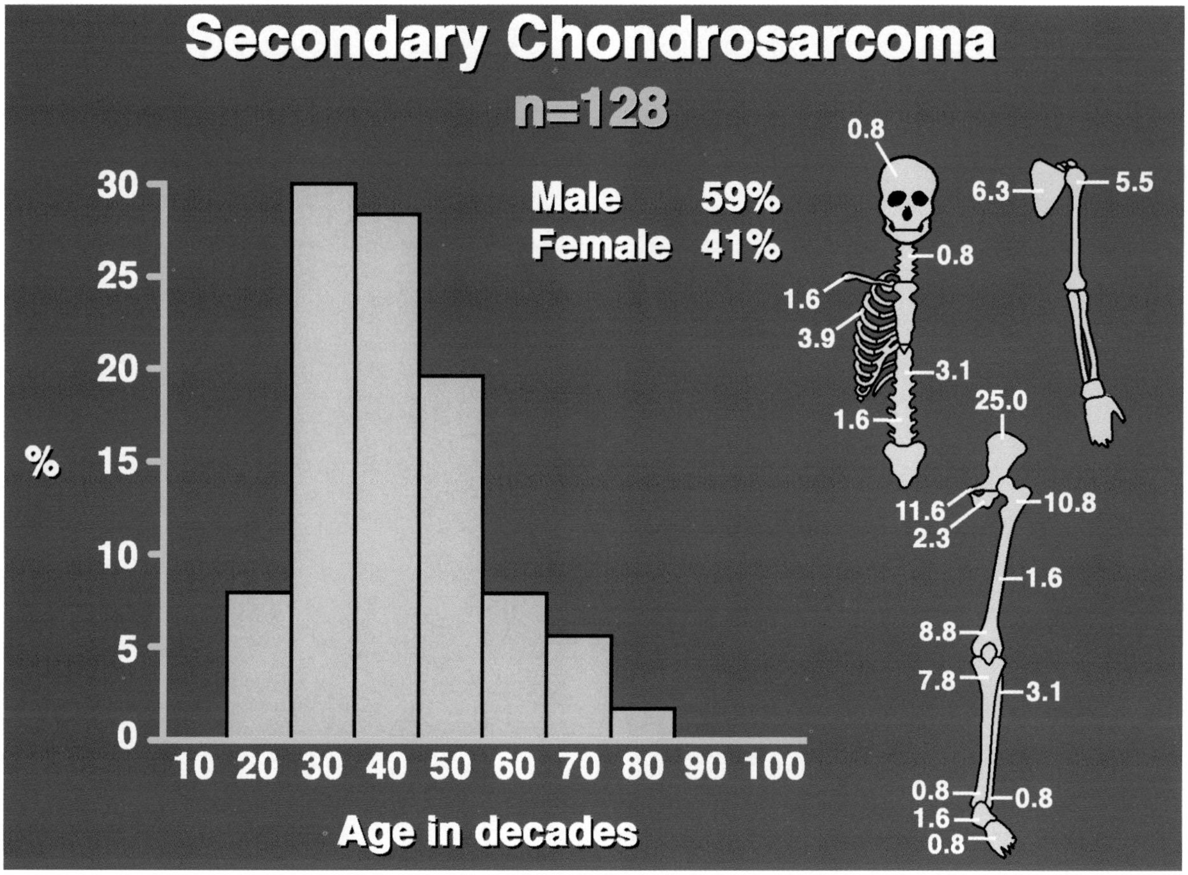

Figure 4-96

SECONDARY CHONDROSARCOMA

The distribution of secondary chondrosarcoma according to the age and sex of the patient and the site of the lesion.

Dedifferentiated Chondrosarcoma

Definition. Dedifferentiated chondrosarcoma is a bimorphic malignant neoplasm of bone in which a well-differentiated chondrosarcoma is juxtaposed to a high-grade spindle cell sarcoma.

General Features. Although Jaffe (233) mentioned the term "dedifferentiation" in his discussion of chondrosarcoma, it was not until the description by Dahlin and Beabout (230) that the concept was formally accepted. The concept proposed at that time was that a high-grade spindle cell sarcoma arose from a preexisting (probably long-standing) low-grade chondrosarcoma. The term "dedifferentiated" has been criticized as being biologically unsound. The term "chondrosarcoma with additional mesenchymal component" has been suggested as an alternative (234,237). However, the term "dedifferentiated" has gained wide acceptance as a clinically useful concept and has been used in other tumor systems such as liposarcoma and chordoma (232,235). The question of whether high-grade sarcoma arises from a chondrosarcoma or from the scar tissue around the cartilage is not settled.

Dedifferentiation can be expected in about 10 percent of chondrosarcomas. However, this may be an underestimation because some high-grade sarcomas arising in older adults may represent dedifferentiated chondrosarcoma in which the underlying cartilage tumor has been completely destroyed. Until the end of the year 2000, the Mayo Clinic files included 130 cases of dedifferentiated chondrosarcoma and 1,151 cases of chondrosarcoma of bone (fig. 4-102). Of the 130 dedifferentiated chondrosarcomas, 123

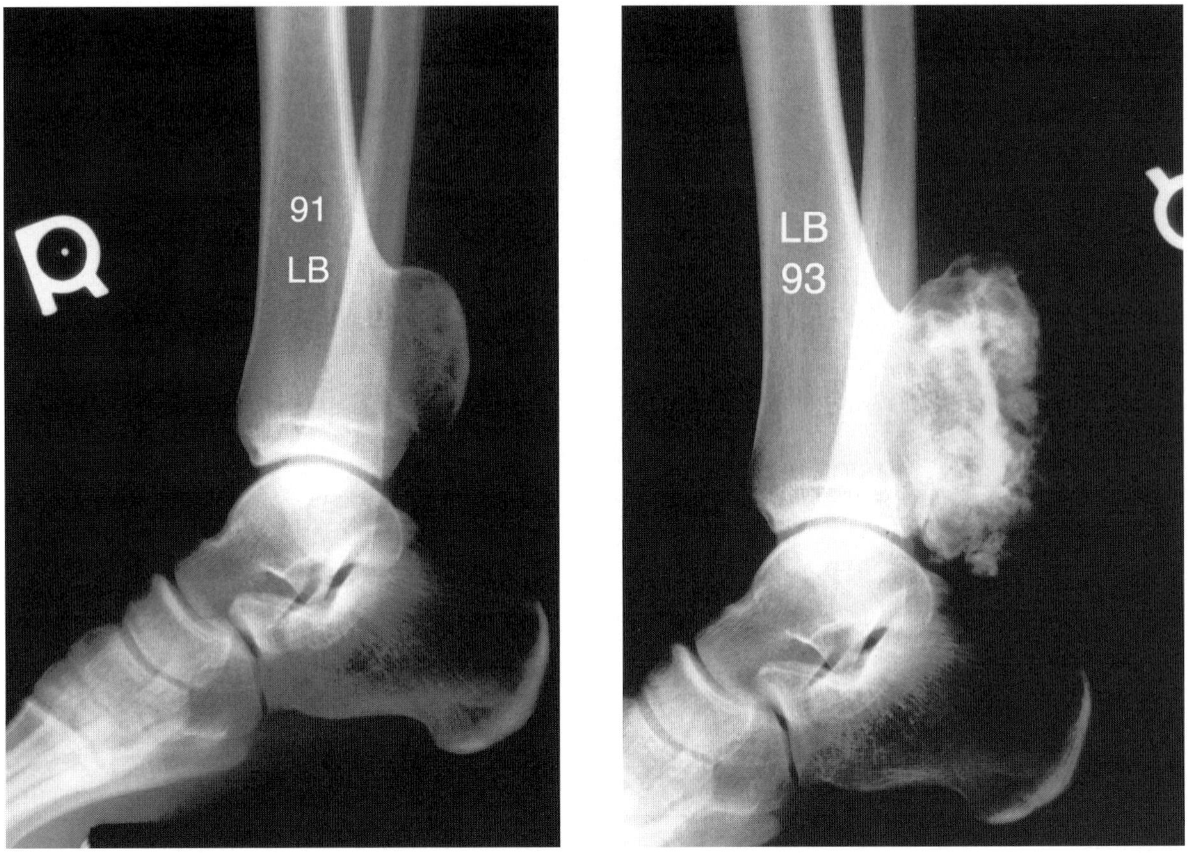

Figure 4-97

SECONDARY CHONDROSARCOMA

Left: The tumor surface is smooth and thin.

Right: Two years later, the cap is irregular and nodular, a change supporting the diagnosis of secondary chondrosarcoma. (Fig. 6-17A,B from Unni KK. Dahlin's bone tumors: general aspects and data on 11,087 cases, 5th ed. Philadelphia: Lippincott-Raven; 1996:28. By permission of Mayo Foundation.)

Figure 4-98

SECONDARY CHONDROSARCOMA

The lesion consists almost entirely of cartilage but clearly arises on the surface of bone. There is gross cystic change. The cystic cavities contain gelatinous material representing myxoid change. (Fig. 6-19 from Unni KK. Dahlin's bone tumors: general aspects and data on 11,087 cases, 5th ed. Philadelphia: Lippincott-Raven; 1996:83. By permission of Mayo Foundation.)

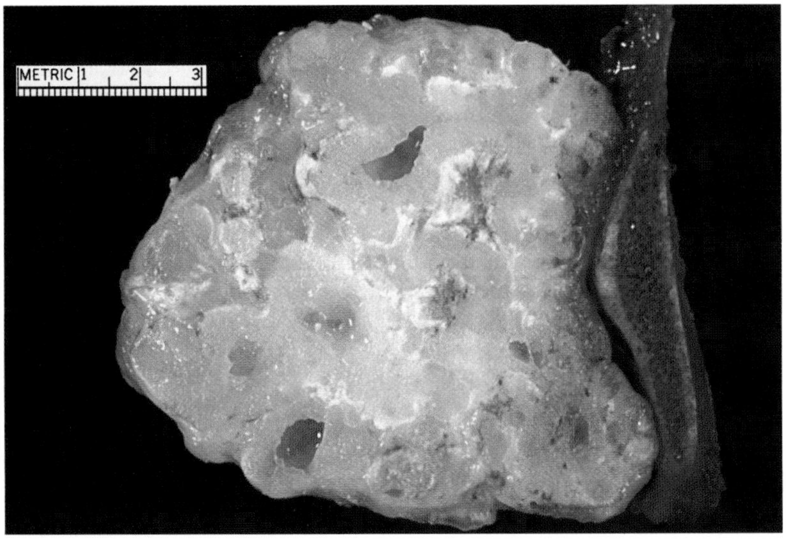

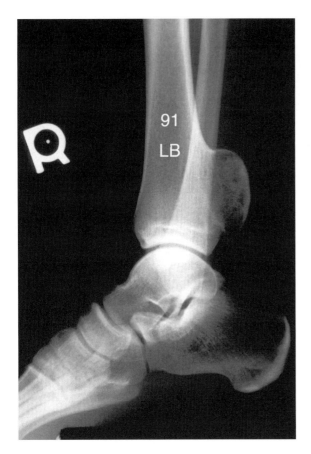

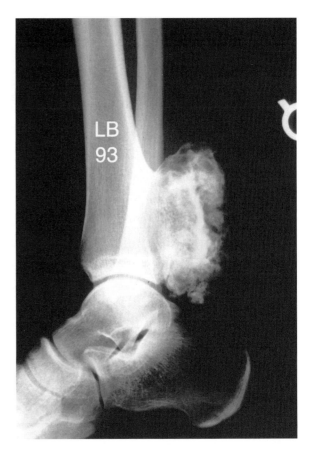

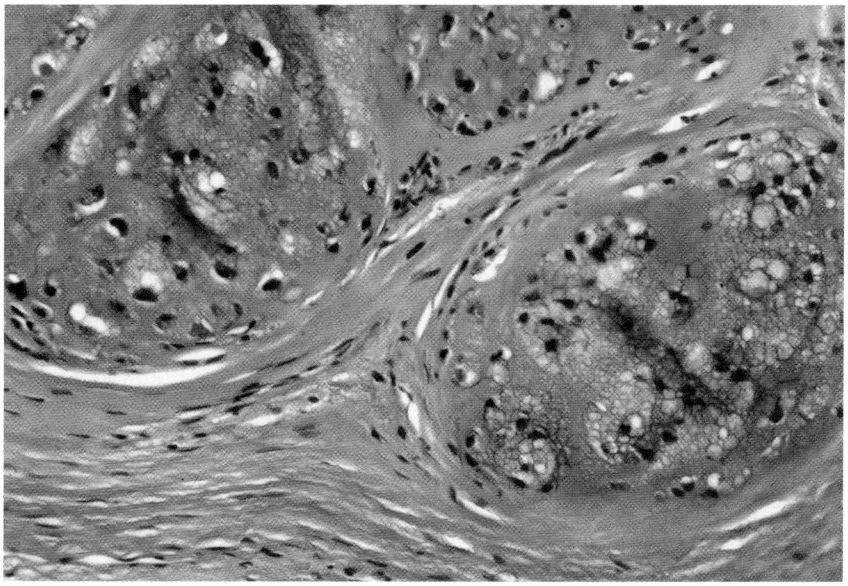

Figure 4-99

SECONDARY CHONDROSARCOMA

The tumor arose in an osteochondroma of the ilium. Usually extremely well differentiated, these lesions are difficult to diagnose cytologically. Peripheral invasion into surrounding soft tissue is a helpful feature.

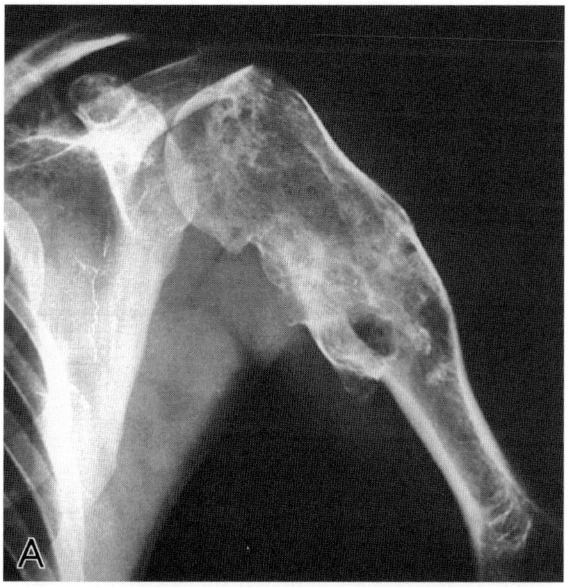

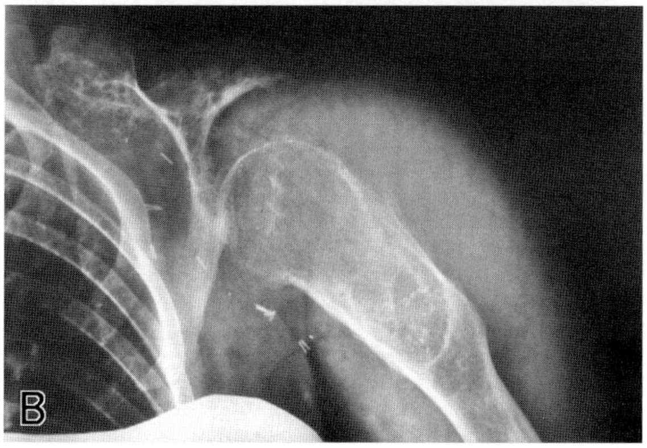

Figure 4-100

SECONDARY CHONDROSARCOMA

A: Radiograph of 32-year-old man with Ollier's disease shows a deformed left proximal humerus with abnormal modeling and calcification. The left glenoid is hypoplastic.

B: Eight years later, a radiograph shows a secondary chondrosarcoma arising in the proximal humerus. The lateral cortex is destroyed, and there is a large soft tissue mass.

C: Corresponding gross specimen. The medullary portion shows dysplastic cartilage, whereas the soft tissue mass shows extensive myxoid and cystic changes.

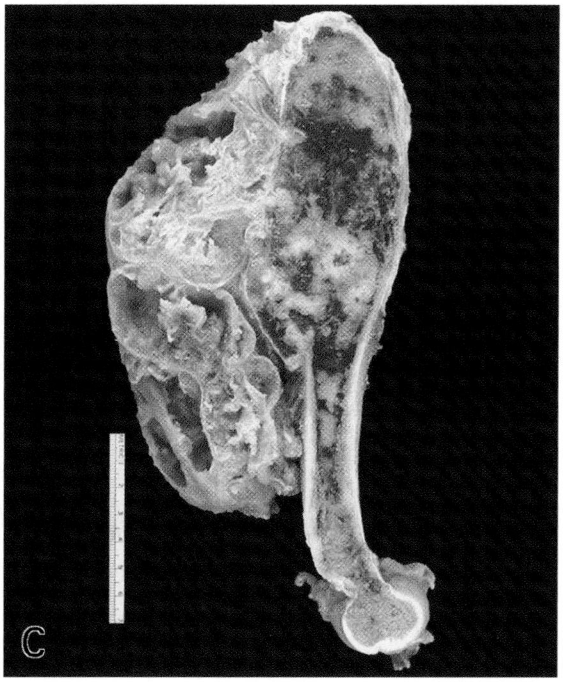

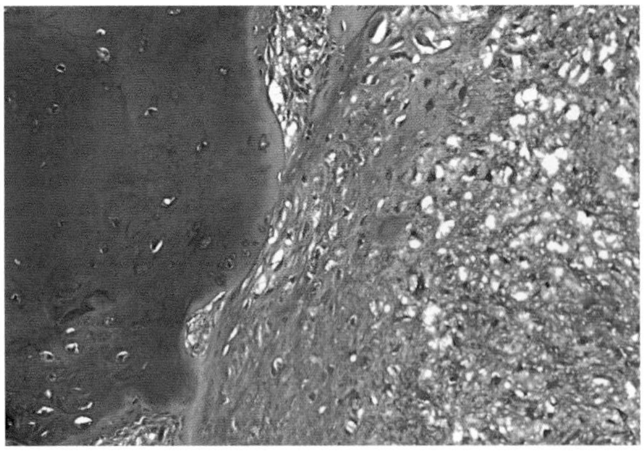

Figure 4-101

SECONDARY CHONDROSARCOMA

The chondrosarcoma on the right is more cellular than the preexisting dysplastic cartilage on the left and has myxoid matrix.

arose from central chondrosarcoma and 7 arose secondary to peripheral chondrosarcoma (4 solitary osteochondromas, 1 with multiple osteochondromas, and 2 with periosteal chondrosarcoma). Two patients had Ollier's disease.

Clinical Features. Patients complain of pain or swelling or both. Symptoms may have been present for months or years. Pathologic fractures are more common than with conventional chondrosarcoma. The majority of patients are older adults, generally a decade older than those with conventional chondrosarcoma. Of the cases in the Mayo Clinic files, the youngest patient was 15 years and the oldest was 92; 71.6 percent were older than 50.

Sites. The bones involved by conventional chondrosarcoma are also the preferred sites for

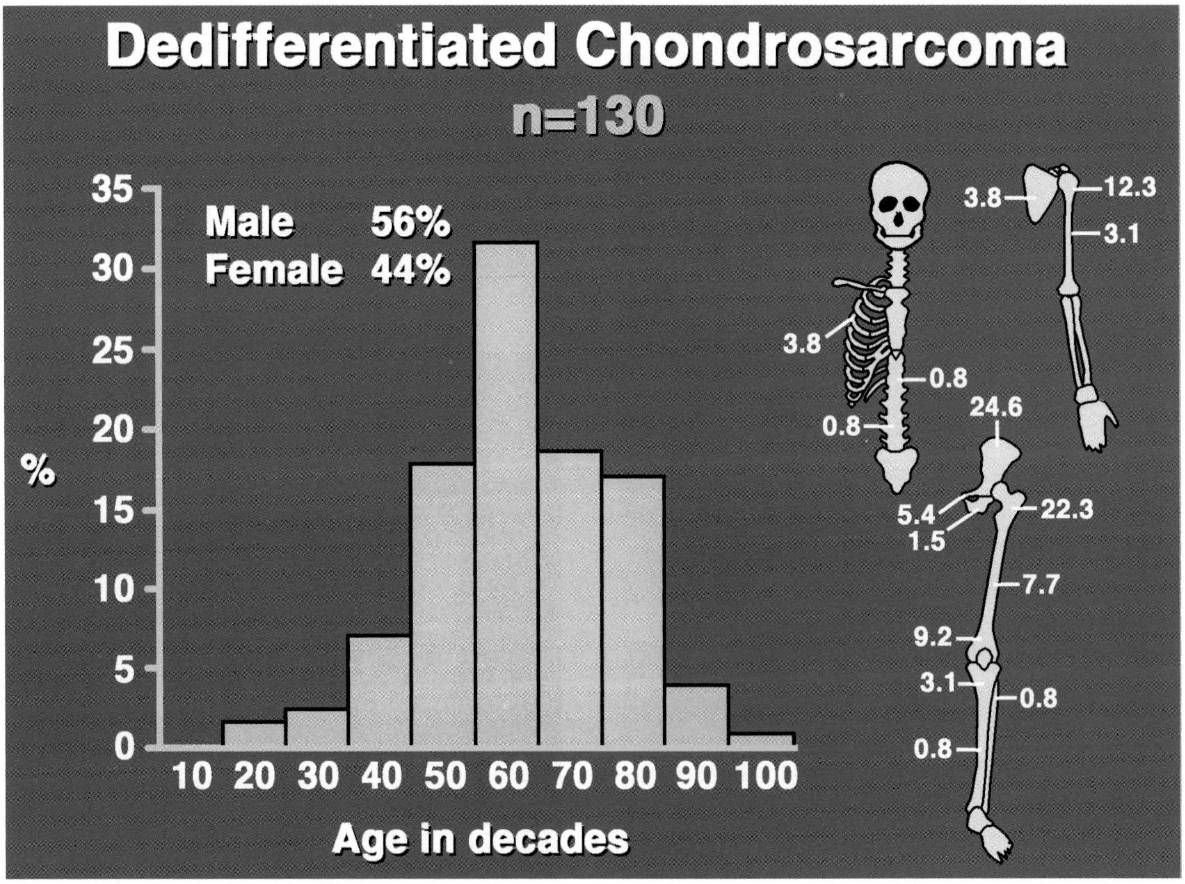

Figure 4-102

DEDIFFERENTIATED CHONDROSARCOMA

The distribution of dedifferentiated chondrosarcoma according to the age and sex of the patient and the site of the lesion.

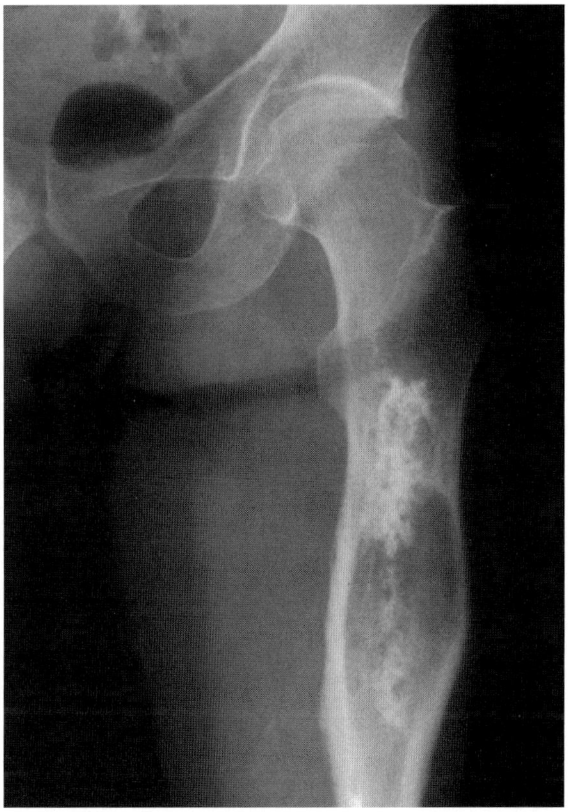

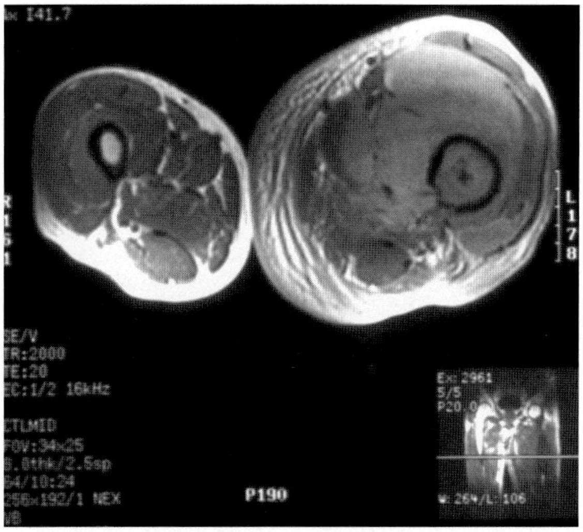

Figure 4-103

DEDIFFERENTIATED CHONDROSARCOMA

Left: The cortical expansion and cortical thickening of this mineralized lesion involving the proximal femur suggests that it is an ordinary chondrosarcoma.

Above: An axial proton density T_2-weighted MRI of the tumor, however, demonstrates a large soft tissue mass, suggesting the diagnosis of dedifferentiated chondrosarcoma.

dedifferentiated chondrosarcoma. The pelvic and shoulder girdles are involved most commonly. There are no examples in the Mayo Clinic files of these tumors involving the skull, facial skeleton, or small bones of the hands and feet.

Radiographic Findings. A dedifferentiated chondrosarcoma arising in a preexisting condition (such as Ollier's disease) has the features of that process as well as those of the malignant neoplasm.

The radiographic appearance of nearly all dedifferentiated chondrosarcomas suggests a high-grade sarcoma: large size, cortical destruction, and a soft tissue mass. About 50 percent of the tumors contain mineralization, suggesting a cartilage tumor. Most show the cortical thickening and expansion of bone typical of chondrosarcoma (fig. 4-103). According to Capanna et al. (229), this appearance suggests high-grade histology of the cartilaginous component. The diagnosis is suggested by the presence of a large area of lysis and cortical destruction associated with a lesion that has the calcification typical of cartilage (fig. 4-104).

Radiographs usually have a bimorphic pattern: the central portion suggests a cartilage tumor and the cortical and especially soft tissue portions appear more aggressive. MRI and CT are especially useful in demonstrating the bimorphic pattern (fig. 4-103, left). In rare instances, radiographs suggest a benign lesion, especially an enchondroma (fig. 4-105).

Gross Findings. The gross appearance of dedifferentiated chondrosarcoma also suggests a bimorphic tumor (fig. 4-106). If the lesion is resected intact, the medullary portion has the typical appearance of chondrosarcoma, that is, blue lobulated cartilage filling the bone marrow cavity, with expansion of bone and erosion and thickening of the cortex. Foci of calcification and cyst formation are common. Juxtaposed to the cartilage is a fleshy white "sarcomatous" tumor that has the appearance of a high-grade sarcoma. Occasionally, the fleshy tumor predominates and only small inconspicuous nodules of cartilage are found. Rarely, the tumor has the gross appearance of a chondrosarcoma, and only microscopy shows the high-grade areas. Rarely, the recurrence or even metastasis shows spindle cell sarcoma; a high-grade sarcoma must have been present in the original tumor, but it was too small to be recognized.

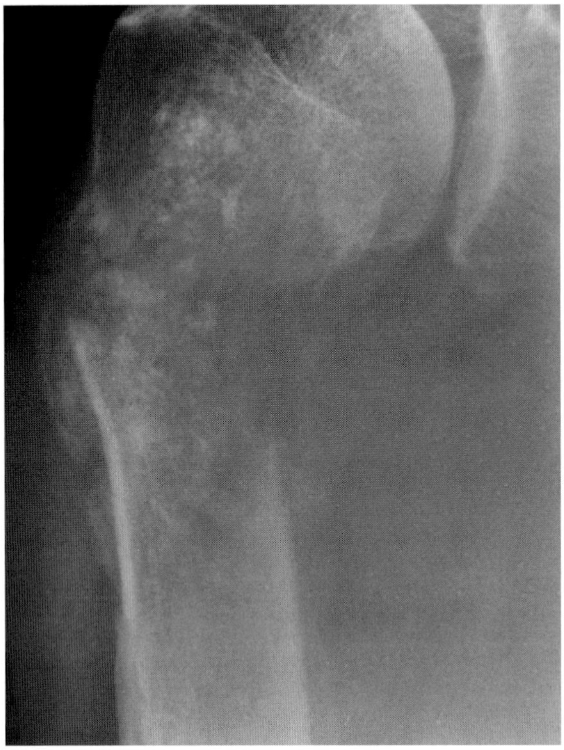

Figure 4-104

DEDIFFERENTIATED CHONDROSARCOMA

A plain radiograph shows an extremely destructive lesion with stippled calcification and pathologic fracture of the right proximal humerus. The radiographic appearance is more aggressive than that typical of a low-grade chondrosarcoma.

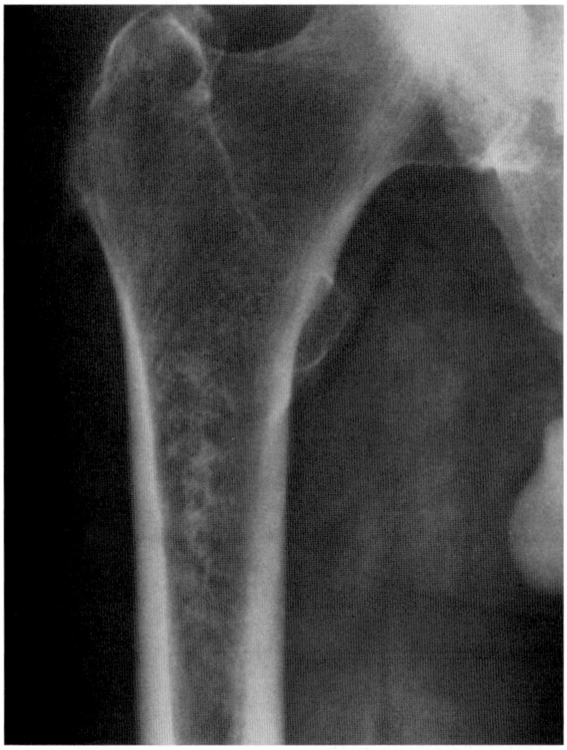

Figure 4-105

DEDIFFERENTIATED CHONDROSARCOMA

The tumor, in the proximal femur of a 78-year-old man, has a radiographic appearance that suggests enchondroma. This is an uncommon radiographic presentation for dedifferentiated chondrosarcoma.

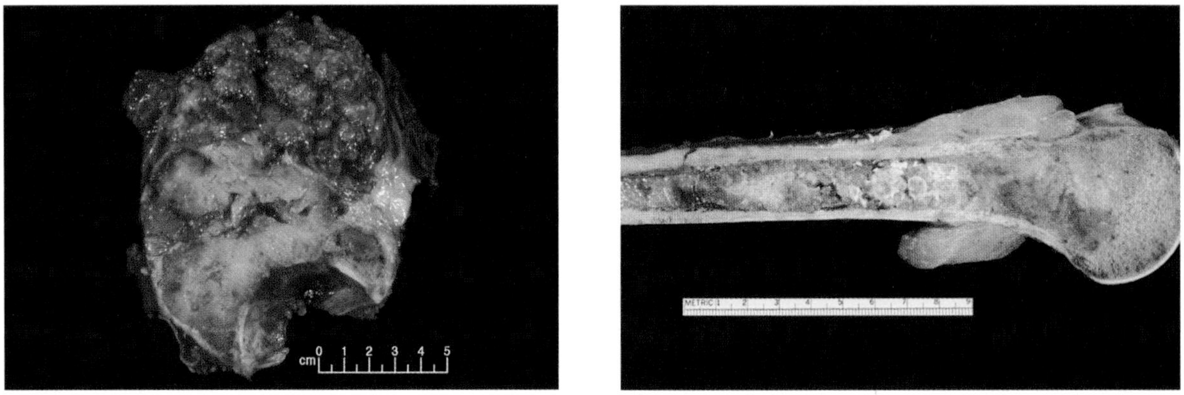

Figure 4-106

DEDIFFERENTIATED CHONDROSARCOMA

Left: The tumor arose in the ilium and has the gross features typical of dedifferentiated chondrosarcoma. The central area contains cartilage with the cystic necrosis and myxoid change characteristic of ordinary chondrosarcoma. However, the extraosseous lobulated mass has a tan-gray fleshy appearance that corresponds to the high-grade spindle cell sarcoma component of the tumor.

Right: The medullary part of this tumor is cartilaginous. It is associated with a solid, light tan soft tissue mass that is wrapped around the proximal portion of the tumor. This mass had microscopic features of a high-grade fibrosarcoma.

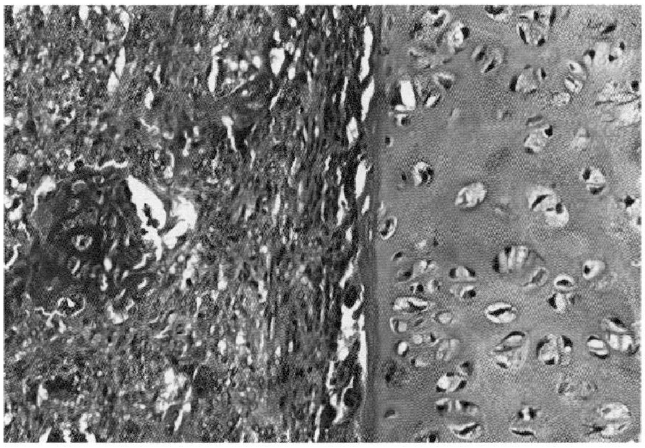

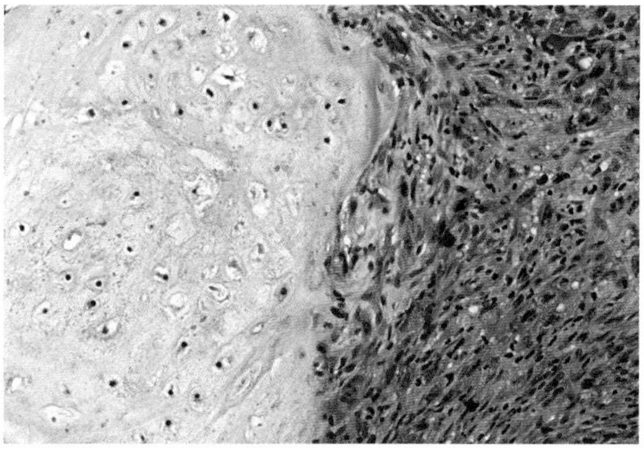

Figure 4-107

DEDIFFERENTIATED CHONDROSARCOMA

Left: The demarcation is sharp between the high-grade osteosarcoma on the left and the low-grade chondrosarcoma on the right. Right: A well-differentiated chondrosarcoma with necrosis of scattered chondrocytes is juxtaposed to a high-grade spindle cell sarcoma.

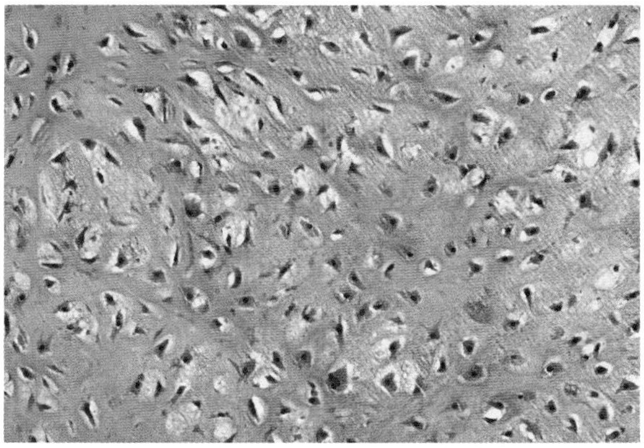

Figure 4-108

DEDIFFERENTIATED CHONDROSARCOMA

The cartilaginous portion of this dedifferentiated chondrosarcoma has features of a grade 2 chondrosarcoma.

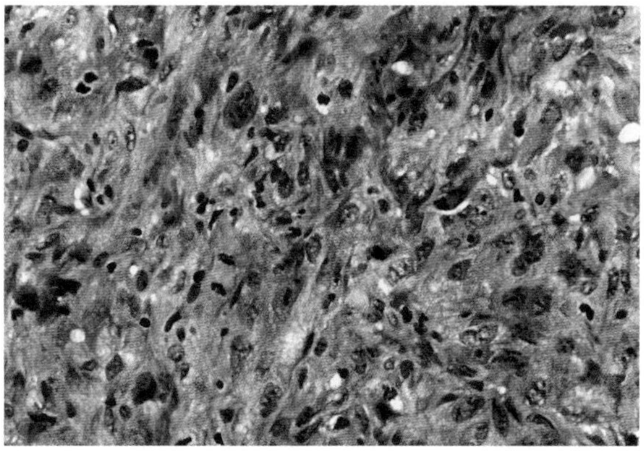

Figure 4-109

HIGH-GRADE SPINDLE CELL SARCOMA WITH FEATURES OF MALIGNANT FIBROUS HISTIOCYTOMA

Sampling error can be a problem with small biopsy specimens, for example, the low-grade chondrosarcoma portion of this dedifferentiated chondrosarcoma is not seen in this field.

Microscopic Findings. Typically, dedifferentiated chondrosarcoma is a bimorphic tumor in which chondrosarcoma is juxtaposed to a high-grade spindle cell sarcoma (fig. 4-107). In the original description, the chondrosarcoma is always considered to be low grade and the spindle cell component is sharply demarcated from the cartilaginous component (230). However, this is not always the case. About 15 percent of dedifferentiated chondrosarcomas have a grade 2 chondrosarcoma associated with a spindle cell component (fig. 4-108) (231). In some cases, however, the cartilage is so bland that an enchondroma is suggested. Although the typical pattern is juxtaposition of the chondrosarcoma and spindle cell sarcoma, some otherwise typical dedifferentiated chondrosarcomas have focal intermingling of the two elements.

The spindle cell sarcoma is always highly malignant, but it may be a fibrosarcoma, a malignant fibrous histiocytoma, or an osteosarcoma (fig. 4-109). Occasionally, rhabdomyosarcomatous differentiation is seen (236). Rarely, the dedifferentiated portion contains a large number of giant cells, simulating the appearance of a

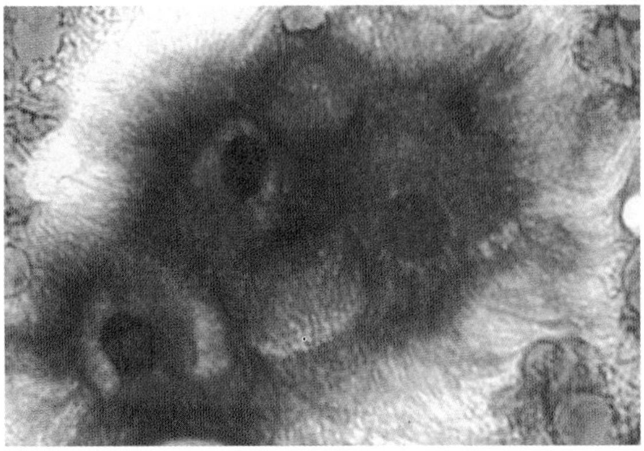

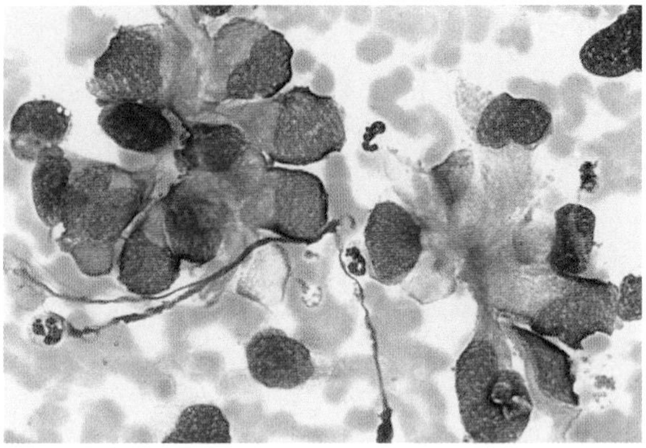

Figure 4-110

FINE-NEEDLE ASPIRATION BIOPSY OF DEDIFFERENTIATED CHONDROSARCOMA

The aspirate on the left contains well-differentiated cartilage fragments that on the right have a high-grade, poorly differentiated sarcomatous component (May-Grünwald-Giemsa stain).

giant cell tumor. In some tumors, the high-grade areas appear distinctly epithelial and there may even be gland formation. If a biopsy specimen from the bone of an older person shows an epithelial-appearing tumor but the radiographs show features typical of cartilage, the diagnosis of dedifferentiated chondrosarcoma is justified.

As pointed out above, dedifferentiated chondrosarcoma is always a high-grade malignancy. We have seen a rare example in which the spindle cell component was better differentiated.

Immunohistochemical Findings. The cartilaginous areas are reportedly positive for S-100 protein but not the spindle cell areas, which have shown variable staining with histiocytic, smooth muscle, and skeletal muscle markers (236).

Ultrastructural Findings. According to electron microscopic studies, the chondroid portion of the tumor has features typical of cartilage and the spindle cell area has fibroblastic or rhabdomyoblastic features (236).

Cytologic Findings. Dedifferentiated chondrosarcoma is recognizable on fine-needle aspiration cytology only when the well-differentiated chondroid and high-grade sarcomatous components are both present in the sample (fig. 4-110). Representative sampling is achieved by directing the aspiration needle toward the areas with different radiographic appearances.

Genetics and Other Special Techniques. The classic dedifferentiated chondrosarcoma consists of two distinct histologic components: a low-grade chondrosarcoma adjacent to a high-grade sarcoma such as a malignant fibrous histiocytoma, osteosarcoma, or rhabdomyosarcoma. A subject of controversy has been whether the low-grade chondrosarcomatous component and the high-grade sarcomatous component are derived from a common precursor cell or whether they represent separate genotypic lineages (collision tumor) (226). Genetic characterization of both components of a dedifferentiated chondrosarcoma showing shared anomalies supports the theory of a common primitive mesenchymal cell progenitor with the ability to differentiate or to express features of more than one line of mesenchymal differentiation (227,228). Not all genetic alterations have been shown to be shared, however, and it has been hypothesized that these alterations arise after the diversion of the two components and are later events in the histogenesis of dedifferentiated chondrosarcoma (227).

Differential Diagnosis. If both the cartilaginous and spindle cell elements are represented in the biopsy specimen, the diagnosis is straightforward. Rarely, chondroblastic osteosarcoma is included in the differential diagnosis. In chondroblastic osteosarcoma, the cartilage component is very malignant-appearing and merges into the spindle cell component, unlike the abrupt change from a low-grade chondrosarcoma to a high-grade spindle cell sarcoma in dedifferentiated chondrosarcoma. Although a mesenchymal chondrosarcoma has a combination of well-differentiated cartilage and high-grade malignancy, the latter consists of small cells.

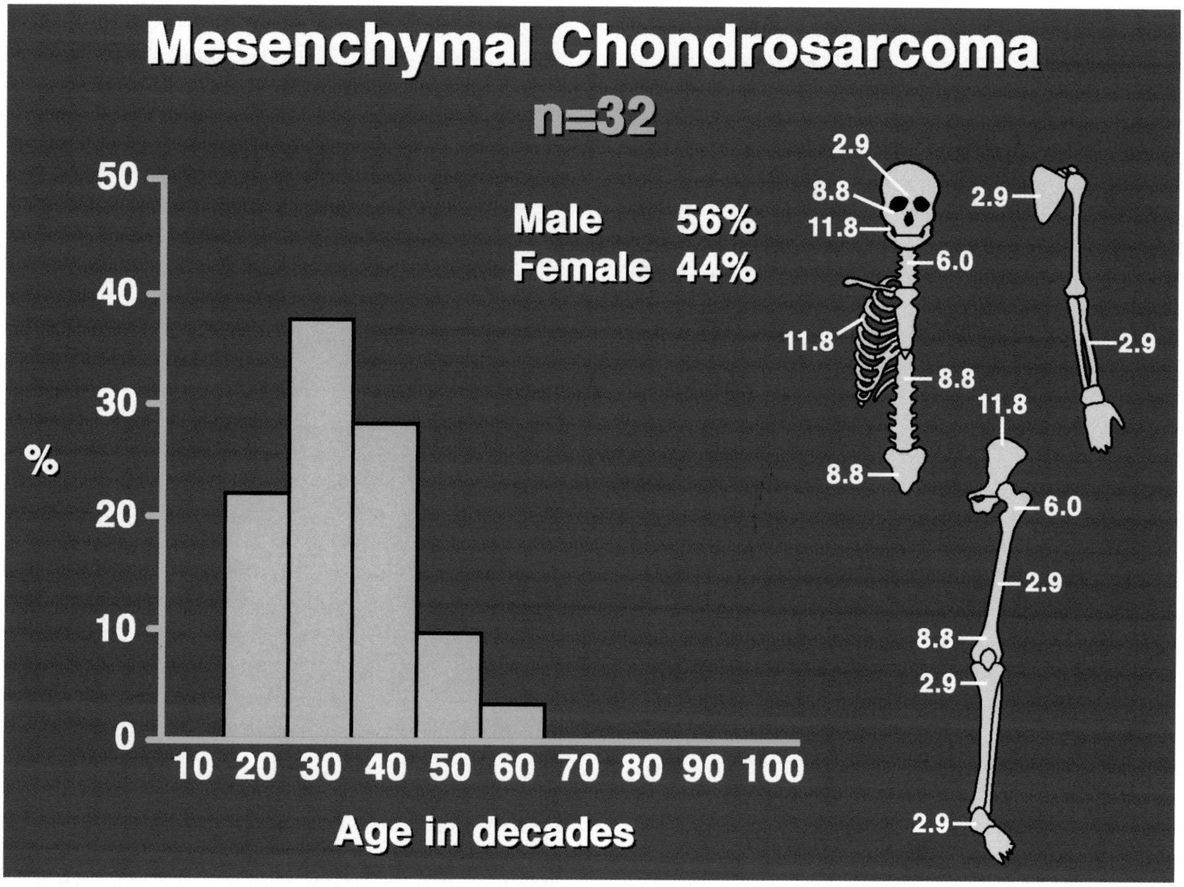

Figure 4-111

MESENCHYMAL CHONDROSARCOMA

The distribution of mesenchymal chondrosarcoma according to the age and sex of the patient and the site of the lesion.

Spread and Metastasis. Metastasis usually affects the lungs, although lymph nodes and other visceral organs also may be involved.

Treatment and Prognosis. Treatment is surgical extirpation. Not enough experience has accrued with chemotherapy to know whether this modality is effective. In the few cases in the Mayo Clinic files treated with preoperative chemotherapy, the response was disappointing. The prognosis is dismal. The 5-year survival rate is less than 10 percent, and of the cases in the Mayo Clinic files, there were no long-term survivors.

Mesenchymal Chondrosarcoma

Definition. Mesenchymal chondrosarcoma is a malignant tumor with a bimorphic growth pattern that consists of islands of more or less differentiated cartilage admixed with a small cell malignancy frequently associated with a hemangiopericytomatous vascular pattern.

General Features. Mesenchymal chondrosarcoma was defined by Lichtenstein and Bernstein (245) in a series of unusual cartilaginous tumors of bone and soft tissue. Some of the tumors described by Hutter et al. (241) in a series of primitive multipotential sarcomas undoubtedly were mesenchymal chondrosarcomas. Jacobson (244) preferred the term "polyhistioma" for small cell malignancies with matrix production; his series also included examples of small cell osteosarcoma. Mesenchymal chondrosarcoma is one of the rarest of bone sarcomas: 32 examples are included in the Mayo Clinic files (compared with 1,023 examples of chondrosarcomas of the usual kind) (fig. 4-111). About one third of the tumors occur in soft tissues. These tumors have

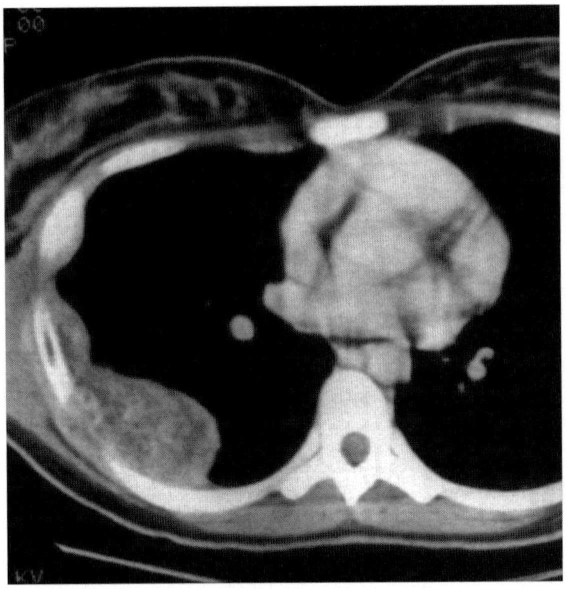

Figure 4-112

MESENCHYMAL CHONDROSARCOMA

CT shows a calcified mesenchymal chondrosarcoma with intrathoracic extension and destruction of a rib. (Courtesy of Dr. A. Vandersteenhoven, Dallas, TX.)

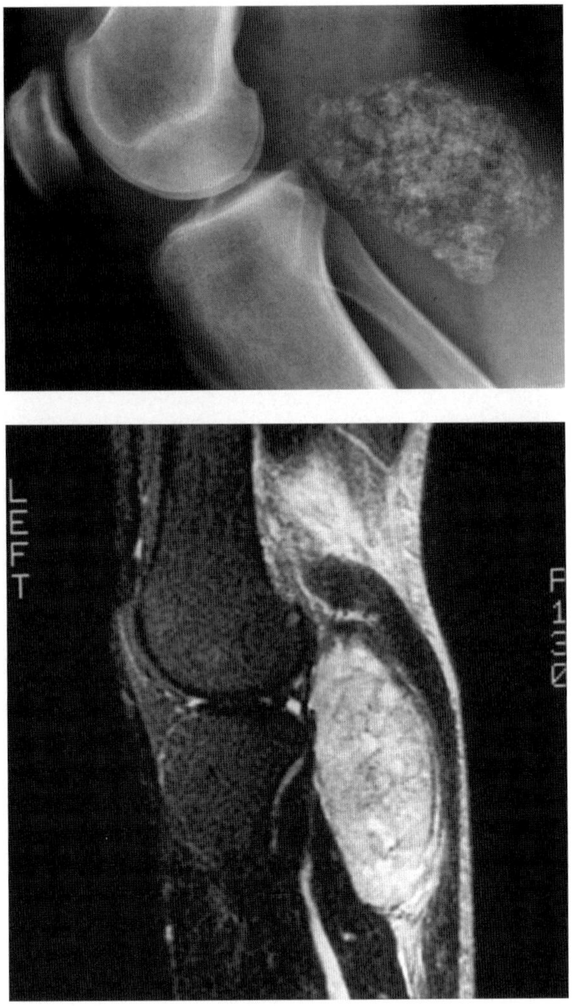

Figure 4-113

MESENCHYMAL CHONDROSARCOMA

Top: Heavily and diffusely mineralized soft tissue mass in the popliteal fossa.

Bottom: Sagittal T_2-weighted MRI shows a heterogeneous high signal intensity mass. The extent of mineralization is difficult to appreciate, but it accurately depicts the size and extent of the soft tissue mass.

clinical and histologic features identical to those of the skeletal counterparts.

Clinical Features. Mesenchymal chondrosarcomas tend to affect young adults, although the age range can be broad (242). About half of the patients are in the second and third decades of life. There is a slight male predominance in Mayo Clinic series, although one large study from Mayo Clinic, including consultation cases, reported a slight female predominance (246). The symptoms are nonspecific and consist of pain, swelling, or both. Symptoms may be longstanding (up to 7 years in the report of Bertoni et al. [239]). A small proportion of tumors are discovered incidentally on radiographs (246,248).

Sites. Any portion of the skeleton may be involved, and rarely, a patient presents with involvement of multiple bones. In the large series reported by Nakashima et al. (246), the jawbones were the most common site. The spine, ilium, and ribs are other relatively common sites.

Radiographic Findings. Radiographs frequently show a lytic destructive process (fig. 4-112). Most of these tumors contain mineral, which has the characteristics of mineral seen in cartilage tumors (fig. 4-113). Many of the lesions have the radiographic features of chondrosarcoma, with expansion of bone and thickening of the cortex. The margins are often poorly defined. An unusual appearance is that of a mineralizing mass arising on the surface of bone, suggesting a periosteal osteosarcoma (fig. 4-114). Although the radiographic features are nonspecific, they nearly always suggest a malignant neoplasm.

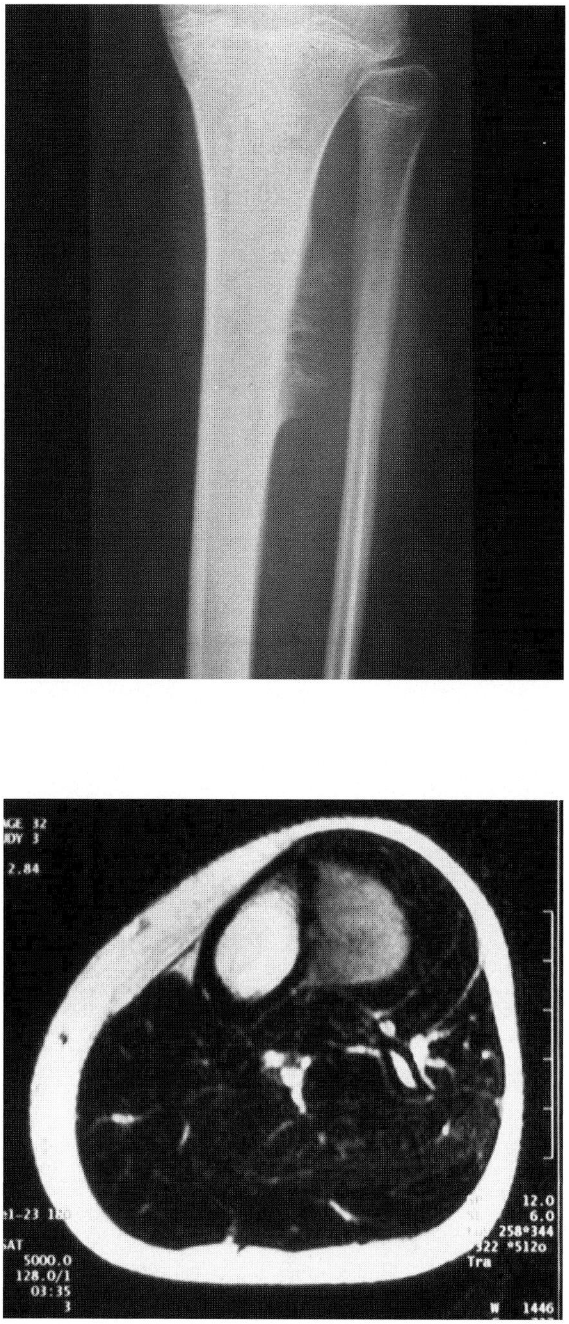

Figure 4-114

MESENCHYMAL CHONDROSARCOMA

Top: Plain radiograph of the left leg shows a mineralized spiculated lesion arising from the lateral cortex of the tibia. The radiographic appearance suggests periosteal osteosarcoma.

Bottom: Axial T_2-weighted MRI clearly shows a surface lesion arising from the lateral cortex of the tibia without intramedullary involvement. (Courtesy of Dr. MacGrogan, Bordeaux, France.)

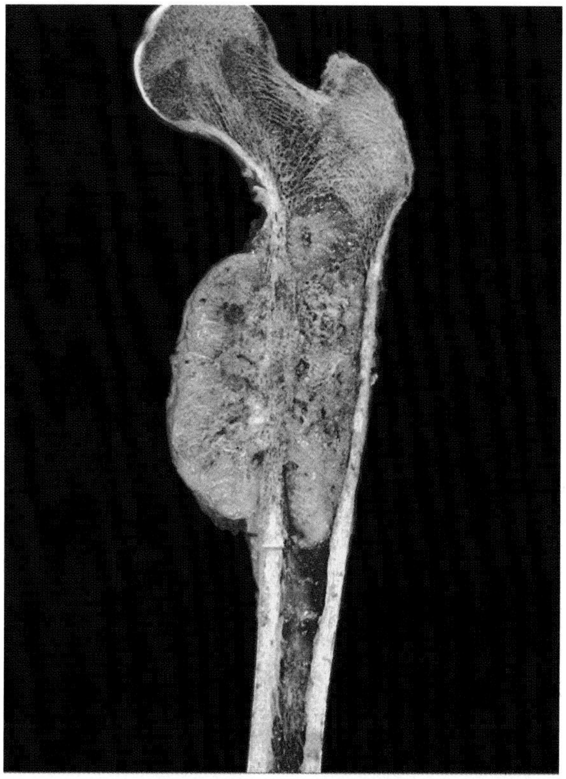

Figure 4-115

MESENCHYMAL CHONDROSARCOMA

Mineralized areas are seen in both the intraosseous and extraosseous components of this tumor involving the proximal femoral shaft of a 19-year-old man. The patient died of metastatic disease within 18 months post surgery. (Fig. 7-2 from Unni KK. Dahlin's bone tumors: general aspects and data on 11,087 cases, 5th ed. Philadelphia: Lippincott-Raven; 1996:111. By permission of Mayo Foundation.)

Gross Findings. The tumor is typically gray to pink, firm to soft, and generally well demarcated. Foci of chalky white calcification are usually seen (fig. 4-115). Areas of hyaline cartilage may be apparent, but are rarely prominent.

Microscopic Findings. Mesenchymal chondrosarcoma consists of two distinct elements: clearly recognizable hyaline cartilage and a proliferation of small malignant cells (fig. 4-116). The proportion of the two elements is variable. Some tumors have small inconspicuous islands of cartilage within sheets of small cells. In other tumors, large islands of cartilage appear juxtaposed to sheets of small cells. Rarely, the chondroid matrix dominates and the small anaplastic cells appear as inconspicuous condensations at the periphery of the chondroid lobules.

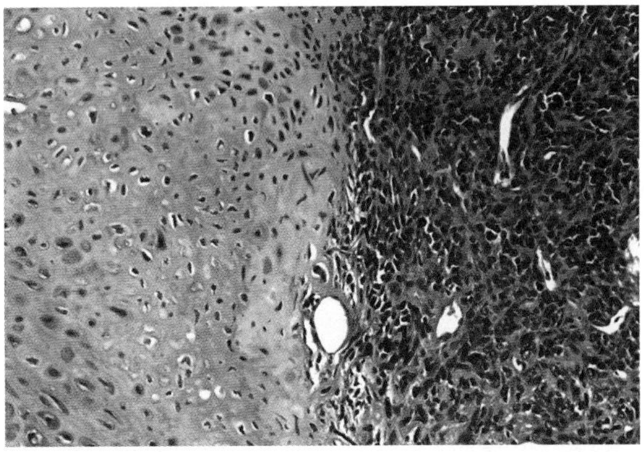

Figure 4-116

MESENCHYMAL CHONDROSARCOMA

The chondroid portion (left) of this mesenchymal chondrosarcoma is juxtaposed to the small blue cell component (right).

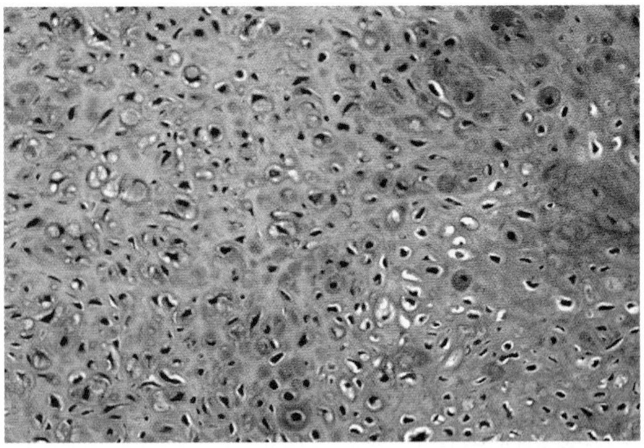

Figure 4-117

MESENCHYMAL CHONDROSARCOMA

Moderately cellular chondroid area with eosinophilic changes in the matrix (right) suggesting ossification.

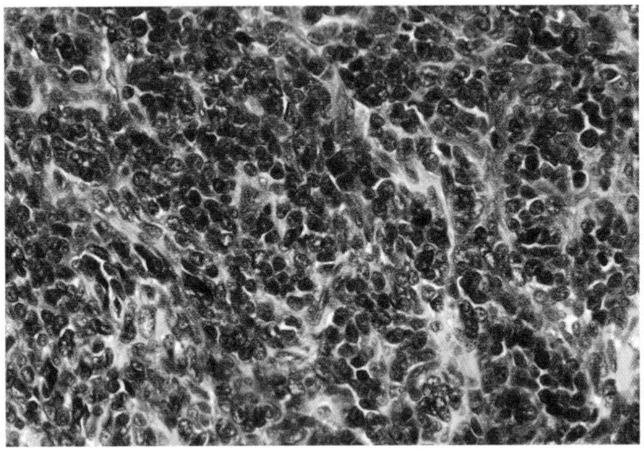

Figure 4-118

MESENCHYMAL CHONDROSARCOMA

Compact sheets of small blue cells with round to oval nuclei.

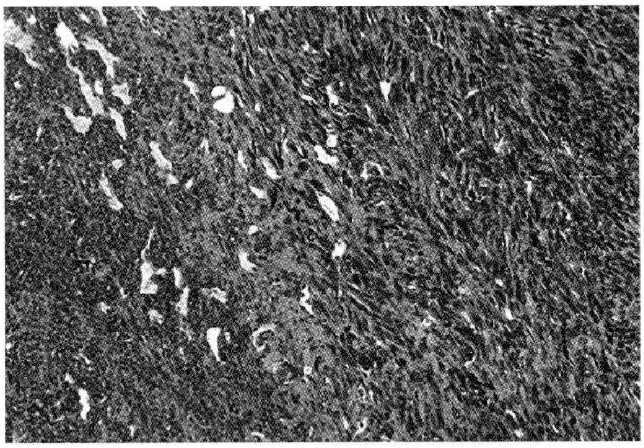

Figure 4-119

MESENCHYMAL CHONDROSARCOMA

The high-grade component of this tumor shows features of a small round cell sarcoma on the left and a spindle cell sarcoma on the right.

The cartilage is well differentiated and suggests a well-differentiated chondrosarcoma (fig. 4-117), although in a small proportion of tumors, it suggests a moderately differentiated malignancy. The change from cartilage to small cells is usually abrupt, but occasionally there is a gradual transition, with cells with the cytologic features of the small cells lying in a chondroid matrix. The high-grade component is composed of small cells whose nuclei are relatively uniform (fig. 4-118). The nuclei are generally round but may be oval or even spindled (fig. 4-119). The nuclei are extremely dense, and the cytoplasm is sparse. The round cells usually are arranged in sheets or they may have an alveolar pattern. Spindle cells may be arranged in a herringbone pattern. The nuclear characteristics are sufficiently unique to be diagnostic.

One of the characteristic features of mesenchymal chondrosarcoma is the vascular proliferation that produces thin-walled vessels with tumor cells outside (which compress the vessels), giving rise to a hemangiopericytomatous pattern (fig. 4-120). This pattern may predominate or it may be focal and inconspicuous.

The islands of cartilage frequently undergo calcification or even ossification. Rarely, fine lines of pink matrix are seen between the small cells. Multinucleated giant cells are rare.

Grading. Mesenchymal chondrosarcomas are always high grade (grade 4) because of the presence of small cells, although the chondroid areas show some variation from tumor to tumor.

Immunohistochemical Findings. The chondroid islands, but not the small cell areas, reportedly stain for S-100 protein (243). CD99 staining has been reported to be positive in the small cell areas of all tumors (240). The type of collagen identified with immunohistochemical staining supports chondrocytic differentiation of the small cells (238). The transcription factor Sox9 has been shown to be helpful in differentiating mesenchymal chondrosarcoma from other small cell malignancies (252).

Ultrastructural Findings. The undifferentiated cells have large nuclei and sparse organelles. The cartilaginous areas have the usual appearance, with dilated endoplasmic reticulum (249).

Cytologic Findings. Cellular smears of the few mesenchymal chondrosarcomas diagnosed on fine-needle aspiration biopsy contain small, primitive cells with sparse, poorly defined cytoplasm and dense nuclei that occur singly or in coherent clusters (fig. 4-121). Also, scattered small osteoclasts and a matrix component ranging from myxoid to hyaline or even osteoid-like may be seen (251). Without the latter two components, differentiating a mesenchymal chondrosarcoma from other small cell malignancies is difficult and requires the use of adjunctive techniques in the analysis of the biopsy material.

Genetics and Other Special Techniques. An identical robertsonian translocation involving chromosomes 13 and 21 [der(13;21)(q10;q10)] has been detected in two mesenchymal chondrosarcomas, one arising skeletally and the other extraskeletally, possibly representing a characteristic rearrangement for this histopathologic entity (fig. 4-122) (247). Both cases also exhibited loss of all or a portion of chromosomes 8 and 20 and gain of all or a portion of chromosome

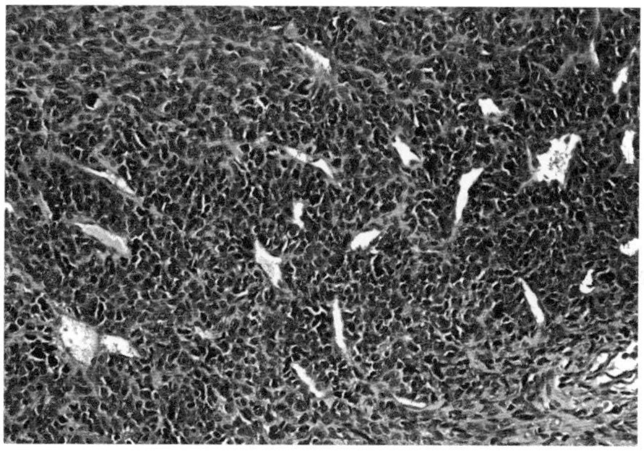

Figure 4-120

MESENCHYMAL CHONDROSARCOMA

Vascular proliferation with a hemangiopericytomatous pattern within a small cell area.

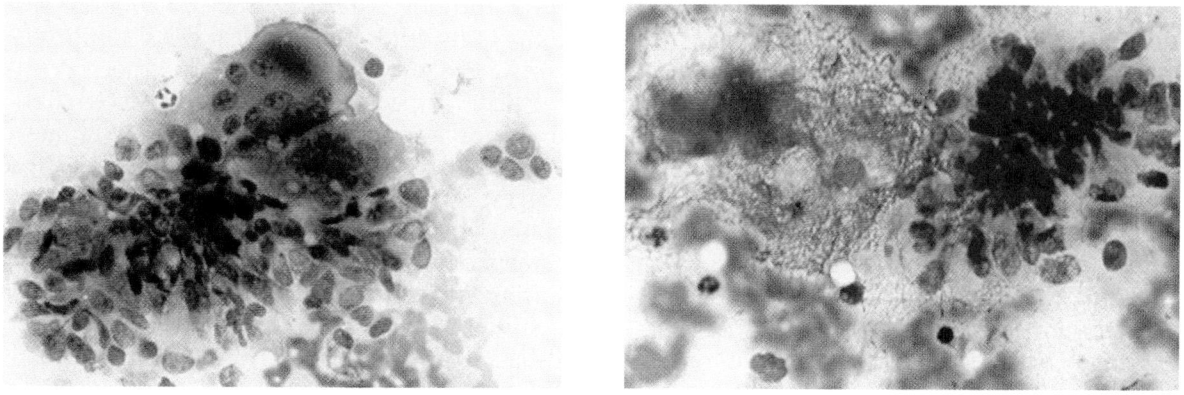

Figure 4-121

FINE-NEEDLE ASPIRATION BIOPSY OF MESENCHYMAL CHONDROSARCOMA

Dense clusters of small primitive-looking tumor cells with compact chromatin and sparse, poorly defined cytoplasm are seen adjacent to osteoclasts (left) and a fibrillary, myxoid chondroid matrix (right) (May-Grünwald-Giemsa stain).

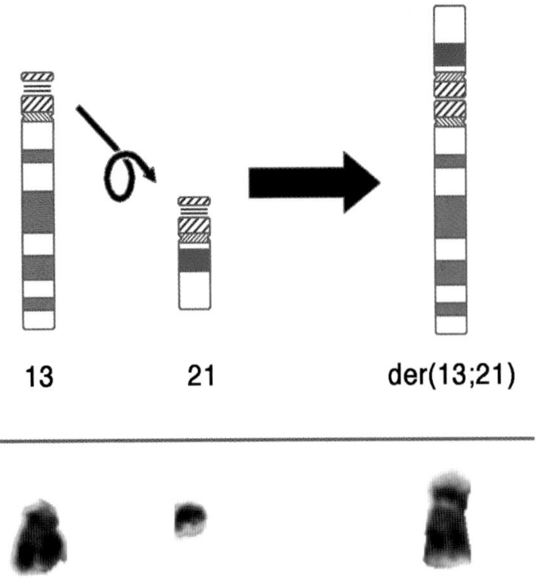

Figure 4-122

MESENCHYMAL CHONDROSARCOMA

Schematic and partial karyotype of the 13;21 translocation [der(13;21)(q10;q10)] detected in mesenchymal chondrosarcoma.

12. The observation of similar chromosomal abnormalities in both skeletal and extraskeletal mesenchymal chondrosarcomas supports a genetic as well as a histopathologic relationship between these anatomically distinct neoplasms.

Differential Diagnosis. Frequently, mesenchymal chondrosarcoma is mistaken for hemangiopericytoma. However, the malignant appearance of the cells and the presence of chondroid matrix help make the distinction. In small samples, the tumor may be mistaken for other small cell malignancies, such as Ewing's sarcoma or malignant lymphoma, but the vascular pattern and the presence of matrix help differentiate these from mesenchymal chondrosarcoma. The highly malignant cells of dedifferentiated chondrosarcoma are large and pleomorphic, unlike the small cells of mesenchymal chondrosarcoma.

Spread and Metastasis. Metastasis usually involves the lungs, but it can include other sites such as visceral organs and skeleton.

Staging. Mesenchymal chondrosarcoma is always at least stage 2; however, it may be present with metastasis (stage 3).

Treatment and Prognosis. The treatment is surgical ablation. Not enough experience has accrued with chemotherapy to know whether it is effective. Huvos et al. (242) have suggested treating tumors that have a predominant hemangiopericytomatous pattern according to an osteosarcoma protocol and treating those with small cells in sheets according to an Ewing's tumor protocol.

The prognosis is unpredictable. Some patients present with disseminated metastasis and die within a year, but others survive for decades. Metastasis may be unexpectedly delayed, and 5-year survival does not mean cure. In the series of Huvos et al. (242), the 5-year survival rate was 42 percent and the 10-year rate was only 28 percent. Nakashima et al. (246) reported a 5-year survival rate of more than 54 percent; the 10-year rate was half of that. It has been suggested that patients with tumors of the orbit (243) and the jaws (250) have a better prognosis.

Clear Cell Chondrosarcoma

Definition. Clear cell chondrosarcoma is a rare variant of chondrosarcoma with a peculiar tendency to involve the ends of long bones. It is composed of cells with clear cytoplasm.

General Features. Clear cell chondrosarcoma has some features in common with chondroblastoma, including a strong tendency to involve the epiphysis and a combination of giant cells scattered among mononuclear cells. Clear cell chondrosarcoma occurs in young adults, whereas chondroblastoma occurs in children and adolescents. Although this may argue for chondroblastoma transforming into a clear cell chondrosarcoma, this transformation has not been documented. The peculiar tendency for clear cell chondrosarcoma to have bony trabeculae intimately associated with the tumor cells has led to the suggestion that it is an osteosarcoma rather than chondrosarcoma. Bosse et al. (255) demonstrated osteonectin immunoreactivity in the tumor cells, further bolstering this argument. Aigner et al. (253) demonstrated type 2 and type 10 but not type 1 collagen in the tumor. These authors believe their results favored a chondrocytic derivation.

Clinical Features. Clear cell chondrosarcoma is the rarest type of chondrosarcoma: until the year 2000, only 20 cases had been reported in the Mayo Clinic files (fig. 4-123). There is a

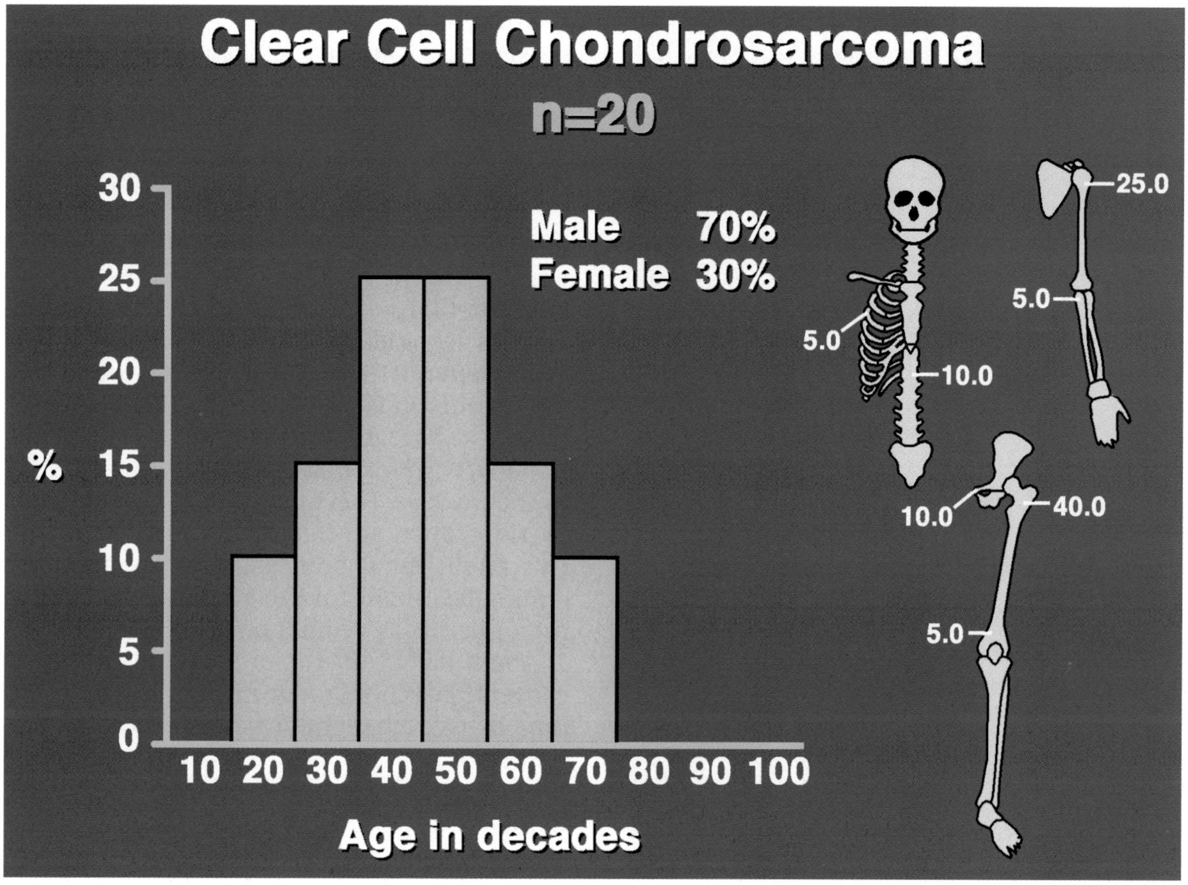

Figure 4-123

CLEAR CELL CHONDROSARCOMA

The distribution of clear cell chondrosarcoma according to the age and sex of the patient and the site of the lesion.

pronounced male predilection, and the majority of patients are in the fourth and fifth decades of life. Pain, sometimes of long duration, is a cardinal symptom. In a study from the Mayo Clinic, 18 percent of the patients had symptoms that lasted longer than 5 years (254).

Sites. Clear cell chondrosarcoma has an unusual propensity to involve the ends of long bones. The femur, particularly the head and neck, is the most common site of involvement. Rarely, the lesion is metaphyseal or even diaphyseal. Some patients have multifocal involvement of the skeleton.

Radiographic Findings. On radiographs, a clear cell chondrosarcoma is a lytic defect that extends to the end of the bone. In the early stages, the lesion tends to be sharply demarcated and may even have a sclerotic border, suggesting that it is benign (fig. 4-124). Over time, the lytic area expands and the margins become less well defined. The cortex is destroyed, and the tumor extends to the soft tissue (fig. 4-125). Less than half of the lesions contain calcification (254). The mineral has a soft fluffy character similar to that seen in chondroblastoma (254). CT demonstrates mineral better than plain radiographs (256).

Gross Findings. Clear cell chondrosarcomas involve the end of a bone, presenting as an expansile mass and extending to the articular cartilage (fig. 4-126). The tumor may have nodules of light blue hyaline cartilage, as in conventional chondrosarcoma. The rest of the tumor appears soft and gray. Small cystic areas are frequently present. Rarely, the major part of the lesion is cystic and the tumor is a mural nodule.

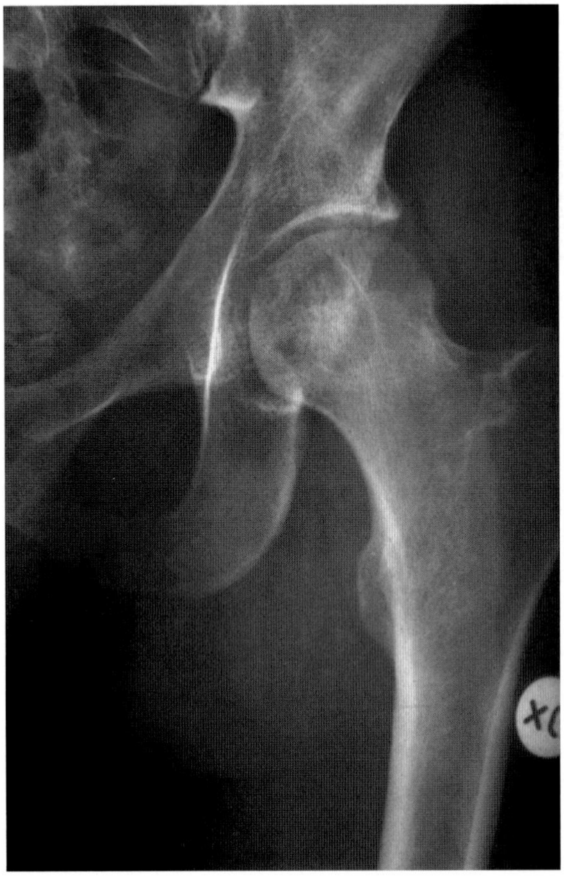

Figure 4-124

CLEAR CELL CHONDROSARCOMA

There is a lytic lesion with a well-defined sclerotic rim in the femoral head of a 23-year-old man. The differential diagnosis includes chondroblastoma and clear cell chondrosarcoma. (Courtesy of Dr. O. Larsson, Stockholm, Sweden.)

Microscopic Findings. Clear cell chondrosarcoma tends to have a lobulated growth pattern. The lobules are small and indistinct, and in among them, there is usually vascular proliferation and a scattering of benign giant cells (fig. 4-127). The centers of the lobules contain short trabeculae of bone (fig. 4-128). The tumor cells have distinct cytoplasmic boundaries, which abut one another, similar to the appearance of plant cells. The centrally located nucleus is vesicular and usually has a single prominent nucleolus. The nucleus is round and the chromatin is evenly distributed. The cytoplasm is abundant and clear (fig. 4-129). Occasionally, wisps of pink cytoplasm are seen close to the nucleus. Foci of cystic spaces, separated by thin septa, are frequently present. Rarely, this aneurysmal bone cyst-like component dominates the histologic appearance, and the tumor occurs as a mural nodule.

About half of the tumors contain nodules of conventional chondrosarcoma (fig. 4-130). These tumors have a bimorphic pattern, with conventional chondrosarcoma juxtaposed to more typical areas of clear cell chondrosarcoma with bone formation and giant cells. The cytologic features of clear cell chondrosarcoma do not have enough variation to permit histologic grading. Conventional chondrosarcoma, if present, is usually grade 1.

Cytologic Findings. There are few reports on the fine-needle aspiration features of clear cell chondrosarcoma (257). The variable presence of epithelioid tumor cells with large, pale-staining, finely vacuolated cytoplasm and a scant

Figure 4-125

CLEAR CELL CHONDROSARCOMA

Left: Expanded osteolytic lesion involves the head and neck of the right humerus, with a fracture through the neck. The lesion extends to the glenohumeral joint surface and is unmineralized. The differential diagnosis includes giant cell tumor.

Right: Coronal T_1-weighted spoiled gradient echo (SPGR) MRI with gadolinium enhancement confirms the radiographic extent of the lesion, which reaches the joint surface medially. (Courtesy of Dr. J. Wejde, Stockholm, Sweden.)

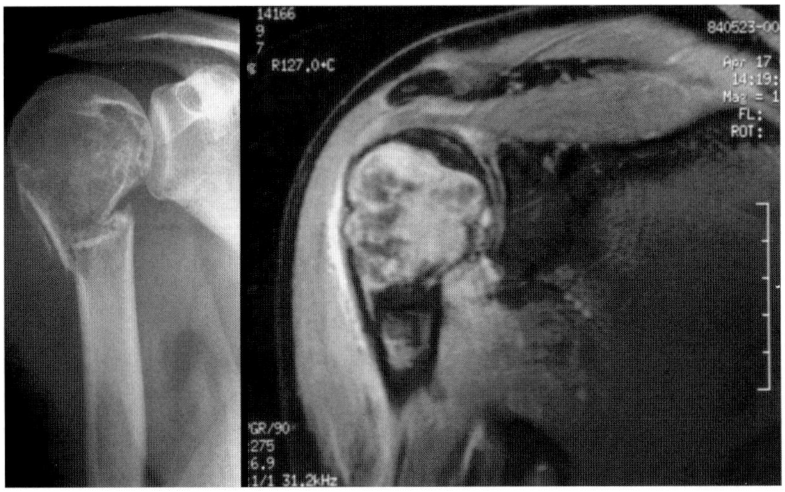

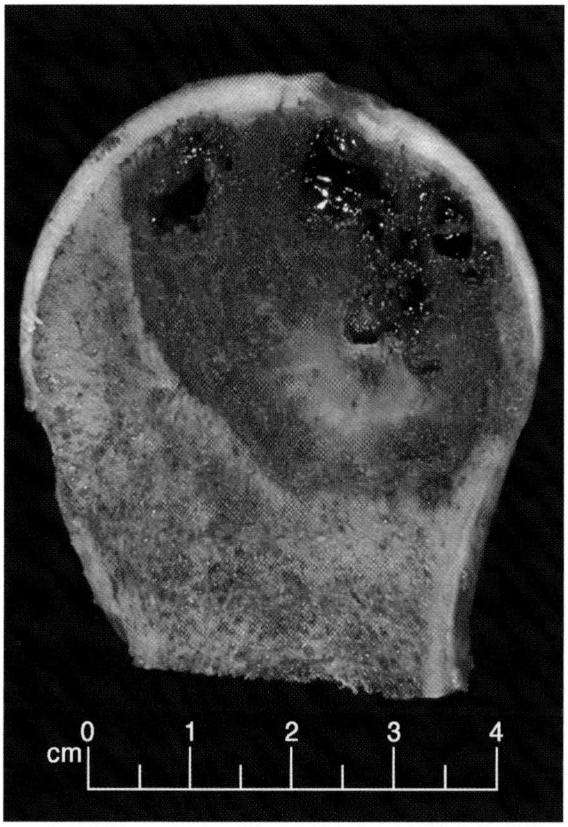

Figure 4-126

CLEAR CELL CHONDROSARCOMA

The tumor extends up to the articular surface and contains cystic changes. The preoperative diagnosis was chondroblastoma with secondary aneurysmal bone cyst.

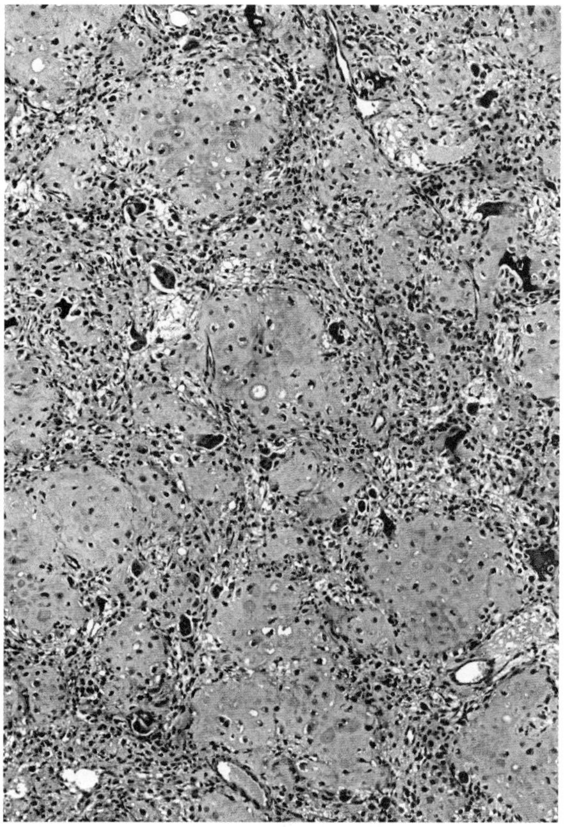

Figure 4-127

CLEAR CELL CHONDROSARCOMA

Low-power view of the lobulated growth pattern. Multinucleated giant cells intermingle with the cells between the lobules.

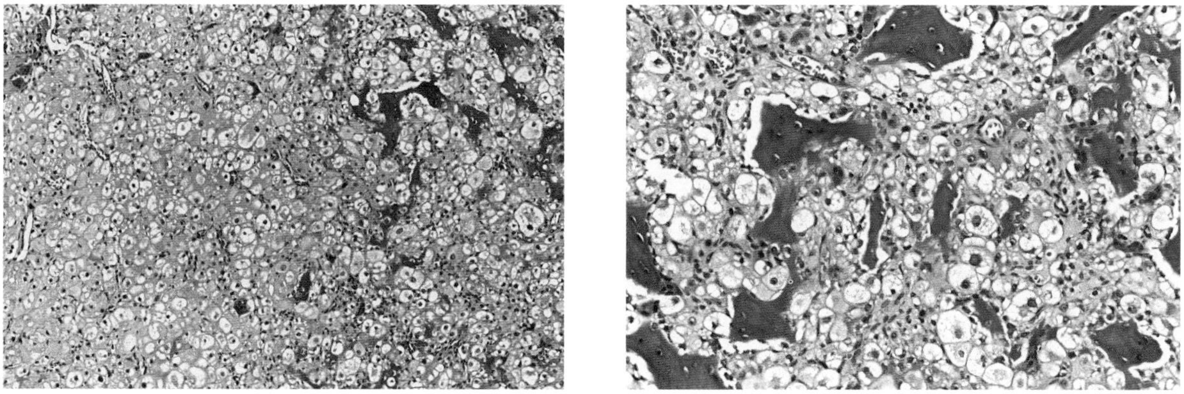

Figure 4-128

CLEAR CELL CHONDROSARCOMA

Left: A compact sheet of clear cells is associated with numerous small trabeculae of bone (right).
Right: The presence of woven bone trabeculae can lead to a mistaken diagnosis of osteosarcoma. With careful attention to the cytologic features of the clear cells, this error can be avoided.

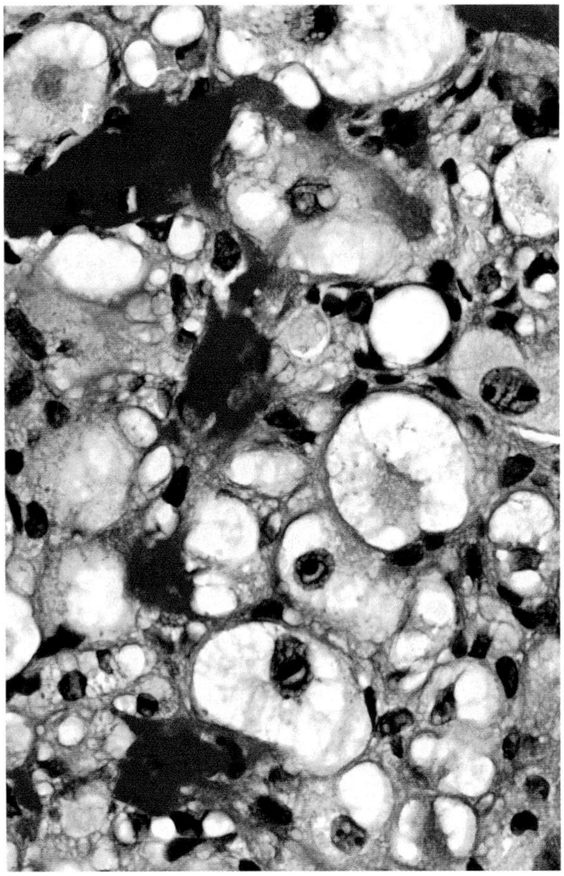

Figure 4-129

CLEAR CELL CHONDROSARCOMA

The tumor cells have distinct cytoplasmic boundaries, clear or pink cytoplasm, and round to oval nuclei with prominent nucleoli.

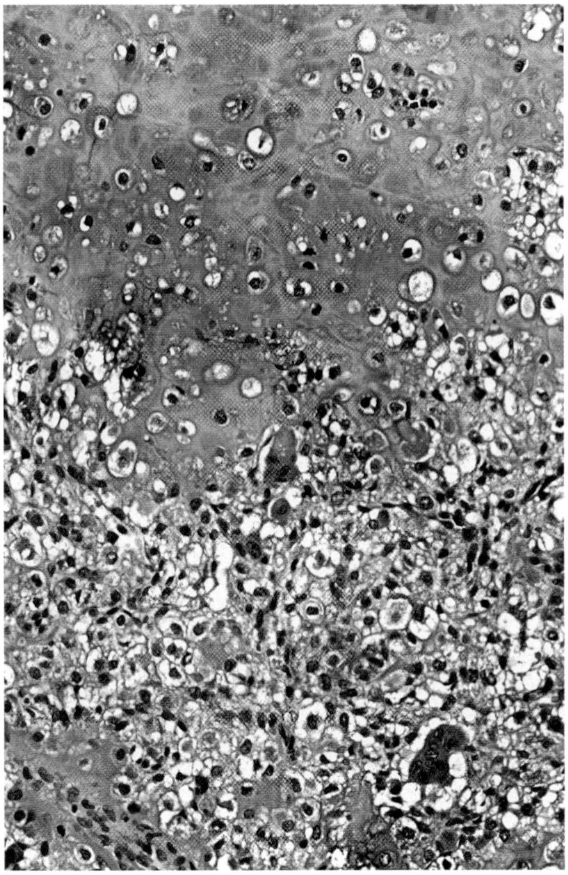

Figure 4-130

CLEAR CELL CHONDROSARCOMA

Hyaline cartilage with features of chondrosarcoma (top) may or may not be present in clear cell chondrosarcoma.

matrix can cause diagnostic difficulties and raise the possibility of metastatic carcinoma.

Differential Diagnosis. Clear cell chondrosarcoma may be mistaken for chondroblastoma, osteoblastoma, osteosarcoma, or aneurysmal bone cyst. The cells of chondroblastoma have elongated nuclei with a central groove, whereas the nuclei in clear cell chondrosarcoma are round. The presence of short bony trabeculae may suggest osteoblastoma, but clear cells are not a feature of that neoplasm. In conventional osteosarcoma, the cells have more pronounced cytologic features of malignancy than those in clear cell chondrosarcoma. Aneurysmal bone cysts usually are metaphyseal, whereas clear cell chondrosarcomas occur at the ends of bones. The presence of clusters of cells in the wall of a cyst confirms the diagnosis of clear cell chondrosarcoma. The clear cell appearance always suggests the diagnosis of metastatic renal cell carcinoma; however, the clinical features, the presence of giant cells, and the typical bone formation help in making the correct diagnosis.

Treatment and Prognosis. Wide resection is the treatment of choice. Recurrences may be long delayed. Metastases are to the lungs and other skeletal sites. Of the 48 patients reported by Bjornsson et al. (254), 7 died of metastatic disease.

REFERENCES

Osteochondroma

1. Ahn J, Ludecke HJ, Lindow S, et al. Cloning of the putative tumour suppressor gene for hereditary multiple exostoses (EXT1). Nat Genet 1995;11:137–43.
2. Amling M, Neff L, Tanaka S, et al. Bcl-2 lies downstream of parathyroid hormone-related peptide in a signaling pathway that regulates chondrocyte maturation during skeletal development. J Cell Biol 1997;136:205–13.
3. Bartsch O, Wuyts W, Van Hul W, et al. Delineation of a contiguous gene syndrome with multiple exostoses, enlarged parietal foramina, craniofacial dysostosis, and mental retardation, caused by deletions in the short arm of chromosome 11. Am J Hum Genet 1996;58:734–42.
4. Bellaiche Y, The I, Perrimon N. Tout-velu is a Drosophila homologue of the putative tumour suppressor EXT-1 and is needed for Hh diffusion. Nature 1998;394:85–8.
5. Bernard MA, Hall CE, Hogue DA, et al. Diminished levels of the putative tumor suppressor proteins EXT1 and EXT2 in exostosis chondrocytes. Cell Motil Cytoskeleton 2001;48:149–62.
6. Borges AM, Huvos AG, Smith J. Bursa formation and synovial chondrometaplasia associated with osteochondromas. Am J Clin Pathol 1981;75:648–53.
7. Bovee JV, Cleton-Jansen AM, Kuipers-Dijkshoorn NJ, et al. Loss of heterozygosity and DNA ploidy point to a diverging genetic mechanism in the origin of peripheral and central chondrosarcoma. Genes Chromosomes Cancer 1999;26:237–46.
8. Bovee JV, Cleton-Jansen AM, Wuyts W, et al. EXT-mutation analysis and loss of heterozygosity in sporadic and hereditary osteochondromas and secondary chondrosarcomas. Am J Hum Genet 1999;65:689–98.
9. Bovee JV, van den Broek LJ, Cleton-Jansen AM, Hogendoorn PC. Up-regulation of PTHrP and Bcl-2 expression characterizes the progression of osteochondroma towards peripheral chondrosarcoma and is a late event in central chondrosarcoma. Lab Invest 2000;80:1925–34.
10. Bridge JA. Cytogenetic and molecular cytogenetic techniques in orthopaedic surgery. J Bone Joint Surg Am 1993;75:606–14.
11. Bridge JA, Bhatia PS, Anderson JR, Neff JR. Biologic and clinical significance of cytogenetic and molecular cytogenetic abnormalities in benign and malignant cartilaginous lesions. Cancer Genet Cytogenet 1993;69:79–90.
12. Bridge JA, Nelson M, Orndal C, Bhatia P, Neff JR. Clonal karyotypic abnormalities of the hereditary multiple exostoses chromosomal loci 8q24.1 (EXT1) and 11p11-12 (EXT2) in patients with sporadic and hereditary osteochondromas. Cancer 1998;82:1657–63.
13. Carroll KL, Yandow SM, Ward K, Carey JC. Clinical correlation to genetic variations of hereditary multiple exostosis. J Pediatr Orthop 1999;19:785–91.
14. Cheung PK, McCormick C, Crawford BE, Esko JD, Tufaro F, Duncan G. Etiological point mutations in the hereditary multiple exostoses gene EXT1. A functional analysis of heparan sulfate polymerase activity. Am J Hum Genet 2001;69:55–66.
15. Chin KR, Kharrazi FD, Miller BS, Mankin HJ, Gebhardt MC. Osteochondromas of the distal aspect of the tibia or fibula. Natural history and treatment. J Bone Joint Surg Am 2000;82:1269–78.
16. Cook A, Raskind W, Blanton SH, et al. Genetic heterogeneity in families with hereditary multiple exostoses. Am J Hum Genet 1993;53:71–9.
17. Erlebacher A, Filvaroff EH, Gitelman SE, Derynck R. Toward a molecular understanding of skeletal development. Cell 1995;80:371–8.
18. Fechner RE, Mills SE. Tumors of the bones and joints. Atlas of Tumor Pathology, 3rd Series, Fascicle 8. Washington, DC: Armed Forces Institute of Pathology; 1993:79–83.
19. Feely MG, Boehm AK, Bridge RS, et al. Cytogenetic and molecular cytogenetic evidence of recurrent 8q24.1 loss in osteochondroma. Cancer Genet Cytogenet 2002;137:102–7.
20. Francannet C, Cohen-Tanugi A, Le Merrer M, Munnich A, Bonaventure J, Legeai-Mallet L. Genotype-phenotype correlation in hereditary multiple exostoses. J Med Genet 2001;38:430–4.
21. Garrison RC, Unni KK, McLeod RA, Pritchard DJ, Dahlin DC. Chondrosarcoma arising in osteochondroma. Cancer 1982;49:1890–7.
22. Goldfarb M. Functions of fibroblast growth factors in vertebrate development. Cytokine Growth Factor Rev 1996;7:311–25.
23. Hecht JT, Hogue D, Wang Y, et al. Hereditary multiple exostoses (EXT): mutational studies of familial EXT1 cases and EXT-associated malignancies. Am J Hum Genet 1997;60:80–6.
24. Herman TE, McAlister WH, Rosenthal D, Dehner LP. Case report 691. Radiation-induced osteochondromas (RIO) arising from the neural arch and producing compression of the spinal cord. Skeletal Radiol 1991;20:472–6.

25. Hou J, Parrish J, Ludecke HJ, et al. A 4-megabase YAC contig that spans the Langer-Giedion syndrome region on human chromosome 8q24.1: use in refining the location of the trichorhinophalangeal syndrome and multiple exostoses genes (TRPS1 and EXT1). Genomics 1995;29:87–97.
26. Jones KB, Morcuende JA. Of hedgehogs and hereditary bone tumors: re-examination of the pathogenesis of osteochondromas. Iowa Orthop J 2003;23:87–95.
27. Kivioja A, Ervasti H, Kinnunen J, Kaitila I, Wolf M, Bohling T. Chondrosarcoma in a family with multiple hereditary exostoses. J Bone Joint Surg Br 2000;82:261–6.
28. Lee JK, Yao L, Wirth CR. MR imaging of solitary osteochondromas: report of eight cases. AJR Am J Roentgenol 1987;149:557–60.
29. Legeai-Mallet L, Margaritte-Jeannin P, Lemdani M, et al. An extension of the admixture test for the study of genetic heterogeneity in hereditary multiple exostoses. Hum Genet 1997;99:298-302.
30. Le Merrer M, Legeai-Mallet L, Jeannin PM, et al. A gene for hereditary multiple exostoses maps to chromosome 19p. Hum Mol Genet 1994;3:717–22.
31. Libshitz HI, Cohen MA. Radiation-induced osteochondromas. Radiology 1982;142:643–7.
32. Lind T, Tufaro F, McCormick C, Lindahl U, Lidholt K. The putative tumor suppressors EXT1 and EXT2 are glycosyltransferases required for the biosynthesis of heparan sulfate. J Biol Chem 1998;273:26265–8.
33. Ludecke HJ, Johnson C, Wagner MJ, et al. Molecular definition of the shortest region of deletion overlap in the Langer-Giedion syndrome. Am J Hum Genet 1991;49:1197–206.
34. McCormick C, Duncan G, Goutsos KT, Tufaro F. The putative tumor suppressors EXT1 and EXT2 form a stable complex that accumulates in the Golgi apparatus and catalyzes the synthesis of heparan sulfate. Proc Natl Acad Sci U S A 2000;97:668–73.
35. McCormick C, Duncan G, Tufaro F. New perspectives on the molecular basis of hereditary bone tumours. Mol Med Today 1999;5:481–6.
36. McCormick C, Leduc Y, Martindale D, et al. The putative tumour suppressor EXT1 alters the expression of cell-surface heparan sulfate. Nat Genet 1998;19:158–61.
37. Mertens F, Rydholm A, Kreicbergs A, et al. Loss of chromosome band 8q24 in sporadic osteocartilaginous exostoses. Genes Chromosomes Cancer 1994;9:8–12.
38. Parrish JE, Wagner MJ, Hecht JT, Scott CI Jr, Wells DE. Molecular analysis of overlapping chromosomal deletions in patients with Langer-Giedion syndrome. Genomics 1991;11:54–61.
39. Porter DE, Simpson AH. The neoplastic pathogenesis of solitary and multiple osteochondromas. J Pathol 1999;188:119–25.
40. Potocki L, Shaffer LG. Interstitial deletion of 11(p11.2p12): a newly described contiguous gene deletion syndrome involving the gene for hereditary multiple exostoses (EXT2). Am J Med Genet 1996;62:319–25.
41. Raskind WH, Conrad EU 3rd, Matsushita M, et al. Evaluation of locus heterogeneity and EXT1 mutations in 34 families with hereditary multiple exostoses. Hum Mutat 1998;11:231–9.
42. Sandberg AA, Bridge JA. The cytogenetics of bone and soft tissue tumors. Austin: R. G. Landes: 1994.
43. Schmale GA, Conrad EU 3rd, Raskind WH. The natural history of hereditary multiple exostoses. J Bone Joint Surg Am 1994;76:986–92.
44. Simmons AD, Musy MM, Lopes CS, Hwang LY, Yang YP, Lovett M. A direct interaction between EXT proteins and glycosyltransferases is defective in hereditary multiple exostoses. Hum Mol Genet 1999;8:2155–64.
45. The I, Bellaiche Y, Perrimon N. Hedgehog movement is regulated through tout velu-dependent synthesis of a heparan sulfate proteoglycan. Mol Cell 1999;4:633–9.
46. Tiet TD, Alman BA. Developmental pathways in musculoskeletal neoplasia: involvement of the Indian Hedgehog–parathyroid hormone-related protein pathway. Pediatr Res 2003;53:539–43.
47. Toyoda H, Kinoshita-Toyoda A, Selleck SB. Structural analysis of glycosaminoglycans in Drosophila and Caenorhabditis elegans and demonstration that tout-velu, a Drosophila gene related to EXT tumor suppressors, affects heparan sulfate in vivo. J Biol Chem 2000;275:2269–75.
48. van der Eerden BC, Karperien M, Gevers EF, Lowik CW, Wit JM. Expression of Indian hedgehog, parathyroid hormone-related protein, and their receptors in the postnatal growth plate of the rat: evidence for a locally acting growth restraining feedback loop after birth. J Bone Miner Res 2000;15:1045–55.
49. Wu YQ, Badano JL, McCaskill C, Vogel H, Potocki L, Shaffer LG. Haploinsufficiency of ALX4 as a potential cause of parietal foramina in the 11p11.2 contiguous gene-deletion syndrome. Am J Hum Genet 2000;67:1327–32.
50. Wu YQ, Heutink P, de Vries BB, et al. Assignment of a second locus for multiple exostoses to the pericentromeric region of chromosome 11. Hum Mol Genet 1994;3:167–71.
51. Wuyts W, Van Hul W, De Boulle K, et al. Mutations in the EXT1 and EXT2 genes in hereditary multiple exostoses. Am J Hum Genet 1998;62:346–54.

52. Wuyts W, Van Hul W, Wauters J, et al. Positional cloning of a gene involved in hereditary multiple exostoses. Hum Mol Genet 1996;5:1547–57.

Multiple Hereditary Exostoses

53. Garrison RC, Unni KK, McLeod RA, Pritchard DJ, Dahlin DC. Chondrosarcoma arising in osteochondroma. Cancer 1982;49:1890–7.
54. Peterson HA. Multiple hereditary osteochondromata. Clin Orthop 1989;239:222–30.
55. Schmale GA, Conrad EU 3rd, Raskind WH. The natural history of hereditary multiple exostoses. J Bone Joint Surg Am 1994;76:986–92.

Enchondroma

56. Bridge JA, Persons DL, Neff JR, Bhatia P. Clonal karyotypic aberrations in enchondromas. Cancer Detect Prev 1992;16:215–9.
57. Buddingh EP, Naumann S, Nelson M, Neff JR, Birch N, Bridge JA. Cytogenetic findings in benign cartilaginous neoplasms. Cancer Genet Cytogenet 2003;141:164–8.
58. Dahlen A, Mertens F, Rydholm A, et al. Fusion, disruption, and expression of HMGA2 in bone and soft tissue chondromas. Mod Pathol 2003; 16:1132–40.
59. Gunawan B, Weber M, Bergmann F, Wildberger J, Niethard FU, Fuzesi L. Clonal chromosome abnormalities in enchondromas and chondrosarcomas. Cancer Genet Cytogenet 2000;120:127–30.
60. Hopyan S, Gokgoz N, Poon R, et al. A mutant PTH/PTHrP type I receptor in enchondromatosis. Nat Genet 2002;30:306–10.
61. Sawyer JR, Swanson CM, Lukacs JL, Nicholas RW, North PE, Thomas JR. Evidence of an association between 6q13-21 chromosome aberrations and locally aggressive behavior in patients with cartilage tumors. Cancer 1998;82:474–83.
62. Shimizu K, Kotoura Y, Nishijima N, Nakamura T. Enchondroma of the distal phalanx of the hand. J Bone Joint Surg Am 1997;79:898–900.
63. Teyssier JR, Ferre D. Frequent clonal chromosomal changes in human non-malignant tumors. Int J Cancer 1989;44:828–32

Multiple Chondromas

64. Fanburg JC, Meis-Kindblom JM, Rosenberg AE. Multiple enchondromas associated with spindle-cell hemangioendotheliomas. An overlooked variant of Maffucci's syndrome. Am J Surg Pathol 1995;19:1029–38.
65. Lewis RJ, Ketcham AS. Maffucci's syndrome: functional and neoplastic significance. Case report and review of the literature. J Bone Joint Surg Am 1973;55:1465–79.
66. Liu J, Hudkins PG, Swee RG, Unni KK. Bone sarcomas associated with Ollier's disease. Cancer 1987;59:1376–85.
67. Schwartz HS, Zimmerman NB, Simon MA, Wroble RR, Millar EA, Bonfiglio M. The malignant potential of enchondromatosis. J Bone Joint Surg Am 1987;69:269–74.
68. Sun TC, Swee RG, Shives TC, Unni KK. Chondrosarcoma in Maffucci's syndrome. J Bone Joint Surg Am 1985;67:1214–9.

Periosteal Chondroma

69. Bauer TW, Dorfman HD, Latham JT Jr. Periosteal chondroma. A clinicopathologic study of 23 cases. Am J Surg Pathol 1982;6:631–7.
70. Buddingh EP, Naumann S, Nelson M, Neff JR, Birch N, Bridge JA. Cytogenetic findings in benign cartilaginous neoplasms. Cancer Genet Cytogenet 2003;141:164–8.
71. deSantos LA, Spjut HJ. Periosteal chondroma: a radiographic spectrum. Skeletal Radiol 1981;6:15–20.
72. Lewis MM, Kenan S, Yabut SM, Norman A, Steiner G. Periosteal chondroma. A report of ten cases and review of the literature. Clin Orthop 1990;256:185–92.
73. Mandahl N, Willen H, Rydholm A, Heim S, Mitelman F. Rearrangement of band q13 on both chromosomes 12 in a periosteal chondroma. Genes Chromosomes Cancer 1993;6:121–3.
74. Nojima T, Unni KK, McLeod RA, Pritchard DJ. Periosteal chondroma and periosteal chondrosarcoma. Am J Surg Pathol 1985;9:666–77.
75. Tallini G, Dorfman H, Brys P, et al. Correlation between clinicopathological features and karyotype in 100 cartilaginous and chordoid tumours. A report from the Chromosomes and Morphology (CHAMP) Collaborative Study Group. J Pathol 2002;196:194–203.

Soft Tissue Chondroma

76. Buddingh EP, Naumann S, Nelson M, Neff JR, Birch N, Bridge JA. Cytogenetic findings in benign cartilaginous neoplasms. Cancer Genet Cytogenet 2003;141:164–8.
77. Cates JM, Rosenberg AE, O'Connell JX, Nielsen GP. Chondroblastoma-like chondroma of soft tissue: an underrecognized variant and its differential diagnosis. Am J Surg Pathol 2001;25:661–6.
78. Chung EB, Enzinger FM. Chondroma of soft parts. Cancer 1978;41:1414–24.
79. Dahlin DC, Salvador AH. Cartilaginous tumors of the soft tissues of the hands and feet. Mayo Clin Proc 1974;49:721–6.

80. Mandahl N, Willen H, Rydholm A, Heim S, Mitelman F. Rearrangement of band q13 on both chromosomes 12 in a periosteal chondroma. Genes Chromosomes Cancer 1993;6:121–3.
81. Shadan FF, Mascarello JT, Newbury RO, Dennis T, Spallone P, Stock AD. Supernumerary ring chromosomes derived from the long arm of chromosome 12 as the primary cytogenetic anomaly in a rare soft tissue chondroma. Cancer Genet Cytogenet 2000;118:144–7.
82. Tallini G, Dorfman H, Brys P, et al. Correlation between clinicopathological features and karyotype in 100 cartilaginous and chordoid tumours. A report from the Chromosomes and Morphology (CHAMP) Collaborative Study Group. J Pathol 2002;196:194–203.
83. Yamada T, Irisa T, Nakano S, Tokunaga O. Extraskeletal chondroma with chondroblastic and granuloma-like elements. Clin Orthop 1995;315:257–61.

Chondroblastoma

84. Bridge JA, Bhatia PS, Anderson JR, Neff JR. Biologic and clinical significance of cytogenetic and molecular cytogenetic abnormalities in benign and malignant cartilaginous lesions. Cancer Genet Cytogenet 1993;69:79–90.
85. Dahlin DC, Ivins JC. Benign chondroblastoma. A study of 125 cases. Cancer 1972;30:401–13.
86. Fanning CV, Sneige NS, Carrasco CH, Ayala AG, Murray JA, Raymond AK. Fine needle aspiration cytology of chondroblastoma of bone. Cancer 1990;65:1847–63.
87. Hazarika D, Kumar RV, Rao CR, Mukherjee G, Pattabhiraman V, Shekar MC. Fine needle aspiration cytology of chondroblastoma and chondromyxoid fibroma: a report of two cases. Acta Cytol 1994;38:592–6.
88. Huang L, Cheng YY, Chow LT, Zheng MH, Kumta SM. Receptor activator of NF-κB ligand (RANKL) is expressed in chondroblastoma: possible involvement in osteoclastic giant cell recruitment. J Clin Pathol: Mol Pathol 2003; 56:116–20.
89. Hudson TM, Hawkins IF Jr. Radiological evaluation of chondroblastoma. Radiology 1981; 139:1–10.
90. Jain M, Kaur M, Kapoor S, Arora DS. Cytological features of chondroblastoma: a case report with review of the literature. Diagn Cytopathol 2000;23:348–50.
91. Kilpatrick SE, Pike EJ, Geisinger KR, Ward WG. Chondroblastoma of bone: use of fine-needle aspiration biopsy and potential diagnostic pitfalls. Diagn Cytopathol 1997;16:65–71.
92. Kurt AM, Unni KK, Sim FH, McLeod RA. Chondroblastoma of bone. Hum Pathol 1989; 20:965–76.
93. Kyriakos M, Land VJ, Penning HL, Parker SG. Metastatic chondroblastoma. Report of a fatal case with a review of the literature on atypical, aggressive, and malignant chondroblastoma. Cancer 1985;55:1770–89.
94. Levine GD, Bensch KG. Chondroblastoma—the nature of the basic cell. A study by means of histochemistry, tissue culture, electron microscopy, and autoradiography. Cancer 1972;29:1546–62.
95. Mark J, Wedell B, Dahlenfors R, Grepp C, Burian P. Human benign chondroblastoma with a pseudodiploid stemline characterized by a complex and balanced translocation. Cancer Genet Cytogenet 1992;58:14–7.
96. McLeod RA, Beabout JW. The roentgenographic features of chondroblastoma. Am J Roentgenol Radium Ther Nucl Med 1973;118:464–71.
97. Oxtoby JW, Davies AM. MRI characteristics of chondroblastoma. Clin Radiol 1996;51:22–6.
98. Ramappa AJ, Lee FY, Tang P, Carlson JR, Gebhardt MC, Mankin HJ. Chondroblastoma of bone. J Bone Joint Surg Am 2000;82:1140–5.
99. Romeo S, Bovee JV, Jadnanansing NA, Taminiau AH, Hogendoorn PC. Expression of cartilage growth plate signalling molecules in chondroblastoma. J Pathol 2004;202:113–20.
100. Schaffler A, Ehling A, Neumann E, et al. Genomic organization, promoter, amino acid sequence, chromosomal localization, and expression of the human gene for CORS-26 (collagenous repeat-containing sequence of 26-kDa protein). Biochem Biophys Acta 2003;1630: 123–9.
101. Schajowicz F, Gallardo H. Epiphyseal chondroblastoma of bone. A clinico-pathological study of sixty-nine cases. J Bone Joint Surg Br 1970;52:205–26.
102. Springfield DS, Capanna R, Gherlinzoni F, Picci P, Campanacci M. Chondroblastoma. A review of seventy cases. J Bone Joint Surg Am 1985;67:748–55.
103. Swarts SJ, Neff JR, Johansson SL, Nelson M, Bridge JA. Significance of abnormalities of chromosomes 5 and 8 in chondroblastoma. Clin Orthop 1998;349:189–93.
104. van Zelderen-Bhola SL, Bovee JV, Wessels HW, et al. Ring chromosome 4 as the sole cytogenetic anomaly in a chondroblastoma: a case report and review of the literature. Cancer Genet Cytogenet 1998;105:109–12.
105. Walaas L, Kindblom LG, Gunterberg B, Bergh P. Light and electron microscopic examination of fine-needle aspirates in the preoperative diagnosis of cartilaginous tumors. Diagn Cytopathol 1990;6:396–408.

106. Weatherall PT, Maale GE, Mendelsohn DB, Sherry CS, Erdman WE, Pascoe HR. Chondroblastoma: classic and confusing appearance at MR imaging. Radiology 1994;190:467–74.

Chondromyxoid Fibroma

107. Dahlin DC. Chondromyxoid fibroma of bone, with emphasis on its morphological relationship to benign chondroblastoma. Cancer 1956;9:195–203.
108. Granter SR, Renshaw AA, Kozakewich HP, Fletcher JA. The pericentromeric inversion, inv (6)(p25q13), is a novel diagnostic marker in chondromyxoid fibroma. Mod Pathol 1998;11:1071–4.
109. Halbert AR, Harrison WR, Hicks MJ, Davino N, Cooley LD. Cytogenetic analysis of a scapular chondromyxoid fibroma. Cancer Genet Cytogenet 1998;104:52–6.
110. Hazarika D, Kumar RV, Rao CR, Mukherjee G, Pattabhiraman V, Shekar MC. Fine needle aspiration cytology of chondroblastoma and chondromyxoid fibroma. A report of two cases. Acta Cytol 1994;38:592–6.
111. Jaffe HL, Lichtenstein L. Chondromyxoid fibroma of bone: a distinctive benign tumor likely to be mistaken especially for chondrosarcoma. Arch Pathol 1948;45:541–51.
112. Kyriakos M. Soft tissue implantation of chondromyxoid fibroma. Am J Surg Pathol 1979;3:363–72.
113. Layfield LJ, Ferreiro JA. Fine-needle aspiration cytology of chondromyxoid fibroma: a case report. Diagn Cytopathol 1988;4:148–51.
114. Rahimi A, Beabout JW, Ivins JC, Dahlin DC. Chondromyxoid fibroma: a clinicopathologic study of 76 cases. Cancer 1972;30:726–36.
115. Robinson LH, Unni KK, O'Laughlin S, Beabout JW, Siegal GP. Surface chondromyxoid fibroma of bone [Abstract]. Mod Pathol 1994;7:10A.
116. Safar A, Nelson M, Neff JR, et al. Recurrent anomalies of 6q25 in chondromyxoid fibroma. Hum Pathol 2000;31:306–11.
117. Sawyer JR, Swanson CM, Lukacs JL, Nicholas RW, North PE, Thomas JR. Evidence of an association between 6q13-21 chromosome aberrations and locally aggressive behavior in patients with cartilage tumors. Cancer 1998;82:474–83.
118. Soder S, Inwards C, Muller S, Kirchner T, Aigner T. Cell biology and matrix biochemistry of chondromyxoid fibroma. Am J Clin Pathol 2001;116:271–7.
119. Tallini G, Dorfman H, Brys P, et al. Correlation between clinicopathological features and karyotype in 100 cartilaginous and chordoid tumours. A report from the Chromosomes and Morphology (CHAMP) Collaborative Study Group. J Pathol 2002;196:194–203.
120. Wu CT, Inwards CY, O'Laughlin S, Rock MG, Beabout JW, Unni KK. Chondromyxoid fibroma of bone: a clinicopathologic review of 278 cases. Hum Pathol 1998;29:438–46.
121. Zillmer DA, Dorfman HD. Chondromyxoid fibroma of bone: thirty-six cases with clinicopathologic correlation. Hum Pathol 1989;20:952–64.

Chondrosarcoma

122. Abdul-Karim FW, Wasman JK, Pitlik D. Needle aspiration cytology of chondrosarcomas. Acta Cytol 1993;37:655–60.
123. Adler CP, Herget GW, Neuburger M. Cartilaginous tumors: prognostic applications of cytophotometric DNA analysis. Cancer 1995;76: 1176–80.
124. Antonescu CR, Argani P, Erlandson RA, Healey JH, Ladanyi M, Huvos AG. Skeletal and extraskeletal myxoid chondrosarcoma: a comparative clinicopathologic, ultrastructural, and molecular study. Cancer 1998;83:1504–21.
125. Asp J, Sangiorgi L, Inerot SE, et al. Changes of the p16 gene but not the p53 gene in human chondrosarcoma tissues. Int J Cancer 2000;85:782–6.
126. Ayala G, Liu C, Nicosia R, Horowitz S, Lackman R. Microvasculature and VEGF expression in cartilaginous tumors. Hum Pathol 2000;31:341–6.
127. Berend KR, Toth AP, Harrelson JM, Layfield LJ, Hey LA, Scully SP. Association between ratio of matrix metalloproteinase-1 to tissue inhibitor of metalloproteinase-1 and local recurrence, metastasis, and survival in human chondrosarcoma. J Bone Joint Surg Am 1998;80:11–7.
128. Bjornsson J, McLeod RA, Unni KK, Ilstrup DM, Pritchard DJ. Primary chondrosarcoma of long bones and limb girdles. Cancer 1998;83:2105–19.
129. Block RS, Burton RI. Multiple chondrosarcomas in a hand: a case report. J Hand Surg [Am] 1977;2:310–3.
130. Bovee JV, Cleton-Jansen AM, Kuipers-Dijkshoorn NJ, et al. Loss of heterozygosity and DNA ploidy point to a diverging genetic mechanism in the origin of peripheral and central chondrosarcoma. Genes Chromosomes Cancer 1999;26:237–46.
131. Bovee JV, Sciot R, Cin PD, et al. Chromosome 9 alterations and trisomy 22 in central chondrosarcoma: a cytogenetic and DNA flow cytometric analysis of chondrosarcoma subtypes. Diagn Mol Pathol 2001;10:228–35.
132. Bovee JV, van Royen M, Bardoel AF, et al. Near-haploidy and subsequent polyploidization characterize the progression of peripheral chondrosarcoma. Am J Pathol 2000;157:1587–95.

133. Bridge JA, Bhatia PS, Anderson JR, Neff JR. Biologic and clinical significance of cytogenetic and molecular cytogenetic abnormalities in benign and malignant cartilaginous lesions. Cancer Genet Cytogenet 1993;69:79–90.
134. Brody RI, Ueda T, Hamelin A, et al. Molecular analysis of the fusion of EWS to an orphan nuclear receptor gene in extraskeletal myxoid chondrosarcoma. Am J Pathol 1997;150:1049–58.
135. Campanacci M, Guernelli N, Leonessa C, Boni A. Chondrosarcoma: a study of 133 cases, 80 with long term follow up. Ital J Orthop Traumatol 1975;1:387–414.
136. Castresana JS, Barrios C, Gomez L, Kreicbergs A. Amplification of the c-myc proto-oncogene in human chondrosarcoma. Diagn Mol Pathol 1992;1:235–8.
137. Clark J, Benjamin H, Gill S, et al. Fusion of the EWS gene to CHN, a member of the steroid/thyroid receptor gene superfamily, in a human myxoid chondrosarcoma. Oncogene 1996;12:229–35.
138. Coughlan B, Feliz A, Ishida T, Czerniak B, Dorfman HD. p53 expression and DNA ploidy of cartilage lesions. Hum Pathol 1995;26:620–4.
139. Day SJ, Nelson M, Rosenthal H, Vergara GG, Bridge JA. Der(16)t(1;16)(q21;q13) as a secondary structural aberration in yet a third sarcoma, extraskeletal myxoid chondrosarcoma. Genes Chromosomes Cancer 1997;20:425–7.
140. Dobashi Y, Sugimura H, Sato A, et al. Possible association of p53 overexpression and mutation with high-grade chondrosarcoma. Diagn Mol Pathol 1993;2:257–63.
141. Dorfman HD, Czerniak B. Bone tumors. St. Louis: Mosby; 1998:353–440.
142. Eisenberg MB, Woloschak M, Sen C, Wolfe D. Loss of heterozygosity in the retinoblastoma tumor suppressor gene in skull base chordomas and chondrosarcomas. Surg Neurol 1997;47: 156–60.
143. Enzinger FM, Weiss SW. Soft tissue tumors, 3rd ed. St. Louis: Mosby; 1995.
144. Evans HL, Ayala AG, Romsdahl MM. Prognostic factors in chondrosarcoma of bone: a clinicopathologic analysis with emphasis on histologic grading. Cancer 1977;40:818–31.
145. Fechner RE, Mills SE. Tumors of the bones and joints. Atlas of Tumor Pathology, 3rd Series, Fascicle 8. Washington, DC: Armed Forces Institute of Pathology; 1993:101-12.
146. Franchi A, Calzolari A, Zampi G. Immunohistochemical detection of c-fos and c-jun expression in osseous and cartilaginous tumours of the skeleton. Virchows Arch 1998;432:515–9.
147. Gitelis S, Bertoni F, Picci P, Campanacci M. Chondrosarcoma of bone. The experience at the Istituto Ortopedico Rizzoli. J Bone Joint Surg Am 1981;63:1248–57.
148. Greenspan A. Orthopedic radiology: a practical approach, 3rd ed. Philadelphia: Lippincott Williams & Wilkins; 2000:673–7.
149. Grigioni WF, Fiorentino M, D'Errico A, et al. Overexpression of c-met protooncogene product and raised Ki67 index in hepatocellular carcinomas with respect to benign liver conditions. Hepatology 1995;21:1543–6.
150. Gunawan B, Weber M, Bergmann F, Wildberger J, Niethard FU, Fuzesi L. Clonal chromosome abnormalities in enchondromas and chondrosarcomas. Cancer Genet Cytogenet 2000;120:127–30.
151. Hackel CG, Krueger S, Grote HJ, et al. Overexpression of cathepsin B and urokinase plasminogen activator is associated with increased risk of recurrence and metastasis in patients with chondrosarcoma. Cancer 2000;89:995–1003.
152. Helio H, Karaharju E, Bohling T, Kivioja A, Nordling S. Chondrosarcoma of bone. A clinical and DNA flow cytometric study. Eur J Surg Oncol 1995;21:408–13.
153. Herget GW, Neuburger M, Adler CP. Prognostic significance of nuclear DNA content in chondrosarcoma. Ann Diagn Pathol 2000;4:11–6.
154. Hinrichs SH, Jaramillo MA, Gumerlock PH, Gardner MB, Lewis JP, Freeman AE. Myxoid chondrosarcoma with a translocation involving chromosomes 9 and 22. Cancer Genet Cytogenet 1985;14:219–26.
155. Hisaoka M, Ishida T, Imamura T, Hashimoto H. *TGF* is a novel fusion partner of *NOR1* in extraskeletal myxoid chondrosarcoma. Genes Chromosomes Cancer 2004;40:325–8.
156. Huvos AG. Chondrosarcoma and its variants. J Orthop Sci 1996;1:90–7.
157. Huvos AG, Marcove RC. Chondrosarcoma in the young. A clinicopathologic analysis of 79 patients younger than 21 years of age. Am J Surg Pathol 1987;11:930–42.
158. Jagasia AA, Block JA, Qureshi A, et al. Chromosome 9 related aberrations and deletions of the CDKN2 and MTS2 putative tumor suppressor genes in human chondrosarcomas. Cancer Lett 1996;105:91–103.
159. Jiang X, Dutton CM, Qi W, et al. Inhibition of MMP-1 expression by antisense RNA decreases invasiveness of human chondrosarcoma. J Orthop Res 2003;21:1063–70.
160. Kanoe H, Nakayama T, Murakami H, et al. Amplification of the CDK4 gene in sarcomas: tumor specificity and relationship with the RB gene mutation. Anticancer Res 1998;18:2317–21.

161. Kawashima A, Okada Y, Nakanishi I, Ueda Y, Iwata K, Roessner A. Immunolocalization of matrix metalloproteinases and tissue inhibitors of metalloproteinases in human chondrosarcomas. Gen Diagn Pathol 1997;142:129–37.
162. Kivioja A, Ervasti H, Kinnunen J, Kaitila I, Wolf M, Bohling T. Chondrosarcoma in a family with multiple hereditary exostoses. J Bone Joint Surg Br 2000;82:261–6.
163. Kleist B, Poetsch M, Lang C, et al. Clear cell chondrosarcoma of the larynx: a case report of a rare histologic variant in an uncommon localization. Am J Surg Pathol 2002;26:386–92.
164. Kreicbergs A, Boquist L, Borssen B, Larsson SE. Prognostic factors in chondrosarcoma: a comparative study of cellular DNA content and clinicopathologic features. Cancer 1982;50:577–83.
165. Kusuzaki K, Murata H, Takeshita H, et al. Usefulness of cytofluorometric DNA ploidy analysis in distinguishing benign cartilaginous tumors from chondrosarcomas. Mod Pathol 1999;12:863–72.
166. Labelle Y, Zucman J, Stenman G, et al. Oncogenic conversion of a novel orphan nuclear receptor by chromosome translocation. Hum Mol Genet 1995;4:2219–26.
167. Larramendy ML, Mandahl N, Mertens F, et al. Clinical significance of genetic imbalances revealed by comparative genomic hybridization in chondrosarcomas. Hum Pathol 1999;30:1247–53.
168. Larsson SE, Borssen B, Boquist L. Chondrosarcoma: a multifactorial clinical and histopathological study with particular regard to therapy and survival. Int Orthop 1979;2:333–41.
169. Lichtenstein L, Jaffe HL. Chondrosarcoma of bone. Am J Pathol 1943;19:553–89.
170. Lin C, Meitner PA, Terek RM. PTEN mutation is rare in chondrosarcoma. Diagn Mol Pathol 2002;11:22–6.
171. Liu J, Hudkins PG, Swee RG, Unni KK. Bone sarcomas associated with Ollier's disease. Cancer 1987;59:1376–85.
172. Mandahl N, Gustafson P, Mertens F, et al. Cytogenetic aberrations and their prognostic impact in chondrosarcoma. Genes Chromosomes Cancer 2002;33:188–200.
173. Mankin HJ, Fondren G, Hornicek FJ, Gebhardt MC, Rosenberg AE. The use of flow cytometry in assessing malignancy in bone and soft tissue tumors. Clin Orthop 2002;397:95–105.
174. Mirra JM, Gold R, Downs J, Eckardt JJ. A new histologic approach to the differentiation of enchondroma and chondrosarcoma of the bones. A clinicopathologic analysis of 51 cases. Clin Orthop 1985;201:214–37.
175. Murata H, Kusuzaki K, Kuzuhara A, et al. DNA ploidy alterations detected during dedifferentiation of periosteal chondrosarcoma. Anticancer Res 1999;19:2285–8.
176. Naka T, Iwamoto Y, Shinohara N, Ushijima M, Chuman H, Tsuneyoshi M. Expression of c-met proto-oncogene product (c-MET) in benign and malignant bone tumors. Mod Pathol 1997;10:832–8.
177. Nawa G, Ueda T, Mori S, et al. Prognostic significance of Ki67 (MIB1) proliferation index and p53 over-expression in chondrosarcomas. Int J Cancer 1996;69:86–91.
178. O'Donovan M, Russell JM, O'Leary JJ, Gillan JA, Lawler MP, Gaffney EF. Abl expression, tumour grade, and apoptosis in chondrosarcoma. Mol Pathol 1999;52:341-4.
179. O'Neill AJ, Cotter TG, Russell JM, Gaffney EF. Abl expression in human fetal and adult tissues, tumours, and tumour microvessels. J Pathol 1997;183:325–9.
180. Oshiro Y, Chaturvedi V, Hayden D, et al. Altered p53 is associated with aggressive behavior of chondrosarcoma: a long term follow-up study. Cancer 1998;83:2324–34.
181. Ozisik YY, Meloni AM, Spanier SS, Bush CH, Kingsley KL, Sandberg AA. Deletion 1p in a low-grade chondrosarcoma in a patient with Ollier disease. Cancer Genet Cytogenet 1998;105:128–33.
182. Panagopoulos I, Mencinger M, Dietrich CU, et al. Fusion of the RBP56 and CHN genes in extraskeletal myxoid chondrosarcomas with translocation t(9;17)(q22;q11). Oncogene 1999;18:7594–8.
183. Park HR, Kim YW, Jung WW, Kim HS, Unni KK, Park YK. Evaluation of HER-2/neu status by real-time quantitative PCR in malignant cartilaginous tumors. Int J Oncol 2004;24:575–80.
184. Pisters LL, Troncoso P, Zhau HE, Li W, von Eschenbach AC, Chung LW. c-met proto-oncogene expression in benign and malignant human prostate tissues. J Urol 1995;154:293–8.
185. Pompetti F, Rizzo P, Simon RM, et al. Oncogene alterations in primary, recurrent, and metastatic human bone tumors. J Cell Biochem 1996;63:37–50.
186. Pritchard DJ, Lunke RJ, Taylor WF, Dahlin DC, Medley BE. Chondrosarcoma: a clinicopathologic and statistical analysis. Cancer 1980;45: 149–57.
187. Ptaszynski K, Ramesh KH, Cannizzaro LA. Clonal chromosome aberrations with monosomy of chromosome 8 in a case of grade III chondrosarcoma. Cancer Genet Cytogenet 1997;97:60–3.
188. Raskind WH, Conrad EU, Matsushita M. Frequent loss of heterozygosity for markers on chromosome arm 10q in chondrosarcomas. Genes Chromosomes Cancer 1996;16:138–43.

189. Rosier RN, O'Keefe RJ, Teot LA, et al. P-glycoprotein expression in cartilaginous tumors. J Surg Oncol 1997;65:95–105.
190. Sakamoto A, Oda Y, Iwamoto Y, Tsuneyoshi M. Expression of membrane type 1 matrix metalloproteinase, matrix metalloproteinase 2 and tissue inhibitor of metalloproteinase 2 in human cartilaginous tumors with special emphasis on mesenchymal and dedifferentiated chondrosarcoma. J Cancer Res Clin Oncol 1999;125:541–8.
191. Sandberg AA, Bridge JA. Updates on the cytogenetics and molecular genetics of bone and soft tissue tumors: osteosarcoma and related tumors. Cancer Genet Cytogenet 2003;145:1–30.
192. Sawyer JR, Swanson CM, Lukacs JL, Nicholas RW, North PE, Thomas JR. Evidence of an association between 6q13-21 chromosome aberrations and locally aggressive behavior in patients with cartilage tumors. Cancer 1998;82:474–83.
193. Schoedel KE, Ohori NP, Greco MA, Steiner GC. Expression of metalloproteinases and tissue inhibitor in cartilaginous neoplasms of bone. Appl Immunohistochem Mol Morphol 1997;5:111–6.
194. Scotlandi K, Baldini N, Oliviero M, et al. Expression of Met/hepatocyte growth factor receptor gene and malignant behavior of musculoskeletal tumors. Am J Pathol 1996;149:1209–19.
195. Scotlandi K, Serra M, Manara MC, et al. Clinical relevance of Ki-67 expression in bone tumors. Cancer 1995;75:806–14.
196. Scully SP, Berend KR, Toth A, Qi WN, Qi Z, Block JA. Marshall Urist Award. Interstitial collagenase gene expression correlates with in vitro invasion in human chondrosarcoma. Clin Orthop 2000;376:291–303.
197. Shakunaga T, Ozaki T, Ohara N, et al. Expression of connective tissue growth factor in cartilaginous tumors. Cancer 2000;89:1466–73.
198. Shih CS, Wang LS, Yang SS, et al. DNA flow cytometric analysis of chest-wall chondroma and chondrosarcoma. Scand J Thorac Cardiovasc Surg 1996;30:157–61.
199. Simms WW, Ordonez NG, Johnston D, Ayala AG, Czerniak B. p53 expression in dedifferentiated chondrosarcoma. Cancer 1995;76:223–7.
200. Sjogren H, Meis-Kindblom J, Kindblom LG, Aman P, Stenman G. Fusion of the EWS-related gene TAF2N to TEC in extraskeletal myxoid chondrosarcoma. Cancer Res 1999;59:5064–7.
201. Sjogren H, Meis-Kindblom JM, Orndal C, et al. Studies on the molecular pathogenesis of extraskeletal myxoid chondrosarcoma—cytogenetic, molecular genetic, and cDNA microarray analyses. Am J Pathol 2003;162:781–92.
202. Sjogren H, Wedell B, Meis-Kindblom JM, Kindblom LG, Stenman G, Kindblom JM. Fusion of the NH2-terminal domain of the basic helix-loop-helix protein TCF12 to TEC in extraskeletal myxoid chondrosarcoma with translocation t(9;15)(q22;q21). Cancer Res 2000;60:6832–5.
203. Skoog L, Pereira ST, Tani E. Fine-needle aspiration cytology and immunocytochemistry of soft-tissue tumors and osteo/chondrosarcomas of the head and neck. Diagn Cytopathol 1999;20:131–6.
204. Springfield DS, Gebhardt MC, McGuire MH. Chondrosarcoma: a review. J Bone Joint Surg Am 1996;78:141–9.
205. Sun TC, Swee RG, Shives TC, Unni KK. Chondrosarcoma in Maffucci's syndrome. J Bone Joint Surg Am 1985;67:1214–9.
206. Swarts SJ, Neff JR, Nelson M, Johansson S, Bridge JA. Chromosomal abnormalities in low grade chondrosarcoma and a review of the literature. Cancer Genet Cytogenet 1997;98:126–30.
207. Tallini G, Dorfman H, Brys P, et al. Correlation between clinicopathological features and karyotype in 100 cartilaginous and chordoid tumours. A report from the Chromosomes and Morphology (CHAMP) Collaborative Study Group. J Pathol 2002;196:194–203.
208. Terek RM, Healey JH, Garin-Chesa P, Mak S, Huvos A, Albino AP. p53 mutations in chondrosarcoma. Diagn Mol Pathol 1998;7:51–6.
209. Terek RM, Schwartz GK, Devaney K, et al. Chemotherapy and P-glycoprotein expression in chondrosarcoma. J Orthop Res 1998;16:585–90.
210. Toriyama M, Rosenberg AE, Mankin HJ, Fondren T, Treadwell BV, Towle CA. Matrix metalloproteinase digestion of aggrecan in human cartilage tumours. Eur J Cancer 1998;34:1969–73.
211. Tunc M, Ekinci C. Chondrosarcoma diagnosed by fine needle aspiration cytology. Acta Cytol 1996;40:283–8.
212. Unni KK. Dahlin's bone tumors: general aspects and data on 11,087 cases, 5th ed. Philadelphia: Lippincott-Raven; 1996:71–108.
213. Uria JA, Balbin M, Lopez JM, et al. Collagenase-3 (MMP-13) expression in chondrosarcoma cells and its regulation by basic fibroblast growth factor. Am J Pathol 1998;153:91–101.
214. van Beerendonk HM, Rozeman LB, Taminiau AH, et al. Molecular analysis of the INK4A/INK4A-ARF gene locus in conventional (central) chondrosarcomas and enchondromas: indication of an important gene for tumour progression. J Pathol 2004;202:359–66.
215. Wadayama B, Toguchida J, Yamaguchi T, Sasaki MS, Yamamuro T. p53 expression and its relationship to DNA alterations in bone and soft tissue sarcomas. Br J Cancer 1993;68:1134–9.

216. Walaas L, Kindblom LG, Gunterberg B, Bergh P. Light and electron microscopic examination of fine-needle aspirates in the preoperative diagnosis of cartilaginous tumors. Diagn Cytopathol 1990;6:396–408.
217. Yamaguchi T, Toguchida J, Wadayama B, et al. Loss of heterozygosity and tumor suppressor gene mutations in chondrosarcomas. Anticancer Res 1996;16:2009–15.
218. Young CL, Sim FH, Unni KK, McLeod RA. Chondrosarcoma of bone in children. Cancer 1990;66:1641–8.
219. Yu C, Le AT, Yeger H, Perbal B, Alman BA. NOV (CCN3) regulation in the growth plate and CCN family member expression in cartilage neoplasia. J Pathol 2003;201:609–15.

Chondrosarcoma of the Small Bones of the Hands and Feet

220. Bovee JV, van der Heul RO, Taminiau AH, Hogendoorn PC. Chondrosarcoma of the phalanx: a locally aggressive lesion with minimal metastatic potential: a report of 35 cases and a review of the literature. Cancer 1999;86:1724–32.
221. Karabela-Bouropoulou V, Patra-Malli F, Agnantis N. Chondrosarcoma of the thumb: an unusual case with lung and cutaneous metastases and death of the patient 6 years after treatment. J Cancer Res Clin Oncol 1986;112:71–4.
222. Mankin HJ. Chondrosarcomas of digits: are they really malignant? Cancer 1999;86:1635-7.
223. Ogose A, Unni KK, Swee RG, May GK, Rowland CM, Sim FH. Chondrosarcoma of small bones of the hands and feet. Cancer 1997;80:50–9.

Periosteal Chondrosarcoma

224. Bertoni F, Boriani S, Laus M, Campanacci M. Periosteal chondrosarcoma and periosteal osteosarcoma. Two distinct entities. J Bone Joint Surg Br 1982;64:370–6.
225. Nojima T, Unni KK, McLeod RA, Pritchard DJ. Periosteal chondroma and periosteal chondrosarcoma. Am J Surg Pathol 1985;9:666–77.

Dedifferentiated Chondrosarcoma

226. Aigner T, Unni KK. Is dedifferentiated chondrosarcoma a 'de-differentiated' chondrosarcoma? J Pathol 1999;189:445–7.
227. Bovee JV, Cleton-Jansen AM, Rosenberg C, Taminiau AH, Cornelisse CJ, Hogendoorn PC. Molecular genetic characterization of both components of a dedifferentiated chondrosarcoma, with implications for its histogenesis. J Pathol 1999;189:454–62.
228. Bridge JA, DeBoer J, Travis J, et al. Simultaneous interphase cytogenetic analysis and fluorescence immunophenotyping of dedifferentiated chondrosarcoma. Implications for histopathogenesis. Am J Pathol 1994;144:215–20.
229. Capanna R, Bertoni F, Bettelli G, et al. Dedifferentiated chondrosarcoma. J Bone Joint Surg Am 1988;70:60–9.
230. Dahlin DC, Beabout JW. Dedifferentiation of low-grade chondrosarcomas. Cancer 1971;28:461–6.
231. Frassica FJ, Unni KK, Beabout JW, Sim FH. Dedifferentiated chondrosarcoma. A report of the clinicopathological features and treatment of seventy-eight cases. J Bone Joint Surg Am 1986;68:1197–205.
232. Henricks WH, Chu YC, Goldblum JR, Weiss SW. Dedifferentiated liposarcoma: a clinicopathological analysis of 155 cases with a proposal for an expanded definition of dedifferentiation. Am J Surg Pathol 1997;21:271–81.
233. Jaffe HL. Tumors and tumorous conditions of the bones and joints. Philadelphia: Lea & Febiger; 1958:314–40.
234. Johnson S, Tetu B, Ayala AG, Chawla SP. Chondrosarcoma with additional mesenchymal component (dedifferentiated chondrosarcoma). I. A clinicopathologic study of 26 cases. Cancer 1986;28:278–86.
235. Meis JM, Dorfman HD, Nathanson SD, Haggar AM, Wu KK. Primary malignant giant cell tumor of bone: "dedifferentiated" giant cell tumor. Mod Pathol 1989;2:541–6.
236. Reith JD, Bauer TW, Fischler DF, Joyce MJ, Marks KE. Dedifferentiated chondrosarcoma with rhabdomyosarcomatous differentiation. Am J Surg Pathol 1996;20:293–8.
237. Tetu B, Ordonez NG, Ayala AG, Mackay B. Chondrosarcoma with additional mesenchymal component (dedifferentiated chondrosarcoma). II. An immunohistochemical and electron microscopic study. Cancer 1986;58:287–98.

Mesenchymal Chondrosarcoma

238. Aigner T, Loos S, Muller S, Sandell LJ, Unni KK, Kirchner T. Cell differentiation and matrix gene expression in mesenchymal chondrosarcomas. Am J Pathol 2000;156:1327–35.
239. Bertoni F, Picci P, Bacchini P, et al. Mesenchymal chondrosarcoma of bone and soft tissues. Cancer 1983;52:533–41.
240. Granter SR, Renshaw AA, Fletcher CD, Bhan AK, Rosenberg AE. CD99 reactivity in mesenchymal chondrosarcoma. Hum Pathol 1996;27:1273–6.
241. Hutter RV, Foote FW Jr, Francis KC, Sherman RS. Primitive multipotential primary sarcoma of bone. Cancer 1966;19:1–25.
242. Huvos AG, Rosen G, Dabska M, Marcove RC. Mesenchymal chondrosarcoma. A clinicopathologic analysis of 35 patients with emphasis on treatment. Cancer 1983;51:1230–7.

243. Jacobs JL, Merriam JC, Chadburn A, Garvin J, Housepian E, Hilal SK. Mesenchymal chondrosarcoma of the orbit. Report of three new cases and review of the literature. Cancer 1994;73:399–405.
244. Jacobson SA. Polyhistioma: a malignant tumor of bone and extraskeletal tissues. Cancer 1977;40:2116–30.
245. Lichtenstein L, Bernstein D. Unusual benign and malignant chondroid tumors of bone: a survey of some mesenchymal cartilage tumors and malignant chondroblastic tumors, including a few multicentric ones, as well as many atypical benign chondroblastomas and chondromyxoid fibromas. Cancer 1959;12:1142–57.
246. Nakashima Y, Unni KK, Shives TC, Swee RG, Dahlin DC. Mesenchymal chondrosarcoma of bone and soft tissue: a review of 111 cases. Cancer 1986;57:2444–53.
247. Naumann S, Krallman PA, Unni KK, Fidler ME, Neff JR, Bridge JA. Translocation der(13;21)(q10;q10) in skeletal and extraskeletal mesenchymal chondrosarcoma. Mod Pathol 2002;15:572–6.
248. Salvador AH, Beabout JW, Dahlin DC. Mesenchymal chondrosarcoma—oberservations on 30 new cases. Cancer 1971;28:605–15.
249. Scheithauer BW, Rubinstein LJ. Meningeal mesenchymal chondrosarcoma: report of 8 cases with review of the literature. Cancer 1978;42:2744–52.
250. Vencio EF, Reeve CM, Unni KK, Nascimento AG. Mesenchymal chondrosarcoma of the jaw bones: clinicopathologic study of 19 cases. Cancer 1998;82:2350–5.
251. Walaas L, Kindblom LG, Gunterberg B, Bergh P. Light and electron microscopic examination of fine-needle aspirates in the preoperative diagnosis of cartilaginous tumors. Diagn Cytopathol 1990;6:396–408.
252. Wehrli BM, Huang W, De Crombrugghe B, Ayala AG, Czerniak B. Sox9, a master regulator of chondrogenesis, distinguishes mesenchymal chondrosarcoma from other small blue round cell tumors. Hum Pathol 2003;34:263–9.

Clear Cell Chondrosarcoma

253. Aigner T, Dertinger S, Belke J, Kirchner T. Chondrocytic cell differentiation in clear cell chondrosarcoma. Hum Pathol 1996;27:1301–5.
254. Bjornsson J, Unni KK, Dahlin DC, Beabout JW, Sim FH. Clear cell chondrosarcoma of bone. Observations in 47 cases. Am J Surg Pathol 1984;8:223–30.
255. Bosse A, Ueda Y, Wuisman P, Jones DB, Vollmer E, Roessner A. Histogenesis of clear cell chondrosarcoma. An immunohistochemical study with osteonectin, a non-collagenous structure protein. J Cancer Res Clin Oncol 1991;117:43–9.
256. Kumar R, David R, Cierney G 3rd. Clear cell chondrosarcoma. Radiology 1985;154:45–8.
257. Walaas L, Kindblom LG, Gunterberg B, Bergh P. Light and electron microscopic examination of fine-needle aspirates in the preoperative diagnosis of cartilaginous tumors. Diagn Cytopathol 1990;6:396–408.

5 BONE-FORMING LESIONS

BENIGN BONE-FORMING TUMORS

Osteoid Osteoma

Definition. Osteoid osteoma is a benign bone-forming neoplasm that is characterized by a limited growth potential. It usually is less than 1 cm in greatest dimension.

General Features. Until 2000, osteoid osteoma accounted for more than 13 percent of all benign tumors in the Mayo Clinic files of bone tumors. These tumors may be over-represented in a surgical series of benign bone lesions because they usually cause symptoms and are likely to be removed surgically.

Clinical Features. Osteoid osteoma is a disease of adolescents and young adults. According to the Mayo Clinic files, more than three fourths of patients are between the ages of 5 and 24 years (fig. 5-1). Patients are rarely older than 30 years (16). The male to female ratio is 2 or 3 to 1 (5,16,17).

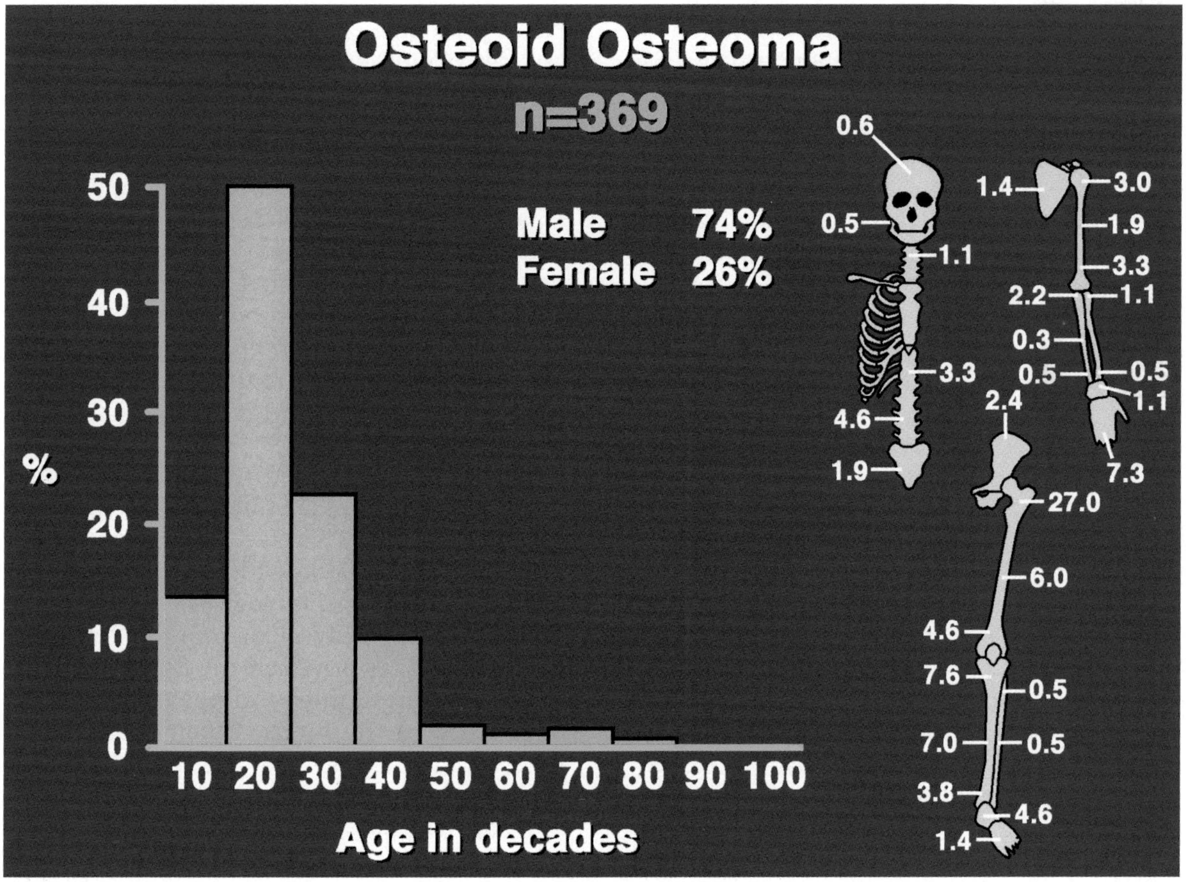

Figure 5-1

OSTEOID OSTEOMA

Distribution of osteoid osteoma according to the age and sex of the patient and the site of the lesion.

Pain, progressive and typically worse at night, is a characteristic symptom of patients with osteoid osteoma. The pain is relieved almost instantly with ingestion of nonsteroidal anti-inflammatory agents. Although this symptom complex is practically diagnostic of patients with osteoid osteoma, other symptoms may predominate. Lesions involving the proximal femur frequently produce referred pain that suggests lumbar disk prolapse (5). Lesions involving the proximal femoral shaft may produce symptoms referred to the knee joint, and those within a joint capsule, as in the femoral neck, may produce symptoms of arthritis. It is extremely unusual for osteoid osteoma to be painless. McDermott et al. (10) described one well-documented osteoid osteoma that involved the rib of an adult and was an incidental finding. In a review of the literature, these authors found 18 examples of painless osteoid osteomas. In the Mayo Clinic files, only four lesions were painless. The cause of the characteristic pain is not clear, but it has been suggested that the presence of nerve fibers in the nidus of an osteoid osteoma (14) and the production of prostaglandins by the nidus (9) are important factors. That the pain is relieved with nonsteroidal anti-inflammatory agents such as aspirin, which is known to suppress prostaglandin production, suggests that the latter theory is correct.

The most common physical finding is tenderness over the site of involvement. The tenderness is usually slight, but may be exquisite. There may be localized swelling, especially when the lesion involves a superficially located bone such as the tibia. The involved extremity may show disuse atrophy, probably because of the pain. Patients with involvement of the spine may have evidence of scoliosis or lordosis. Additional site-related symptoms depend on the location of the tumor (4). Tumors that grow near the epiphyseal plate may accelerate growth in the affected bone, leading to skeletal asymmetry. Epiphyseal lesions are often associated with joint effusion, and this may result in the misdiagnosis of arthritis.

Sites. The long bones, particularly the femur and the tibia, are the most common sites; however, any portion of the skeleton may be involved. In long bones, the lesion may involve the diaphysis or metaphysis. The proximal femur, including the femoral neck, is by far the most common location of the tumors recorded in the Mayo Clinic files. The phalanges of the hands and tarsal bones are commonly involved.

There are very few examples of multicentric involvement with osteoid osteoma. In one case in the Mayo Clinic files, a patient who had an osteoid osteoma of the distal phalanx of the index finger removed presented 14 years later with a typical osteoid osteoma of the femoral neck. In two other cases in the Mayo Clinic files, patients had multicentric disease involving one site.

Radiographic Findings. The lesions involve the cortex, medulla, subcortical bone, or even the bone surface. Radiographic findings depend to a great extent on the location of the lesion. If the lesion is in the spine, the neural arch is involved. In a long bone, the classic location is in the cortex, with the nidus appearing as a well-demarcated oval lucency with variable mineralization (fig. 5-2). The central lucency may undergo calcification, appearing as a central area of calcification with a lucent halo. Although this appearance is unusual, it is practically diagnostic of osteoid osteoma. The associated sclerosis in cortical bone varies, but usually appears as a tapering or fusiform thickening of the cortex, which is thickest overlying the nidus. The reactive sclerosis may be 3 to 4 cm in thickness. If the lesion involves the spongy bone or is in an intracapsular location, there may be no associated sclerosis (fig. 5-3). If there is marked sclerosis of the cortical bone, it may be difficult to localize the nidus.

Swee et al. (16) studied 100 osteoid osteomas on plain radiographs: 75 tumors were typical, 17 were equivocal, and 8 were negative radiographically. Of the 17 patients with equivocal findings, 14 had computerized tomography (CT) scans of which 11 were positive. Radionuclide scans were also generally positive. Of the 8 patients with normal radiographic findings, tomography demonstrated the nidus. When the findings were typical on plain radiographs, tomograms did not add to the preoperative diagnosis.

Helms (7) described the "double density" finding as a useful adjunct to the study of osteoid osteoma. All osteoid osteomas show uptake of the radionuclide on bone scans. In a typical osteoid osteoma, there is an increased focus of uptake over the nidus. This increased

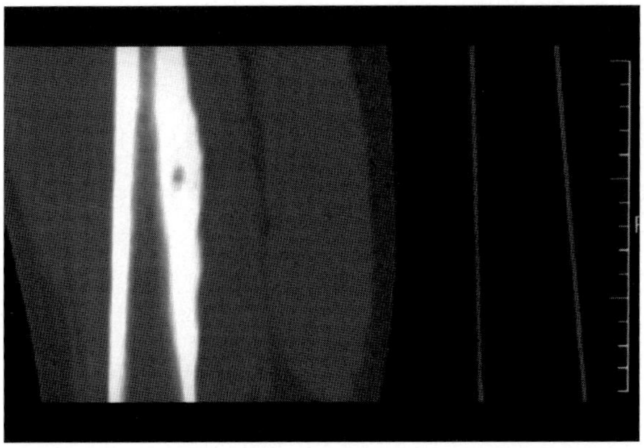

Figure 5-2

OSTEOID OSTEOMA

Computerized tomography (CT) shows a small intracortical osteoid osteoma with extensive associated cortical thickening in the mid-shaft of the femur.

uptake is not present in other conditions, for example, osteomyelitis. CT is sensitive in detecting the nidus of an osteoid osteoma. In anatomic locations where the nidus may be difficult to detect, as in the femoral neck and spine, CT is considered the ideal radiographic technique. This is of more than academic interest because when a nidus is associated with pronounced reactive sclerosis, it may be difficult for the surgeon to identify the nidus (fig. 5-4). Three-dimensional localization with CT is extremely helpful in preoperative planning to ensure that the nidus is localized correctly (fig. 5-5).

Gross Findings. An osteoid osteoma is usually recognized by an experienced surgeon. When the thickened cortical bone is chiseled away, a red granular area is exposed, which is the nidus of osteoid osteoma. It is not necessary to remove the entire sclerotic bone. If the nidus is removed, the sclerotic bone is remodeled over months or years.

The gross features of a nidus depend on the site of involvement. If the lesion is situated in the medullary cavity, there usually is no associated sclerosis. The lesion is well demarcated and resembles a red marble (figs. 5-6, 5-7). If the lesion is in cortical bone or is subcortical, reactive sclerosis may be extensive. If the surgeon resects a segment of sclerotic bone, the nidus usually is identified as a well-demarcated red granular area within a bone that has the appearance of ivory. Rarely, the nidus is heavily

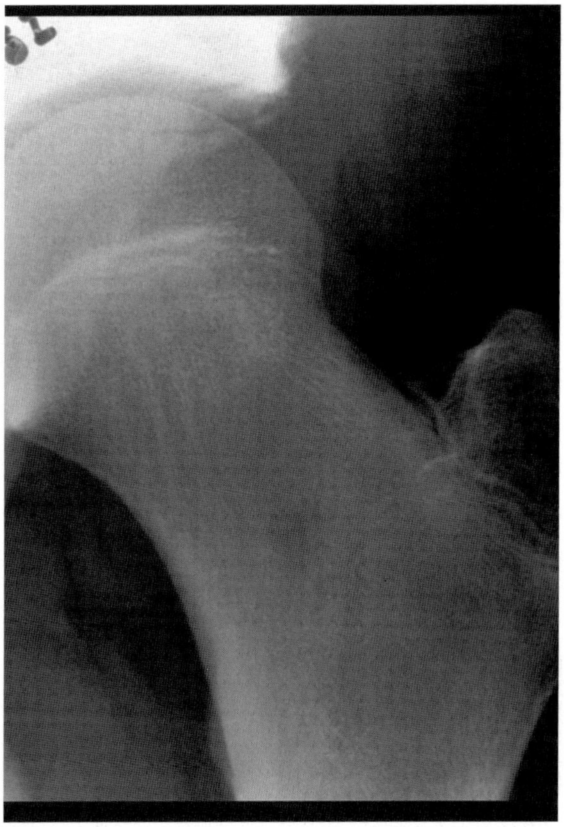

Figure 5-3

OSTEOID OSTEOMA

Osteoid osteomas located within the medullary bone often have no associated sclerosis.

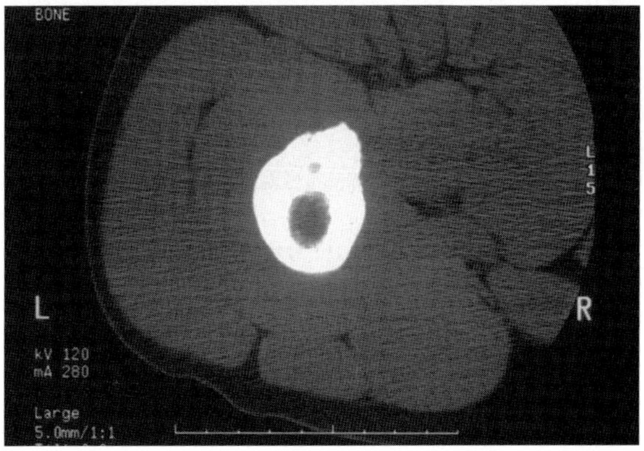

Figure 5-4

OSTEOID OSTEOMA

CT shows cortical thickening and thick periosteal new bone formation surrounding the small lytic nidus within the posterior cortex of the mid-femoral diaphysis.

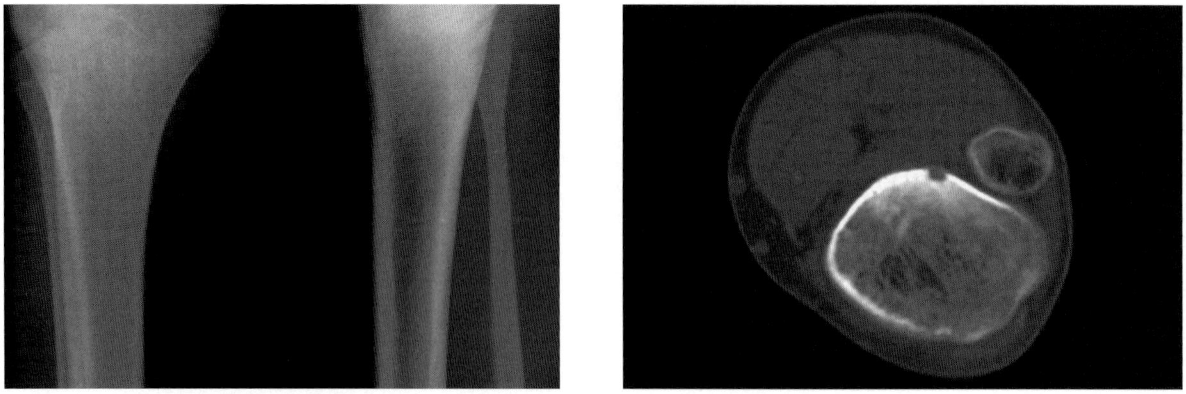

Figure 5-5

OSTEOID OSTEOMA

Left: The lesion is not well visualized on a plain radiograph, which shows nonspecific reactive sclerosis involving the proximal tibia.

Right: The lucent cortical nidus in the tibial metaphysis posteriorly is clearly depicted on CT.

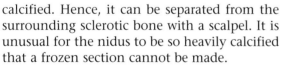

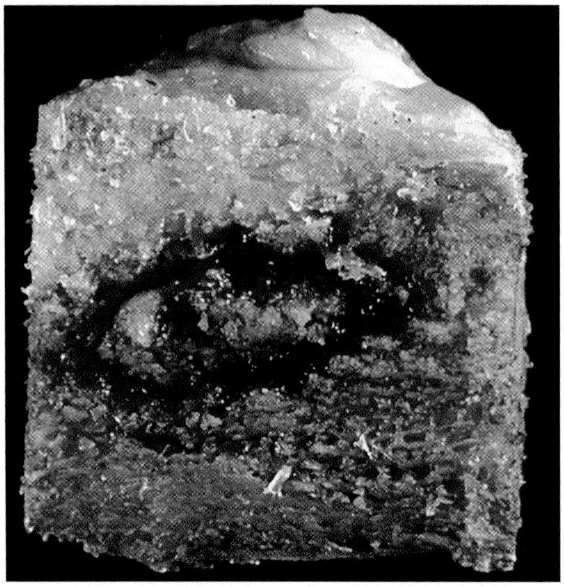

Figure 5-6

OSTEOID OSTEOMA

The nidus of this osteoid osteoma is a nodular mass surrounded by hemorrhage. It is situated between the cortex and medulla.

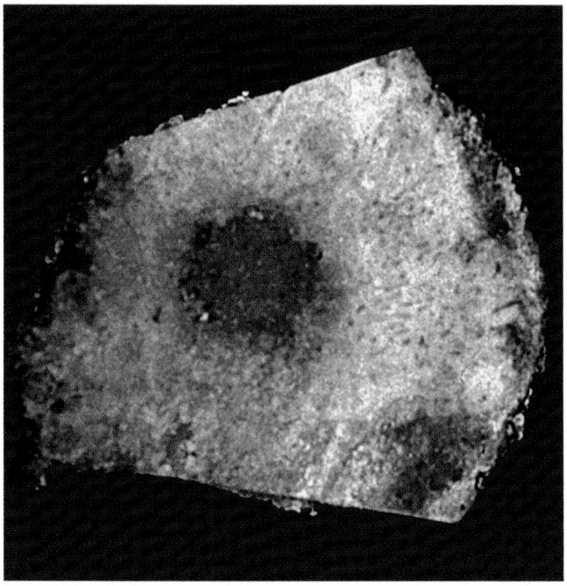

Figure 5-7

OSTEOID OSTEOMA

Reactive sclerosis surrounds the central tan nidus.

calcified. Hence, it can be separated from the surrounding sclerotic bone with a scalpel. It is unusual for the nidus to be so heavily calcified that a frozen section cannot be made.

It is important for the pathologist to examine the gross specimen in order to inform the surgeon whether the nidus has indeed been removed. If a large segment of sclerotic bone is received intact, it may be necessary to slice the bone with a band saw into several slices to identify the nidus. It is not useful to decalcify the entire specimen indiscriminately and look for

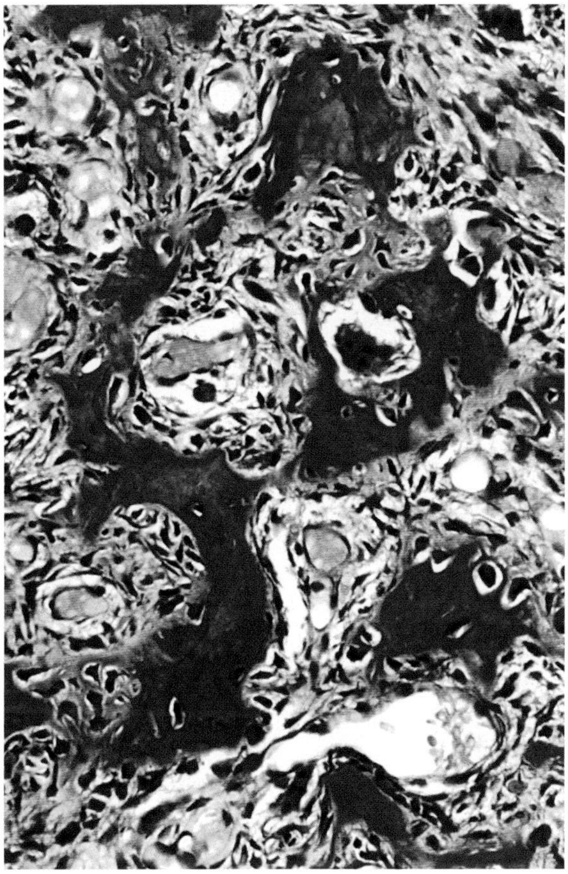

Figure 5-8

OSTEOID OSTEOMA

This nidus contains numerous irregular bony trabeculae with variable mineralization.

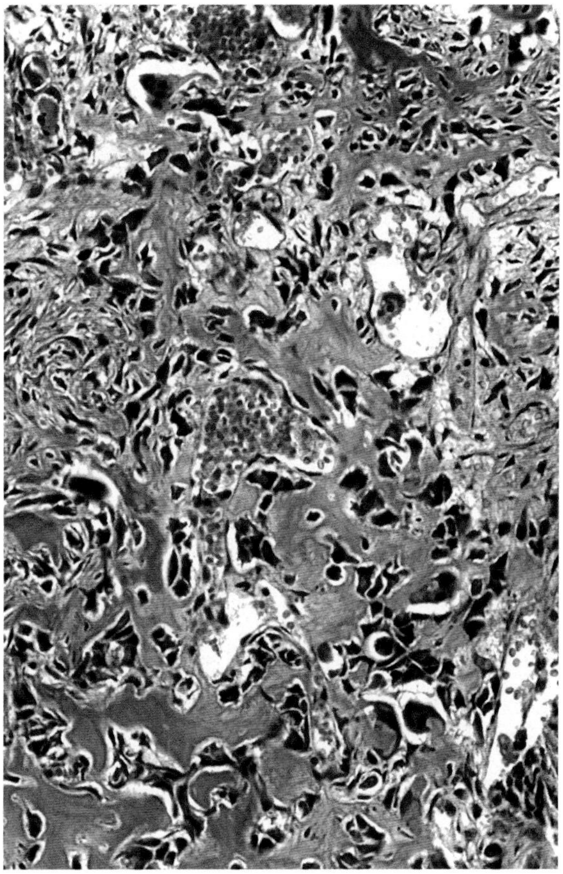

Figure 5-9

OSTEOID OSTEOMA

Trabeculae of woven bone are distributed haphazardly in a loose fibrovascular stroma.

the nidus with the microscope. If the nidus is not found on inspection, the gross specimen can be radiographed in an attempt to identify the area of lucency. Ayala et al. (1) recommended using tetracycline labeling to identify the nidus grossly. Patients are given 750 to 4,000 mg of tetracycline preoperatively. The gross specimen is examined with fluorescent light to identify the nidus. If the nidus still cannot be identified, the surgeon should be informed and radiographs obtained to ensure that the area of involvement has been removed. The patient usually is able to tell whether the lesion has been removed surgically because of the prompt relief of pain.

Microscopic Findings. The nidus of an osteoid osteoma consists of an interlacing network of osteoid and bony trabeculae, with variable mineralization (fig. 5-8). The trabeculae are usually thin and arranged in a random tangle of anastomoses (fig. 5-9). The central part of the nidus is usually more mineralized than the peripheral part. The bony trabeculae have a rim of a single layer of osteoblasts, which are small, polygonal, and not cytologically atypical (fig. 5-10). The intertrabecular spaces contain a proliferation of capillaries and scattered spindled fibroblasts. The bony trabeculae may be thickened, showing cement lines that suggest pagetoid bone (fig. 5-11). The nidus is demarcated sharply from the surrounding sclerotic bone (fig. 5-12) and does not permeate into it. Cartilaginous differentiation may be present but is unusual within the nidus. A biopsy specimen of synovium from a patient who has an osteoid

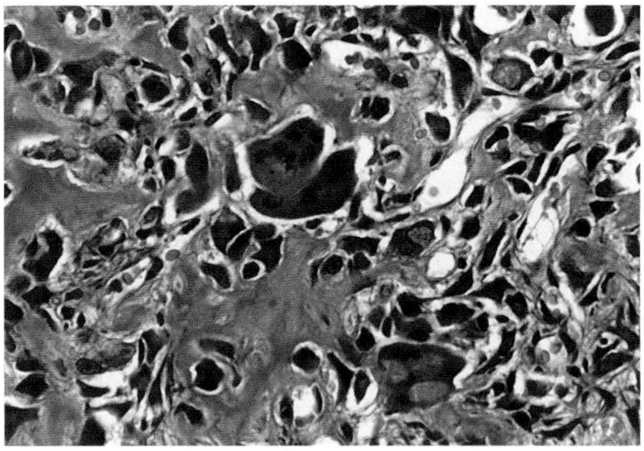

Figure 5-10

OSTEOID OSTEOMA

Plump osteoblasts without cytologic atypia are located between the intertrabecular spaces.

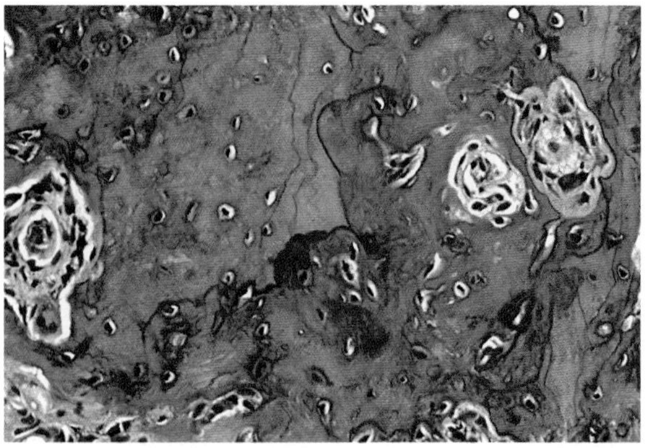

Figure 5-11

OSTEOID OSTEOMA

This sclerotic nidus contains thick bony trabeculae that have prominent cement lines, producing a pagetoid appearance.

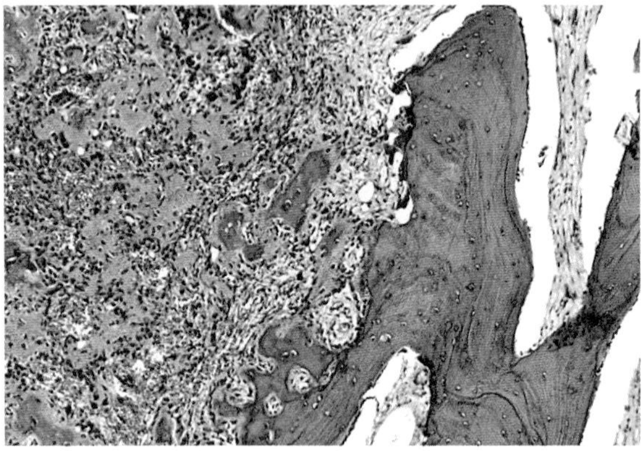

Figure 5-12

OSTEOID OSTEOMA

A low-power magnification view typically shows a well-circumscribed nidus surrounded by reactive sclerosis.

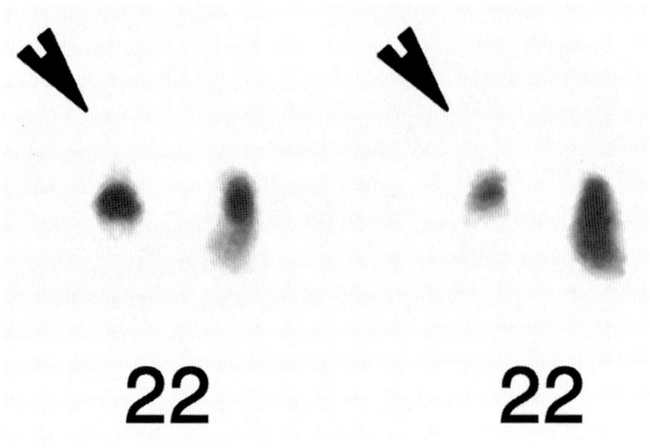

Figure 5-13

CHROMOSOME 22 ALTERATIONS IN OSTEOID OSTEOMA

Partial karyotypes from two metaphase cells of an osteoid osteoma exhibit a del(22)(q13.1) (arrowheads). (Fig. 3B from Baruffi MR, Volpon JB, Neto JB, Casartelli C. Osteoid osteomas with chromosome alterations involving 22q. Cancer Genet Cytogenet 2001;124:127–31.)

osteoma within the capsule of a joint may show a proliferation of lymphocytes and plasma cells, suggesting the diagnosis of synovitis, especially the rheumatoid type.

Cytologic Findings. A fine-needle aspiration (FNA) diagnosis of osteoid osteoma may be a problem for technical reasons. Diagnostic material is difficult to obtain if dense sclerotic bone surrounds the nidus, which usually is small.

The cytologic features of osteoid osteoma are similar to those of osteoblastoma (see Osteoblastoma).

Genetics and Other Special Techniques. Immunohistochemical analysis for c-fos and c-jun expression demonstrated low or moderate immunoreactivity in three of six osteoid osteomas analyzed (6). Diffuse and intense immunoreactivity for these oncoproteins appears to be confined to high-grade osteosarcomas. Chromosomal abnormalities have been observed in only three osteoid osteomas (2,3); a partial deletion of the long arm of chromosome 22 [del(22)(q13.1)] and loss of the distal long arm of chromosome 17 were seen in two of these (fig. 5-13).

Differential Diagnosis. It is well recognized that the histologic features of osteoid osteoma and osteoblastoma overlap. The nidus of an osteoid osteoma is usually more tightly woven than that of an osteoblastoma, which has a loose arrangement. However, this feature cannot be used to distinguish confidently between the two. Currently, it generally is accepted that osteoid osteoma and osteoblastoma represent two ends of the spectrum of a benign bone-forming neoplasm. Osteoid osteoma has a limited growth potential, and its greatest dimension rarely exceeds 1 cm. Osteoblastomas are always larger than 2 cm. If the lesion is between 1 and 2 cm, other features, such as radiographic and clinical features, are used for distinction.

Diagnosing osteosarcoma is not usually difficult. Because osteoid osteomas are extremely well demarcated, they appear rounded at low-power magnification, an appearance never seen in an osteosarcoma because of its tendency to permeate adjacent bone. The loose arrangement of the tissue also argues against the diagnosis of osteosarcoma.

Chronic osteomyelitis, or Brodie's abscess, is typically considered in the radiographic differential diagnosis of osteoid osteoma. However, microscopically, Brodie's abscess shows the characteristic features of osteomyelitis.

Stress fractures may simulate osteoid osteoma clinically and radiographically. Stress fractures show reactive new bone formation in the form of a fracture callus and lack the rounded nidus-like characteristic of osteoid osteomas.

Treatment and Prognosis. Treatment is complete surgical removal or ablation of the nidus. This generally is accomplished by block excision of the nidus and some of the surrounding bone. At the time of excision, the nidus may be difficult to localize, especially in anatomically difficult locations such as the femoral neck and spine. In a study by Sim et al. (15), multiple surgical procedures occasionally were required before a nidus was found. These authors emphasized that excision sometimes produced pain relief even when a nidus was not identified microscopically. Possibly in these patients, a small nidus was lost at the time of the surgery or during handling in the surgical pathology laboratory.

Several alternative methods for the management of osteoid osteoma have been suggested.

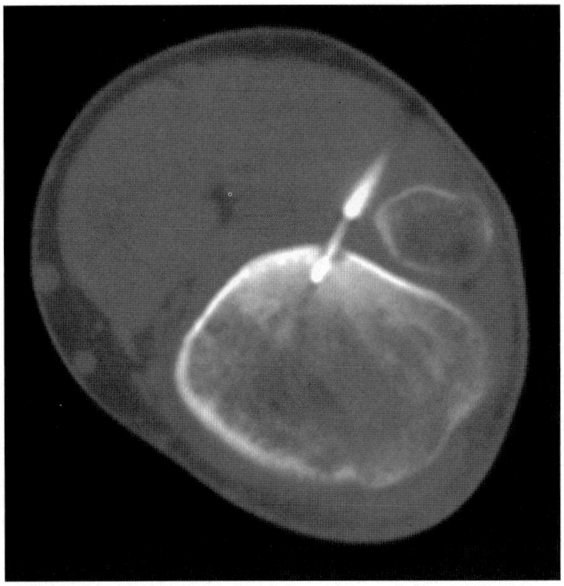

Figure 5-14

OSTEOID OSTEOMA

CT-guided radiofrequency ablation was used in treating this patient with osteoid osteoma. A radiofrequency probe is placed in the lesion so that the tip of the probe traverses the lytic nidus.

In a study by Kneisl and Simon (8), all patients with osteoid osteomas who received surgical treatment were relieved of their symptoms; nine patients given nonsteroidal anti-inflammatory agents had relief of pain, and six of them discontinued taking the medication after 33 months and did not have a recurrence of symptoms. The authors suggest that medical management is a good option if surgical treatment is contraindicated. Several authors have described percutaneous resection of an osteoid osteoma. Muscolo et al. (11) used CT-guided percutaneous resection to treat seven patients (fig. 5-14). In five patients, the lesion was identified microscopically. All patients had relief of pain. Roger et al. (12) described 16 patients in whom percutaneous CT-guided ablation was performed; the procedure was successful in 14. Rosenthal et al. (13) described a method of radiofrequency ablation of osteoid osteoma, which they performed in 18 patients. They were able to confirm the diagnosis of osteoid osteoma microscopically in all the patients before destroying the nidus with a thermal electrode. Of the 18 patients, 16 had complete relief of their symptoms.

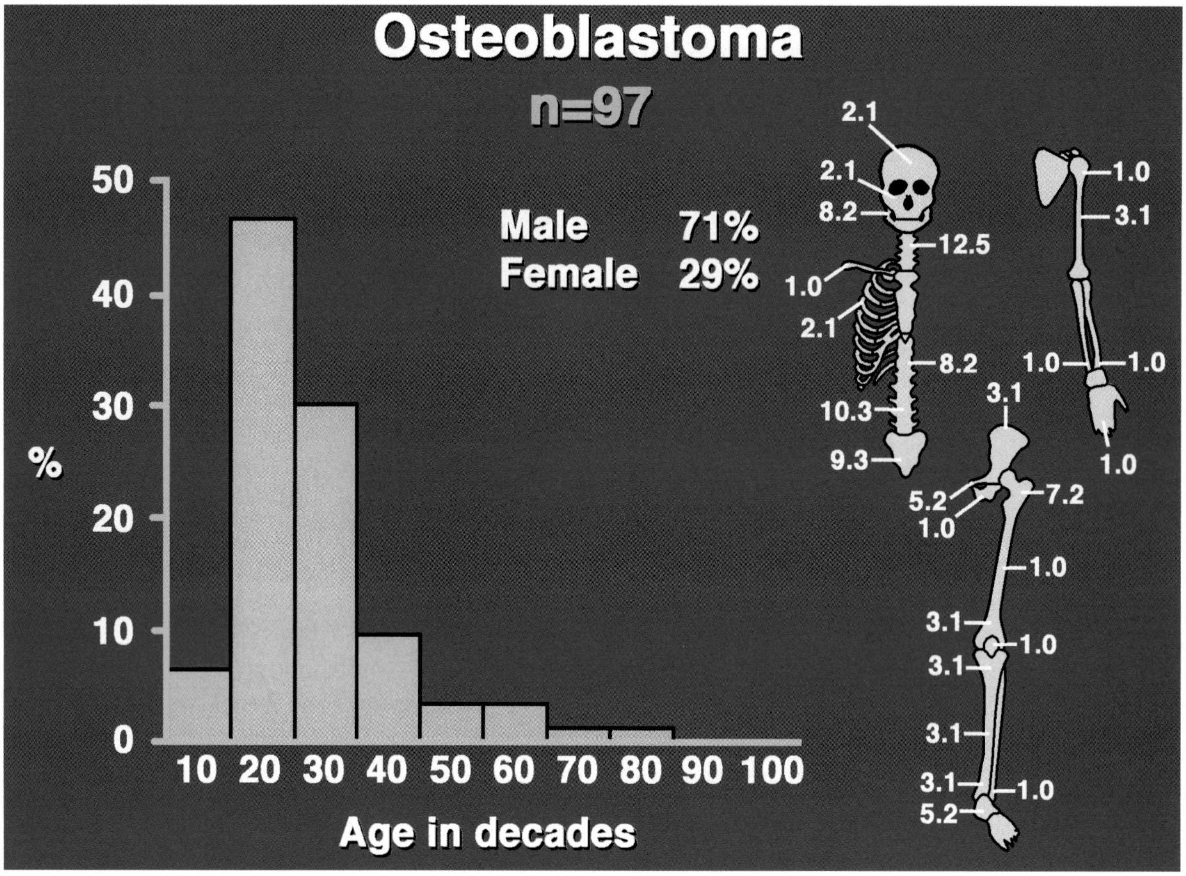

Figure 5-15

OSTEOBLASTOMA

Distribution of osteoblastoma according to the age and sex of the patient and the site of the lesion.

Complete removal of the nidus results in cure. Incomplete removal may lead to recurrence. Seven recurrences are documented in the Mayo Clinic series. However, these lesions were treated with simple re-excision. We have not seen an example of malignant change in osteoid osteoma.

Osteoblastoma

Definition. Osteoblastoma is a benign bone-forming neoplasm with histologic features similar to those of osteoid osteoma but with a potential for progressive growth.

General Features. Osteoid osteoma and osteoblastoma have many similarities, especially histologically, as emphasized by the term "giant osteoid osteoma" used to describe osteoblastoma (21). However, the two tumors also have many differences, which make it important to distinguish them. The characteristic symptom complex of osteoid osteoma is not nearly so consistently present with osteoblastoma. Radiographically, osteoblastoma rarely has a nidus like that of osteoid osteoma. Osteoblastoma involves the vertebral column more often than osteoid osteoma does. Most important, the pathologic distinction between osteoblastoma and osteosarcoma can be difficult or almost impossible to make in some cases, whereas osteoid osteoma is rarely confused histologically with osteosarcoma.

Osteoblastoma is a rare tumor, accounting for only 1 percent of all bone tumors seen at Mayo Clinic. Until the beginning of 2000, the surgical files of Mayo Clinic included only 97 cases.

Clinical Features. Osteoblastoma is predominantly a disease of childhood and adolescence. In the Mayo Clinic files, the patient age has ranged from 4 to 75 years (fig. 5-15), with 80 percent of cases occurring in the first three decades of life. In the large study reported by Lucas et al. (10), the patient age ranged from 6 months to 75 years, with a mean of 20 years, and 75 percent of the patients were 25 years or younger.

As with most bone tumors, osteoblastoma has a predilection for males. The male to female ratio is 2 to 1 (27,29).

The predominant symptom is pain, usually mild and long-standing (27,29). Patients with spinal tumors frequently present with neurologic complaints (24,29). Mirra et al. (30) described on a 7-year-old boy with a tumor of the proximal femur, eventually diagnosed as osteoblastoma, and who presented with severe systemic symptoms. The results of multiple biopsies were nondiagnostic, and the boy was given long-term treatment with intravenous antibiotics for a presumptive diagnosis of osteomyelitis. The symptoms consisted of fever, loss of appetite, cachexia, clubbing of the toes and fingers, and extensive periosteal new bone formation. Because of the severity of the symptoms, hemipelvectomy was performed, and postoperatively the boy had complete symptomatic relief. He was alive 2 years later without evidence of disease. Such dramatic clinical symptoms are uncommon with osteoblastoma.

Patients with osteoblastoma commonly present with localized swelling, tenderness, and warmth in the region of the tumor. The physical examination findings are nonspecific.

Sites. Osteoblastoma can involve virtually any bone in the skeleton. The spinal column reportedly is involved in 21 (24) to 33 percent (27) of cases. The long tubular bones are reported to be involved in from 26 (26) to 38 percent (29) of cases. The jaws are involved in approximately 10 percent of cases.

The location of the lesion can be quite variable, depending on the bone involved. It is useful to divide the location into three distinct anatomic sites: the appendicular skeleton, vertebrae, and jawbones.

Appendicular Skeleton. In the long bones, the diaphysis reportedly is involved in 36 (27) to 76 percent (29) of cases; in a large series reported by Kroon and Schurmans from the Netherlands Tumor Registry (26), the diaphysis was involved in 58 percent. The rest of the osteoblastomas in the series reported by McLeod et al. (29) and Kroon and Schurmans were in the metaphyses. However, in the report of Lucas et al. (27), 22 percent of the lesions were epiphyseal. McLeod et al. found that 60 percent of the tumors were cortical and 40 percent were medullary. In contrast, Kroon and Schurmans documented 58 percent in the medulla and only 42 percent in the cortex. In the report by Lucas et al., 65 percent were cortical and 35 percent were medullary; six tumors occurred on the bone surface.

Vertebrae. Osteoblastoma of the spine has a pronounced tendency to involve the posterior elements. In the series of McLeod et al. (29), 62 percent of the tumors were dorsal and 24 percent involved both the body and dorsal elements; only 14 percent involved the body of the vertebra exclusively. In the report from the Netherlands Tumor Registry (26), only 6 percent were exclusively in the body of the vertebra, 66 percent were purely dorsal, and 28 percent involved both the body and dorsal elements. In the study by Lucas et al. (27), 65 percent were purely dorsal and 32 percent involved both the body and dorsal elements; only 3 percent involved the body of the vertebra only.

Jawbones. In the jawbones, osteoblastoma has a tendency to involve the root of the tooth, where it produces a sclerotic mass. In the oral pathology literature, these lesions are referred to as *cementoblastomas*. Because of the histologic similarity of these tumors with those of the appendicular skeleton and vertebrae, we have included them in the series with osteoblastoma.

Radiographic Findings. The radiographic findings of osteoblastomas vary according to the bone involved by the tumor.

Appendicular Skeleton. In long tubular bones, the interior of the osteoblastoma usually is lucent, with varying amounts of ossification (fig. 5-16). In the series of McLeod et al. (29), 64 percent of the tumors were purely lucent and the rest showed various degrees of ossification. In contrast, Kroon and Schurmans (26) reported that only 35 percent were lucent and the rest had ossification. Lucas et al. (27) described ossification in about 50 percent of all lesions.

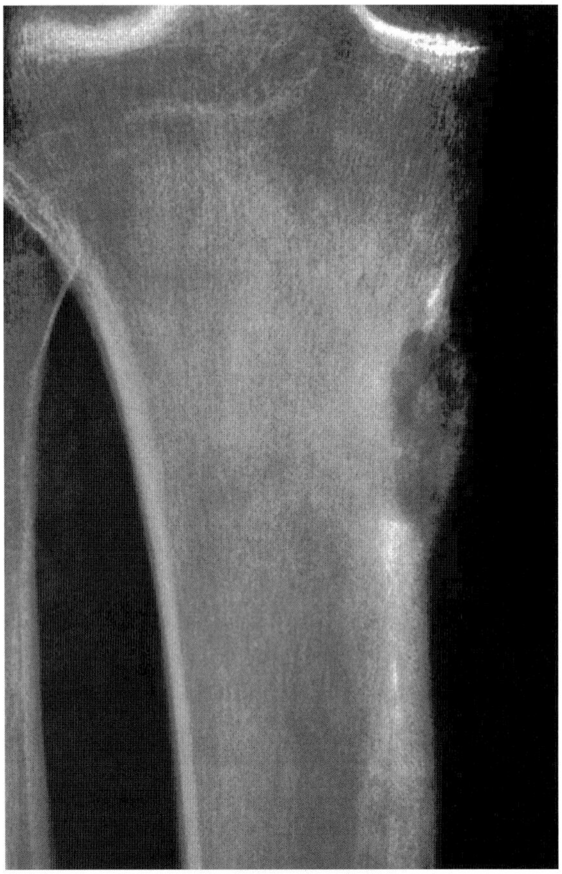

Figure 5-16

OSTEOBLASTOMA

The tumor involves the proximal tibia and has varying degrees of mineralization.

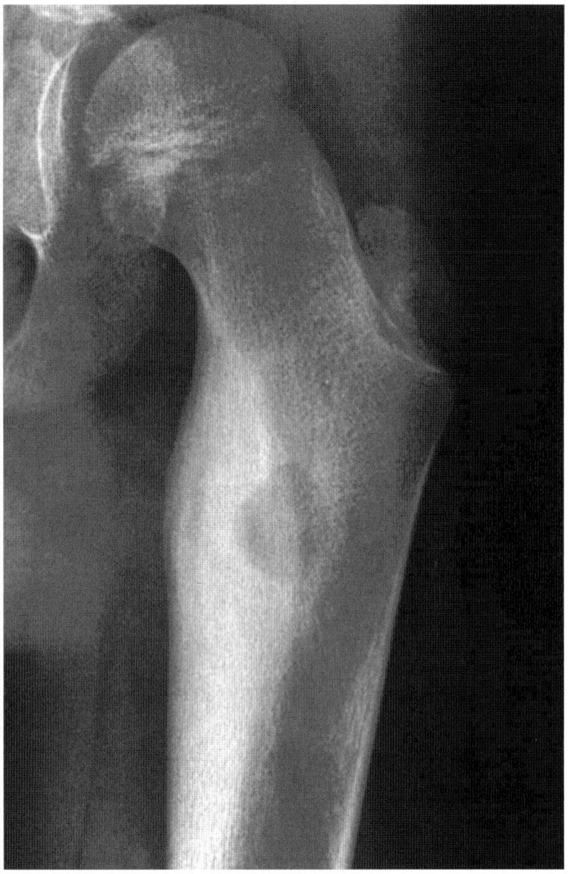

Figure 5-17

OSTEOBLASTOMA

This plain film shows a circumscribed lucent osteoblastoma surrounded by reactive sclerosis and abundant cortical thickening, similar to that seen in osteoid osteoma.

The margin of the tumor usually is well defined and distinct. Only 17 percent of the tumors in the series of McLeod et al. (29) had indistinct margins. Approximately half of the lesions show considerable reactive sclerosis (fig. 5-17). A central nidus is seen in only a small portion of cases. The cortex remains intact in most cases (fig. 5-17). However, about a fifth of cases have frank cortical destruction. Approximately half of the lesions are associated with periosteal new bone formation. Because of the cortical destruction and periosteal new bone formation, a diagnosis of malignancy may be suggested in about a fourth of cases.

Vertebrae. In the spine, the radiographic margin of the tumor usually is well defined. Approximately half of the lesions have surrounding sclerosis (fig. 5-18), and a purely lucent interior (fig. 5-19). Because of the more typical radiographic features, the diagnosis of osteoblastoma is suggested in about two thirds of the cases involving the spine, and in only 15 percent is the diagnosis of malignancy suggested.

Jawbones. Radiographically, osteoblastoma of the jawbone is a well-demarcated mineralizing mass that surrounds the roots of a tooth (fig. 5-20).

Kroon and Schurmans (26) described the results of CT studies of 15 osteoblastomas. In their experience, CT was superior to plain radiography in defining the extent of the lesion, the precise origin of the tumor, and the presence of mineralization, and it also was superior in demonstrating a peripheral bony shell. On magnetic resonance imaging (MRI), the lesion

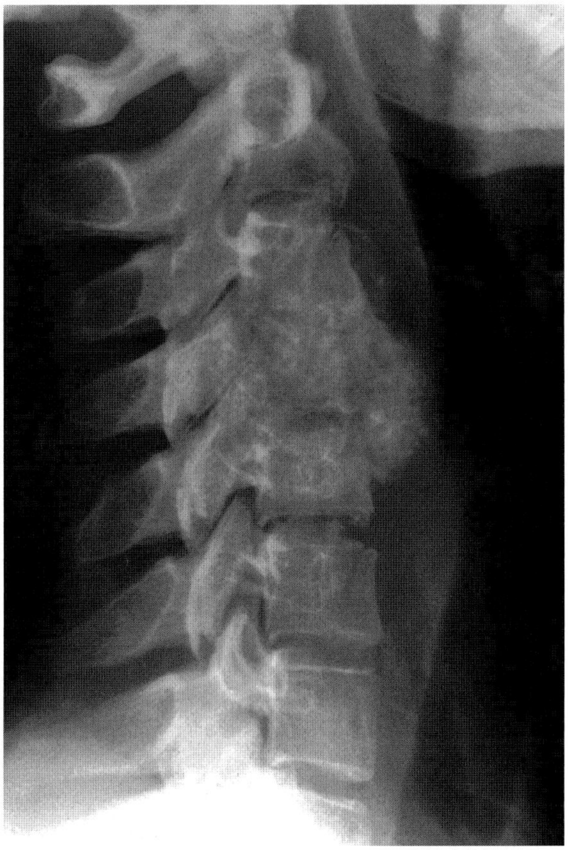

Figure 5-18

OSTEOBLASTOMA

This heavily mineralized osteoblastoma is replacing the fourth cervical vertebra in a 14-year-old girl.

shows low or intermediate signal intensity on T_1-weighted images and a mixed intermediate and high signal intensity on T_2-weighted images (fig. 5-21). Indistinct areas of high signal intensity in the soft tissues suggest edema.

Gross Findings. Most osteoblastomas are treated with curettage. Curetted fragments of osteoblastoma are red to tan, gritty, and friable. When osteoblastomas are removed intact, they are extremely well demarcated (fig. 5-22), red

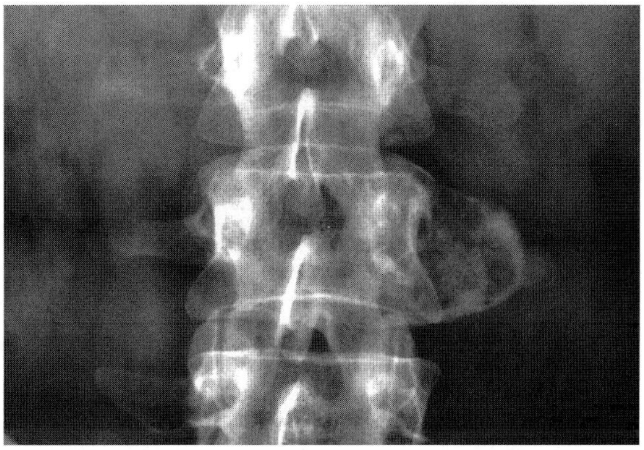

Figure 5-19

OSTEOBLASTOMA

This osteoblastoma involves the pedicle and transverse process of a lumbar vertebra. The lesion is lytic and expansile, with tiny foci of central calcification. There is less obvious evidence of mineralization than in the tumor in figure 5-18.

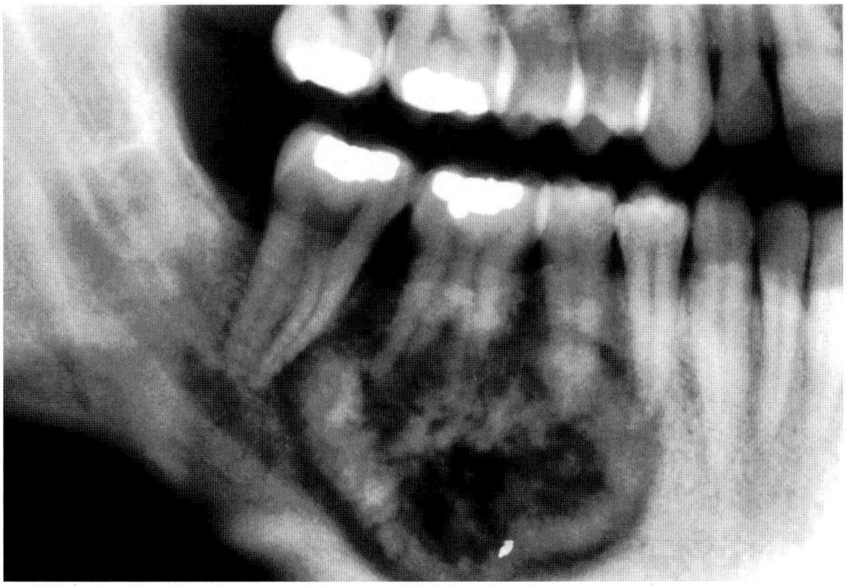

Figure 5-20

OSTEOBLASTOMA

Heavily mineralized osteoblastoma forms a circumscribed mass surrounding the roots of a tooth.

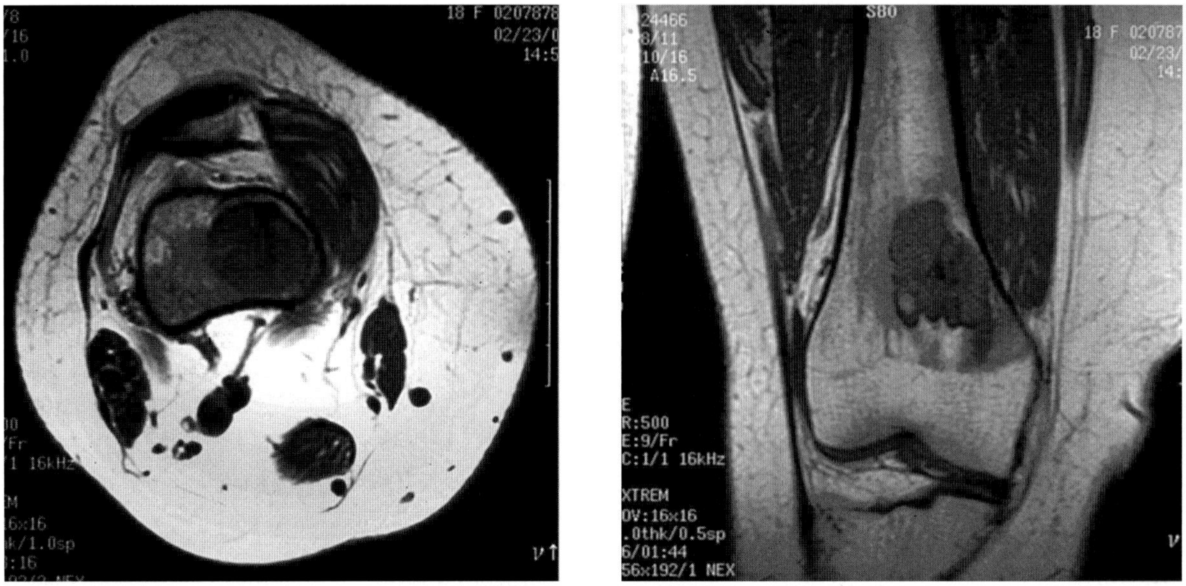

Figure 5-21

OSTEOBLASTOMA

Axial (left) and coronal (right) T_1-weighted magnetic resonance imaging (MRI) studies aid in delineating the extent of this metaphyseal osteoblastoma.

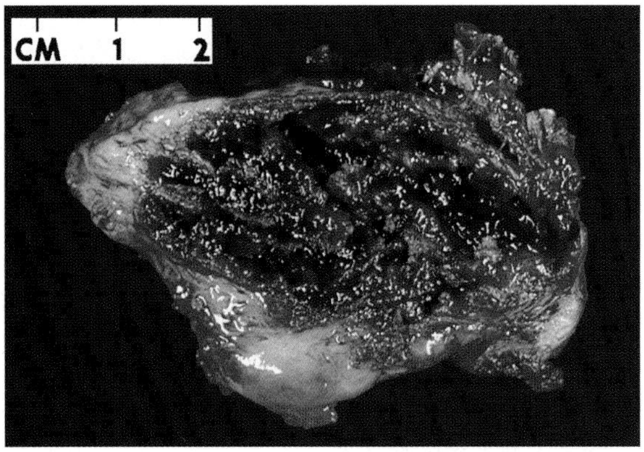

Figure 5-22

OSTEOBLASTOMA

The tissue of this osteoblastoma involving the superior pubic ramus of a 28-year-old woman is hemorrhagic and friable. The gross and preoperative needle biopsy specimens showed features suggestive of an aneurysmal bone cyst.

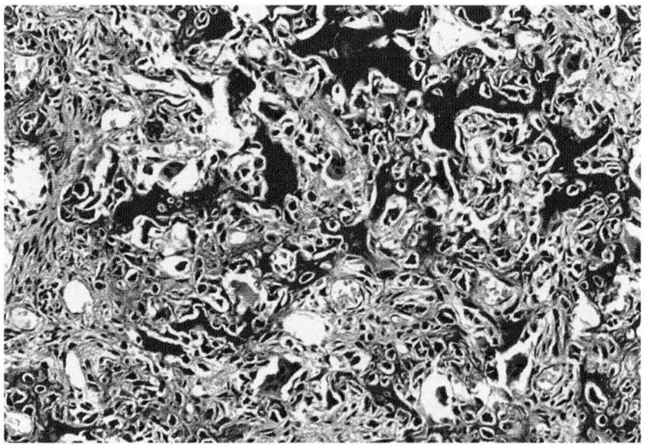

Figure 5-23

OSTEOBLASTOMA

The typical histologic appearance of osteoblastoma, with anastomosing bony trabeculae surrounded by a loose fibrovascular stroma, is seen.

granular lesions with surrounding thick ivory-like bone. The lesion can be large, growing up to 11 cm in its greatest dimension.

Microscopic Findings. Most osteoblastomas have a classic pattern of anastomosing bony trabeculae irregularly arranged in a loose fibrovascular stroma (fig. 5-23). A single layer of osteoblasts rim the trabeculae (fig. 5-24). The tumors tend to be sharply demarcated and may connect with cortical bone, suggesting maturation (fig. 5-25). The amount of bone and osteoid in the tumor is variable. Occasionally, solid sheets

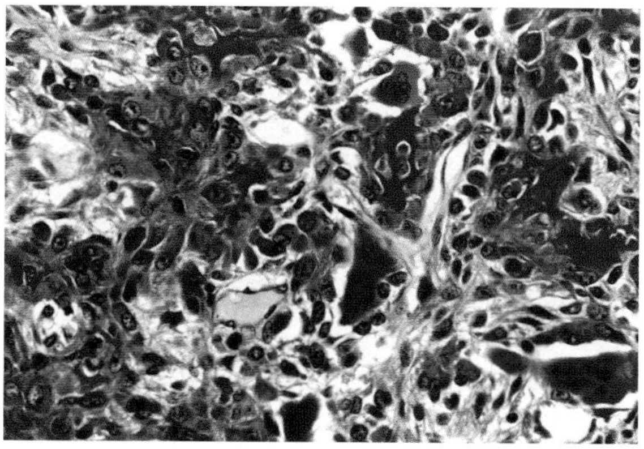

Figure 5-24

OSTEOBLASTOMA

A prominent rim of osteoblasts is commonly seen bordering bony trabeculae.

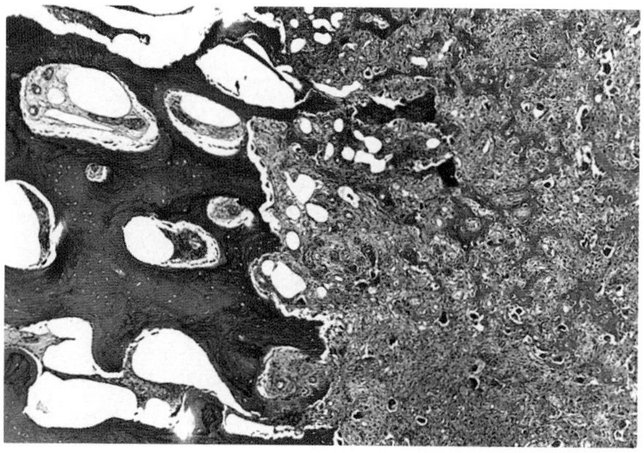

Figure 5-25

OSTEOBLASTOMA

The interface between the tumor and adjacent host bone is well demarcated. This is in contrast to the destructive and permeative growth pattern typically seen in osteosarcomas.

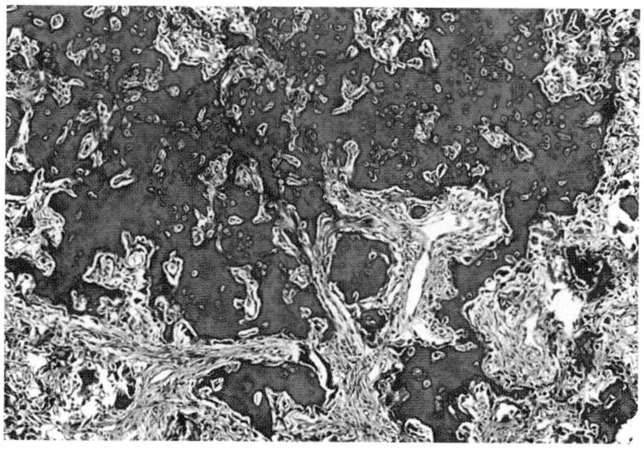

Figure 5-26

OSTEOBLASTOMA

Thick well-mineralized bony trabeculae merge into thinner trabeculae.

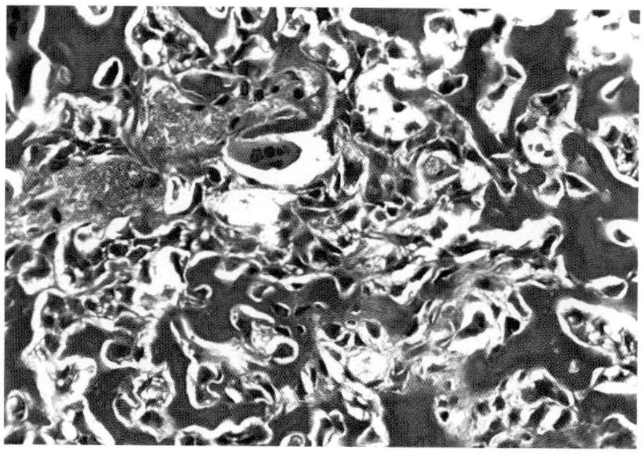

Figure 5-27

OSTEOBLASTOMA

At high-power magnification, a lace-like pattern of osteoid can lead to a mistaken diagnosis of osteosarcoma. However, note the lack of cytologic atypia within the intertrabecular stroma.

of densely calcified matrix radiate from a central focus (fig. 5-26). Lace-like osteoid may be present in a small proportion of cases, but it is focal and generally not a dominant histologic feature (fig. 5-27). Spiculated blue bone (irregular, densely calcified, immature bone), as in osteosarcoma, may be seen in about one fifth of the cases. Although some authors have suggested that chondroid matrix never occurs in osteoblastoma, Lucas et al. (27) found clear-cut chondroid differentiation in 6 percent of the tumors they reviewed (fig. 5-28).

Although the osteoblasts usually lie along the bony trabeculae, rarely they form small clusters without central matrix formation. Osteoblasts usually are polygonal, with moderate cytoplasm, round to oval nuclei, and a single nucleolus (fig. 5-29). Large epithelioid osteoblasts (cells that usually are larger than those seen in common osteoblastoma, with prominent pink cytoplasm, a round vesicular nucleus, and a prominent nucleolus) may be seen in one fifth of osteoblastomas; they are the predominant cell type in only a few cases. A small fraction of

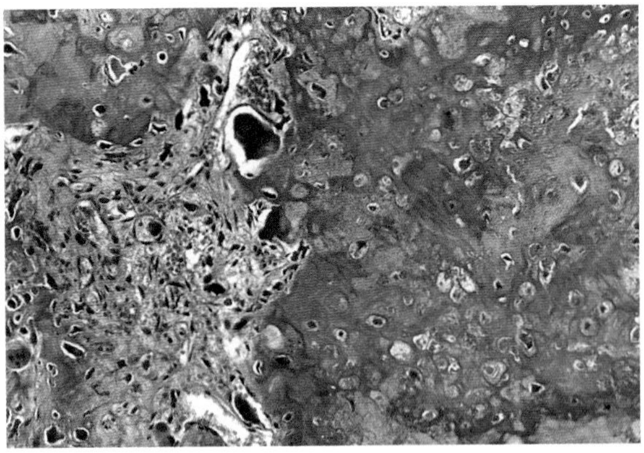

Figure 5-28

OSTEOBLASTOMA

Evidence of cartilaginous differentiation should not exclude the diagnosis of osteoblastoma. Occasionally, it can be seen focally or it can involve the lesion more extensively.

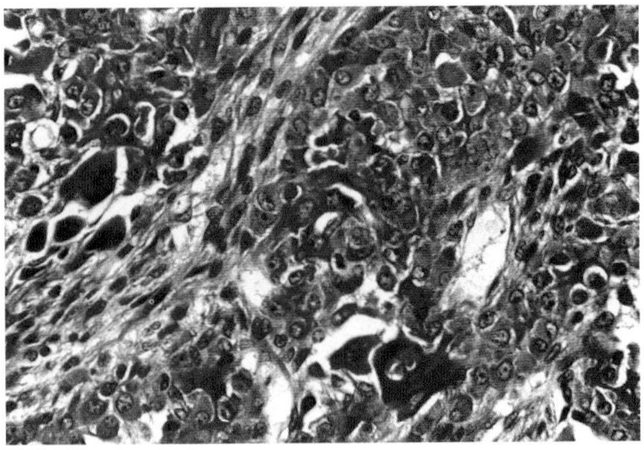

Figure 5-29

OSTEOBLASTOMA

Osteoblasts typically have an epithelioid appearance, with a low nucleus to cytoplasm ratio. Occasionally, they fill the intertrabecular spaces completely.

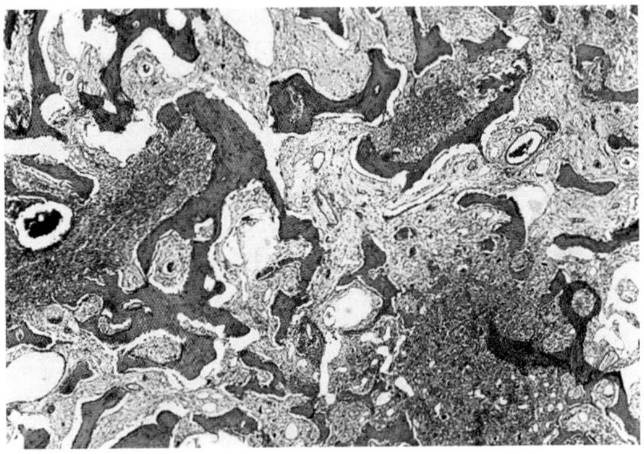

Figure 5-30

OSTEOBLASTOMA

At low-power microscopy, the appearance of a multifocal osteoblastoma should not be mistaken for a permeative growth pattern.

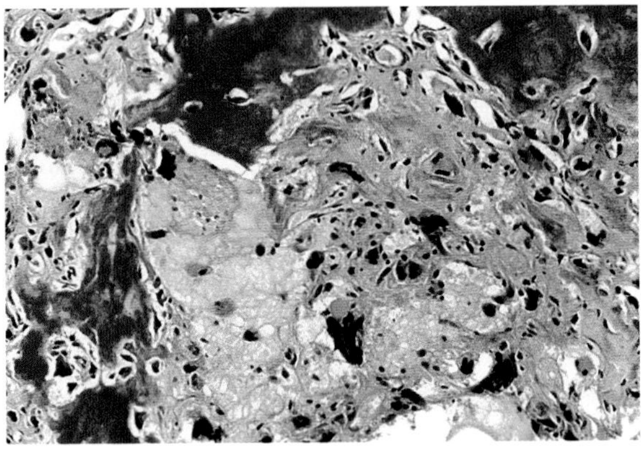

Figure 5-31

OSTEOBLASTOMA

In pseudomalignant osteoblastoma, atypical osteoblasts contain large, hyperchromatic, smudged nuclei surrounded by an abundance of cytoplasm, which is occasionally vacuolated. These cells may be seen rimming trabeculae or scattered throughout a fibrous stroma, which commonly has areas of degenerative fibrosis.

osteoblastomas have a multifocal growth pattern (fig. 5-30).

Small foci of typical osteoblastoma are separated by proliferating bone and fibrous tissue. The lesion may reach a considerable size, suggesting malignancy. Mirra et al. (31) described bizarre pleomorphic nuclei in atypical osteoblasts in otherwise typical osteoblastomas. These nuclei are enlarged and densely hyperchromatic but do not have crisp nuclear features (fig. 5-31). The cells are similar to degenerated cells in neurilemomas. The large hyperchromatic nuclei do not show mitotic activity. Often, these pleomorphic nuclei are scattered in a loose fibrotic background, unlike the typical loose vascular pattern seen in typical osteoblastomas.

Malignant Osteoblastoma. In 1976, Schajowicz and Lemos (33) described eight osteoblastomas that they termed "malignant osteoblastoma." They considered these lesions to be borderline between osteoblastoma and osteosarcoma because of the cellular pleomorphism of the osteoblasts, the large number of giant cells, and the spiculated blue bone, similar to that found in osteosarcoma. One patient died, probably because of local extension of the tumor. Four lesions recurred (including in the patient who died of tumor). However, half of the lesions did not recur and none metastasized. We do not believe that the criteria used for diagnosing "malignant osteoblastoma" are reproducible.

Aggressive Osteoblastoma. Dorfman and Weiss (24) described 102 benign osteoblastic tumors, which they classified as osteoid osteoma, osteoblastoma, and aggressive osteoblastoma. In their study, approximately one fourth of the osteoblastomas were considered aggressive and were characterized by epithelioid osteoblasts, sheet-like osteoid, and osteoclastic resorption. The patients were older than those who had a conventional osteoblastoma. However, the radiographic findings were not distinctive. Histologically, aggressive osteoblastomas showed "larger" osteoid trabeculae. In about half of the cases, the osteoid occurred in a nontrabecular fashion. Epithelioid osteoblasts, defined as osteoblasts at least twice the size of those seen in conventional osteoblastomas, with a round nucleus and one or more prominent nucleoli, were present in all tumors. The cytoplasm was abundant and either clear or slightly eosinophilic. Dorfman and Weiss believe that aggressive osteoblastoma is a reproducible entity that is important prognostically because in about half of their cases surgical treatment was followed by recurrence. No patient died of the tumor, and none of the tumors metastasized.

Dorfman and Czerniak (23) subsequently defined aggressive osteoblastoma as a rare tumor, borderline between osteoblastoma and osteosarcoma, usually larger than conventional osteoblastoma and characterized by epithelioid osteoblasts. These authors did not identify cartilage in any of the lesions. It is debatable whether local recurrence can be used to designate a tumor as "distinctly different." Local recurrence probably reflects the surgical procedure more than the biologic features of the neoplasm. We are unconvinced of the validity of the concept of aggressive osteoblastoma.

Cytologic Findings. In contrast to osteoid osteoma, FNA cell yields are often abundant and allow a diagnosis to be made on the basis of the presence of cytologically benign osteoblasts (34,35). The osteoblasts of osteoblastoma may vary in size and are occasionally large and epithelioid. The nuclei typically are round or oval and occasionally binucleated. The chromatin is evenly distributed, and the nucleoli are distinct and small or intermediate in size. The cytoplasm is homogeneous and fairly dense, with perinuclear clear areas that probably correspond to Golgi zones (fig. 5-32). Mitotic figures are scarce. The osteoblasts are either dissociated or arranged in cellular fragments, with a vascular spindle cell stroma that contains osteoclasts (figs. 5-32, 5-33). The osteoblasts may be enclosed in a fibrillary collagenous matrix that, based on ultrastructural studies of FNA material, corresponds to mineralized osteoid (fig. 5-34).

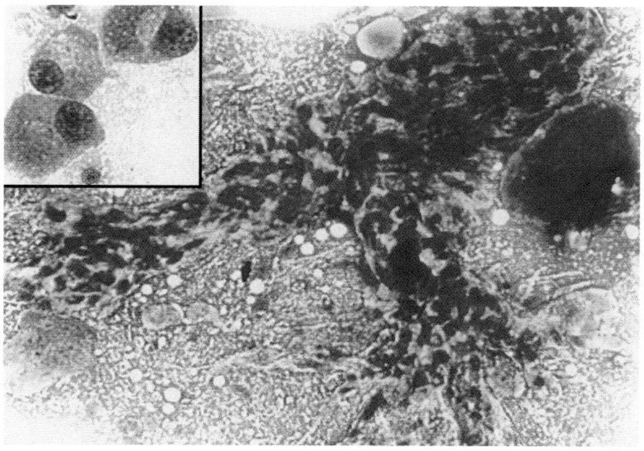

Figure 5-32

OSTEOBLASTOMA

Coherent clusters of uniform osteoblastic tumor cells (inset, high-power magnification), spindle cells, and osteoclasts are seen in a background matrix of stromal mucins (May-Grünwald-Giemsa–stained fine-needle aspiration [FNA] smear).

Genetics and Other Special Techniques. Osteoblastomas have a wide clinical and radiographic spectrum, and this may cause diagnostic difficulties in differentiating an osteoblastoma from an osteosarcoma. It would be useful to establish genetic markers that could be used in classifying osteoblastic bone tumors. Studies of *RB* or *TP53* gene mutations, *c-fos* and *c-jun* expression, or *HDM2 (MDM2)* gene amplification have shown, with rare exception, an absence of genetic alterations in osteoblastoma (19,25, 32). Osteosarcomas, however, frequently exhibit abnormalities of one or more of these genes.

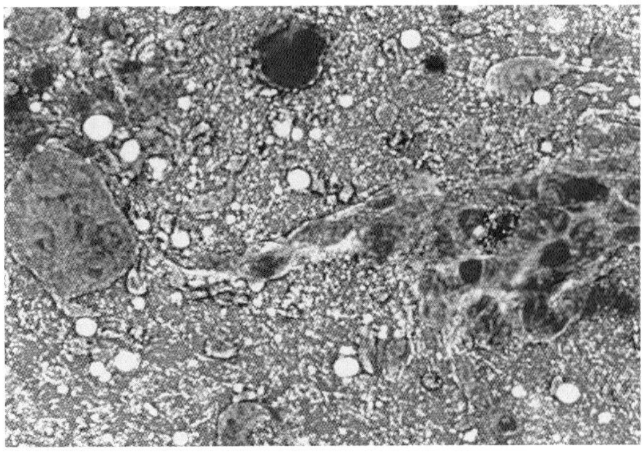

Figure 5-33

OSTEOBLASTOMA

Spindle cells and osteoclasts in a background matrix (May-Grünwald-Giemsa–stained FNA smear).

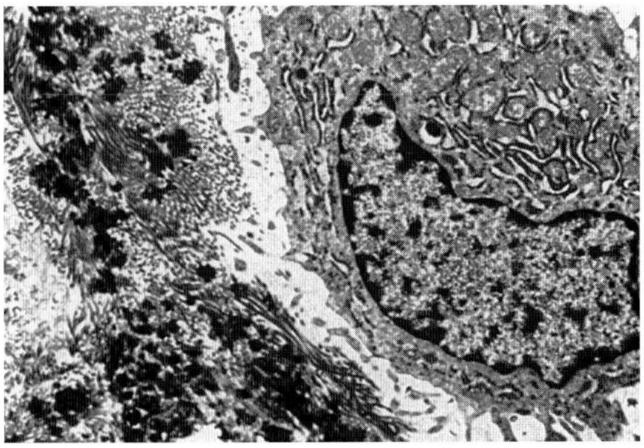

Figure 5-34

OSTEOBLASTOMA

Electron microscopy of FNA specimen shows tumor cells with features of osteoblasts as well as mineralized osteoid.

Table 5-1

CYTOGENETIC FINDINGS IN OSTEOBLASTOMA

Diagnosis	Age (yr)/Sex	Location	Chromosomal Complement	Reference
Osteoblastoma	7/M	Vertebra	46,XY,+der(15)t(15;20)(p11;p11), der(17)t(17;20)(p11-12;q11),-20	28
Aggressive osteoblastoma	34/M	Ilium	52,Y,t(X;11)(q22;p14),+2,del(5)(q22), der(6;8)(p10;q10),+del(9)(q31q33), add(12)(q24),-13,add(13)(p11), add(14)(p22),+16,add(18)(p11),+19, +add(19)(p13),-21,+3mar	22
Large cell epithelioid telangiectatic osteoblastoma	14/F	Mandible	46,XX,del(1)(q42),t(1;5;17;22) (p32-33;p13;q21;q12)	18

Cytogenetic studies performed on an osteoblastoma, an aggressive osteoblastoma, and a large cell, epithelioid, telangiectatic osteoblastoma have demonstrated unrelated rearrangements (Table 5-1) (18,22,28).

Differential Diagnosis. The differential diagnosis of osteoblastoma includes osteoid osteoma, osteosarcoma, giant cell tumor, and aneurysmal bone cyst. As pointed out above, osteoid osteomas and osteoblastomas are similar histologically. The only distinction between the two is the size of the nidus.

The distinction between osteoblastoma and osteosarcoma is usually relatively straightforward. Although, the radiographic features of osteoblastoma can appear worrisome, rarely does a radiograph of osteosarcoma suggest a benign lesion. Histologically, osteoblastoma can be impossible to differentiate from osteosarcoma, especially with limited biopsy material. The most important criterion for differentiating osteoblastoma from osteosarcoma is permeation. Osteoblastomas are well-demarcated lesions with no tendency to permeate between preexisting bony trabeculae. If the edge of the lesion is contained in the biopsy sample, a permeative histologic pattern will always be seen in an osteosarcoma. Osteoblastomas have a loose arrangement of tissue, with fibrovascular stroma between the bony trabeculae. Osteosarcomas can be vascular; however, they usually show a proliferation of cells between the bony trabeculae. Osteoblastomas characteristically have bony trabeculae rimmed by a single layer of osteoblasts, whereas osteosarcomas have many layers of osteoblasts surrounding the bony trabeculae and spindle cell proliferation. In limited biopsy material, this distinction can be nearly impossible to recognize.

When osteoblastoma involves the vertebrae, it tends to involve the posterior elements, the site also preferred by aneurysmal bone cysts. Aneurysmal bone cysts can have large amounts of reactive new bone formation, and, conversely, osteoblastomas may have features of secondary aneurysmal bone cyst. Hence, distinguishing between the two can be difficult, especially with limited biopsy material. However, if enough material is obtained, a characteristic loosely arranged proliferation of spindle cells is seen in aneurysmal bone cysts.

Generally, radiographs of giant cell tumors do not show mineralization; however, rare typical giant cell tumors do contain mineral. Histologically, giant cell tumors have a proliferation of mononuclear cells and giant cells without matrix formation. It has been recognized recently that bone, especially trabeculae, may form in typical giant cell tumors. If the lesion involves the end of a long bone or the body of a vertebra, a giant cell tumor should be considered before the diagnosis of osteoblastoma is made.

Treatment and Prognosis. Osteoblastomas are treated generally with curettage. Small lesions involving long bones may be resected. Recurrence after curettage is uncommon. Radiotherapy and chemotherapy are not indicated, although according to one report an osteoblastoma responded to chemotherapy (20).

MALIGNANT BONE-FORMING TUMORS

Osteosarcoma of Bone

Definition. Osteosarcoma is a malignant tumor in which osteoid or bone is produced directly by the tumor cells. Sanerkin (170) has pointed out that sampling may be a problem in identifying osteoid and has suggested that alkaline phosphatase positivity be used as the defining feature. However, this definition has not been accepted universally.

It is now recognized that, on the basis of clinical, radiographic, and histologic features, osteosarcoma includes several different clinicopathologic entities. Some of these entities are associated with prognostic significance, others are not. The terms *osteosarcoma* and *osteogenic sarcoma* both have been used to describe tumors that produce bone and tumors that arise from bone.

General Features. Except for myeloma, osteosarcoma is the most common primary malignant neoplasm of the skeleton, although only about 900 new cases occur annually in the United States (91). Dorfman and Czerniak (72), reporting on the incidence of bone tumors collected under the auspices of the Surveillance, Epidemiology and End Results (SEER) program, found osteosarcoma to be the most common type of bone sarcoma, accounting for 35 percent of all cases.

The cause of osteosarcoma is not known. A small percentage of these tumors arise in association with a preexisting condition. Included in the Mayo Clinic files are 169 postradiation sarcomas and 70 Paget sarcomas. Osteosarcomas arising in other benign conditions are so rare they may be coincidental and not causally related. Trauma has been suggested as a cause of sarcomas, but it is more likely that trauma only calls attention to the preexisting tumor. The Mayo Clinic files contain one well-documented example of osteosarcoma that developed at the site of a previous fracture sustained from a gunshot wound. Whether the trauma or the bullet fragments gave rise to the tumor is not clear. Brien et al. (56) reported an example of osteosarcoma arising at the site of a previous total hip arthroplasty, suggesting a relationship with metallic ions. No comparable case is included in the Mayo Clinic files.

Genetic abnormalities may be associated with the development of osteosarcoma. As well recognized, patients with the hereditary form of bilateral retinoblastoma are at high risk for the development of osteosarcoma. Mohney et al. (142), using the Mayo Clinic files, reported on the long-term follow-up of 82 children with the hereditary form of retinoblastoma. Nonocular malignancies developed in 15 of these patients, including osteosarcoma in 3 (the lower extremity in 2 and the mandible in 1). This incidence seems to be much less than that suggested in the literature (91). In the Mayo Clinic series, osteosarcoma developed in two patients (a brother and sister) with Rothmund-Thompson syndrome and in two (brothers) with Bloom's syndrome. One patient had Li-Fraumeni syndrome. Another patient (female) had multiple metachronous osteosarcoma, which she survived, but died of bilateral breast carcinoma. This patient's daughter has a rhabdomyosarcoma of the temporal region and may also have a genetic syndrome.

Classification. Osteosarcomas are classified into different types depending on the location and the clinical, radiographic, and microscopic features. They are broadly characterized into those occurring primarily in the medullary cavity and those situated predominantly on the surface of bone (Table 5-2).

The general features of medullary osteosarcomas are described in the following section. Special features associated with the different subtypes are considered in the respective sections.

Table 5-2

CLASSIFICATION OF OSTEOSARCOMAS

Medullary Osteosarcoma	Surface Osteosarcoma
Conventional	Parosteal osteosarcoma
Osteosarcoma of jawbones	Periosteal osteosarcoma
Postradiation sarcoma	High-grade surface osteosarcoma
Osteosarcoma in Paget's disease	
Osteosarcoma in other benign conditions	
Telangiectatic osteosarcoma	
Small cell osteosarcoma	
Low-grade osteosarcoma	
Multicentric osteosarcoma	

MEDULLARY OSTEOSARCOMAS

Conventional Osteosarcoma

Clinical Features. The peak incidence for osteosarcoma is in the second decade of life (46 percent of patients) (fig. 5-35). Of the cases in the Mayo Clinic files, only eight patients were younger than 5 years. In the Mayo Clinic series, there is a steady decrease in incidence after the second decade of life. Dorfman and Czerniak (72) reported a second small peak near age 70. In this series and one from the Memorial Hospital (104), older patients were more likely to have involvement of the axial skeleton. In the Mayo Clinic series, 183 patients were older than 60 years, and 45 percent of them had a preexisting condition such as Paget's disease or previous irradiation. In the Memorial Hospital series, 56 percent of tumors were considered secondary.

Osteosarcoma has a slight but definite predilection for males. In the Mayo Clinic series, 58 percent of patients were males.

Pain, which initially may be intermittent, and swelling are the cardinal symptoms. Pathologic fracture is uncommon; even more uncommon is the detection of tumor as an incidental finding on radiographs. The duration of symptoms before diagnosis varies from a few weeks to months, rarely for longer than 1 year. A flare-up of symptoms in a patient with a known predisposing condition, such as Paget's disease, should arouse suspicion of malignant change. One patient in the Mayo Clinic series had an osteosarcoma of the tibia and radiographic evidence of rickets (oncogenic osteomalacia). Cheng et al. (62) also reported a case of oncogenic osteomalacia associated with osteosarcoma.

A painful mass is usually apparent in the affected region. With large masses, overlying veins may be prominent and edema may occur distal to the lesion. Patients with advanced disease may present with an ulcerating mass lesion.

Sites. The metaphyseal region of long bones is the site of predilection. Almost half of all osteosarcomas arise in the region of the knee; the distal femoral metaphysis is the most common site. Osteosarcomas distal to the ankle and wrist joints are rare. In the Mayo Clinic files, three osteosarcomas involved the phalanges of the foot and only one affected those of the hand. In a series of 4,214 osteosarcomas, Mirra et al. (141) found only 1 involving the phalanx of a toe. Okada et al. (150) reported on 12 patients (13 tumors) who had osteosarcoma involving the small bones of the hand: 7 in the phalanges and 6 in the metacarpals. Only one patient died of metastatic disease. About 10 percent of the tumors involve the diaphyses. Kyriakos (122) described an osteosarcoma arising in the cortex of the shaft of the tibia and found only two other similar cases reported. Radiographic findings may suggest a benign process, especially an osteoblastoma, when the tumor involves the cortex (fig. 5-36).

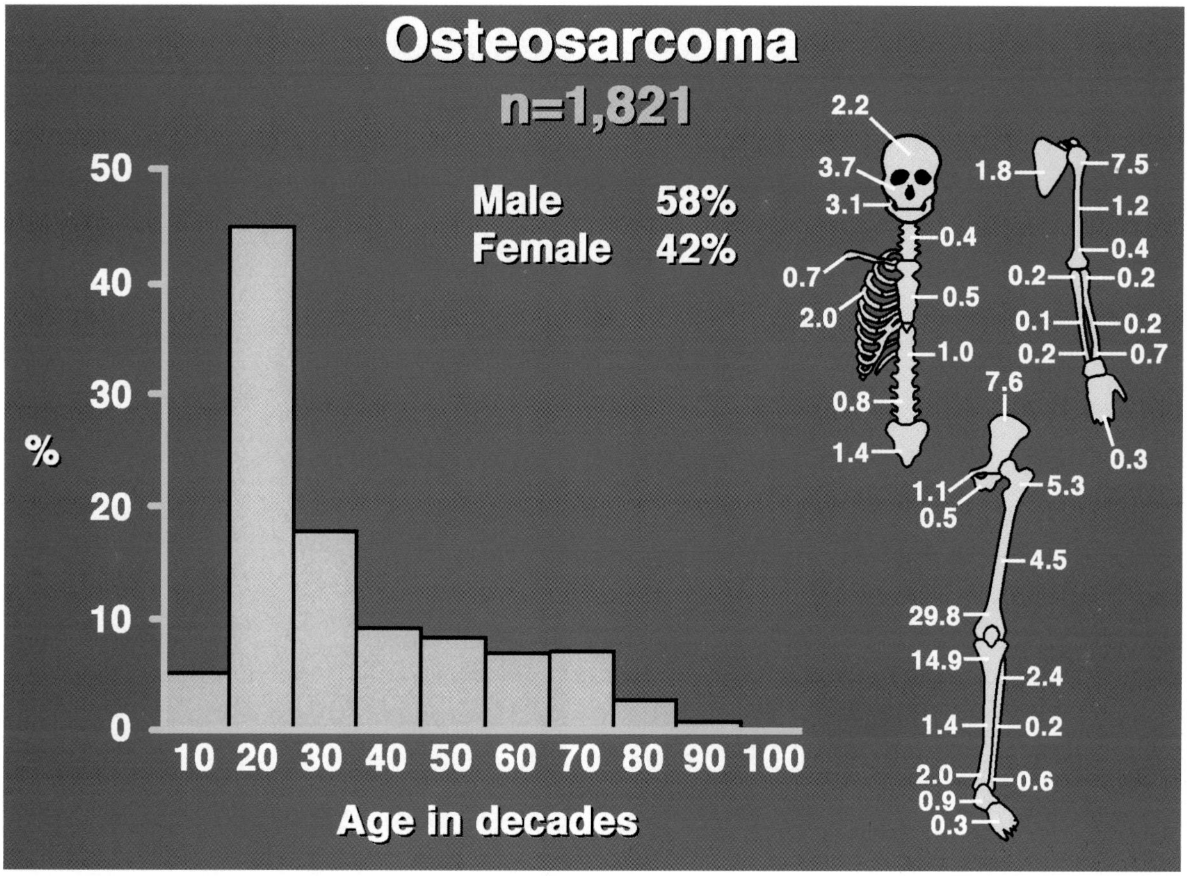

Figure 5-35

OSTEOSARCOMA

Distribution of osteosarcoma according to the age and sex of the patient and the site of the lesion.

Radiographic Findings. The radiographic appearance depends on the amount of mineralization in the lesion. Campanacci and Cervellati (57) found that 47 percent of osteosarcomas were sclerotic, 43 percent were lytic, and 10 percent were mixed.

At presentation, osteosarcoma usually appears as a geographic area of destruction in the metaphyseal region of long bones (fig. 5-37). The margins of the tumor are poorly demarcated. The cortex is almost always destroyed, and the tumor extends into soft tissues. During this process of tumor growth, the periosteum is lifted from the underlying cortex. This gives rise to periosteal new bone formation, usually proximal to the tumor, which has been termed Codman's triangle (fig. 5-38). A biopsy specimen from this area shows only layers of periosteal new bone, not tumor.

Because an osteosarcoma produces a calcifying and ossifying osteoid substance, various degrees of density are seen within the lesion (fig. 5-39). The matrix has been termed cloud-like. The densities may be present in the soft tissue extension, a feature virtually diagnostic of osteosarcoma. Soft tissue mineralization may be in the form of striations perpendicular to the involved bone, giving rise to a "sunburst" pattern (fig. 5-38). Although the radiographic appearance of most osteosarcomas suggests a malignant neoplasm, a few appear deceptively benign (fig. 5-40).

Radioisotope bone scans can be useful in demonstrating multicentric osteosarcoma. In most centers that care for patients with osteosarcoma,

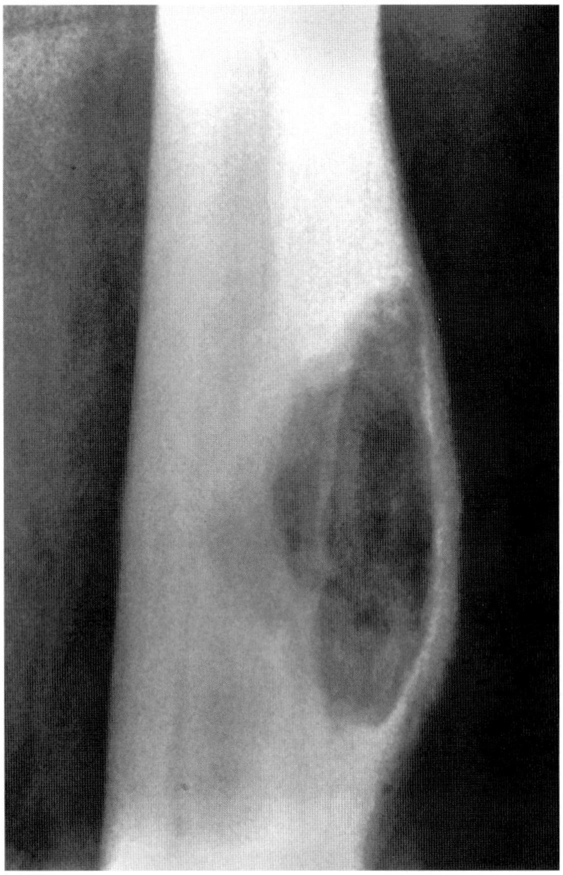

Figure 5-36

OSTEOSARCOMA

When osteosarcomas involve primarily the cortex, the radiographic differential diagnosis is broad and includes both benign and malignant lesions.

CT and MRI are used routinely for preoperative evaluation (fig. 5-37, bottom). With the advent of chemotherapy, most patients have tumor resection instead of amputation; hence, an accurate assessment of the extent of the tumor is essential. McLeod and Berquist (137) have emphasized the superiority of CT and MRI over plain radiographs for delineating the extent of the tumor: CT appears to be superior for the axial skeleton, but MRI is superior for the extremities. Both T_1- and T_2-weighted sequences are necessary. Several studies have emphasized the superiority of MRI over CT for preoperative staging of osteosarcoma (87,154,164).

Efforts are being made to predict the effectiveness of chemotherapy preoperatively.

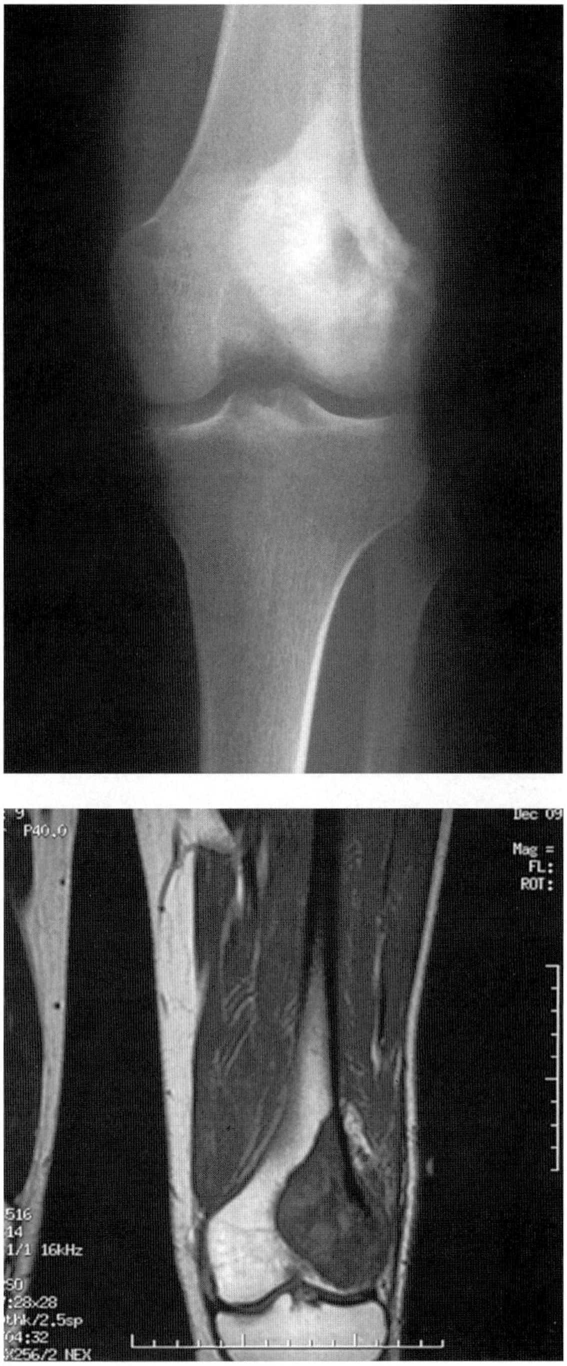

Figure 5-37

OSTEOSARCOMA

Top: A large, mixed sclerotic and lytic lesion involves the metaphyseal region of the left distal femur and extends to the lateral condyle near the articular surface. Note the associated periosteal reaction.

Bottom: MRI defines more clearly the extent of the osteosarcoma, and shows destruction of the lateral cortex and extension into soft tissue.

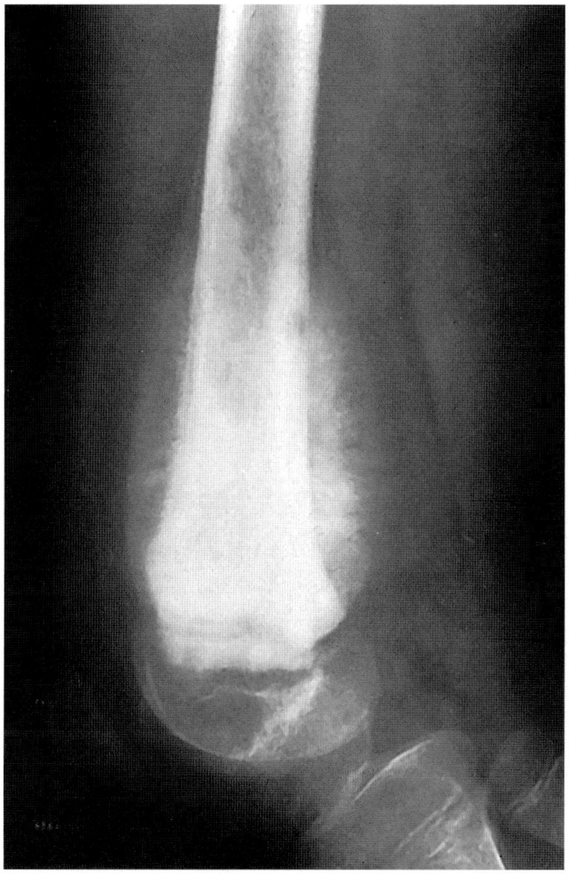

Figure 5-38

OSTEOSARCOMA

A large, malignant, destructive sclerotic lesion in the distal femur has features typical of an osteosarcoma: a mineralized soft tissue mass, malignant periosteal reaction with a spiculated hair-on-end pattern, and formation of Codman's triangle.

Carrasco et al. (58) performed serial angiographic studies and defined response as complete disappearance of neovascularity. They found that this method was sensitive but not very specific and tended to overestimate responders but not nonresponders. Kunisada et al. (119) found that thallium 201 scintigraphy was superior to angiography, especially in recognizing nonresponders.

Gross Findings. The gross appearance of conventional osteosarcoma is highly variable and depends largely on the predominant matrix. By the time therapy is instituted, most osteosarcomas are large and have an extraosseous extension. The tumor usually is situated in the metaphysis; the epiphyseal plate acts as a relative

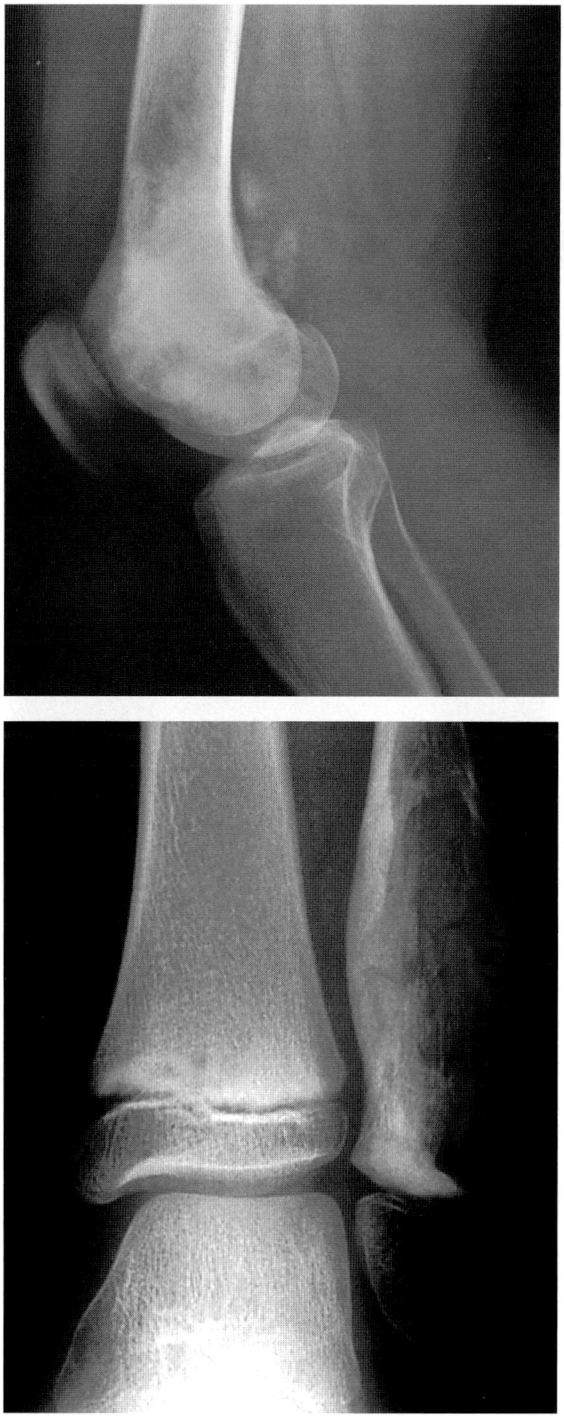

Figure 5-39

OSTEOSARCOMA

Top: A heavily mineralized, destructive osteosarcoma involves the distal femur of a 24-year-old woman and extends posteriorly into soft tissue.

Bottom: This predominantly lytic and destructive tumor involves the distal fibula of an 8-year-old boy.

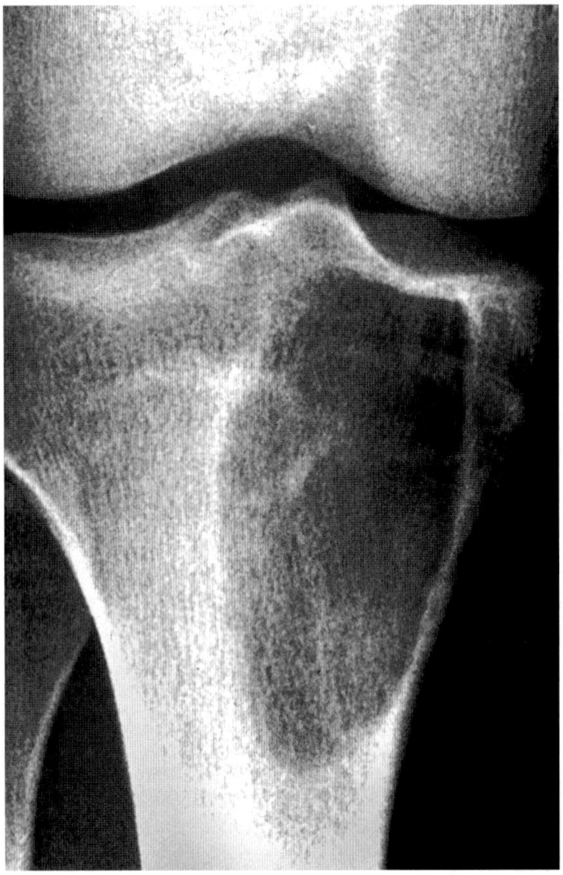

Figure 5-40

OSTEOSARCOMA

Occasionally, the radiographic features of osteosarcoma are misleading. Biopsy tissue from this relatively circumscribed benign-appearing lytic lesion of the proximal tibia showed a grade 3 fibroblastic osteosarcoma.

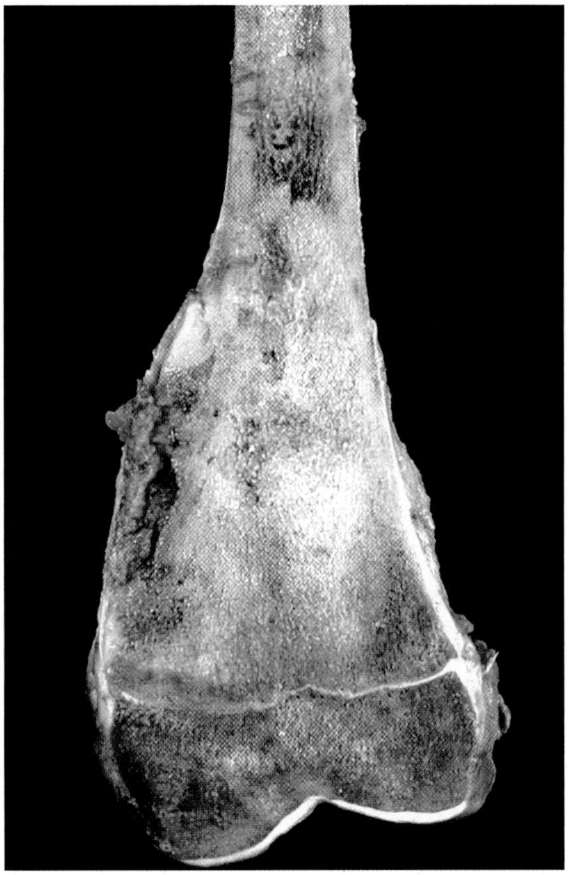

Figure 5-41

OSTEOSARCOMA

This osteosarcoma involves the distal femoral metaphysis and shows a destructive growth pattern, with extension through the cortex and epiphyseal plate.

barrier to its growth, and the tumor may stop abruptly at the plate (fig. 5-41). However, microscopic examination generally shows that the tumor extends into the epiphysis, and it is probably dangerous to perform a resection assuming that the epiphyseal plate is spared. The tumor may extend into the bone marrow cavity for a considerable distance beyond the mass seen in the soft tissue. The margin between the tumor and normal bone marrow is usually sharp.

Most osteosarcomas have the fleshy white appearance typical of high-grade sarcomas. Rarely, the tumor is extremely sclerotic and may simulate ivory (fig. 5-42). These osteosclerotic osteosarcomas nearly always contain some soft fleshy areas, especially in the soft tissue extension. A biopsy of the intraosseous component is rarely necessary to obtain diagnostic material. Decalcification of the biopsy specimen should not be necessary if the surgeon samples the soft area of the tumor. Usually, the type of matrix produced by the tumor cannot be predicted from its gross appearance. A chondroblastic osteosarcoma rarely suggests a cartilaginous tumor (fig. 5-43). Necrosis may be seen microscopically, but it is not prominent grossly.

Currently, most patients with osteosarcoma are treated with chemotherapy preoperatively and the tumor is then resected (figs. 5-44, 5-45). The specimen is handled essentially in the same way whether it is from a resection or amputation. Bone marrow from the resection

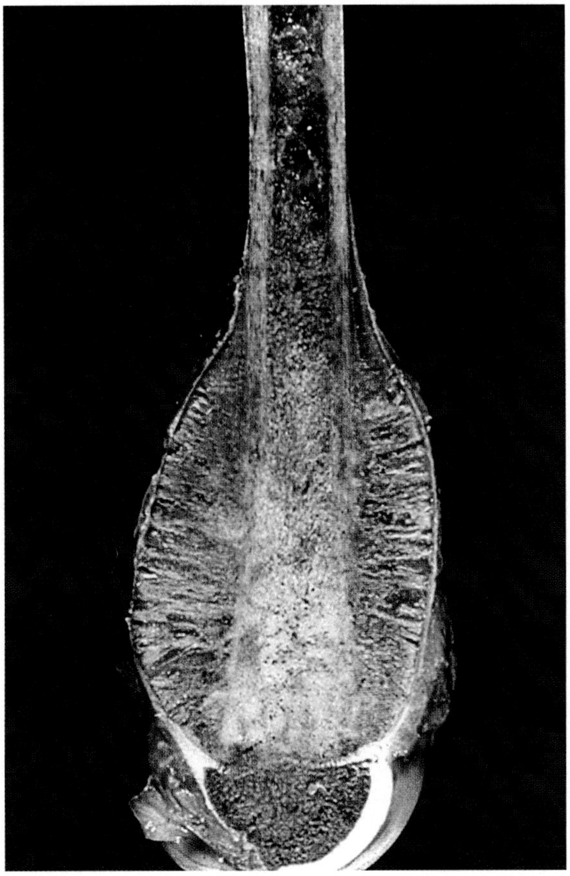

Figure 5-42

OSTEOSARCOMA

A homogeneous, gray-white, densely sclerotic osteosarcoma.

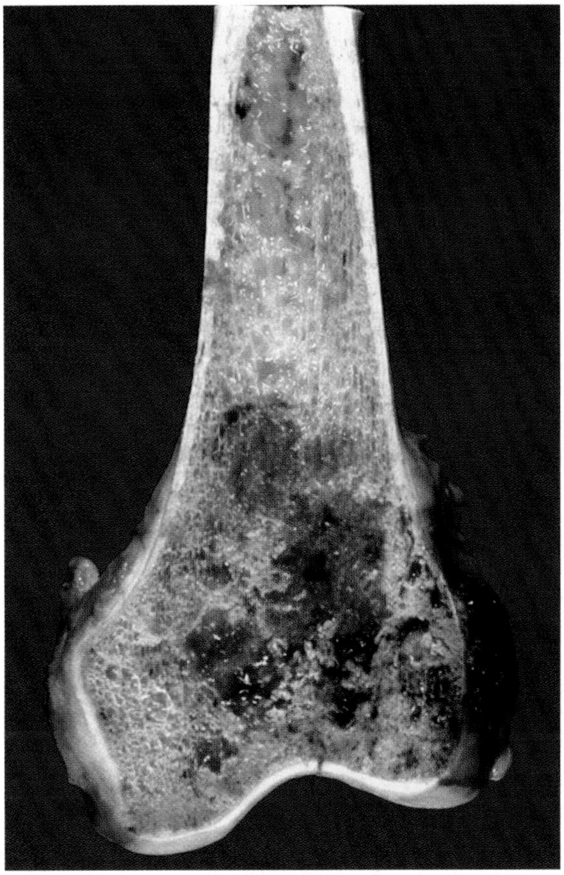

Figure 5-43

OSTEOSARCOMA

The gray-white lobules with myxoid change within the tumor correspond to areas of cartilage production in this grade 3 chondroblastic osteosarcoma.

margin can be removed and checked on a frozen section preparation. The soft tissues, including the skeletal muscles, are dissected to leave the tumor and involved bone. Willen (201) and Raymond and Ayala (163) have described the techniques for evaluating the effect of chemotherapy using preoperative arteriograms. With the arteriogram as a guide, the bone is cut with a bandsaw in a plane to identify maximum viable tumor. Slices 4-mm thick are cut with an Isomet saw. The entire slab is cut into pieces, reassembled, photographed, and decalcified. The sections are evaluated for viable and necrotic tumor, and with the photograph, viable tumor can be mapped.

Skip metastases, as described by Enneking and Kagan (77), have not been a significant problem in most other series (fig. 5-46). These authors found foci of tumor separated from the main mass in 25 percent of cases. This seemed to be associated with a worse prognosis. However, with modern imaging techniques, it is unlikely that skip lesions will be missed.

Microscopic Findings. The histopathologic features of osteosarcoma vary greatly. Lichtenstein (128) considered the following two features to be diagnostic: 1) the presence of frankly sarcomatous stroma and 2) direct formation of osteoid and bone by this malignant connective tissue (fig. 5-47).

Conventional osteosarcoma can be divided into osteoblastic, chondroblastic, and fibroblastic types depending on the predominant matrix produced. Most osteosarcomas show foci

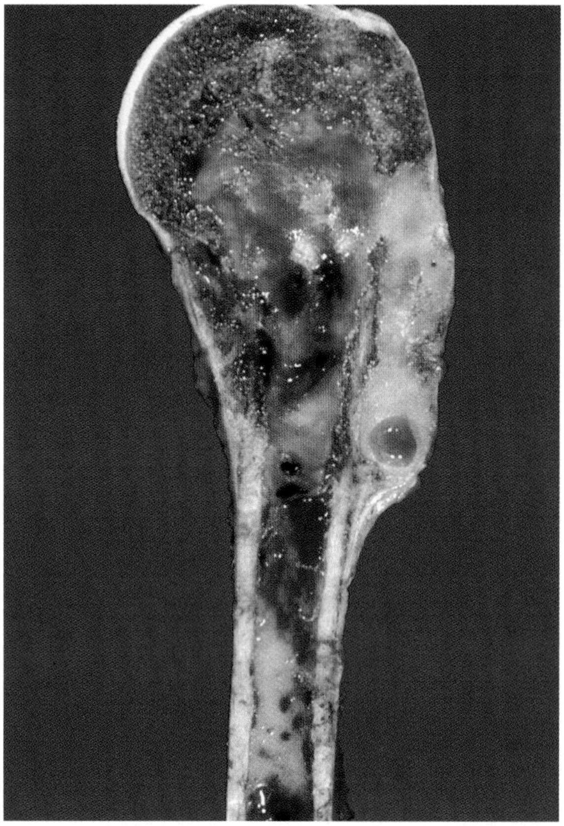

Figure 5-44

OSTEOSARCOMA

The tumor was resected after preoperative chemotherapy. Microscopic sections showed a good response (99 percent necrosis) to chemotherapy. Grossly, the necrotic tumor contains a firm and somewhat gelatinous red-brown and gray area with focal infarct and cystic changes.

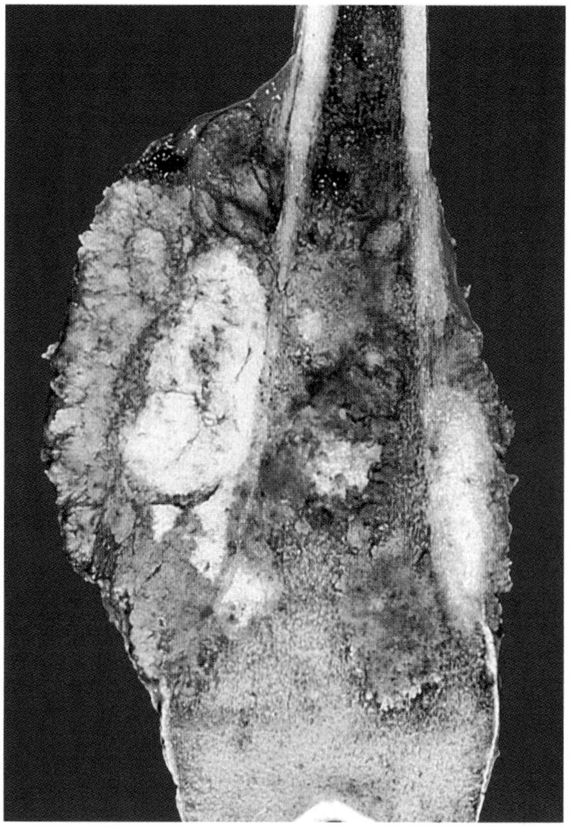

Figure 5-45

OSTEOSARCOMA

The tumor did not respond well to preoperative chemotherapy (40 percent necrosis in the resected specimen). Grossly, there are scattered nodules of viable yellow-gray tumor.

with varying differentiation, but the classification is based on the predominant matrix. Also, it is not unusual for one type of osteosarcoma (e.g., chondroblastic) to metastasize as another (e.g., osteoblastic). This subclassification almost surely has no prognostic significance, although it has been suggested that osteoblastic osteosarcoma is associated with a worse prognosis (186). Currently, most osteosarcomas are diagnosed with an FNA aspirate, and this would make subclassification difficult. However, we believe that it is still important to continue to subclassify osteosarcomas because this emphasizes the variability in the tumor.

About 50 percent of osteosarcomas may be termed *osteoblastic*. Typically, the osteoid appears as pink-staining hyaline material that forms an anastomosing network among individual tumor cells, producing a lace-like pattern (fig. 5-48). Although this pattern is typical of osteosarcoma, it is not diagnostic. "Malignant osteoid" should be diagnosed only if malignant cells are identified adjacent to the matrix. The matrix may undergo various degrees of calcification (fig. 5-49). Mineralized matrix may be arranged as trabeculae; rarely, the matrix of high-grade osteosarcomas forms thick "normal"-appearing bony trabeculae (fig. 5-50). Rarely, an osteosarcoma (osteosclerotic) produces so much mineralizing matrix that tumor cells are not visible. Osteosarcoma can be diagnosed confidently if the matrix fills the bone marrow spaces, entrapping preexisting medullary bone (fig. 5-51).

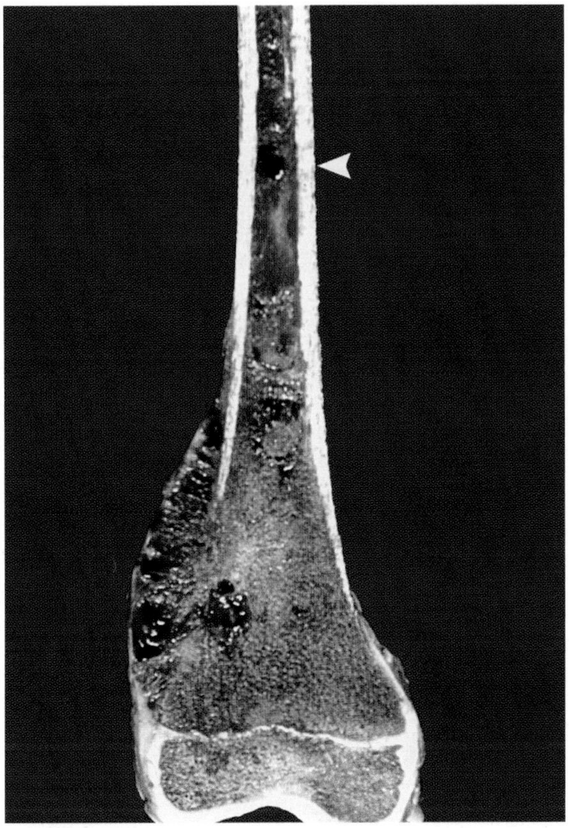

Figure 5-46

OSTEOSARCOMA

A skip metastasis (arrowhead) was identified 3 cm proximal to the main mass in this osteosarcoma involving the distal femur of a 9-year-old boy, in whom pulmonary metastasis developed 4 months after an above-knee amputation.

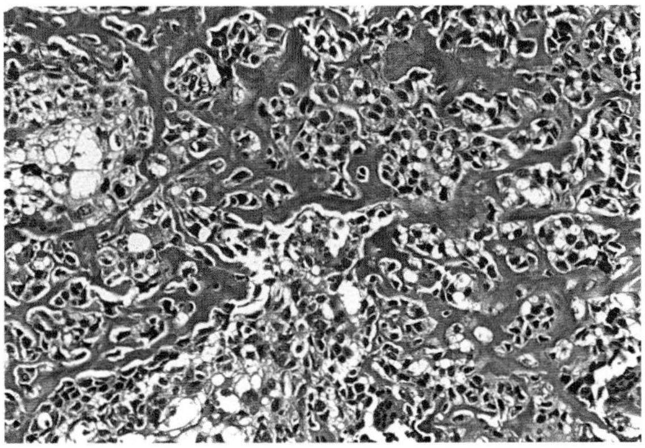

Figure 5-47

OSTEOSARCOMA

Trabeculae of immature bone are produced by tumor cells that have malignant cytologic features.

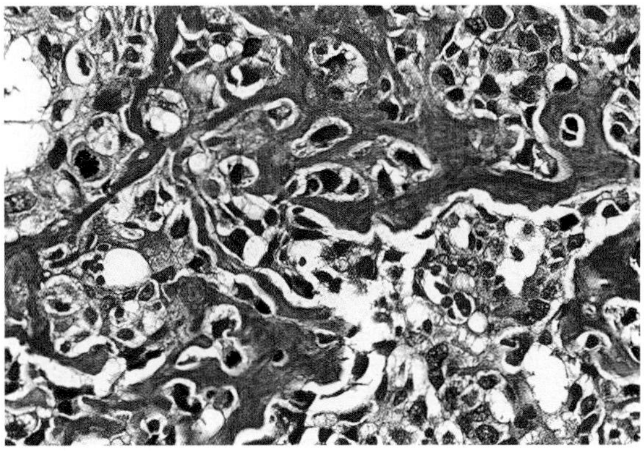

Figure 5-48

OSTEOSARCOMA

A lace-like pattern of osteoid is produced by eosinophilic matrix entrapping anaplastic tumor cells.

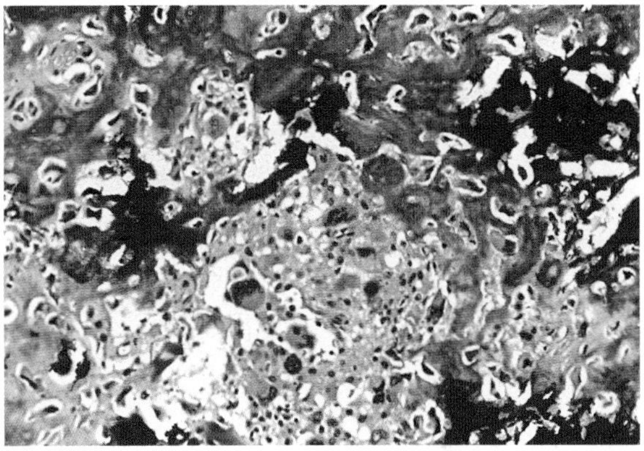

Figure 5-49

OSTEOSARCOMA

The extent of dark blue-purple matrix calcification can vary from focal to diffuse.

Approximately 25 percent of osteosarcomas show prominent cartilage differentiation and are termed *chondroblastic*. The tumor is composed of lobules of cartilage. The cells in the lacunae have the cytologic features of a high-grade malignancy, with increasing cellularity and sheets of spindle cells toward the periphery of the nodules (fig. 5-52). There is a gradual transition from the chondroid areas to the spindle cell areas. Lace-like osteoid is usual between the spindle cells (fig. 5-53). A high-grade cartilage tumor with spindle cells but without clear-cut osteoid production should still be classified as an osteosarcoma. The lack of osteoid is assumed to

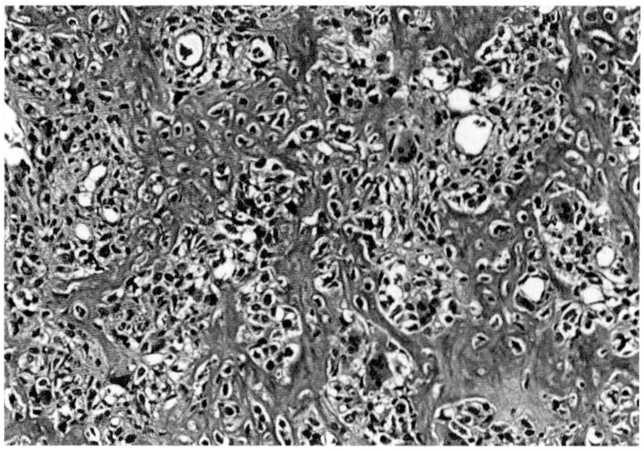

Figure 5-50

OSTEOSARCOMA

Occasionally, heavy amounts of matrix are produced, forming thick sclerotic bony trabeculae.

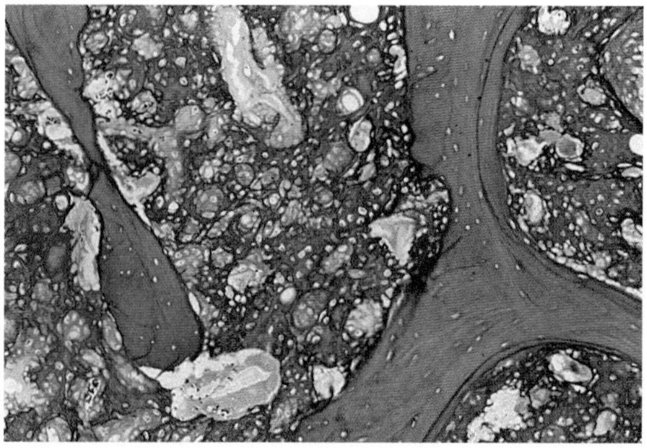

Figure 5-51

OSTEOSARCOMA

Although individual tumor cells are hard to identify in this osteosclerotic osteosarcoma, the pattern of permeation through preexisting medullary bone is sufficient to support the diagnosis.

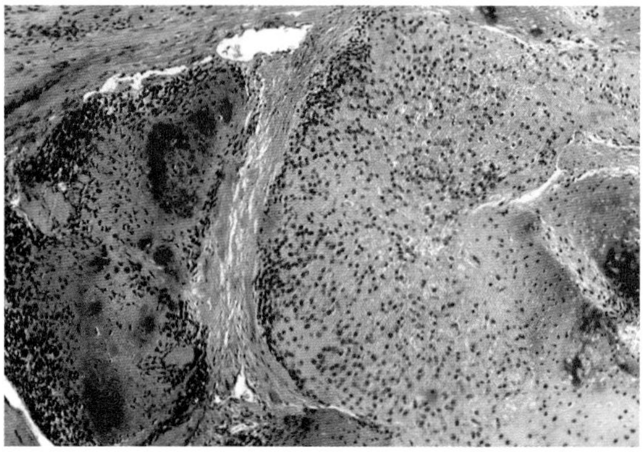

Figure 5-52

OSTEOSARCOMA

Chondroblastic osteosarcoma shows a condensation of spindle cells at the periphery of cartilaginous nodules.

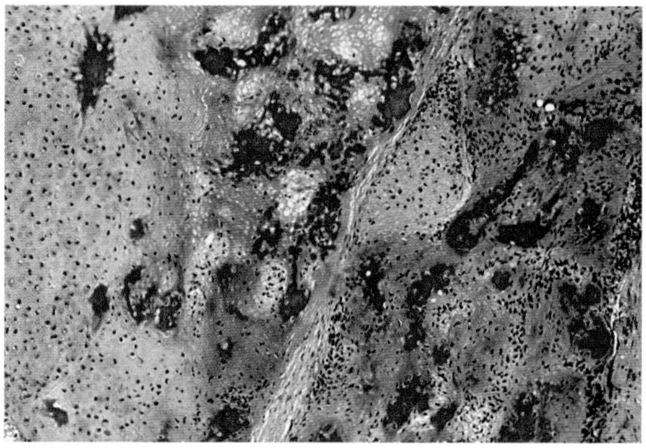

Figure 5-53

OSTEOSARCOMA

Pink osteoid production is evident between the hyperchromatic spindle-shaped tumor cells in this chondroblastic osteosarcoma.

be a sampling problem. It is common to see bony trabeculae in the center of the lobules (fig. 5-54).

The rest of the tumors are classified as *fibroblastic*. The tumor cells are spindle shaped and arranged in interlacing fascicles, suggesting the diagnosis of fibrosarcoma. Generally, the tumor cells are cytologically atypical, which suggests a high-grade sarcoma (Broders grade 3 or 4) (fig. 5-55). In some cases, the spindle cells are arranged in a storiform pattern and associated with pleomorphic nuclei and benign and malignant giant cells, thus simulating the appearance of malignant fibrous histiocytoma (fig. 5-56). In both types, osteoid is seen only focally. It is not uncommon for matrix to be present only in the metastases. Clearly, the diagnosis depends on sampling. This problem has been highlighted by the term *osteosarcoma-malignant fibrous histiocytoma type* (40). It is not clear whether it is important to distinguish between fibroblastic osteosarcoma, on the one hand, and fibrosarcoma and malignant fibrous histiocytoma, on the other, particularly because the distinction can be arbitrary.

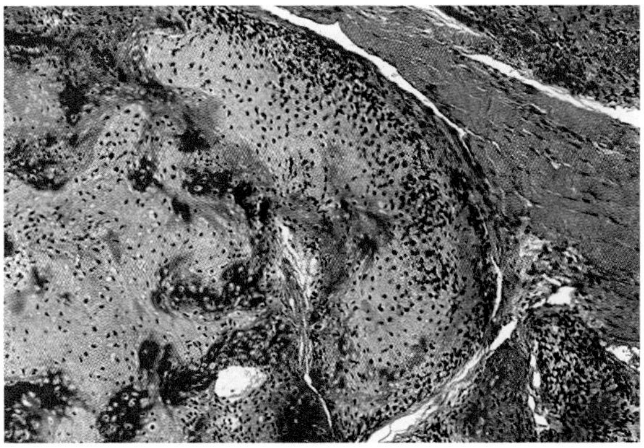

Figure 5-54

OSTEOSARCOMA

Obvious foci of bone production are scattered throughout several chondroblastic lobules.

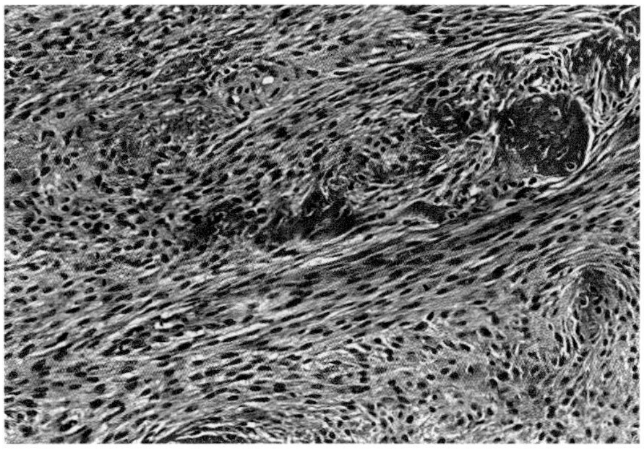

Figure 5-55

OSTEOSARCOMA

This fibroblastic osteosarcoma has the typical appearance of interlacing fascicles of hyperchromatic spindle-shaped stromal cells associated with matrix production.

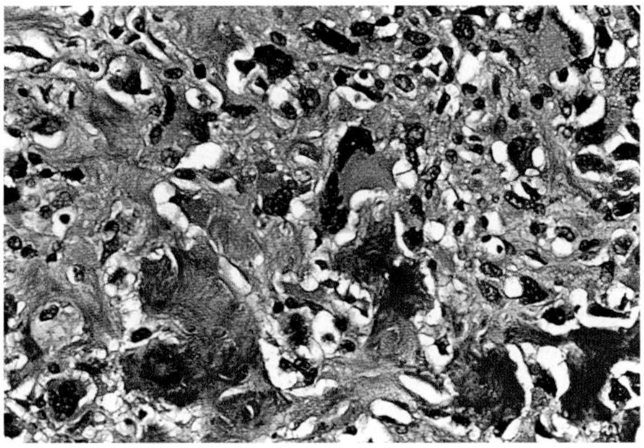

Figure 5-56

OSTEOSARCOMA

Fibroblastic osteosarcoma with a striking degree of cytologic pleomorphism resembles a malignant fibrous histiocytoma. The presence of matrix production associated with tumor cells confirms the diagnosis of osteosarcoma.

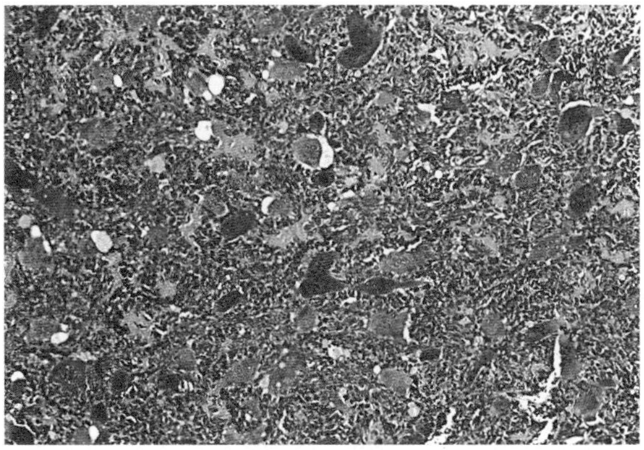

Figure 5-57

OSTEOSARCOMA

The low-power microscopic appearance of this osteosarcoma is similar to that of a giant cell tumor.

Many osteosarcomas contain benign giant cells similar to those seen in giant cell tumor (fig. 5-57). Troup et al. (190) identified collections of giant cells in approximately 25 percent of osteosarcomas. In these cases, the giant cells are not a dominant feature; moreover, clinical features such as the age of the patient and the location in the metaphysis clearly point to the correct diagnosis. In a small proportion of cases, the giant cells may dominate and obscure the nature of the neoplasm. Bathurst et al. (41) named these tumors *osteoclast-rich osteosarcoma*. Of the nine tumors they described, six were diaphyseal, two metadiaphyseal, and one epiphyseal. The presence of a giant cell–rich neoplasm in an unusual location should suggest the possibility of *giant cell–rich osteosarcoma*. Extensive spindling of the mononuclear cells, prominent nucleoli, and other features of atypia (fig. 5-58), and the presence of lace-like osteoid are also helpful in diagnosing osteosarcoma (fig. 5-59). The cytologic features of malignancy in the mononuclear cells can be extremely subtle and the diagnosis of osteosarcoma difficult. In the

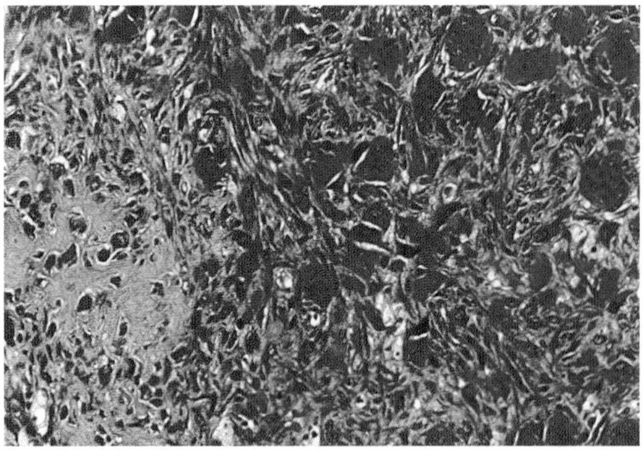

Figure 5-58

OSTEOSARCOMA

The malignant cytologic features of the stromal cells are obvious in this osteosarcoma containing numerous multinucleated giant cells.

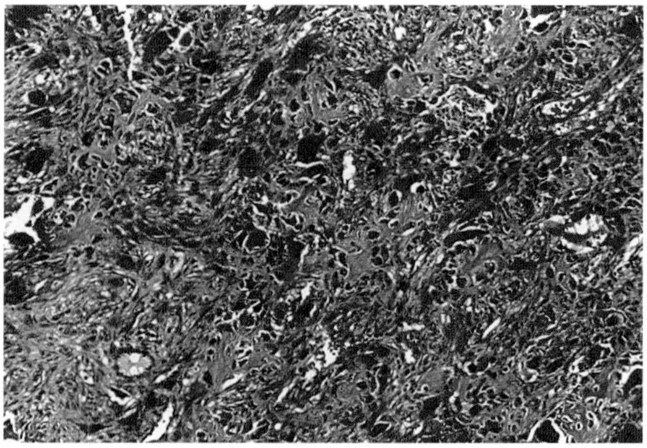

Figure 5-59

OSTEOSARCOMA

Abundant matrix production is evident in this giant cell–rich osteosarcoma.

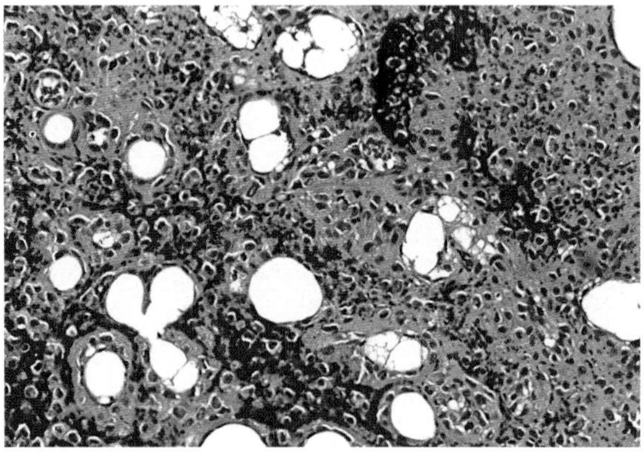

Figure 5-60

OSTEOSARCOMA

Although the cytologic features and calcified matrix are suggestive of chondroblastoma, the permeation of bone marrow fat seen in this osteosarcoma is not.

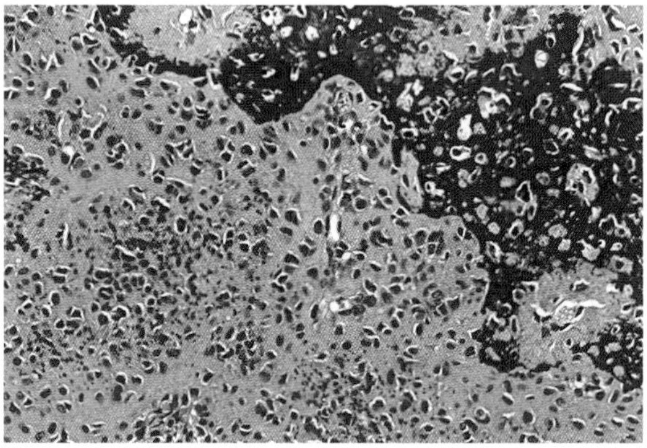

Figure 5-61

OSTEOSARCOMA

The coarse pattern of calcified matrix deposition supports the diagnosis of osteosarcoma rather than chondroblastoma.

series of Bathurst et al. 50 percent of the patients died of disease.

Some osteosarcomas produce trabecular-appearing bone, simulating the appearance of osteoblastoma (49). The distinction between osteosarcoma and osteoblastoma can be difficult to make and is based on the presence of permeation and multiple layers of osteoblasts in the former.

Rarely, an osteosarcoma has tumor cells that are oval and have cleaved nuclei, simulating the appearance of chondroblastoma (171). Osteosarcoma should be suspected if the lesion is not epiphyseal, the tumor cells are arranged in sheets, preexisting structures have been permeated (fig. 5-60), and the matrix is mineralized osteoid (fig. 5-61) rather than the "chicken wire" calcification typical of chondroblastoma.

Some osteosarcomas have epithelioid-appearing cells (fig. 5-62). This is not unexpected because osteoblasts frequently appear epithelioid. Kramer et al. (116) and Hasegawa et al. (98) reported on epithelioid-appearing osteosarcomas in which immunohistochemical stains also

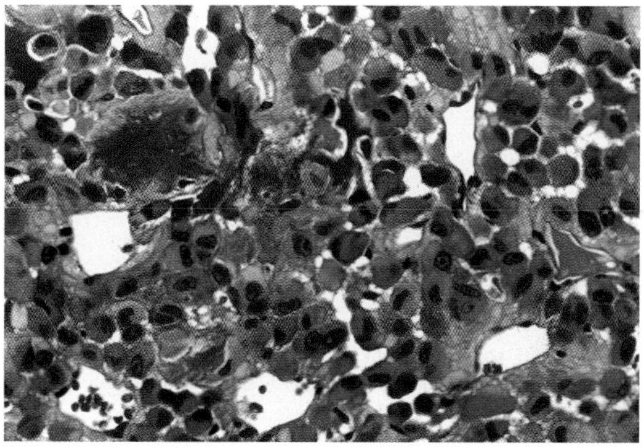

Figure 5-62

OSTEOSARCOMA

A lace-like pattern of matrix production is associated with epithelioid cells that have round nuclei and abundant eosinophilic cytoplasm.

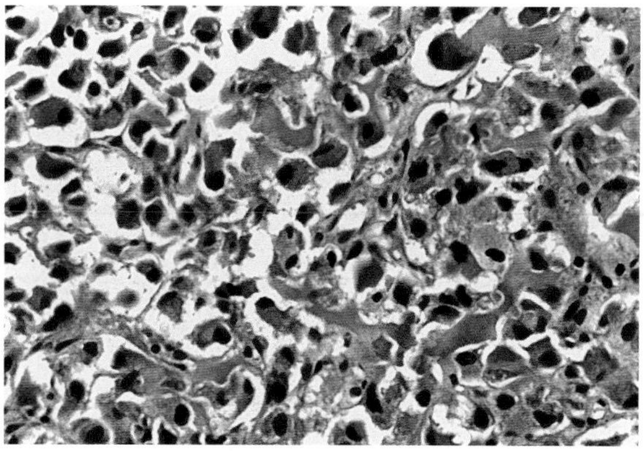

Figure 5-63

OSTEOSARCOMA

Occasionally, the plump tumor cells of epithelioid osteosarcoma have cytologic features resembling those of a signet ring cell carcinoma.

showed epithelial differentiation. True gland formation and squamous differentiation are extremely unusual. However, the osteoblasts may cluster, with central matrix production suggesting gland formation. The tumor cells may have a signet ring appearance and focal osteoid production (fig. 5-63). The presence of an epithelial-appearing malignancy but with clinical features that favor osteosarcoma should suggest the diagnosis of osteosarcoma.

Cytologic Findings. For most high-grade osteosarcomas, the FNA diagnosis of a primary malignant bone tumor is usually straightforward (124,146,196,198,200). The aspirate is typically cellular and consists of mesenchymal cells with prominent atypia and frequent mitoses. Some of the cellular and matrix features depend on the type of osteosarcoma. Six types of high-grade osteosarcoma can be recognized cytologically: osteoblastic (frequently with epithelioid features), chondroblastic, pleomorphic (malignant fibrous histiocytoma–like), spindle cell–fibroblastic, small cell, and giant cell (osteoclast)–rich types. Also, mixed types are encountered frequently.

Osteoblastic and Pleomorphic Types. Most high-grade osteosarcomas are either osteoblastic or pleomorphic, with most cases demonstrating features of both. At one end of the spectrum, the majority of tumor cells have prominent osteoblastic and epithelioid features, closely resembling an osteoblastoma (fig. 5-64). However,

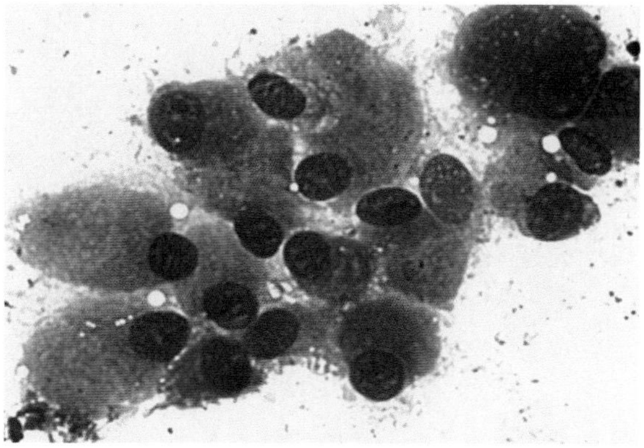

Figure 5-64

OSTEOSARCOMA

This osteoblastic osteosarcoma shows moderate atypia (May-Grünwald-Giemsa–stained FNA smear).

compared with osteoblastoma, nuclear size and shape are more variable, the chromatin is dispersed more irregularly, and the nucleoli are larger (fig. 5-65). Also, multinucleated tumor cells are seen. At the other end of the spectrum, bizarre large multinucleated tumor cells predominate, with few or no osteoblastic cells (fig. 5-66). In some cases, clusters of tumor cells are enclosed in a delicate, fibrillary collagenous matrix (figs. 5-67, 5-68) that is mineralized osteoid (compare with fig. 5-65). The osteoblastic nature of the tumor cells is demonstrated by staining the aspirates for alkaline phosphatase (fig. 5-69).

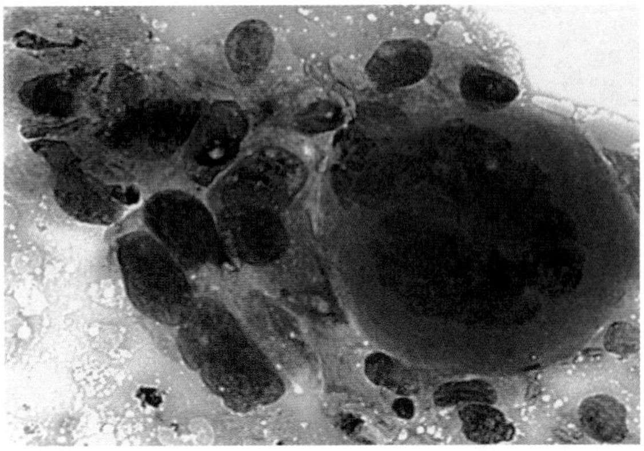

Figure 5-65

OSTEOSARCOMA

The osteoblastic osteosarcoma shows severe atypia and scattered, bizarre multinucleated tumor cells (May-Grünwald-Giemsa–stained FNA smear).

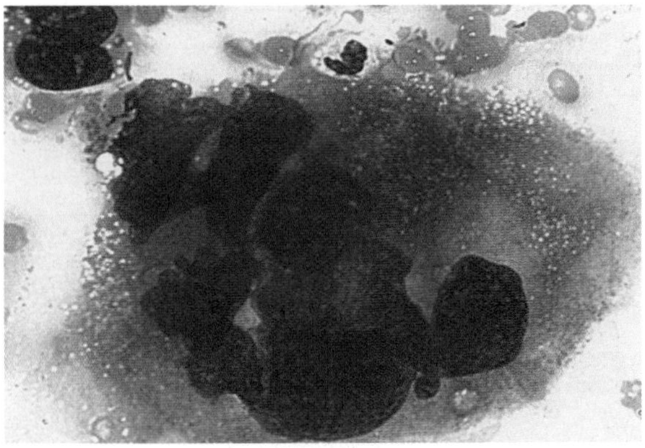

Figure 5-66

OSTEOSARCOMA

A pleomorphic high-grade osteosarcoma with predominantly giant tumor cells resembles malignant fibrous histiocytoma (May-Grünwald-Giemsa–stained FNA smear).

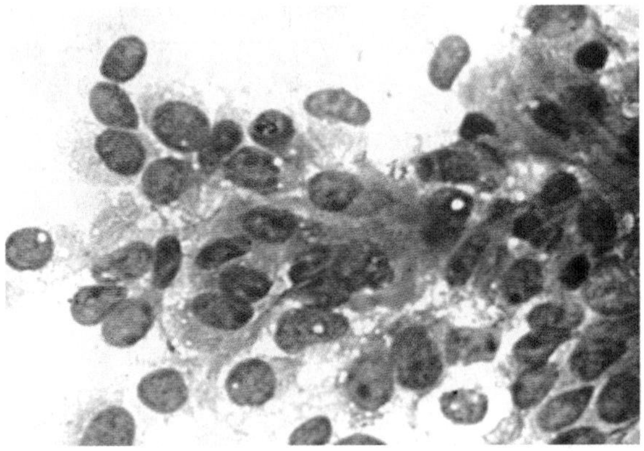

Figure 5-67

OSTEOBLASTIC OSTEOSARCOMA

There is a tendency toward spindling (May-Grünwald-Giemsa–stained FNA smear).

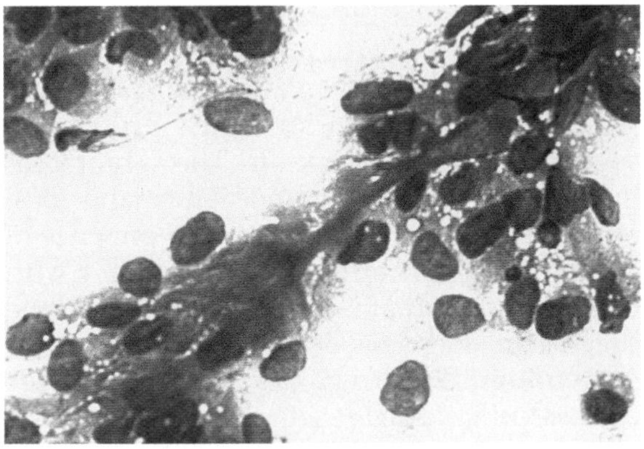

Figure 5-68

OSTEOBLASTIC OSTEOSARCOMA

The delicate, fibrillary collagenous matrix corresponds to osteoid (May-Grünwald-Giemsa–stained FNA smear).

Chondroblastic Osteosarcoma. Cytologically, most chondroblastic osteosarcomas are high-grade, with chondroblastic and osteoblastic components as well as a chondroid matrix that stains intensely purple with the May-Grünwald-Giemsa stain (figs. 5-70, 5-71). The chondroblastic cells have abundant pale cytoplasm, one or more rounded central nuclei, and relatively small nucleoli.

Fibrosarcoma-like Osteosarcoma. The FNA characteristics of fibroblastic osteosarcoma may be impossible to distinguish from those of other primary malignant spindle cell tumors of bone (figs. 5-72, 5-73).

Giant Cell–Rich Osteosarcoma. Benign giant cells or osteoclasts are common in the FNA samples of all types of osteosarcoma. Osteoclasts are particularly abundant in giant cell–rich osteosarcomas. An erroneous diagnosis of giant cell tumor may be made if the malignant nature of the accompanying cell population is not recognized.

FNA analysis is particularly useful in the diagnosis of local recurrences and metastases of osteosarcoma (65,71). Ancillary useful techniques include alkaline phosphatase stains and ultrastructural studies, as well as DNA ploidy analysis, tissue culture, karyotyping, and fluorescence

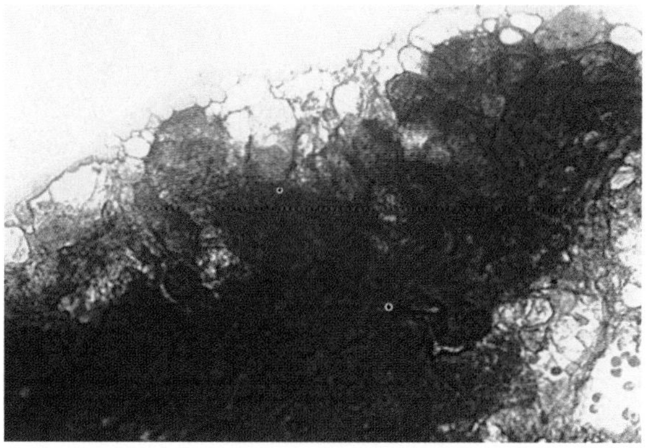

Figure 5-69

OSTEOBLASTIC OSTEOSARCOMA

The FNA fragment is strongly positive for alkaline phosphatase.

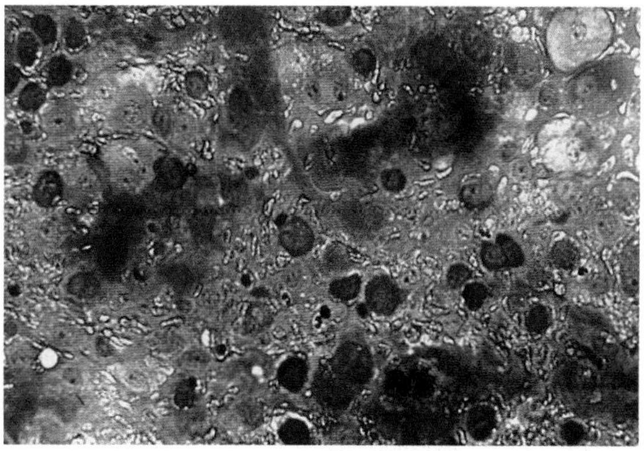

Figure 5-70

OSTEOSARCOMA

High-grade chondroblastic osteosarcoma with abundant, purple-staining chondroid matrix (May-Grünwald-Giemsa stain).

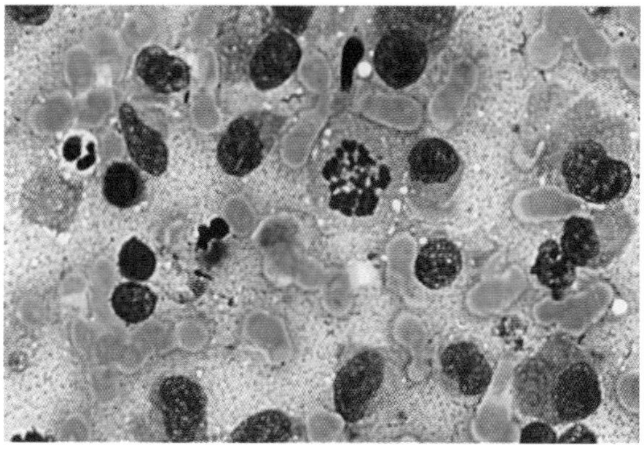

Figure 5-71

OSTEOSARCOMA

Tumor cells with chondroblastic, osteoblastic, and mixed features as well as mitotic figures in a high-grade chondroblastic osteosarcoma (May-Grünwald-Giemsa stain).

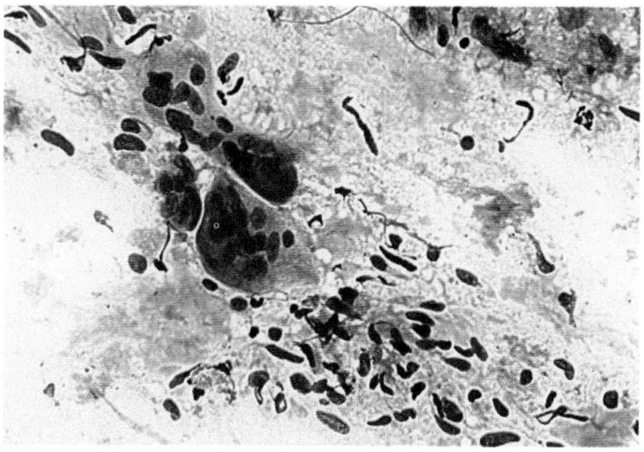

Figure 5-72

OSTEOSARCOMA

Fibroblastic osteosarcoma with an atypical spindle cell component and benign osteoclasts.

in situ hybridization (FISH)– and polymerase chain reaction (PCR)–based investigations.

Osteosarcoma of Jawbones

Osteosarcomas involving the jawbones are rare, accounting for only 6 percent of osteosarcomas in the Mayo Clinic series. The mandible and maxilla are involved almost equally. Most of the patients are young adults, about a decade older than those with conventional osteosarcoma. Symptoms consist of pain or swelling (or both) and numbness. The interpretation of radiographs can be difficult. The lesions are destructive and poorly marginated, and may be lytic or sclerotic (or both). Grossly, the tumor may be fleshy or lobulated, with a distinctly cartilaginous appearance (fig. 5-74).

Microscopically, approximately 50 percent of osteosarcomas of the jawbones are chondroblastic and, thus, often mistaken for chondrosarcoma (fig. 5-75). The cartilage is hypercellular and arranged in lobules. Osteoid is present in the center of the lobules as short, poorly formed bony trabeculae or within spindle cells at the periphery of the lobules. The rest of the tumors show osteoblastic or fibroblastic differentiation.

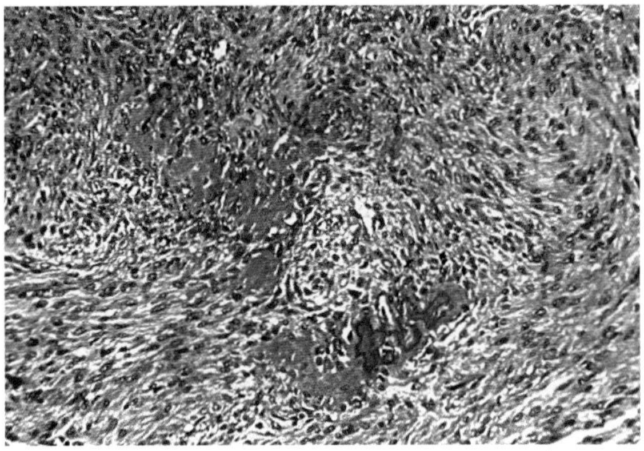

Figure 5-73

OSTEOSARCOMA

The FNA smear in figure 5-72 corresponds histologically to a high-grade spindle cell malignancy with focal osteoid production.

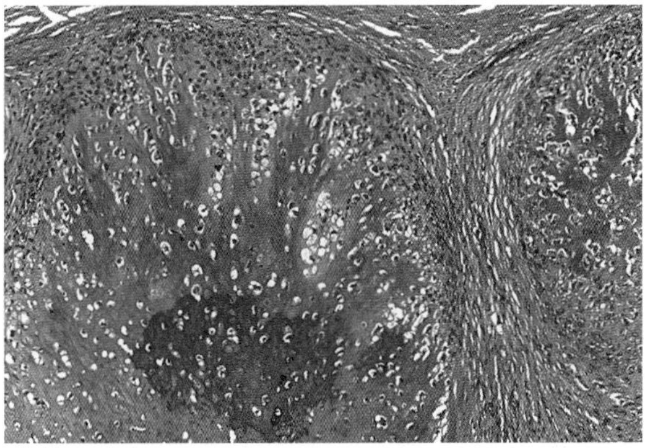

Figure 5-75

OSTEOSARCOMA OF JAWBONES

Chondroblastic osteosarcoma is the most common histologic type of osteosarcoma involving jawbones.

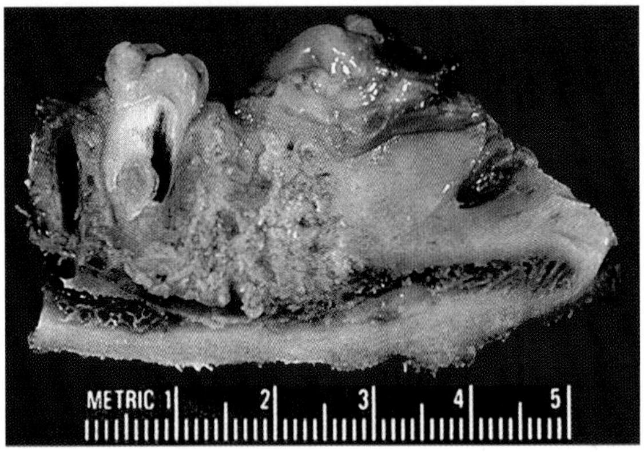

Figure 5-74

OSTEOSARCOMA

This osteosarcoma in the mandible forms a destructive mass that displaces the teeth. The blue-gray nodules seen throughout the tumor confirm the histologic diagnosis of chondroblastic osteosarcoma.

Osteosarcomas of the jaws tend to be better differentiated than conventional osteosarcomas (grade 2 or 3).

Treatment is predominantly surgical. The role of chemotherapy is not clear. There is not enough experience to know whether surgical treatment is sufficient or if adjunctive therapy is necessary. Two studies from Mayo Clinic have shown that the prognosis for patients with osteosarcoma of the jawbones after surgery alone is considerably better than for those with conventional osteosarcoma (64,115). However, this has not been the experience of others (48).

Osteosarcoma of the jaws illustrates the importance of tumor location for prognosis. Although the prognosis for patients with jaw osteosarcomas has been relatively good (at least in the Mayo Clinic experience), the prognosis for those with osteosarcoma of the skull has been bleak (107,148).

Osteosarcoma in Paget's Disease

The true incidence of osteosarcoma arising in patients with Paget's disease is not known. The Mayo Clinic files contain 70 cases of sarcoma associated with Paget's disease (fig. 5-76). However, no accurate information is available about the number of patients with Paget's disease who were evaluated during the same period. The risk of sarcoma in those with Paget's disease is higher when the disease is extensive.

When a patient with an established diagnosis of Paget's disease complains of increasing localized pain, sarcomatous change should be suspected. Radiographs show features typical of Paget's disease, with thickening of the cortex and medullary bone almost invariably extending to the end of the bone. The demarcation between involved and uninvolved bone is always sharp and resembles a flame. Areas of bone lysis may be present and may represent active areas of Paget's disease or Paget's sarcoma, especially if the lesion destroys the cortex and extends into

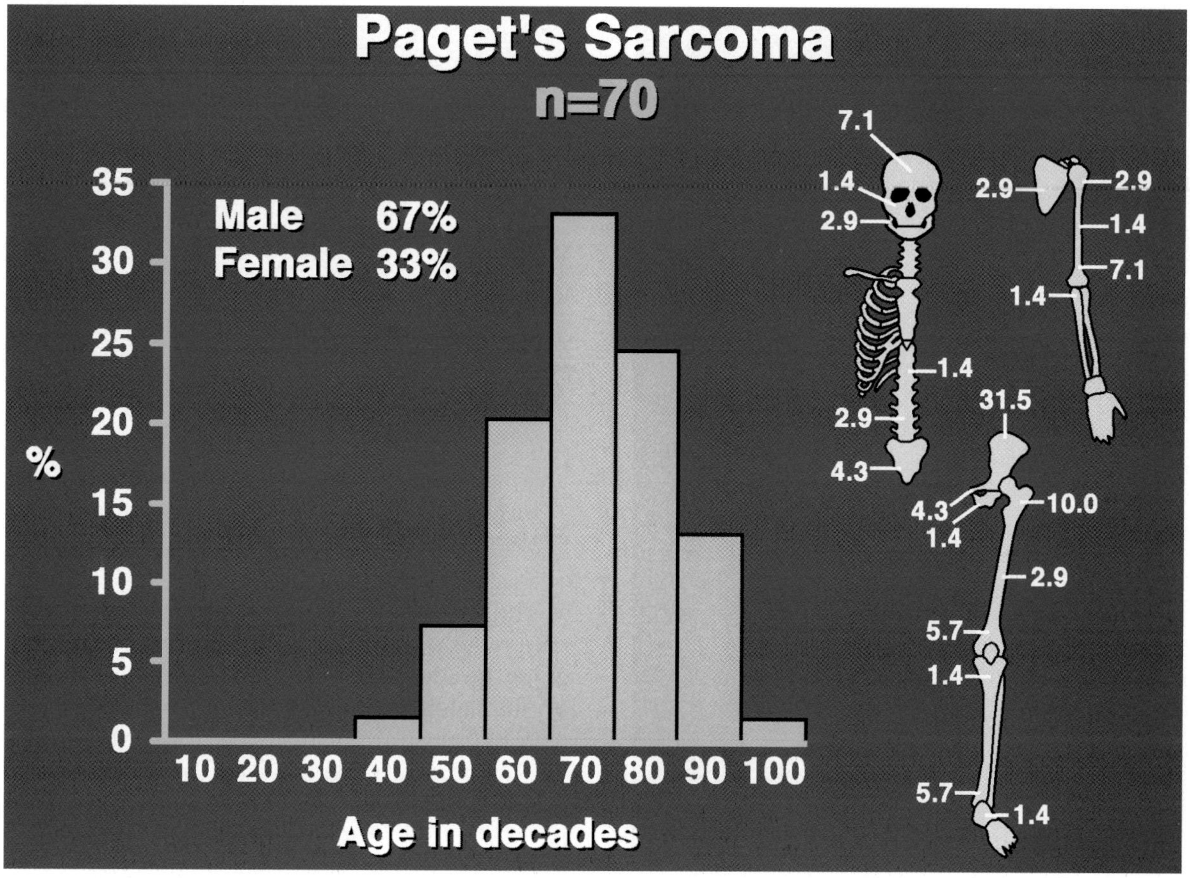

Figure 5-76

PAGET'S SARCOMA

Distribution of Paget's sarcoma according to the age and sex of the patient and the site of the lesion.

soft tissue (figs. 5-77, 5-78). The histologic features of Paget's osteosarcoma are not distinctive, except that they are almost always high grade. Features of the underlying Paget's disease may or may not be present (fig. 5-79). The prognosis for patients with Paget's sarcoma is uniformly bad, and there are few long-term survivors (105,199).

Postradiation Sarcoma

To make the diagnosis of postradiation sarcoma, the following conditions have to be met: 1) there has to be a history of irradiation to the site involved by the sarcoma; 2) there has to be a latent period between the delivery of irradiation and the development of sarcoma. In the Mayo Clinic series, the average latent period is

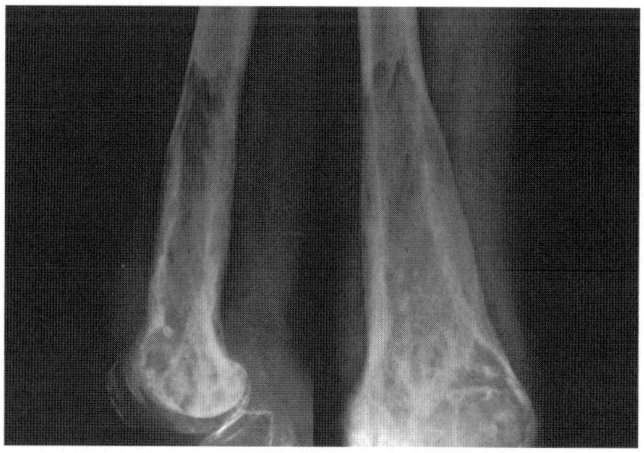

Figure 5-77

SARCOMA IN PAGET'S DISEASE

Radiographic features of a destructive osteosarcoma arising in Paget's disease.

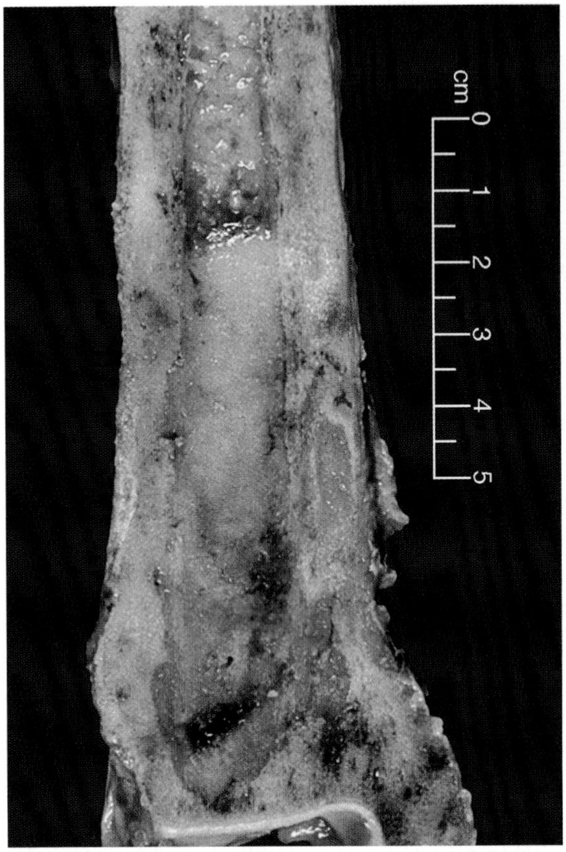

Figure 5-78

OSTEOSARCOMA IN PAGET'S DISEASE

The thick cortical bone suggests underlying Paget's disease in this fibroblastic osteosarcoma that forms a fleshy yellow-gray mass in the distal tibia of a 74-year-old man.

15.6 years (range, 1 to 55 years). The consensus is that the latent period should be at least 5 to 7 years, but there is no reason why it cannot be shorter. Also, the addition of chemotherapy may shorten the latent period; and 3) there has to be histologic verification of the sarcoma, which should be different from the original process for which irradiation was administered.

Until the beginning of 2000, the Mayo Clinic files contained 169 cases of postradiation sarcoma. Patients with postradiation sarcoma are older than those with conventional osteosarcoma; the largest group was in the sixth decade of life. The skeletal distribution is also different, with preferential involvement of the pelvic and shoulder girdles because of the use of radiotherapy in the management of breast carcinoma and gynecologic malignancies (fig. 5-80).

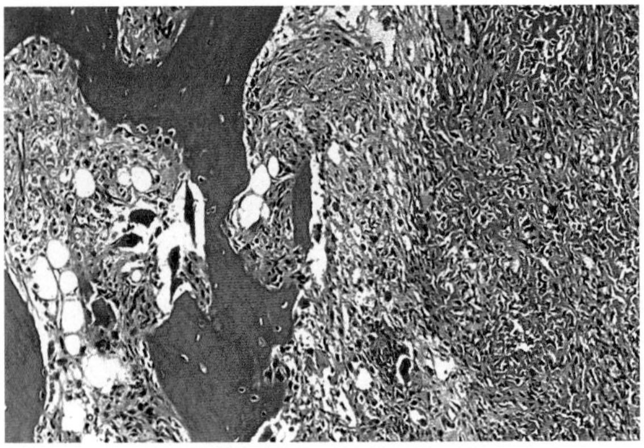

Figure 5-79

OSTEOSARCOMA IN PAGET'S DISEASE

High-grade osteoblastic osteosarcoma (right) merging into preexisting bone shows features of Paget's disease (left).

The histologic features of postradiation sarcomas are not distinctive. They tend to be high grade (grade 3 or 4) (fig. 5-81). Foci of amorphous calcification, as seen in bone infarcts, may be found, indicating previous irradiation.

The literature suggests that the prognosis for patients with postradiation sarcoma is poor, in part because of the tendency for these tumors to involve unfavorable sites such as the pelvic or shoulder girdle, the spine, and the sternum. A recent study from Mayo Clinic (108) has shown that the prognosis for those with postradiation sarcoma in surgically accessible sites, such as the appendicular skeleton, is the same as that for conventional sarcoma. Thus, it is important to treat these tumors aggressively.

Osteosarcoma in Other Benign Conditions

Osteosarcomas arising in preexisting benign conditions, other than those mentioned above, are so rare they may be considered medical curiosities. The benign precursor lesions may be coincidental and not causally related. In the Mayo Clinic series, three osteosarcomas arose in association with osteochondromas (one patient had multiple exostoses), two in infarcts of bone, and one each in Ollier's disease, in the sinus tract of a patient with chronic osteomyelitis, in osteoblastoma, and in osteopoikilosis. Seventeen patients had osteosarcoma in fibrous dysplasia. Of these, 12 had previous radiotherapy, and the tumors may be considered postradiation sarcomas. In a larger series, approximately half

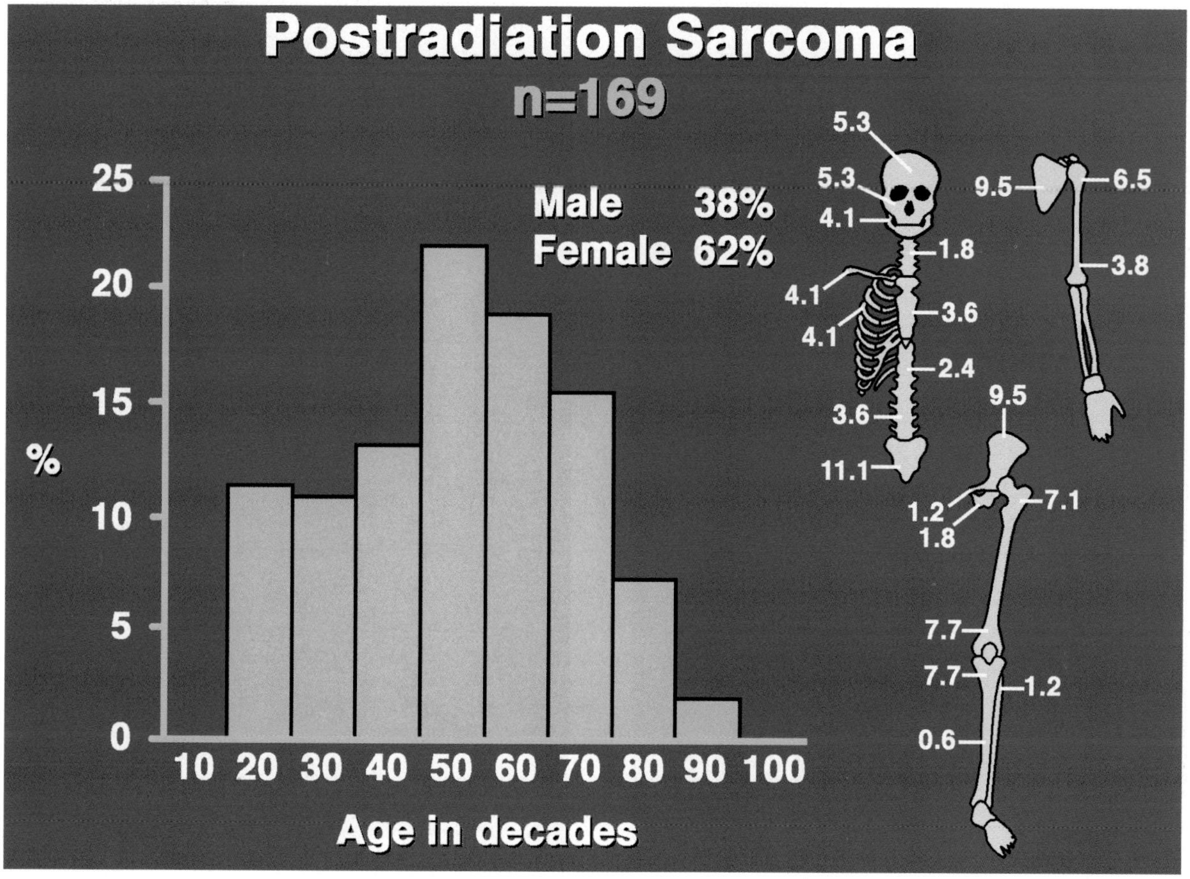

Figure 5-80

POSTRADIATION SARCOMA

Distribution of postradiation sarcoma according to the age and sex of the patient and the site of the lesion.

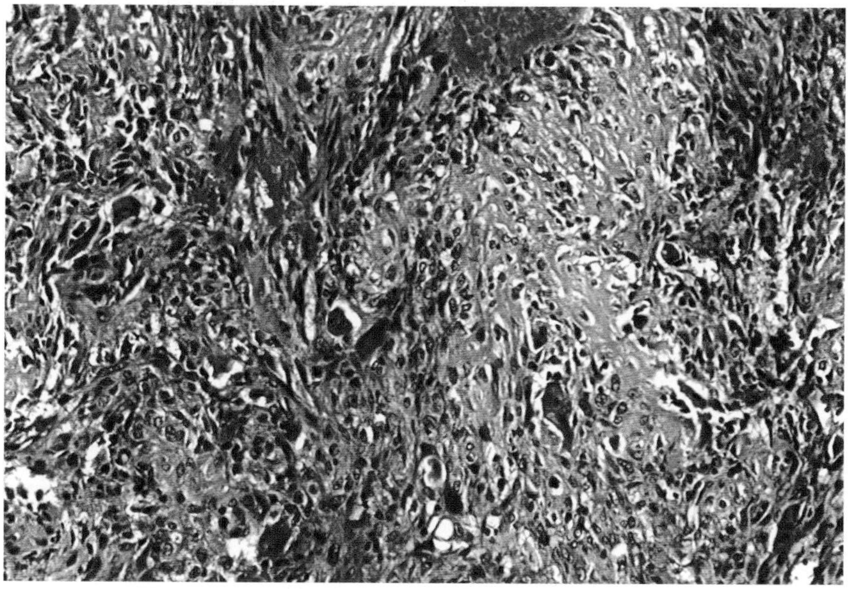

Figure 5-81

POSTRADIATION SARCOMA

High-grade osteosarcoma arising in the tibia of an 18-year-old woman who had received radiotherapy for Ewing's sarcoma 5 years earlier.

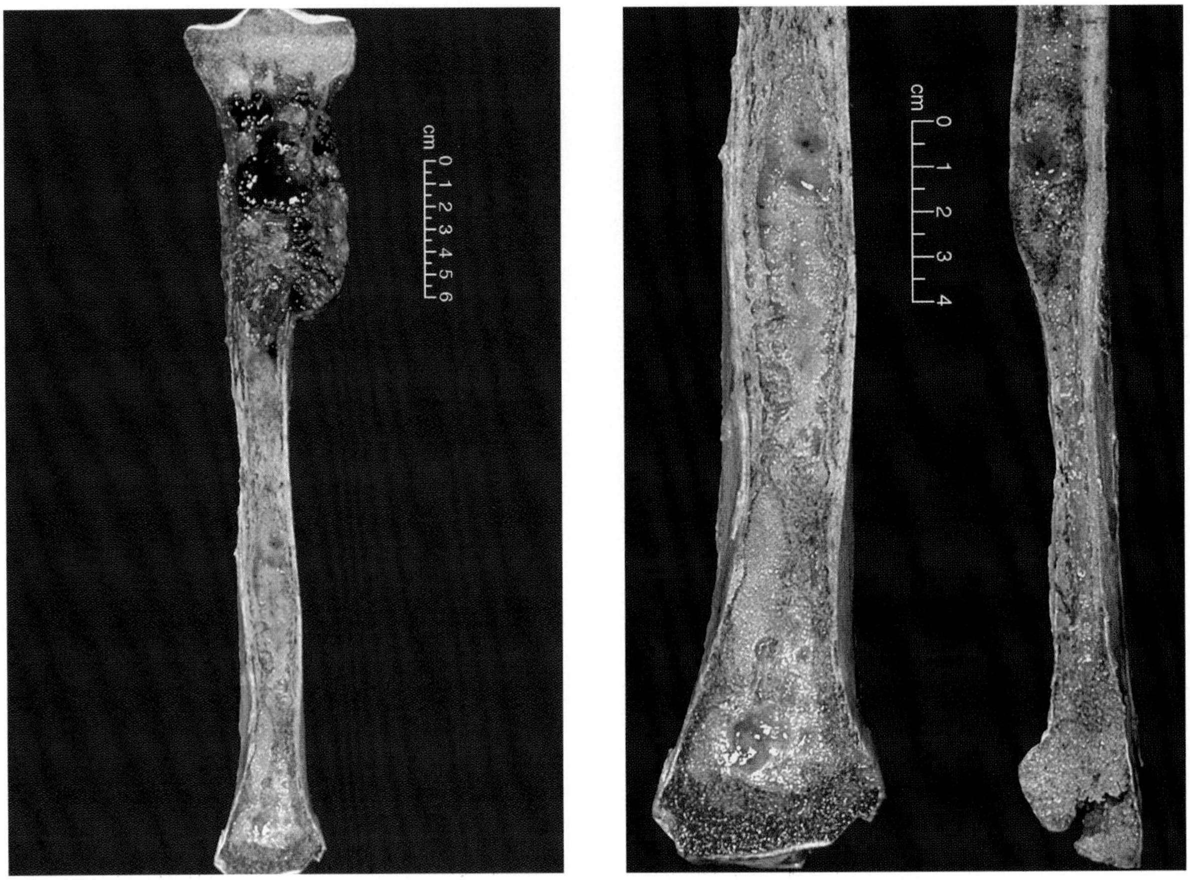

Figure 5-82

POLYOSTOTIC FIBROUS DYSPLASIA AND ALBRIGHT'S SYNDROME

Left: The proximal tibia of a 41-year-old man contains a destructive mass that histologically showed features of high-grade fibroblastic osteosarcoma.

Right: Close-up view of the distal tibia shows intramedullary, solid, gray-white tissue that histologically showed features of fibrous dysplasia.

of the patients had no previous exposure to irradiation (fig. 5-82) (166).

Multicentric Osteosarcoma

Rarely, a patient presents with osteosarcoma involving multiple skeletal sites but not the viscera. These multicentric tumors may be synchronous or metachronous. Whether they represent true multicentricity or skeletal metastases from a dominant site is not known. It seems reasonable to consider true multicentricity when there are no visceral lesions. The radiographic and microscopic features of each tumor are no different from those of solitary osteosarcomas. The prognosis for patients with the synchronous type is predictably bad; however, some patients with metachronous osteosarcomas become long-term survivors (82).

Telangiectatic Osteosarcoma

Definition. Telangiectatic osteosarcoma is an unusual variant of osteosarcoma that resembles an aneurysmal bone cyst radiographically, grossly, and microscopically. Both tend to occur in the metaphysis of long bones and to have a similar age distribution.

General Features. The incidence of telangiectatic osteosarcoma varies in different series. In a Mayo Clinic series, these tumors formed less than 3 percent of all osteosarcomas (136), but in a report from Memorial Hospital, they accounted for more than 10 percent (106). This discrepancy

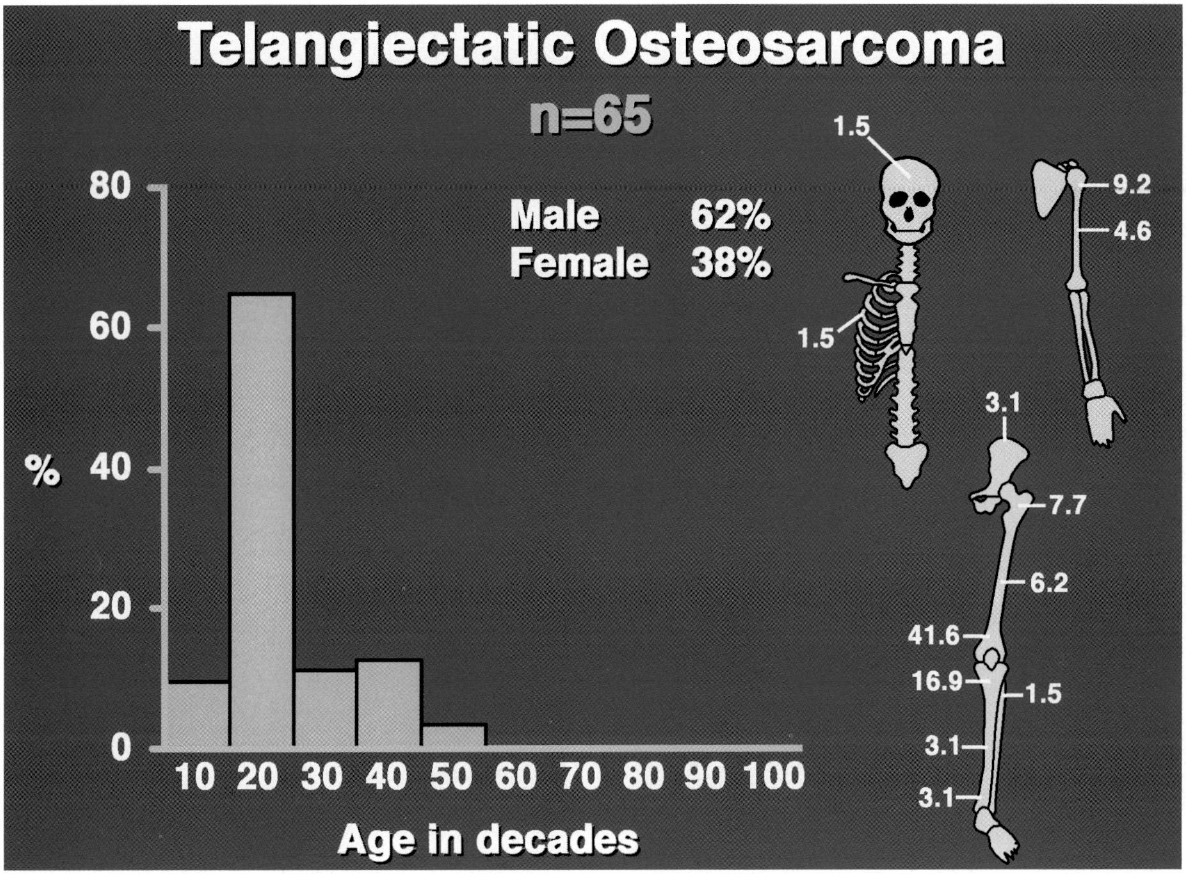

Figure 5-83

TELANGIECTATIC OSTEOSARCOMA

Distribution of telangiectatic osteosarcoma according to the age and sex of the patient and the site of the lesion.

may be explained by the different criteria for diagnosis used by different institutions.

Clinical Features. Patients present with pain, swelling, or both, usually of short duration. The lesion may be rapidly progressive. Pathologic fractures are more common than with conventional osteosarcoma. The patient age and skeletal distribution are the same as for conventional osteosarcoma (fig. 5-83).

Radiographic Findings. Radiographs show a purely lytic destructive lesion that involves the metaphysis of a long bone (fig. 5-84). The margins are poorly demarcated, and there is no appreciable sclerosis. If untreated, the lesion may progress rapidly. The cortex is destroyed, and a significant soft tissue mass may be seen. CT may show fluid-fluid levels, as in aneurysmal bone cysts. MRI is better than CT for showing the extent of the lesion and may show septation and fluid-fluid levels. Rarely, the lesion is permeative and destructive, suggesting the diagnosis of a small cell malignancy (fig. 5-85).

Gross Findings. Telangiectatic osteosarcoma lacks the "fish-flesh" appearance of the usual high-grade sarcoma. Rather, the gross appearance is that of a cyst filled with blood clot (figs. 5-86, 5-87). If the blood is washed away, cystic spaces that are separated by thin fibrous septa, suggesting a honeycomb, are apparent in most instances. Rarely, the blood clot appears to be in a large "simple" cyst.

Microscopic Findings. In most cases of telangiectatic osteosarcoma, the low-power microscopic appearance suggests the diagnosis of aneurysmal bone cyst (fig. 5-88). The septa vary in thickness but usually are thin and membranous.

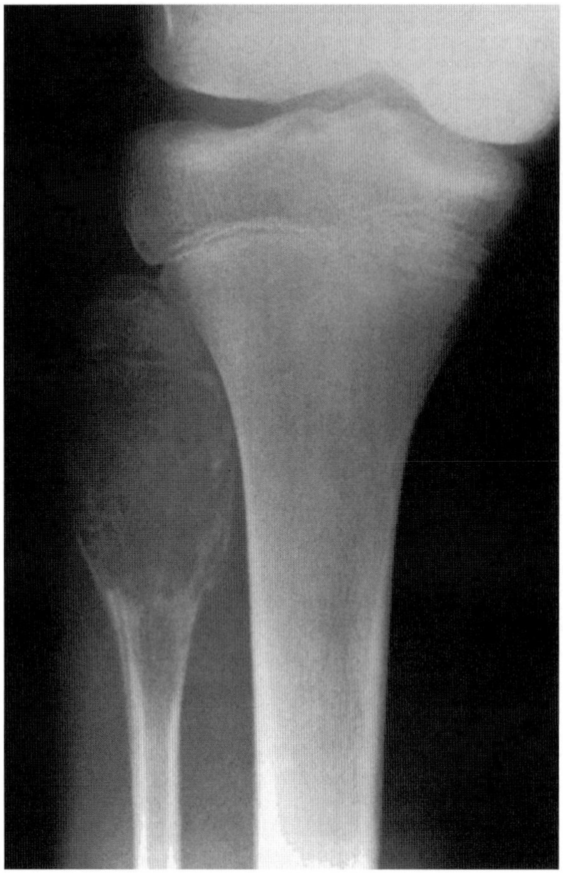

Figure 5-84

TELANGIECTATIC OSTEOSARCOMA

This purely lytic lesion involves the proximal fibula. Occasionally, the radiographic features of telangiectatic osteosarcoma simulate those of aneurysmal bone cyst.

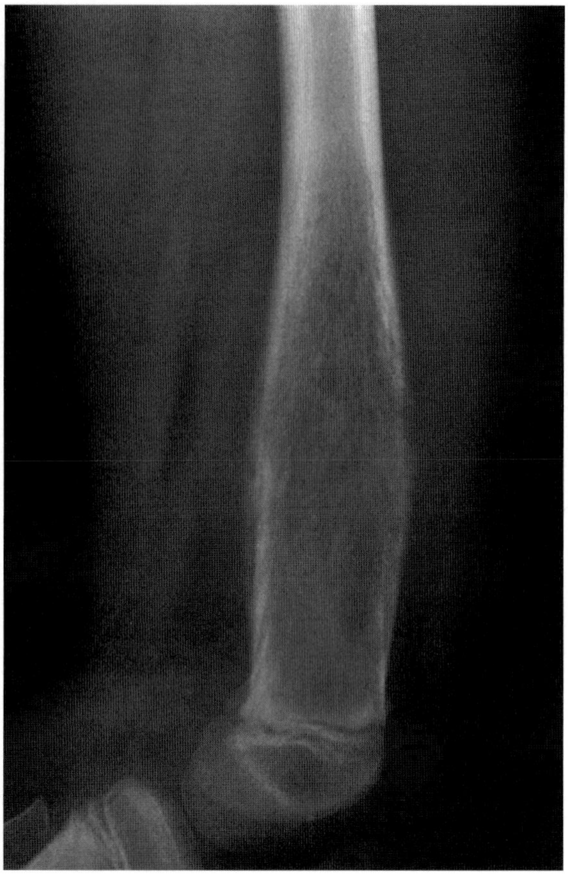

Figure 5-85

TELANGIECTATIC OSTEOSARCOMA

This telangiectatic osteosarcoma shows evidence of cortical destruction and had a permeative appearance.

Benign giant cells are almost always present. The septa are composed of very pleomorphic cells (fig. 5-89). Typical and atypical mitoses are abundant. Rarely, there is no organization in the tumor, and the diagnosis is made by identifying atypical cells floating in the blood clot. Matrix formation is minimal and present as thin wisps of unmineralized osteoid. On occasion, extensive sampling may not reveal matrix; however, if the pattern is that of an aneurysmal bone cyst but with pleomorphic nuclei, the diagnosis of telangiectatic osteosarcoma is justified.

Cytologic Findings. The aspirates of most telangiectatic osteosarcomas are hemorrhagic and paucicellular. Otherwise, the cytologic features are similar to those of osteoblastic osteosarcoma (figs. 5-90, 5-91). Benign osteoclasts may be seen.

Differential Diagnosis. The differential diagnosis includes aneurysmal bone cyst and giant cell tumor. The location in the metaphysis, the radiographic appearance, the gross appearance, and the low-power microscopic appearance may all suggest the diagnosis of aneurysmal bone cyst. However, the clear-cut and obvious anaplasia in the cells in telangiectatic osteosarcoma is absent in aneurysmal bone cysts, making the distinction easy. Giant cell tumors occur in the ends of long bones in skeletally mature patients. Moreover, the mononuclear cells in giant cell tumors do not have the cytologic features of malignancy.

Treatment and Prognosis. Most patients with telangiectatic osteosarcoma receive neoadjuvant chemotherapy before surgery. The

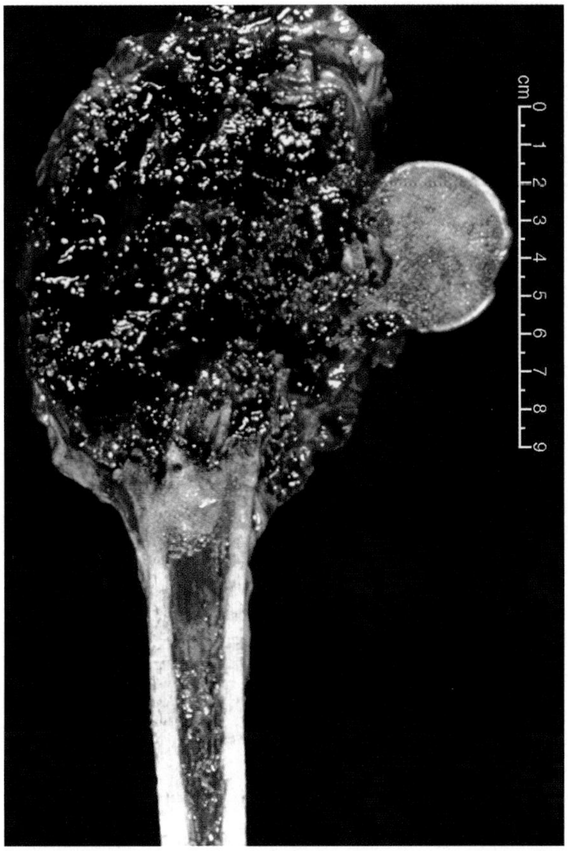

Figure 5-86

TELANGIECTATIC OSTEOSARCOMA

The entire proximal femur is destroyed by a large tumor composed predominantly of numerous cystic spaces filled with clotted blood.

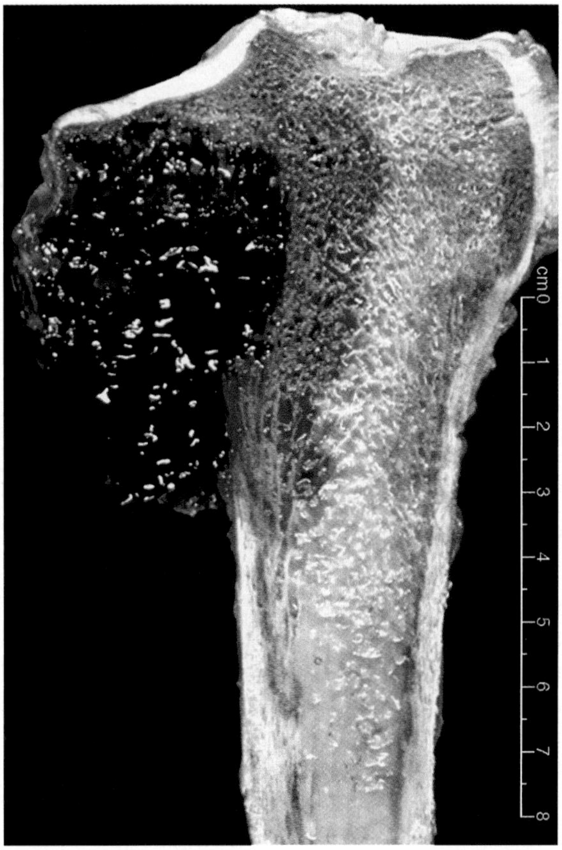

Figure 5-87

TELANGIECTATIC OSTEOSARCOMA

In this hemorrhagic telangiectatic osteosarcoma in the proximal tibia, there is no gross evidence of solid tumor tissue forming a destructive mass.

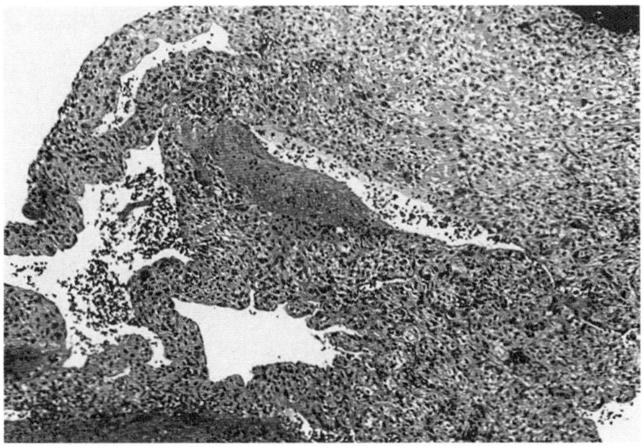

Figure 5-88

TELANGIECTATIC OSTEOSARCOMA

At low-power magnification, it is difficult to determine whether this lesion is an aneurysmal bone cyst or telangiectatic osteosarcoma.

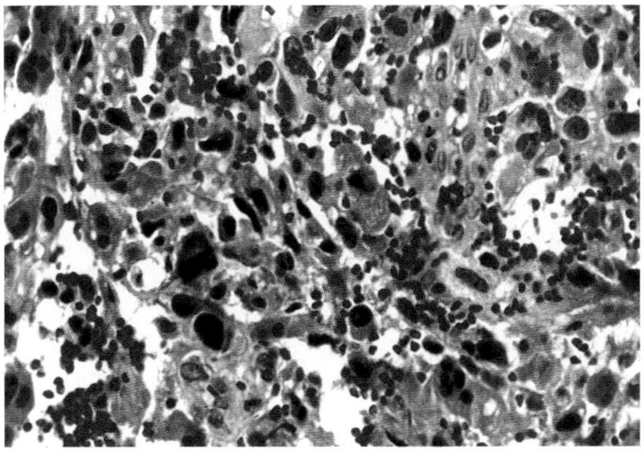

Figure 5-89

TELANGIECTATIC OSTEOSARCOMA

This high-power microscopic view of the fibrous septa clearly shows tumor cells that have malignant cytologic features.

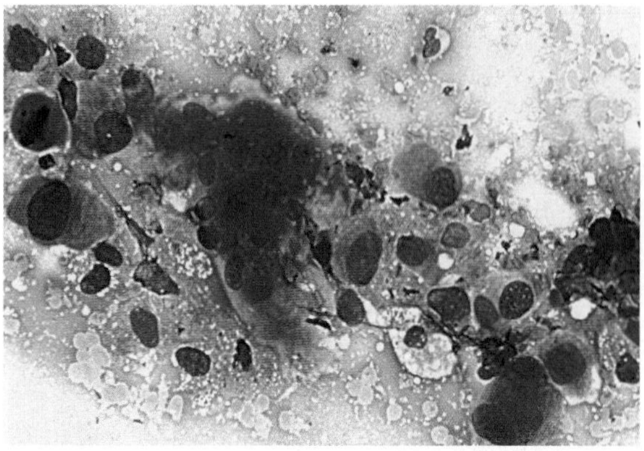

Figure 5-90

TELANGIECTATIC OSTEOSARCOMA

FNA specimen of a telangiectatic osteosarcoma (May-Grünwald-Giemsa–stained FNA smear).

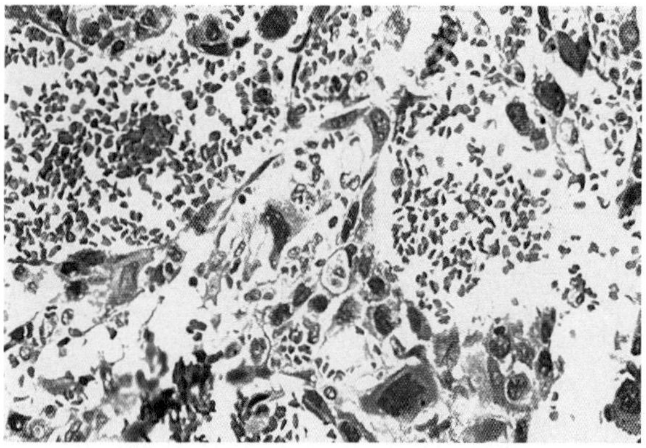

Figure 5-91

TELANGIECTATIC OSTEOSARCOMA

The FNA specimen seen in figure 5-90 corresponds histologically with the surgical specimen.

tumor appears to be exquisitely sensitive to chemotherapy and often undergoes complete necrosis. Before the advent of chemotherapy, a study from Mayo Clinic suggested that the prognosis for patients with telangiectatic osteosarcoma was significantly worse than for those with conventional osteosarcoma (136). However, a study from Memorial Hospital found no difference in survival (106). The latest study from Mayo Clinic found no prognostic difference for those with telangiectatic osteosarcoma (138).

Small Cell Osteosarcoma

Definition. Small cell osteosarcoma is a sarcoma composed of small round or spindled cells that produce osteoid matrix.

General Features. Small cell osteosarcoma is extremely rare, accounting for less than 1 percent of all cases of osteosarcoma in the Mayo Clinic files (fig. 5-92). Patients present with pain, swelling, or both. The age, sex, and skeletal distribution are similar to those of conventional osteosarcoma.

Radiographic Findings. Radiographs may or may not show mineral within the lesion. Ewing's sarcoma frequently contains abundant mineral, and it may be impossible to differentiate this tumor from osteosarcoma. The presence of mineral within a soft tissue extension strongly favors the diagnosis of osteosarcoma. Rarely, radiographs show a permeative pattern that suggests a small cell malignancy.

Gross Findings. Small cell osteosarcomas have the fleshy white appearance common to all high-grade sarcomas.

Microscopic Findings. Implicit in the diagnosis is the feature that separates small cell osteosarcoma from conventional osteosarcoma, namely, the size of the tumor cells (fig. 5-93). Whereas a conventional osteosarcoma is usually a spindle cell sarcoma with pleomorphic nuclei, a small cell osteosarcoma has tumor cells that are predominantly small and round (but may be spindled) and contain hyperchromatic nuclei, suggesting at first glance a diagnosis of Ewing's sarcoma or malignant lymphoma. The osteoid matrix needs to be identified focally to confirm the diagnosis (fig. 5-94). If the matrix is mineralized, the identification is easy. A focal hemangiopericytomatous pattern may be identified. Chondroid matrix may be seen, but it is not a dominant feature.

Cytologic Findings. There is little experience with the FNA findings of this rare variant of osteosarcoma. Large coherent tumor fragments, increased nuclear pleomorphism, and a tendency for tumor cell elongation have all been reported to aid in the distinction between small cell osteosarcoma and Ewing's sarcoma (198).

Differential Diagnosis. It may be difficult to distinguish between Ewing's sarcoma and small cell osteosarcoma. Ewing's sarcoma frequently shows a fibrinous exudate that simulates osteoid. Any true spindling rules out the diagnosis of Ewing's sarcoma. CD99 is usually

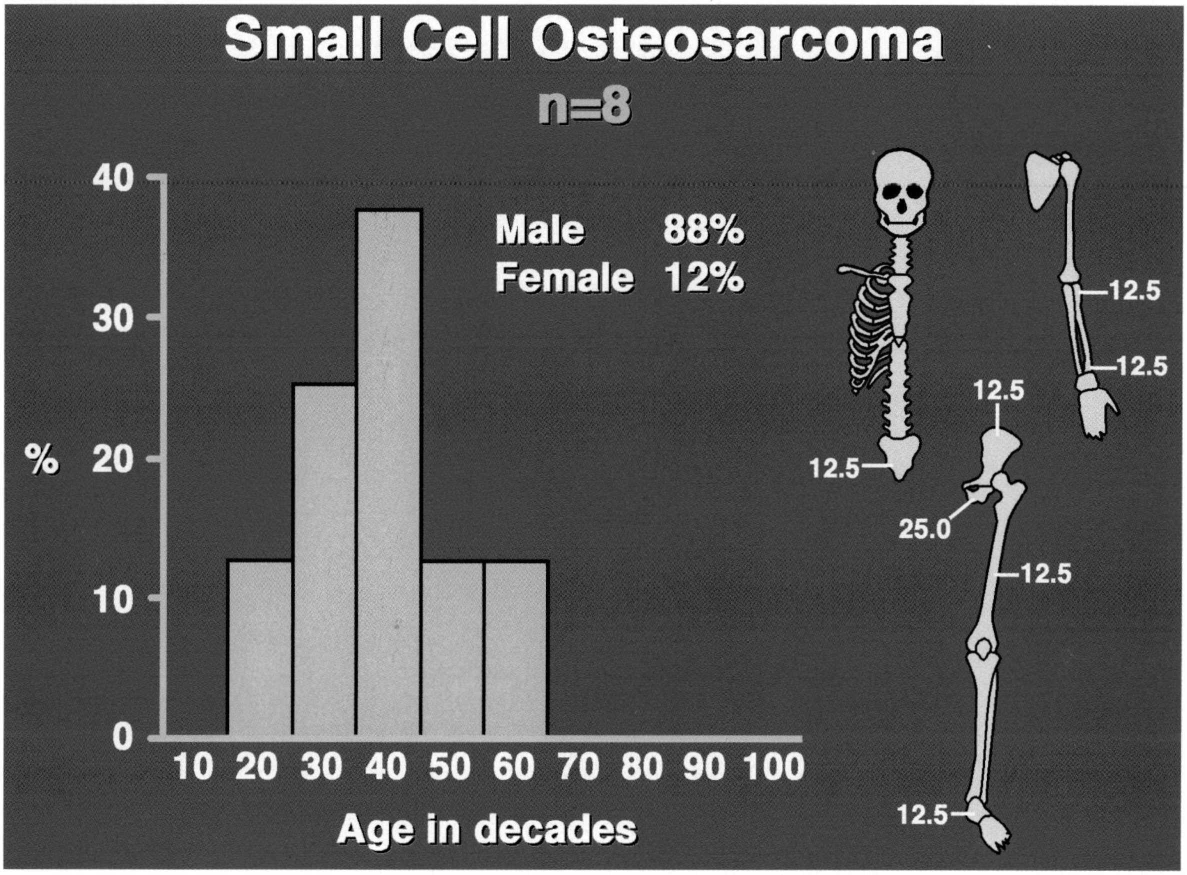

Figure 5-92

SMALL CELL OSTEOSARCOMA

Distribution of small cell osteosarcoma according to the age and sex of the patient and the site of the lesion.

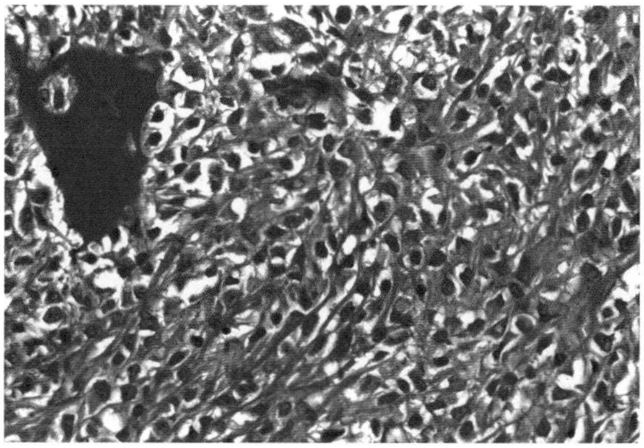

Figure 5-93

SMALL CELL OSTEOSARCOMA

Round to oval-shaped tumor cells are associated with osteoid production.

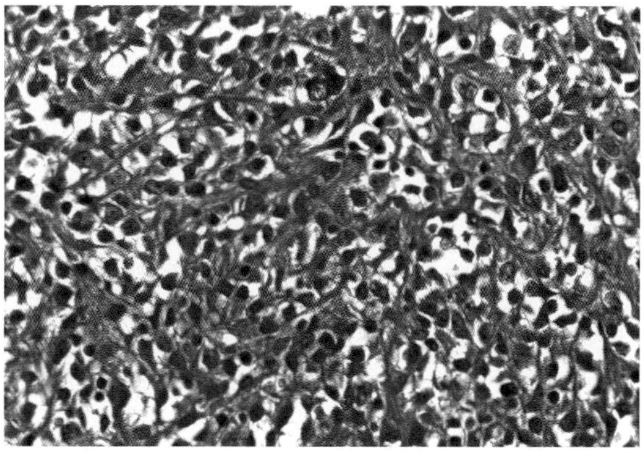

Figure 5-94

SMALL CELL OSTEOSARCOMA

Sheets of small round tumor cells were seen throughout this osteosarcoma, which also shows a lace-like pattern of osteoid production.

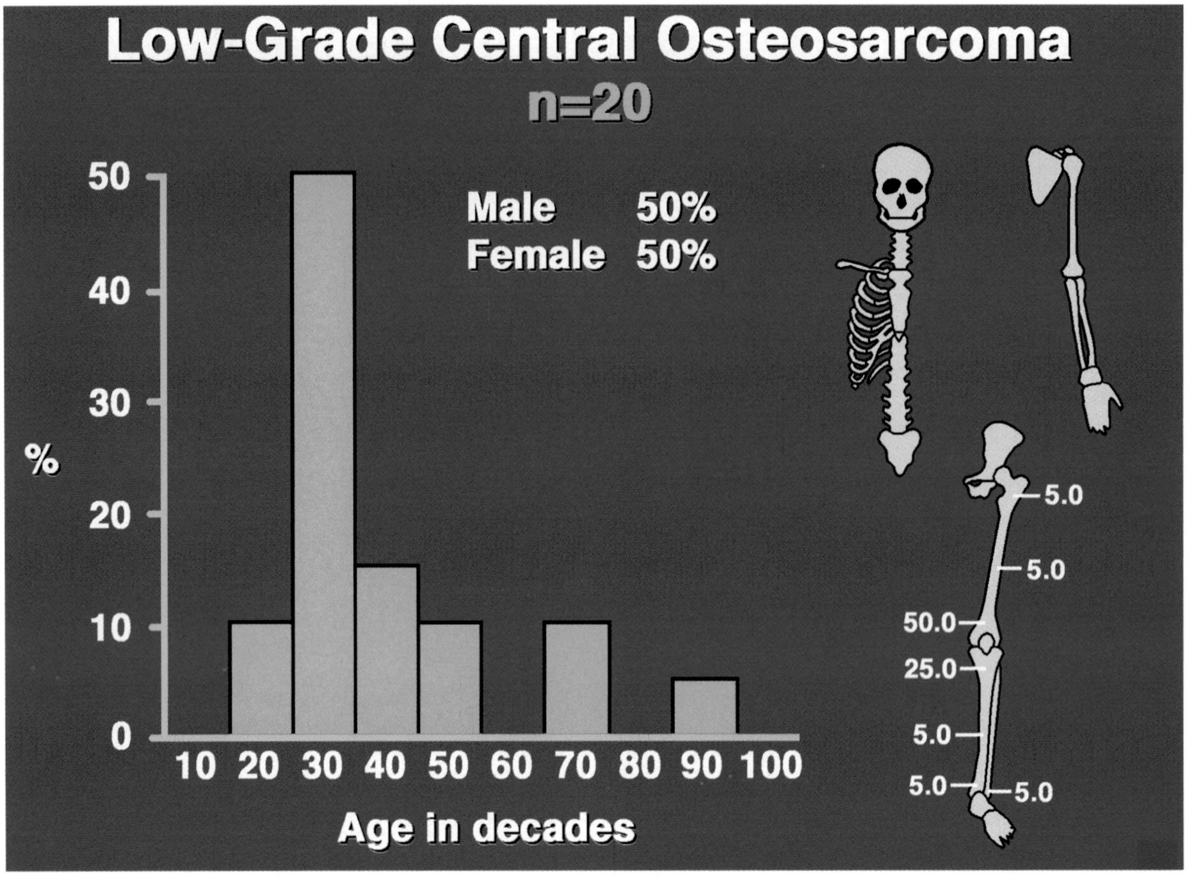

Figure 5-95

LOW-GRADE OSTEOSARCOMA

Distribution of low-grade osteosarcoma according to the age and sex of the patient and the site of the lesion.

positive in Ewing's sarcoma but also has been reported to be positive in small cell osteosarcoma. Malignant lymphoma is less of a problem because of its cytologic features and polymorphism. Positive staining for common leukocyte antigen, a feature of malignant lymphoma, is not a feature of small cell osteosarcoma. Mesenchymal chondrosarcoma has a distinctly bimorphic pattern, with relatively prominent islands of cartilage juxtaposed to a small cell malignancy.

Treatment and Prognosis. Because of the rarity of the neoplasm, information about treatment and prognosis is limited. Nakajima et al. (143) reported a 5-year survival rate of 28 percent. They suggested that cases with a questionable diagnosis be treated as Ewing's sarcoma.

Low-Grade Osteosarcoma

Definition. Low-grade (well-differentiated) osteosarcoma is a malignant, bone-forming, intramedullary neoplasm in which the tumor cells are so well differentiated that it is difficult to make a diagnosis of malignancy.

General Features. Low-grade osteosarcoma is very rare: until 2000, only 20 cases were reported in the Mayo Clinic files, accounting for 1 percent of the total number of osteosarcomas (fig. 5-95). Patients present with intermittent pain, with or without swelling, usually of long duration. The male to female ratio is about equal. The patients are young adults who are about a decade older than those who have conventional osteosarcoma. The distal femur and the proximal tibia are involved most commonly. Kurt et

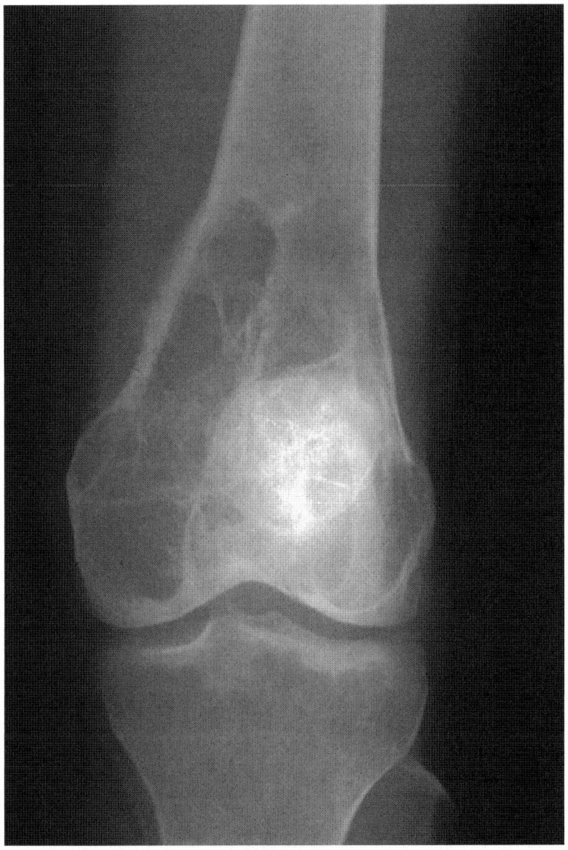

Figure 5-96

LOW-GRADE OSTEOSARCOMA

An expansile, mixed lytic and sclerotic lesion with trabeculation.

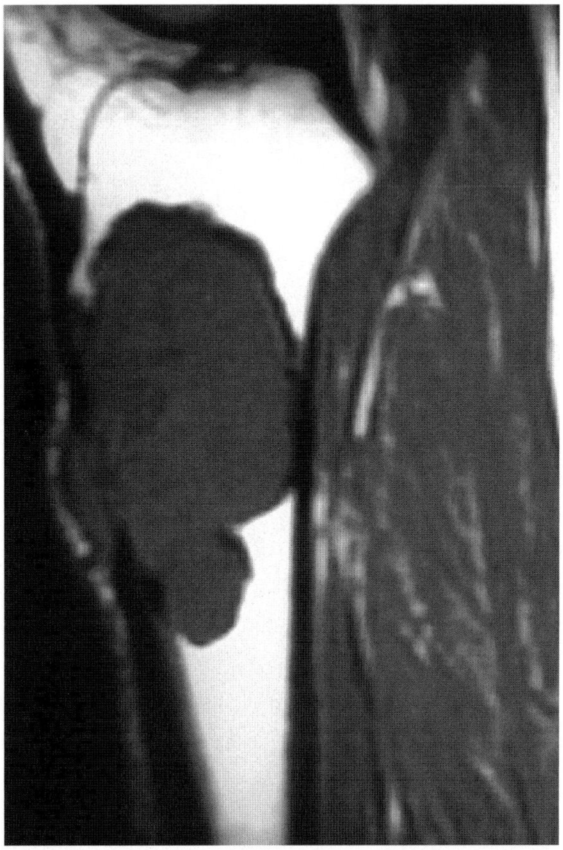

Figure 5-97

LOW-GRADE OSTEOSARCOMA

MRI shows cortical destruction anteriorly and a small soft tissue mass.

al. (120) found that more than 80 percent of these tumors involved long tubular bones.

Radiographic Findings. Radiographs show a large lytic process with poor margination involving the meta-diaphyseal region of long bones. Many of the lesions have a trabeculated appearance that represents the residual bony trabeculae of the host bone (fig. 5-96). Frequently, the lesions show sharp margination about much of the tumor, with only focal cortical destruction suggesting an aggressive process. MRI and CT may show cortical destruction and soft tissue extension, features that may not be obvious on plain radiographs (fig. 5-97).

Gross Findings. Low-grade osteosarcomas are well-demarcated, firm, white masses with a whorled appearance that suggests a desmoid tumor (fig. 5-98). These tumors do not have the fleshy appearance of high-grade sarcomas.

Microscopic Findings. Low-grade osteosarcoma is a hypocellular, spindle cell neoplasm in which the tumor cells are arranged in interlacing fascicles. The spindle cells show only slight atypia, and mitotic figures are rare (fig. 5-99). The tumor permeates into the surrounding bone marrow or entraps preexisting bony trabeculae. The matrix is produced as well-formed bony trabeculae (fig. 5-100); lace-like osteoid is not present. The amount of bone is variable, and large areas of the tumor may only show spindle cell proliferation. About 15 percent of low-grade osteosarcomas dedifferentiate into high-grade osteosarcomas.

Cytologic Findings. Diagnosing low-grade surface and intramedullary osteosarcomas by FNA analysis may be difficult. The few reports of the FNA features of parosteal osteosarcoma mention spindle cells with minimal or moderate atypia,

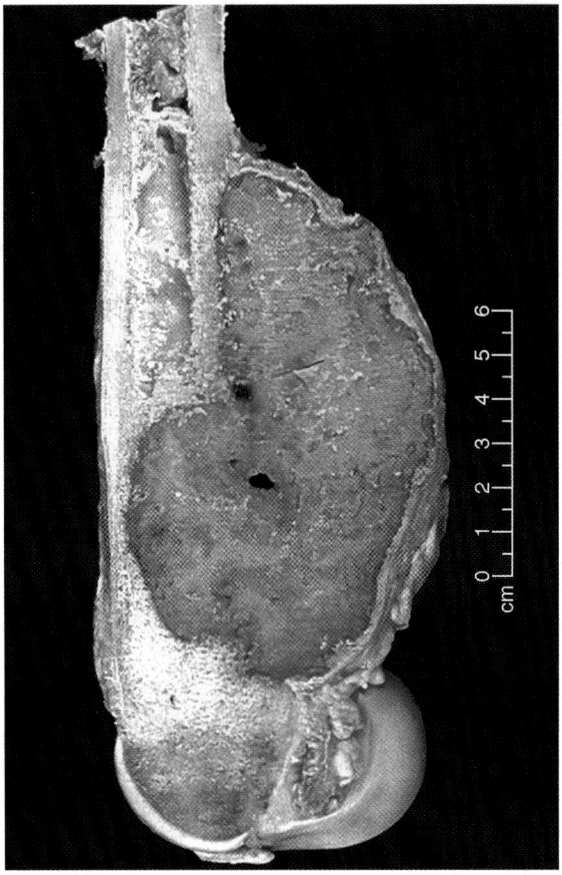

Figure 5-98

LOW-GRADE OSTEOSARCOMA

This homogeneous, firm, gray-white tumor shows extensive medullary and extramedullary involvement.

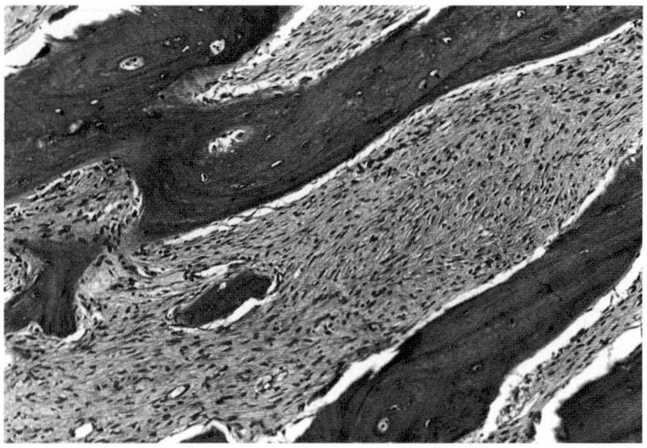

Figure 5-99

LOW-GRADE OSTEOSARCOMA

The minimal cytologic atypia in a low-grade osteosarcoma can make the diagnosis difficult or impossible if it is based on the histologic appearance of the center of the tumor. It is more helpful to review tissue at the interface with the surrounding tissue to determine whether there is a permeative growth pattern.

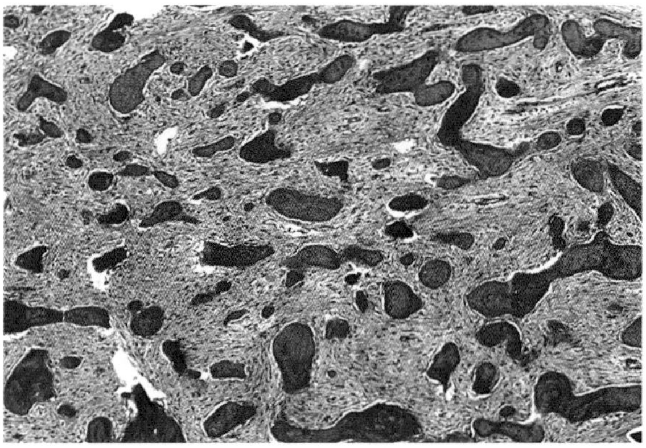

Figure 5-100

LOW-GRADE OSTEOSARCOMA

In some cases, the low-power microscopic appearance is similar to that of a parosteal osteosarcoma or fibrous dysplasia.

scattered osteoclasts, and occasional fragments of cartilage with minimal atypia (154).

Differential Diagnosis. The differential diagnosis of low-grade osteosarcoma includes desmoplastic fibroma and fibrous dysplasia. The only feature that differentiates desmoplastic fibroma from osteosarcoma is the production of matrix in the latter. Fibrous dysplasia has benign radiographic features and does not permeate surrounding tissues.

Treatment and Prognosis. Complete surgical removal is the treatment of choice. Because low-grade osteosarcomas rarely metastasize (in the absence of dedifferentiation), chemotherapy is not indicated.

GENETICS AND OTHER SPECIAL TECHNIQUES

Genetic Predisposition to Osteosarcoma

Osteosarcoma in siblings occurs in fewer than 1 in 1,000 patients. An underlying genetic predisposition is seen in many families with two or more affected siblings. An autosomal dominant disorder is most likely responsible when siblings in multiple generations are affected.

Table 5-3

CONDITIONS THAT PREDISPOSE TO OR MAY BE ASSOCIATED WITH THE DEVELOPMENT OF OSTEOSARCOMA

Paget's disease
Fibrous dysplasia
Osteoblastoma
Hereditary multiple exostosis
Ollier's disease
Hereditary retinoblastoma
Li-Fraumeni syndrome
Rothmund-Thomson syndrome
Werner's syndrome
Congenital hypoplastic or absent thumbs
Chemotherapy
Radiotherapy

Conditions associated with an increased risk of osteosarcoma are listed in Table 5-3.

Two autosomal dominant disorders predisposing persons to an increased risk of the development of osteosarcoma are the hereditary form of retinoblastoma and the Li-Fraumeni syndrome (73,84,126). The incidence of osteosarcoma among patients with heritable retinoblastoma has been reported to be 300 times greater than that of the general population (99). This risk is heightened by the inclusion of radiotherapy in the primary treatment of retinoblastoma (202). Osteosarcomas develop in approximately 6 percent of patients with Li-Fraumeni syndrome, a cancer predisposition syndrome associated with osteosarcomas, soft tissue sarcomas, premenopausal breast cancer, brain tumors, leukemia, adrenal cortical tumors, and other malignant neoplasms (133).

The development of retinoblastoma is the result of the loss of function of the *RB* gene, which has been localized to chromosomal band 13q14. The development of retinoblastoma follows the "two-hit" kinetic model proposed by Knudson (114) and serves as a model for the class of genes designated as tumor suppressor genes or antioncogenes. Tumor suppressor genes cause malignant change through loss of function rather than overexpression. For heritable retinoblastoma, the primary mutation in one *RB* locus occurs in germinal (ovum, sperm) cells, and for sporadically occurring retinoblastoma, the primary mutation transpires in somatic cells. Subsequently, the second "hit" responsible for malignant transformation is the loss of function of the remaining normal (wild-type) allele in somatic cells by a chromosomal rearrangement or mutation of the *RB* gene (fig. 5-101) (74,96). Similarly, germline mutations of a different tumor suppressor gene, *TP53*, localized to chromosome 17p13, are an underlying cause of the Li-Fraumeni syndrome (195). (Germline mutations of *CHK2* [checkpoint kinase 2] have also been detected in a subset of Li-Fraumeni patients who do not have *TP53* mutations [45], and somatic *CHK2* mutations have been observed in some sporadic osteosarcomas [140].) The offspring of a person affected with hereditary retinoblastoma or Li-Fraumeni syndrome have a 50 percent chance of inheriting the disease-causing *RB* or *TP53* mutations. *TP53* germline mutations are also present in some osteosarcoma patients with no apparent family history of Li-Fraumeni syndrome (189).

***RB* Mutations.** Mutation of the *RB* gene has an essential role in the development of osteosarcoma (both of a sporadic nature or in patients with a hereditary predisposition). The *RB* gene encodes an approximately 105-kDa nuclear phosphoprotein (pRB) that regulates cell cycle progression from the G_1 phase to the S phase. In part, pRB exerts its function by controlling a family of heterodimeric transcription factors, collectively referred to as E2F, that are known to promote cellular proliferation. The growth-suppressive activity of pRB is inactivated by phosphorylation, a process catalyzed by D-type cyclins and cyclin-dependent kinases (CDK4 and 6), or cyclin E/CDK2, cyclin A/CDK2, or both in response to extracellular signals. The activity of these cyclin/CDK complexes is, in turn, regulated by the INK4 (inhibitors of CDK4) and CIP/KIP (CDK-inhibitory protein/kinase-inhibitory protein) families of CDK-inhibitory molecules. Members of these families, capable of blocking pRB phosphorylation by inhibiting cyclin/CDK, include $p15^{INK4b}$, $p16^{INK4a}$, $p18^{INK4c}$, $p19^{INK4d}$, $p21^{CIP1}$, $p27^{KIP1}$, and $p57^{KIP2}$ (66,165,177).

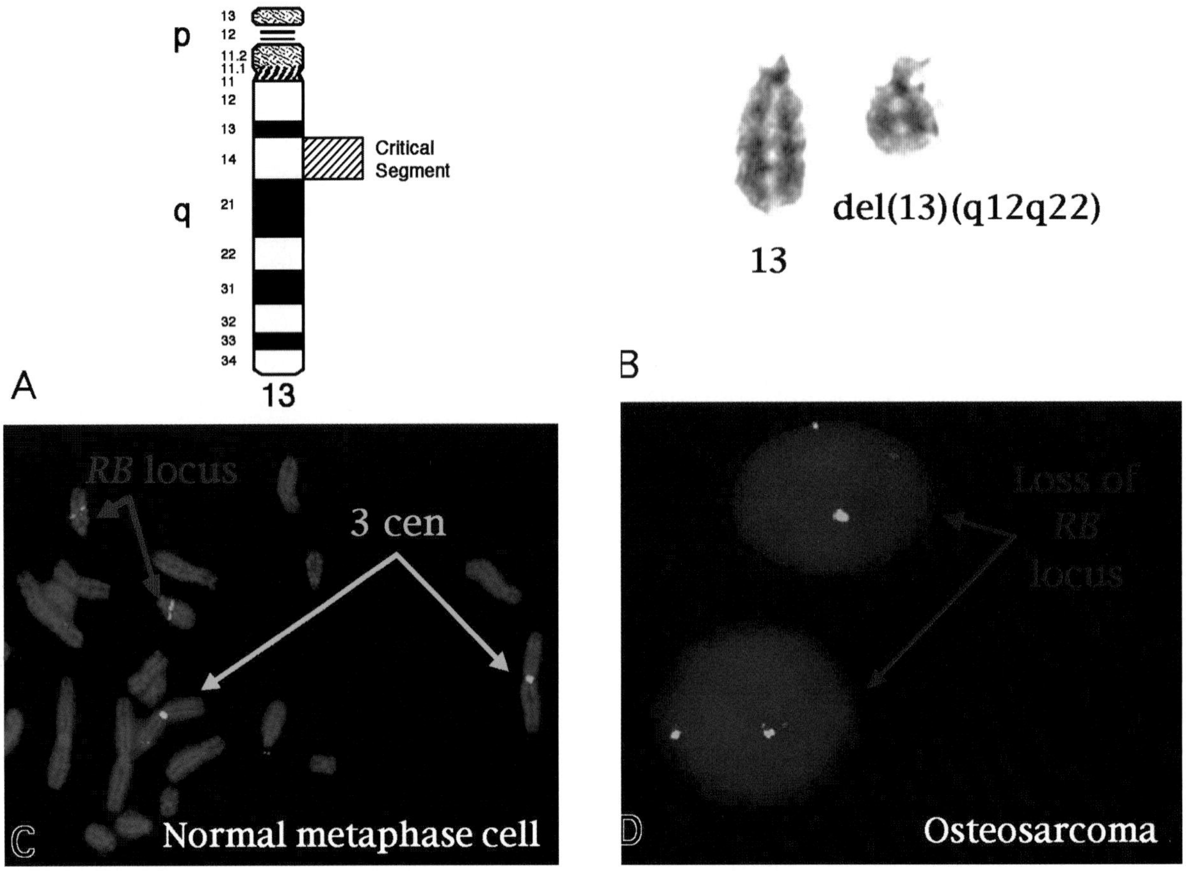

Figure 5-101

LOSS OF RETINOBLASTOMA GENE LOCUS IN OSTEOSARCOMA

A: Schema of chromosome 13 illustrating the critical region of loss that includes the retinoblastoma gene locus in osteosarcoma.

B: Partial karyotype of a conventional osteosarcoma exhibiting an interstitial deletion of the long arm of chromosome 13, including band q14.

C: Fluorescence in situ hybridization (FISH) analysis of a normal metaphase control cell with *RB* gene locus (red) and chromosome 3 centromere (green) probes.

D: Similar FISH studies performed on a cytologic touch preparation of a conventional osteosarcoma shows loss of the *RB* gene locus signal (red). (The chromosome 3 centromeric probe in green is used as a control for ploidy level.)

The interplay between the CKI (CDK-inhibitory) group, cyclin/CDK, and pRB/E2F constitutes the so-called pRB pathway. The mutational profiles of the *RB* gene in osteosarcoma are basically the same as for retinoblastoma; almost all alter or eliminate the functional internal protein receptor or "pocket" domain of pRB. Studies of osteosarcoma show that alterations affecting the *RB* locus (loss of heterozygosity, microsatellite instability, or both) are present in 63 to 78 percent of primary osteosarcoma samples (44). Alterations of members of this pathway, other than pRB, may be present in other osteosarcomas. For example, amplification of *CDK4* or homozygous *CDKN2/p16*^{INK4a} gene deletions or loss of p16^{INK4a} expression have been shown in osteosarcomas with and without *RB* mutations (46,47,112,147,197).

Accumulating evidence points to the pRB pathway as a candidate obligatory target in multistep oncogenesis of possibly all human tumor types (not restricted to retinoblastoma and osteosarcoma) (132). This concept has inspired considerable effort to develop novel cancer therapeutics targeting the G_1/S control, including gene therapy approaches aimed at correction of *RB* gene defects or inhibition of cyclin/CDK activities and induction of apoptosis (110,169). Reintroduction of functional pRB into tumor cells lacking this protein results in both reduced tumorigenicity in nude mice and growth arrest in culture (due in part to transcriptional repression of genes required for the S phase) (54,101,188). Overexpression of CDK inhibitory protein $p21^{CIP1}$ in cells lacking functional pRB has been shown to mediate sensitivity to anticancer drugs by inhibiting E2F1 phosphorylation, which may contribute to increased S/G_2 cell cycle delay and increased cell susceptibility to apoptosis (127).

***TP53* Mutations**. The *TP53* gene is the most commonly mutated gene in nonhereditary human cancer. Somatic mutations of *TP53* have been found in approximately 50 percent of tumors (125). More than 80 percent of cancers display functional inactivation of the p53 pathway when mutations in genes that interact with *TP53,* such as the *HDM2* (also known as *MDM2*) and *p14^ARF^* genes, are taken into account (111, 151,176).The *TP53* gene encodes a 53-kD nuclear phosphoprotein that complexes with the large T antigen of SV40 (123). Induction of the p53 tumor suppressor protein in cells can lead to either G_1 cell cycle arrest or apoptosis. In response to DNA damage, increased wild-type p53 protein leads to transcriptional activation of different genes, including *$p21^{CIP1}$, HDM2, GADD45, BAX, IGF-BP,* and *CCNG1 (cyclin-G),* to repair the damaged DNA or signals a "sensor" molecule that confirms the damage and initiates apoptosis. The ability to arrest the cell cycle, a key regulatory function, occurs with proper activation of the RB pathway, which is *TP53* mediated. The p53 protein functions as a tetramer, which is actually a dimer of dimers (195). This homotetrameric complex renders the p53 protein function vulnerable to numerous mutations.

The majority of *TP53* mutations are missense mutations (amino acid change in the encoded protein) within the DNA-binding domain at the so-called hot spots (exons 5 to 8); 20 percent of mutations may be outside this region, for example, within the tetramerization domain (61,63,94). Alterations of the DNA-binding domain incapacitate *TP53* as a tumor suppressor because the function of p53 to transcriptionally regulate target genes involved in growth arrest and apoptosis is dependent on its ability to bind DNA. Mutations of the DNA-binding domain also create proteins with oncogenic properties. Different authors have reported that the *TP53* mutation rate obtained by direct sequencing is approximately 20 percent in osteosarcoma (162). In contrast to *RB* mutations, which usually are confined to high-grade osteosarcomas, *TP53* mutations have been observed in variant histologic types of low-grade osteosarcoma as well as in high-grade osteosarcoma (161). Loss of heterozygosity at the *TP53* locus has been found in approximately 75 percent of osteosarcomas analyzed.

A second mechanism of inactivating p53 involves proteins that interact with or modify p53, such as HDM2. The HDM2 oncoprotein has the ability to bind to both p53 and pRB and to abrogate the p53 response to DNA damage by inhibiting its transcriptional activity and facilitating its degradation. HDM2 is subject to negative control by the ARF tumor-suppressor protein ($p14^{ARF}$). Amplification of the *HDM2* oncogene, which results in the constitutive inhibition of wild-type p53, has been detected with low frequency (4 to 7 percent) in osteosarcomas. Amplification of *HDM2* in osteosarcoma does not appear to be a major predictor of stage or prognosis (fig. 5-102) (130). Osteosarcomas with *HDM2* amplification do not display high levels of genomic instability, in contrast to osteosarcomas with mutation of *TP53* which do (155).

Analogous to *RB*, reconstitution of wild-type p53 expression inhibits in vitro cell proliferation, in vitro soft agar colony formation, and tumorigenicity in immunodeficient mice (158). These findings raise possibilities for developing drugs that restore the tumor suppressor function of mutant p53 proteins, thus selectively eliminating tumor cells (174). Altered *TP53* gene product is detectable immunohistochemically on routine tissue sections of osteosarcomas (52).

Prognostic Markers

Several studies have been conducted to identify genetic alterations that may serve as prognostic markers in osteosarcoma. The presence of 13q14 loss of heterozygosity and DNA alterations of the *RB* gene have been shown to correlate with the histopathologic grade of osteosarcoma,

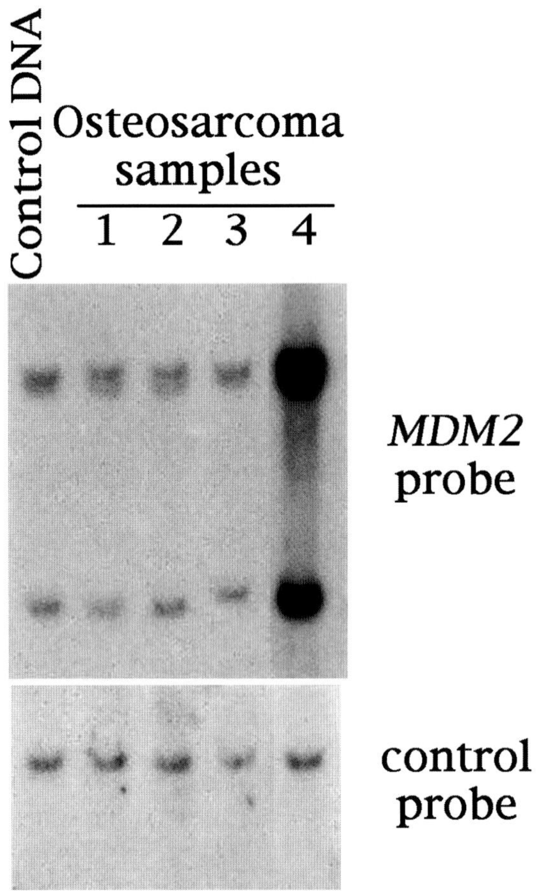

Figure 5-102

AMPLIFICATION OF THE *MDM2* GENE AT 12q13 IN OSTEOSARCOMA

Sequential hybridization of a Southern blot analysis of osteosarcoma and control DNA with an *MDM2* probe followed by a control probe from 12p shows approximately an 18-fold amplification of *MDM2* in one of four osteosarcoma tumor samples, in comparison with control DNA. The other cases showed no amplification. The control DNA is from normal placenta. (Modified from Ladanyi M, Cha C, Lewis R, Jhanwar SC, Huvos AG, Healey JH. *MDM2* gene amplification in metastatic osteosarcoma. Cancer Res 1993;53:16–8.)

a higher probability of metastasis, and an unfavorable outcome (46,81,157,203).

The p-glycoprotein, encoded by the multidrug resistance gene, *MDR1*, is a member of the adenosine triphosphate–dependent transporter superfamily that confers multidrug resistance (MDR) by promoting efflux of important cytotoxins from resistant cells. *MDR1* and p-glycoprotein expression have been detected in osteosarcomas before exposure to chemotherapeutic agents and have been shown in some studies to correlate with an adverse prognosis and resistance to cytotoxic drugs such as doxorubicin (39,59,175). The data are contradictory about an association between p-glycoprotein expression and histologic necrosis after chemotherapy (93). An explanation for the discrepant findings is the unreliability of immunohistochemistry in detecting p-glycoprotein expression (particularly in paraffin-embedded material). In some MDR osteosarcomas, increased expression of a novel human gene that can induce *RB*, the *RB1CC1* (retinoblastoma 1-inducible coiled-coil 1) gene, has been detected in response to doxorubicin-induced cytotoxic stress and remains elevated for the duration of the drug treatment (60).

The *c-fos* and *c-jun* proto-oncogenes are associated with many biologic processes, including transcription regulation of gene expression, cell growth, and cell differentiation (particularly in the differentiation of osteoblasts and chondrocytes). A comparison of *c-fos* and *c-jun* expression, as detected immunohistochemically, showed that high-grade osteosarcomas had a significantly higher expression of both oncoproteins than did low-grade osteosarcomas (83,156). Moreover, alterations of *c-fos* have been shown to occur more frequently in patients with recurrent or metastatic disease, and *c-fos* overexpression may correspond to a poor chemotherapeutic response (109,159). A synchronous overexpression of both *c-myc* and *c-fos* oncogenes has been shown to be highly significant for the metastatic potential of primary osteosarcomas (85).

In some studies, *HER2/erbB2* expression in osteosarcoma has been shown to be associated with a poor prognosis (poor histologic response to preoperative chemotherapy and decreased event-free survival) (80,93,153). Other authors, however, have reported an absence of *HER2/erbB2* gene expression in osteosarcomas (187). These discrepancies have been attributed mainly to technical issues concerning immunohistochemical analysis. Fellenberg et al. (79) demonstrated the reliability of laser microdissection in combination with real-time quantitative reverse transcriptase polymerase chain reaction (RT-PCR) to assess *HER2/erbB2* gene expression in osteosarcoma. These authors determined that *HER2/*

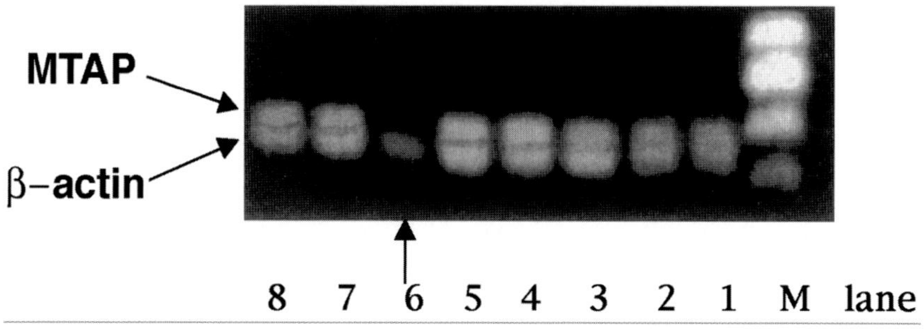

Figure 5-103

MTAP GENE DELETION IN OSTEOSARCOMA

A representative gel for exon 6 of the *MTAP* gene is shown from polymerase chain reaction analysis of genomic DNA in osteosarcoma patient samples. In each lane, *MTAP* and β-actin products are present, with the lower band representing the β-actin. In lane 6, there is clear absence of *MTAP* product. M is the DNA marker. *MTAP* gene deletions with associated loss of detectable mRNA and protein appear common in osteosarcoma. (Fig. 2 from Garcia-Castellano JM, Villanueva A, Healey JH, et al. Methylthioadenosine phosphorylase gene deletions are common in osteosarcoma. Clin Cancer Res 2002;8:782–7.)

erbB2 gene expression in laser-microdissected osteosarcoma cells correlated significantly with the response to preoperative chemotherapy.

It is unclear whether p53 inactivation has an effect on osteosarcoma progression or whether it confers resistance or sensitivity to irradiation and chemotherapy (70,78,162). It has been suggested that p53 pathway alterations may arise early in the pathogenesis of osteosarcoma based on the observation of concordance of *TP53* status in paired primary and metastatic osteosarcoma samples (89).

Deletion or loss of the *MTAP* gene, localized to 9p21, is frequently associated with deletion of the tumor suppressor genes $p15^{INK4b}$ and $p16^{INK4a}$. MTAP is an essential enzyme in the salvage pathway of adenine and in methionine synthesis. Examination of 96 high-grade osteosarcomas revealed *MTAP* gene deletions with loss of protein expression in 37.5 percent of the samples analyzed (fig. 5-103) (86). These findings suggest that inhibitors of de novo purine synthesis or methionine depletion may be effective therapeutically for patients whose osteosarcomas fail to express MTAP.

An inverse relationship between cellular L/B/K ALP (liver/bone/kidney alkaline phosphatase) expression and osteosarcoma aggressiveness exists (134). Further characterization of the gene expression profile of L/B/K ALP-transfected osteosarcoma cells by cDNA microarray analysis has also shown upregulation of two genes involved in cell-cell adhesion and cell growth, cadherin 13 (*CDH13*) and caveolin 1 (*CAV1*), that could explain, at least in part, the lower levels of malignancy found in osteosarcoma cells with high L/B/K ALP activity (204).

CYP3A4/5 is a p450 isoenzyme that is involved in metabolic activation and detoxification of a number of anticancer drugs, several of which are used in the treatment of osteosarcoma. Expression of CYP3A4/5 has been shown to be significantly higher in primary osteosarcoma biopsies of patients who developed distant metastatic disease compared with biopsies from patients with localized disease ($P = 0.0004$) (69). As a potential biomarker of outcome in osteosarcoma, high cytochrome P450 CYP3A4/5 expression may have therapeutic implications for this neoplasm (69).

Cell surface low density lipoprotein (LDL) receptor-related protein 5 (LRP5) is a Wnt (Wingless-type) coreceptor that has been implicated in human skeletal development. Expression of LRP5, as detected by RT-PCR analysis, is a common event in osteosarcoma and correlates significantly with tumor metastasis (decreased event-free survival) (100).

Gene expression profile studies of osteosarcoma using cDNA microarray analysis are few, but they suggest that this may be a useful approach for predicting prognosis and determining therapeutic responsiveness or resistance (149,173,182).

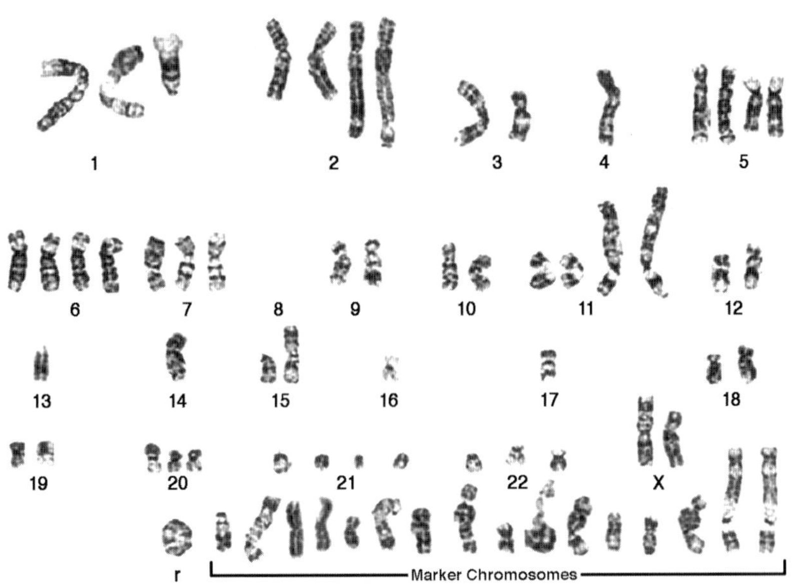

Figure 5-104

REPRESENTATIVE COMPLEX KARYOTYPE TYPICAL OF A HIGH-GRADE OSTEOSARCOMA

Numerous marker chromosomes are seen.

Other Potential Genetic Lesions

Studies aimed at the identification of allelic loss in osteosarcomas have shown involvement of chromosomal loci 3q26, 4q32-34, and 18q21-22, in addition to 13q14 and 17p13, suggesting that these loci may also harbor tumor suppressor genes important in the pathogenesis of osteosarcoma (118,152,181). The 3q26, 4q32-34, and 18q21-22 loci have not been characterized, although a linkage between Paget's disease of bone and the 18q21-23 locus has been seen in some families (90,144). Patients with Paget's disease of bone, a common condition characterized by bone pain and deformity, have a several thousandfold higher risk of developing osteosarcoma than the general population. Loss of heterozygosity of 18q has been seen in both pagetic and sporadic osteosarcoma tumors (97). Two additional genes that appear to have a pathophysiologic role in Paget's disease are the antiapoptotic gene *BCL2* and the proto-oncogene *c-fos* (43,55).

Tumor Cytogenetics

Cytogenetic studies have demonstrated that the majority of osteosarcomas are characterized by complex chromosomal abnormalities with pronounced cell-to-cell variation or heterogeneity (fig. 5-104). Cytogenetic manifestations of gene amplification, including ring chromosomes, homogeneously staining regions, and double minutes are common in osteosarcoma and have been shown to correlate with the amplification of certain oncogenes such as *c-myc* (95). According to a review of the literature that included 161 osteosarcoma specimens (both primary and metastatic lesions), chromosomal bands or regions of 1p11-13, 1q11-12, 1q21-22, 11p14-15, 14p11-13, 15p11-13, 17p, and 19q13 are most frequently rearranged and +1, -9, -10, -13, and -17 are the most common numerical abnormalities (53). An entirely accurate assessment of the frequency of various aberrations in osteosarcoma is limited by the high percentage of marker chromosomes (a marker chromosome is a structurally altered chromosome in which no part can be identified).

Related genetic approaches, such as DNA flow cytometry, FISH, spectral karyotyping (SKY) or multifluor FISH (M-FISH), and comparative genomic hybridization (CGH), have served as important adjuncts in uncovering unidentifiable chromosomal rearrangements and imbalances, and in assessing the prognostic value of some of these anomalies. Gain of 8q21.3-23 as detected with CGH may be present in up to 50 percent of osteosarcomas and, in high-grade osteosarcoma, has been shown to be associated with a statistically significant poor distant disease-free survival rate and a trend toward a short overall survival rate (182–184). Amplification of 17p11-12 also has been identified by CGH in

20 to 30 percent of high-grade osteosarcomas and appears to correspond with aggressive clinical behavior (103,180). Genes *PMP22* and *COPS3*, and possibly three ESTs (expressed sequence tags), are candidate amplification targets in 17p11-12 (194). In addition to confirming the frequent presence of 17p11-12 and 8q23-24 gain in osteosarcoma, SKY analyses have revealed recurrent rearrangements of 20q13 (42). Although the prognostic significance of DNA aneuploidy in osteosarcomas is relatively small because nearly all tumors show aneuploidy, assessment of nuclear DNA content with DNA image cytophotometry appears to be of prognostic value (117,145). Also, a correlation has been observed between RNA content and patient survival (76).

Telomeres are nucleoprotein structures found at the end of linear eukaryotic chromosomes. With cell division, telomeres gradually shorten to a critical size, at which point senescence results through a p53-dependent process (92). Cancer cells use one of two mechanisms, telomerase activation (TA) and alternative lengthening of telomeres (ALT), to maintain telomere length, elude critical telomere shortening, and permit cells to divide indefinitely. In contrast to carcinomas, these two telomere maintenance mechanisms occur with near equal frequency in osteosarcoma (37,172). Molecular analysis of TA and ALT in 71 osteosarcoma specimens from 62 patients demonstrated that the absence of both TA and ALT (in 18 percent) was more strongly associated with improved survival ($P = 0.05$) than were stage ($P = 0.16$) or chemotherapy response ($P = 0.18$) in this group of patients with osteosarcoma (192).

TREATMENT AND PROGNOSIS FOR PATIENTS WITH OSTEOSARCOMAS

There is considerable debate about important prognostic factors in osteosarcoma. Treatment options also have changed dramatically. Whereas 15 years ago immediate amputation was considered the treatment of choice, it is rarely performed now. Most patients with osteosarcoma receive preoperative chemotherapy and a limb salvage procedure if technically feasible. With this regimen, the prognosis has improved considerably.

The following features have been studied in relation to prognosis in osteosarcoma.

Age. Although many studies have suggested that children have a worse prognosis than young adults (36,167,185,186), other studies have not found any correlation between age and prognosis (68,75,102).

Sex. Some studies have reported that the prognosis is worse for males than females (167, 185,186), but others have found that sex does not affect prognosis (68,75,102).

Site. In a landmark study, Dahlin and Coventry (67) showed that the overall 5-year survival rate for patients with osteosarcoma was 20 percent, and those with tumors distal to the knee and elbow had a better prognosis (35.8 percent). Several studies have confirmed that patients with tumors located proximally have a worse prognosis (167,185,186,193). However, Hudson et al. (102) and Davis et al. (68) did not think that the site of the tumor was important prognostically. Still, it seems clear that the site of the osteosarcoma has a significant effect on prognosis. In 1983, Nora et al. (148) reported on 21 patients with osteosarcoma of the skull bones: only two patients survived 5 years and one of them died 65 months after diagnosis. Hence, only one patient survived in this series of osteosarcomas of the skull. Huvos et al. (107) found that those with primary tumors of the skull had a better prognosis than patients with secondary tumors, and Salvati et al. (168) reported improved survival for patients with osteosarcoma of the skull with the institution of chemotherapy. In 1986, Shives et al. (178) reported on 30 patients who had osteosarcoma of the spine. There was only one long-term survivor in this group. In comparison, Okada et al. (150) reported that only 1 of 12 patients with osteosarcoma of the hand died of disease. Possibly, there may not be a significant difference between different bones of the appendicular skeleton. Clearly, however, osteosarcoma involving the axial skeleton is a different treatment problem.

Size. The results of nearly all studies agree that large tumor size is associated with a worse prognosis (50,68,102,167,185,186).

Duration of Symptoms. Two studies from Mayo Clinic suggested that patients with symptoms of short duration had a worse prognosis (185,186).

Histology. Some studies have suggested that histologic subtyping is important for determining

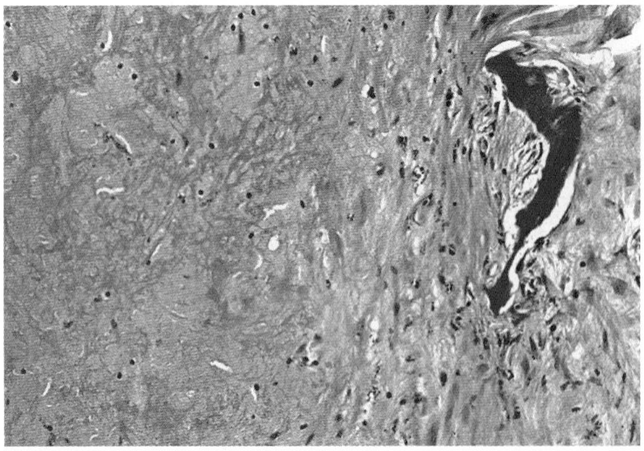

Figure 5-105

CHEMOTHERAPY EFFECT IN OSTEOSARCOMA

Osteosarcoma after preoperative chemotherapy, with nearly complete (99 percent) necrosis. Dense fibrous tissue with scattered histiocytes and hemosiderin-laden macrophages has replaced the bone marrow spaces. There is no evidence of viable tumor.

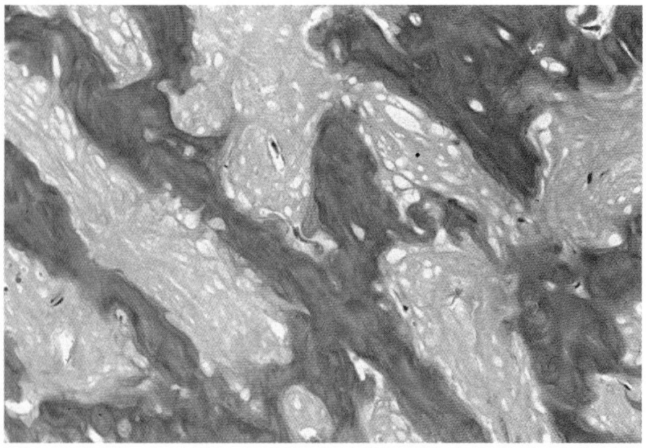

Figure 5-106

CHEMOTHERAPY EFFECT IN OSTEOSARCOMA

Cellular pale pink fibrous tissue devoid of tumor cells surrounds necrotic bony trabeculae. There was 98 percent tumor cell necrosis after preoperative chemotherapy.

prognosis (185,193), but others have found no correlation (167).

Calendar Period. Osteosarcoma was considered an almost certainly lethal disease until Dahlin and Coventry (67) and Marcove et al. (135) showed that the 5-year survival rate is 20 percent. This has since been considered the "gold standard" survival rate. Results from the more recent era have been compared with this, and most studies of the effect of chemotherapy used historical controls, which may not be valid.

In 1976, Rab et al. (160) used prophylactic lung radiation in 53 patients with osteosarcoma and compared them with a control group that did not receive any irradiation. There was no difference in survival: both groups had a 2-year survival rate of 40 percent. This almost doubling of the survival rate (which might have been attributed to therapy if historical controls were used) was almost completely ignored.

For the 181 patients with osteosarcoma in the study of Taylor et al. (185), the survival rate was 25 percent until 1969, and in the 1970s, it was 50 percent. The prognosis did not improve in the later seventies. The authors suggested that the biologic characteristics of the tumor may have changed. Subsequently, Taylor et al. (186) enlarged the study to 330 patients, and the calendar period was still important prognostically. These two studies questioned the validity of historical controls in the evaluation of the effect of chemotherapy.

In a multi-institutional study, Link et al. (129) compared surgery alone with surgery and chemotherapy for osteosarcoma. For the surgery alone group, overall survival was 17 percent and for the surgery and chemotherapy group, 60 percent. The authors concluded that there was no change in the biologic characteristics of the tumor in the newer era. These results were supported by a study of Eilber et al. (75).

Necrosis. Studies have confirmed the correlation between necrosis from chemotherapy and prognosis (figs. 5-105, 5-106) (38,50,68,88, 102,163). However, Bjornsson et al. (51) found that spontaneous necrosis was an adverse prognostic factor.

OSTEOSARCOMAS OF THE SURFACE OF BONE

Parosteal Osteosarcoma

Definition. Parosteal osteosarcoma is a well-differentiated osteosarcoma that arises on the surface of bone and, on radiographs, appears as a heavily mineralized mass.

General Features. All osteosarcomas of the surface of bone are rare; however, parosteal osteosarcoma is the most common of these. It is the earliest type described (207), and its histologic blandness is emphasized by the term parosteal osteoma. The rarity of the tumor is emphasized

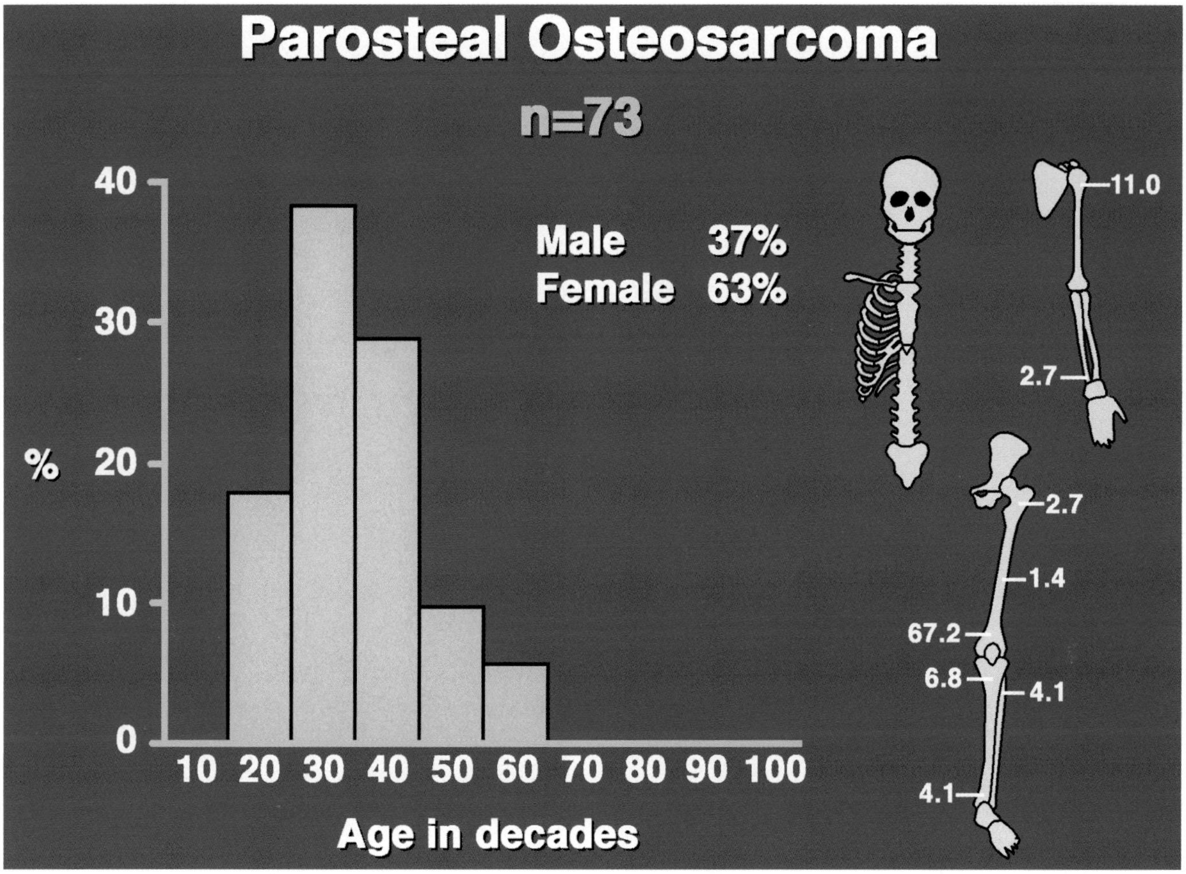

Figure 5-107

PAROSTEAL OSTEOSARCOMA

Distribution of parosteal osteosarcoma according to the age and sex of the patient and the site of the lesion.

by Okada et al. (210), who identified 226 parosteal osteosarcomas in a series of 4,270 osteosarcomas. Parosteal osteosarcomas accounted for 4 percent of all osteosarcomas recorded in the Mayo Clinic files and 6 percent in the consultation files. This may be an overestimation of the incidence because patients with parosteal osteosarcoma are more likely to be treated at major medical centers or to be evaluated in consultation.

The etiology is not known. A history of trauma is elicited in less than 5 percent of patients. Until the beginning of the year 2000, 73 cases of parosteal osteosarcoma were included in the Mayo Clinic files.

Clinical Features. Parosteal osteosarcoma affects young adults; the patients are about a decade older than those with conventional osteosarcoma (fig. 5-107). In the series of Okada et al. (210), about one third of all tumors occurred in the third decade of life. The tumor has a slight but definite predilection for females.

Patients generally complain of a painless swelling of usually longer than 1 year duration; pain with or without swelling may be present. Typically, a patient has a mass in the popliteal fossa that prevents the knee from bending.

Physical examination usually demonstrates a firm to hard mass. Limitation of movement of the adjacent joint may also be noted.

Sites. Parosteal osteosarcoma has a peculiar propensity to involve the posterior cortex of the distal femoral metaphysis. In the Mayo Clinic files, about 70 percent of these tumors involved the distal femur. Okada et al. (210), found 64 percent of the tumors in the posterior distal femur. The proximal tibia and proximal humerus are the next most common sites. Flat bones are rarely involved; moreover, in these sites it may

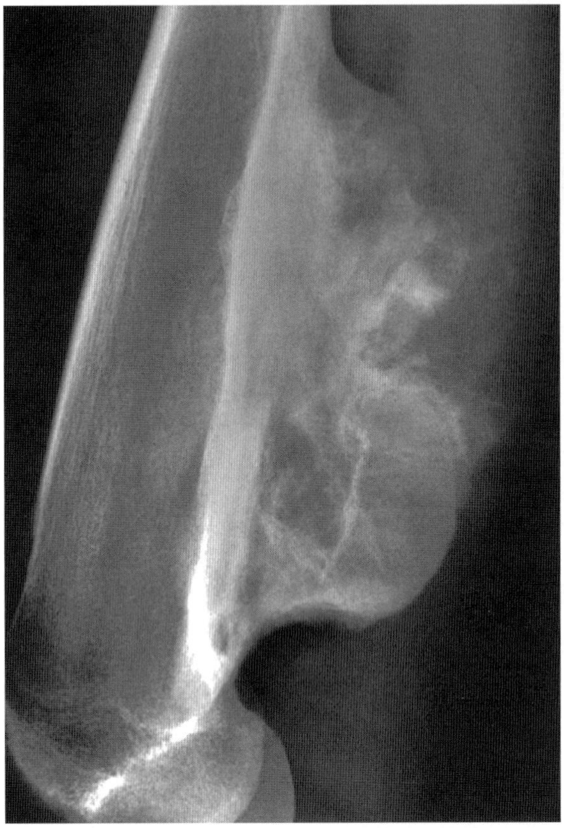

Figure 5-108

PAROSTEAL OSTEOSARCOMA

The lesion is lobulated and heavily mineralized, and has a broad-based attachment to the underlying bone.

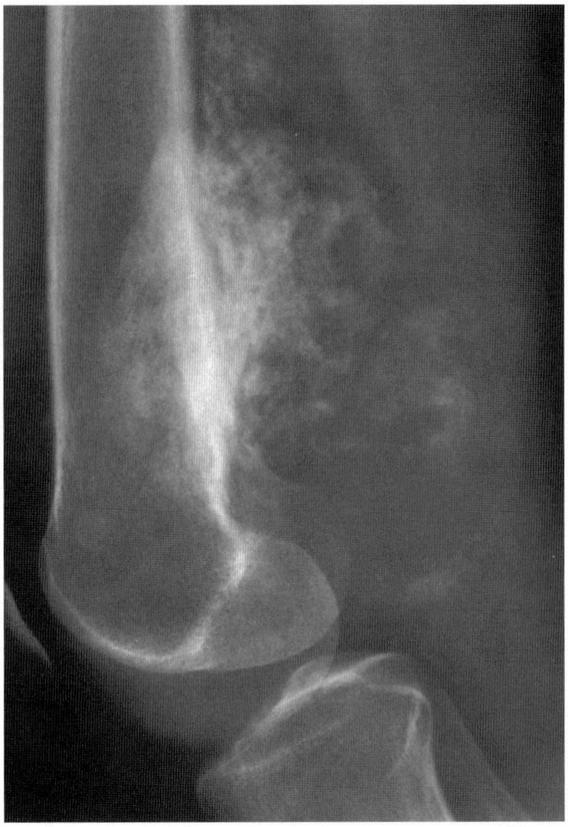

Figure 5-109

PAROSTEAL OSTEOSARCOMA

This densely mineralized parosteal osteosarcoma wraps around the distal femur, but an area of lucency is maintained between the tumor and underlying bone.

be impossible to determine whether the lesion arose on the surface of the bone.

Radiographic Findings. Plain radiographs are almost always diagnostic of parosteal osteosarcoma. The tumor appears as a heavily mineralized mass attached by a broad base to the underlying cortex (fig. 5-108). As the tumor grows, it tends to surround the involved bone; however, because the growing portion is not attached to the bone, there is a lucency between the tumor and the underlying cortex (fig. 5-109). When the involved bone is surrounded with tumor, it may not be possible to discern whether the tumor arises from the surface or bone marrow cavity. The outermost portion is usually less well mineralized.

Lucencies may be seen within the lesion (fig. 5-110). Bertoni et al. (206) suggested that lucencies in the substance of the tumor (but not on the surface) indicate dedifferentiation; Okada et al. (210) did not confirm this. Periosteal new bone formation is unusual, but remodeling of the cortex may be identified in approximately 20 percent of cases.

CT and MRI are helpful in identifying medullary involvement or the lack of it (fig. 5-111). Cross-sectional images show that approximately one fifth of all tumors have medullary involvement. The cross-sectional images also frequently show unmineralized soft tissue tumor masses, and these may affect surgical planning.

Gross Findings. Parosteal osteosarcoma is a lobulated, hard, white mass attached to the underlying cortex (fig. 5-112). Nodules of cartilage may be seen grossly; occasionally, they form plates on the surface, simulating the appearance of osteochondroma (fig. 5-113). The periphery of the lesion may appear fibrous and invade skeletal muscle. Invasion of the underlying bone is seen in fewer than one fourth of tumors (fig. 5-114).

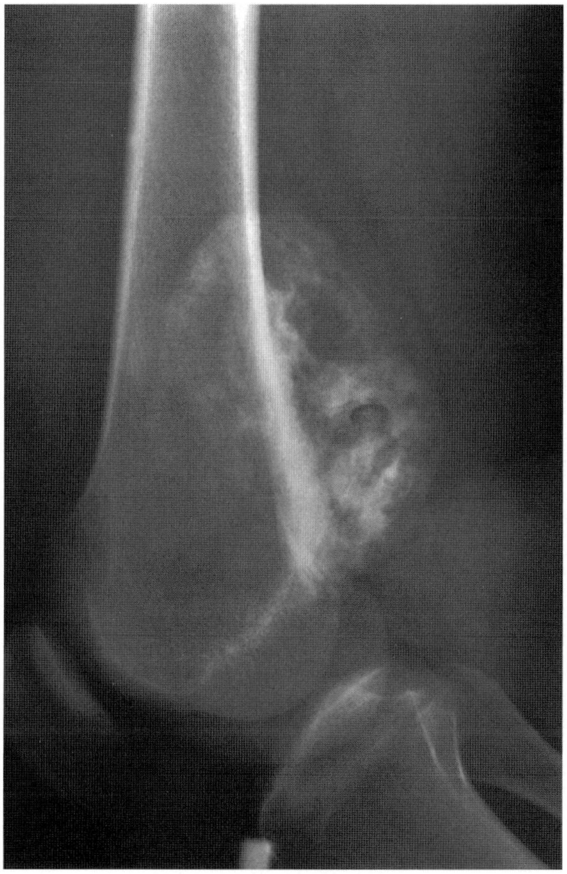

Figure 5-110

PAROSTEAL OSTEOSARCOMA

The lucency posteriorly in this lesion is nondiagnostic and not necessarily indicative of dedifferentiation.

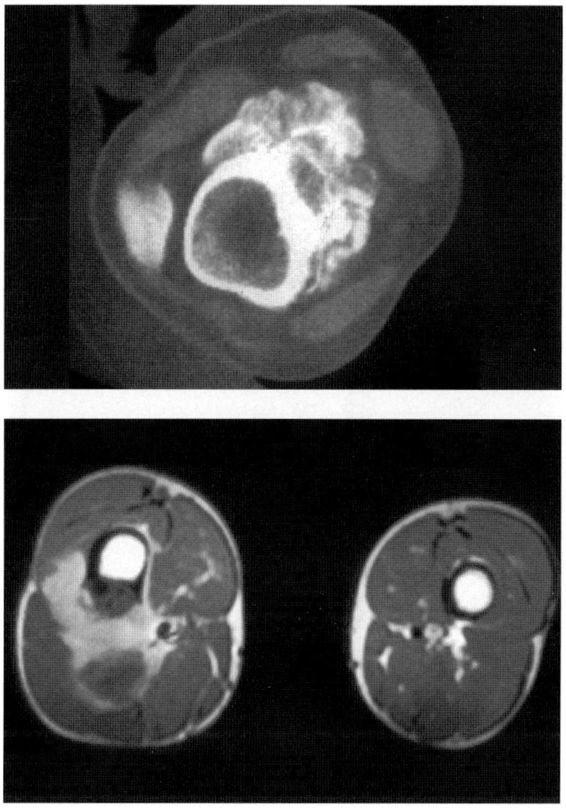

Figure 5-111

PAROSTEAL OSTEOSARCOMA

CT (top) and MRI (bottom) confirm the lack of medullary involvement in two examples of parosteal osteosarcoma.

Microscopic Findings. The cardinal microscopic features are the relatively hypocellular stroma and the well-formed bony trabeculae (fig. 5-115). The spindle cells show minimal cytologic atypia, and mitotic figures are rare (fig. 5-116). Broad trabeculae of bone are arranged in parallel arrays. The bone may be irregular and have cement lines, producing a pagetoid appearance. In about one fifth of cases, the stroma is more cellular and the cells have more obvious features of anaplasia (Broders grade 2) (fig. 5-117). Ahuja et al. (205) graded parosteal osteosarcomas; it seems to us that at least some of these cases are high-grade surface osteosarcomas.

Invasion of the medullary cavity may not be obvious on gross examination but may be seen histologically (fig. 5-118). Cartilaginous differentiation is present in about half of the tumors, usually as hypercellular nodules interspersed among the bony trabeculae (fig. 5-119); the cartilage is at the periphery, forming "caps" in half of these cases (fig. 5-120). These cartilage caps show an irregular arrangement of chondrocytes and lack the columnar arrangement of osteochondroma.

About 15 percent of the tumors have foci of high-grade sarcoma (dedifferentiation) either at the time of initial presentation or at recurrence (figs. 5-121, 5-122) (215). The areas of dedifferentiation may contain osteosarcoma, fibrosarcoma, or malignant fibrous histiocytoma (fig. 5-123). Even microscopic foci of high-grade sarcoma are associated with a grave prognosis.

Genetics and Other Special Techniques. Parosteal osteosarcoma can be differentiated from conventional osteosarcoma by the presence of ring chromosomes as either the sole

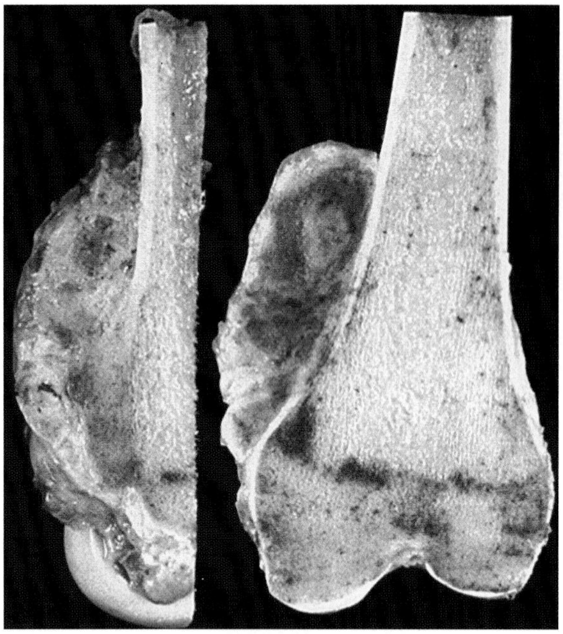

Figure 5-112

PAROSTEAL OSTEOSARCOMA

Typical gross appearance of parosteal osteosarcoma showing a firm mass attached to the surface of the distal femur. There is no evidence of medullary involvement.

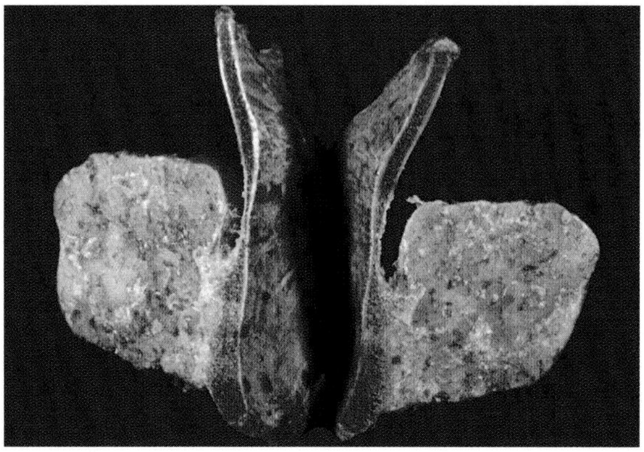

Figure 5-113

PAROSTEAL OSTEOSARCOMA

Blue-gray lobules of cartilage can be seen throughout this parosteal osteosarcoma. More commonly, the cartilage forms a cap, resembling an osteochondroma.

anomaly or accompanied by a few other abnormalities (fig. 5-124) (212). CGH analyses of parosteal osteosarcoma and low-grade central osteosarcomas have demonstrated a gain of 12q13-15 material, which has been shown to correlate with the presence of ring chromosomes

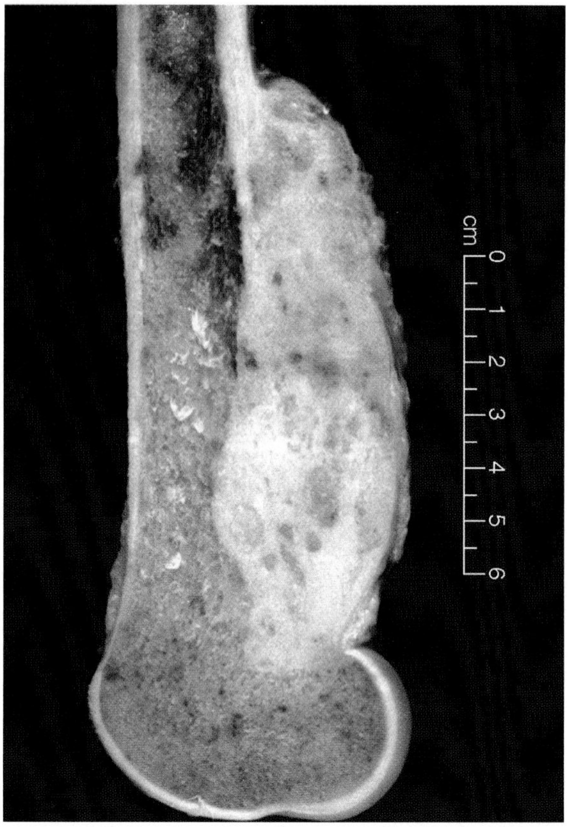

Figure 5-114

PAROSTEAL OSTEOSARCOMA

Evidence of medullary involvement is seen in this parosteal osteosarcoma, which predominantly involves the bone surface.

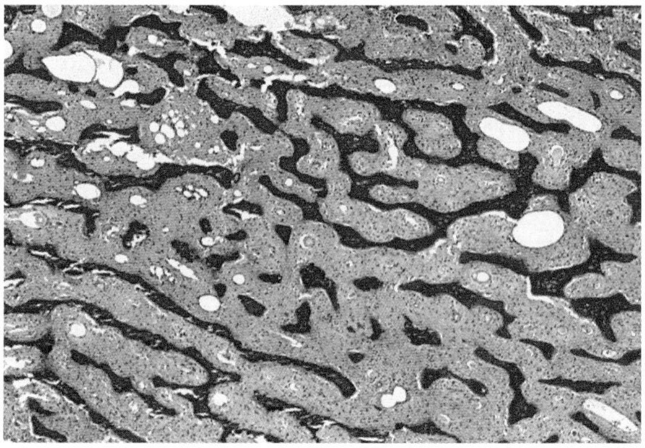

Figure 5-115

PAROSTEAL OSTEOSARCOMA

Typical low-power microscopic appearance of parosteal osteosarcoma shows anastomosing trabecular-appearing bone surrounded by a hypocellular spindle cell stroma.

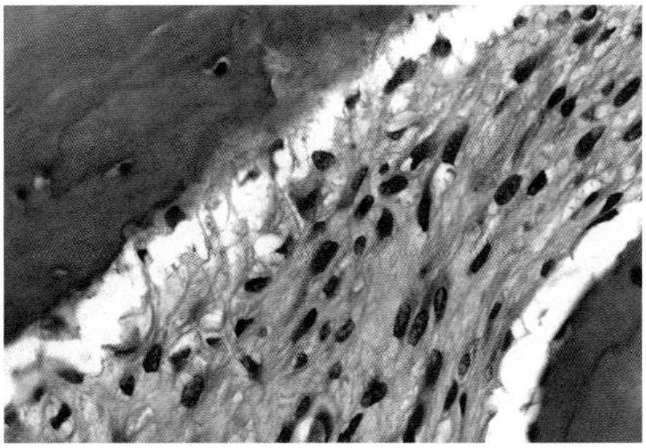

Figure 5-116

PAROSTEAL OSTEOSARCOMA

The spindle-shaped cells do not have features typical of malignancy.

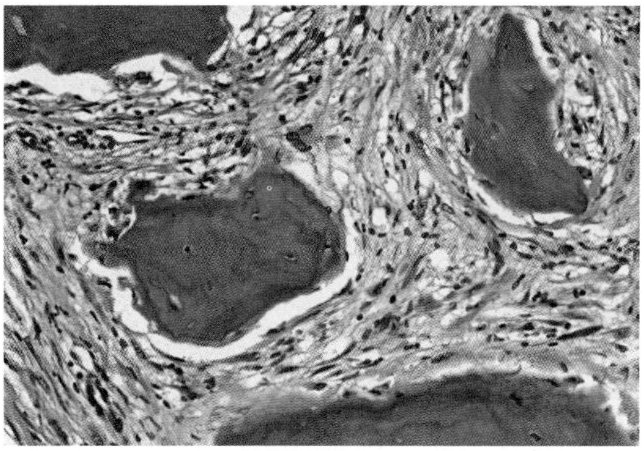

Figure 5-117

PAROSTEAL OSTEOSARCOMA

Although some tumors have more obvious evidence of cytologic anaplasia, this does not appear to be prognostically important.

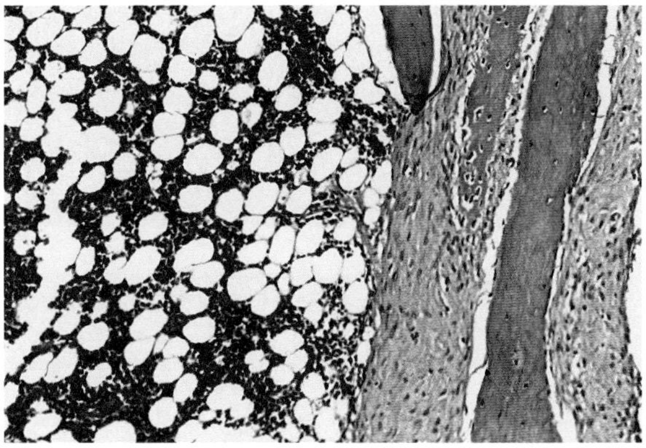

Figure 5-118

PAROSTEAL OSTEOSARCOMA

This parosteal osteosarcoma invades the medullary cavity.

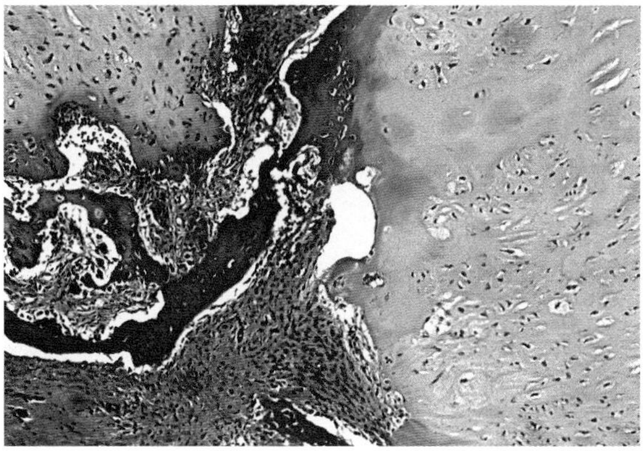

Figure 5-119

PAROSTEAL OSTEOSARCOMA

Cartilaginous nodules within a parosteal osteosarcoma.

(213,214). Several authors have also shown amplification or coamplification and coexpression of *HDM2*, *CDK4*, and *SAS* (all localized to 12q13-15) in a high percentage of parosteal osteosarcomas and central low-grade osteosarcomas (209,211,216). These same oncogenes have been shown to be amplified in high-grade osteosarcomas, but in a smaller subset. In contrast, an overrepresentation of 12p sequences (including one or more of the following regions: *CCND2, ETV6, KRAS2, D12S85*) is more common in high-grade osteosarcomas with ring chromosomes than low-grade osteosarcomas (fig. 5-125). This suggests that gain of sequences from the short arm of chromosome 12 could be a genetic pathway in the development of aggressive osteosarcoma (208). It has been proposed that the low number of DNA sequence copy number alterations and "simple" karyotypes in low-grade osteosarcoma reflects the relatively low rate of metastasis, compared with higher copy number alterations and complex karyotypes seen in higher-grade osteosarcomas (209,211,214).

Differential Diagnosis. The differential diagnosis of parosteal osteosarcoma includes heterotopic ossification, osteochondroma, osteoma, and periosteal and high-grade surface osteosarcomas. Heterotopic ossification is not

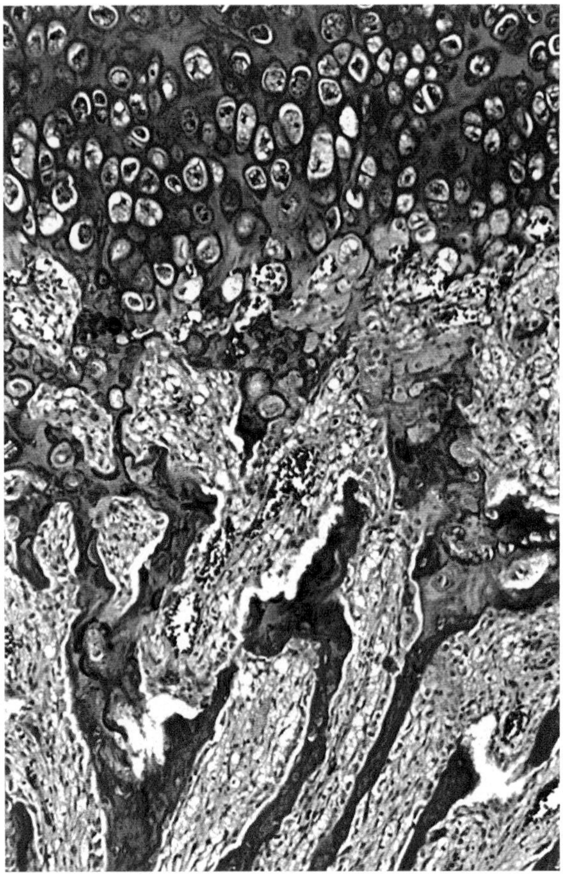

Figure 5-120

PAROSTEAL OSTEOSARCOMA

The cartilaginous caps seen in several parosteal osteosarcomas can simulate the appearance of an osteochondroma. However, the underlying bony trabeculae are surrounded by fibrous stroma and not hematopoietic bone marrow, which is what would be expected in an osteochondroma.

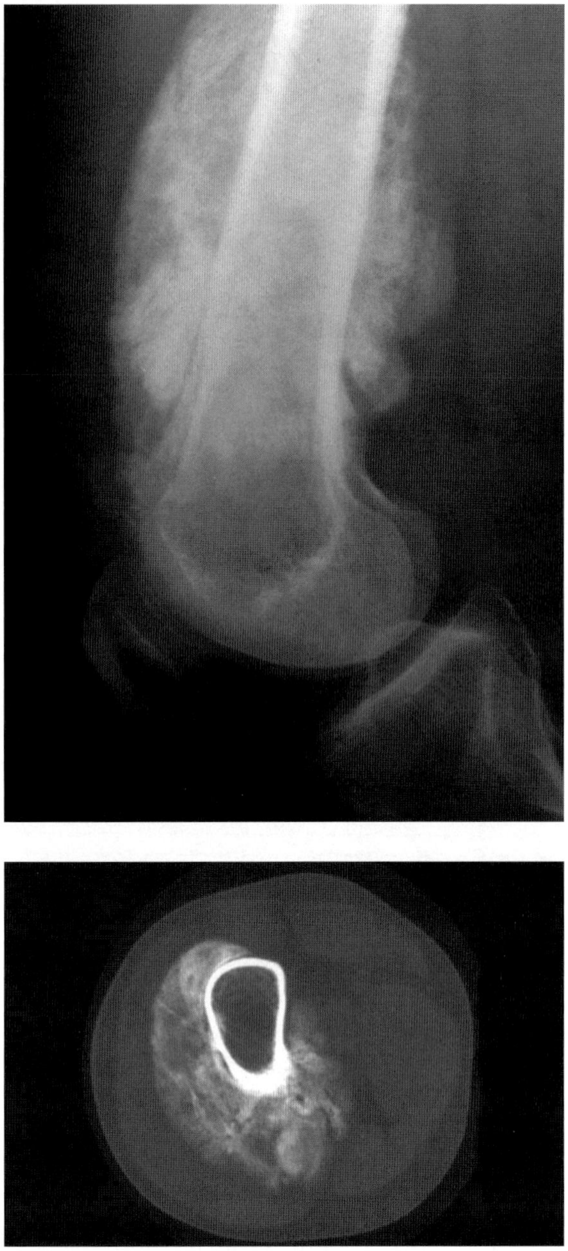

Figure 5-121

DEDIFFERENTIATED PAROSTEAL OSTEOSARCOMA

Plain radiograph (top) and CT (bottom) of a dedifferentiated parosteal osteosarcoma.

attached to bone, and the stroma is more cellular than in parosteal osteosarcoma. In osteochondroma, the cap has a columnar arrangement of chondrocytes and the spaces between bony trabeculae contain fatty or hematopoietic marrow. In contrast, the cartilage cap of parosteal osteosarcoma has an irregular arrangement of chondrocytes and a proliferation of spindle cells between the bony trabeculae. Moreover, in osteochondroma, radiographs show continuity between the lesion and the underlying bone, which is not a feature of parosteal osteosarcoma. Periosteal osteosarcomas are lucent on radiographs and do not have the heavy mineralization typical of parosteal osteosarcoma. They are less well differentiated and predominantly chondroblastic. High-grade surface osteosarcomas show pronounced cytologic atypia, which is not a feature of parosteal osteosarcoma without dedifferentiation.

Treatment and Prognosis. Parosteal osteosarcoma is a locally aggressive tumor with limited potential for distant spread. Hence, surgical resection is the treatment of choice, and there is no role for chemotherapy. The resection needs to be planned so that the entire tumor with an envelope of normal tissue is removed. The prognosis is excellent. The advent of dedifferentiation heralds a prognosis similar to that for conventional osteosarcoma.

Periosteal Osteosarcoma

Definition. Periosteal osteosarcoma is a predominantly chondroblastic, moderately differentiated osteosarcoma situated on the surface of bone without any medullary involvement.

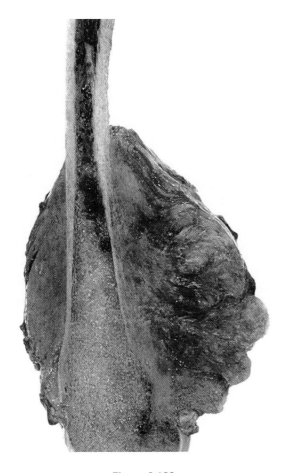

Figure 5-122

DEDIFFERENTIATED PAROSTEAL OSTEOSARCOMA

This tumor was excised from the distal femur of a 21-year-old woman, at which time the diagnosis was "classic parosteal osteosarcoma." Six years after amputation, pulmonary metastasis developed.

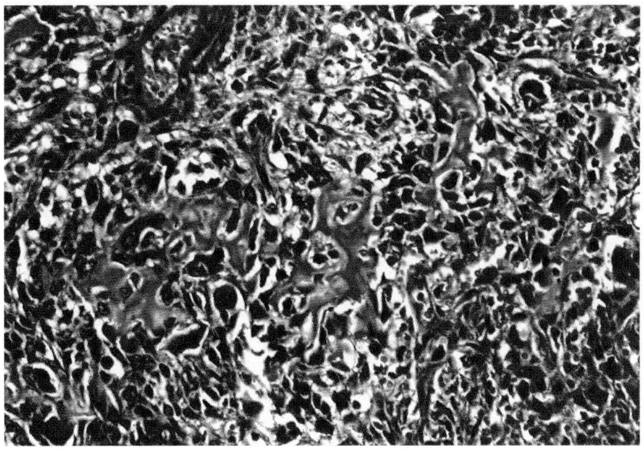

Figure 5-123

PAROSTEAL OSTEOSARCOMA

The area of dedifferentiation in this parosteal osteosarcoma has features of a high-grade osteosarcoma.

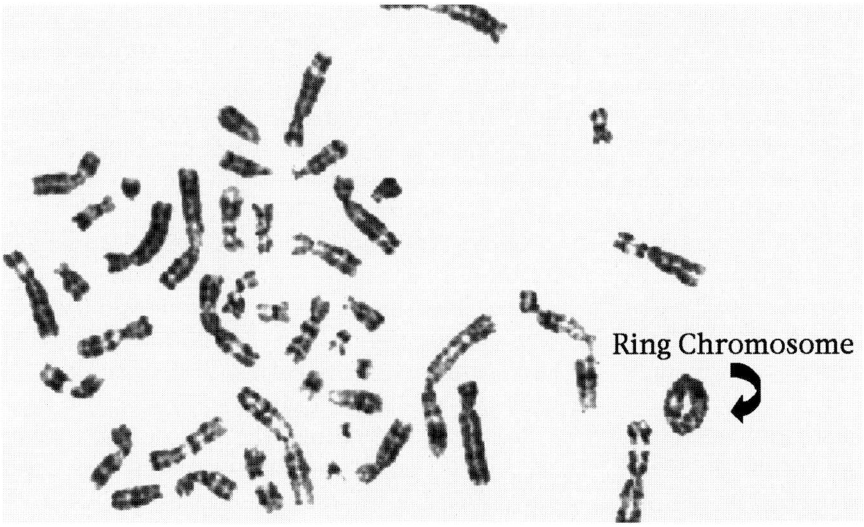

Figure 5-124

REPRESENTATIVE METAPHASE CELL FROM A PAROSTEAL OSTEOSARCOMA

Note the supernumerary ring chromosome (arrow).

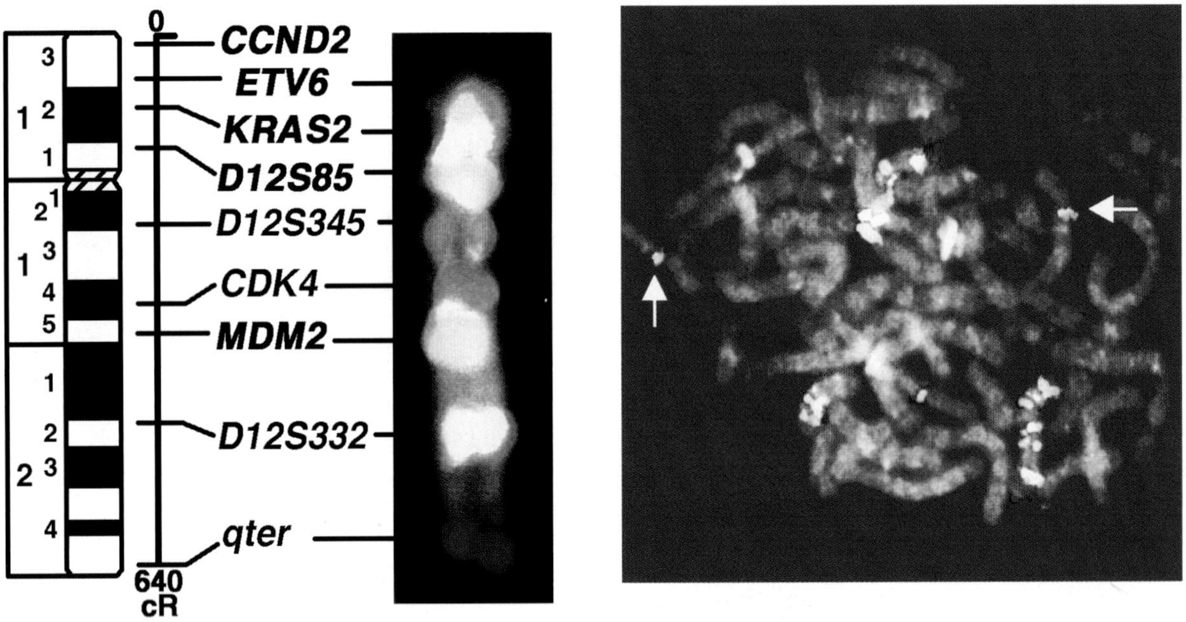

Figure 5-125

DIFFERENTIALLY AMPLIFIED CHROMOSOME 12 SEQUENCES IN LOW- AND HIGH-GRADE OSTEOSARCOMAS

Left: The chromosome 12-probe set (*ETV6, KRAS2, D12S85, D12S345, CDK4, MDM2, D12S332*, and *qter*) used to examine a series of low- and high-grade osteosarcomas is shown positioned in relation to a G-band ideogram (left).

Right: A high-grade osteosarcoma shows complex rearrangements of chromosome 12 leading to gain of *ETV6* (arrows, green-yellow); two normal chromosomes 12 and two other structural rearrangements are also seen. The authors of this study found that an over-representation of 12p sequences was more frequent in high-grade than low-grade osteosarcomas, suggesting that gain of sequences from the short arm of chromosome 12 could be a possible genetic pathway in the development of aggressive osteosarcoma. (Modified from Gisselsson D, Palsson E, Hoglund M, et al. Differentially amplified chromosome 12 sequences in low- and high-grade osteosarcoma. Genes Chromosomes Cancer 2002;33:133-40.)

General Features. Periosteal osteosarcoma was first described as a distinct entity in 1976 (221). These tumors are not half as common as parosteal osteosarcoma but are twice as common as high-grade surface osteosarcomas. They account for only 1.5 percent of osteosarcomas reported in the Mayo Clinic files. Until the beginning of 2000, the Mayo Clinic files included 29 cases of periosteal osteosarcoma.

Clinical Features. Periosteal osteosarcoma occurs in children and adolescents, with the highest incidence in the second decade of life. Similar to parosteal osteosarcoma, there is a slight but definite female predominance.

The symptoms are nonspecific, consisting of pain, swelling, or both. Because of the tendency to involve the surface of the tibia, a mass may be palpable.

Sites. The femur and tibia are involved most commonly, and the lesion has the unusual tendency to involve the diaphysis (fig. 5-126).

Radiographic Findings. Plain radiographs show a lucency in a saucer-shaped depression in the cortex (fig. 5-127). The tumor is usually small, and the surface is not well demarcated and tends to fade out into the soft tissues. Calcified spiculations, which are variable in amount (218), typically produce a sunburst pattern (fig. 5-128). It is rare for periosteal new bone to form Codman's triangle. By definition, the bone marrow cavity is free of involvement. CT and MRI are helpful in ruling out bone marrow disease (fig. 5-129).

Gross Findings. Periosteal osteosarcoma is a lobulated, white, chondroid-appearing neoplasm that appears to be plastered onto the cortical surface (fig. 5-130). The tumor is situated in a concavity of the cortex, but it does not invade the medullary cavity.

Microscopic Findings. The microscopic appearance is typical but not diagnostic. A low-power view shows a lobulated, chondroid-appearing

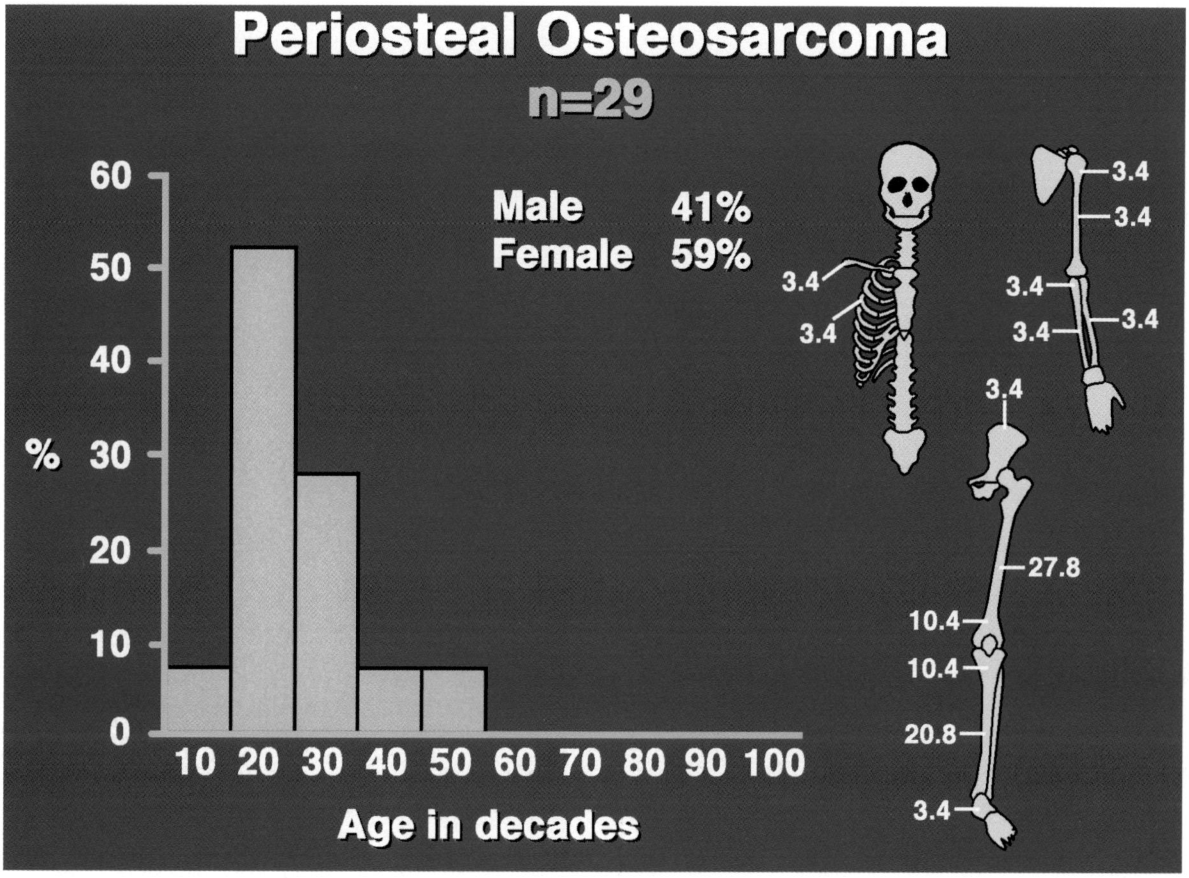

Figure 5-126

PERIOSTEAL OSTEOSARCOMA

Distribution of periosteal osteosarcoma according to the age and sex of the patient and the site of the lesion.

neoplasm; the "spines" of bone in the center of a lobule produce a "feathery" appearance (fig. 5-131). A higher-power view shows moderate cytologic atypia of the tumor cells, which reside within lacunae (fig. 5-132). There is a condensation of the nuclei toward the periphery of the lobules, with sheets of spindle cells that have foci of fine lace-like osteoid (fig. 5-133).

Differential Diagnosis. The differential diagnosis of periosteal osteosarcoma includes osteochondroma, parosteal osteosarcoma, conventional osteosarcoma, and high-grade surface osteosarcoma. In periosteal osteosarcoma, well-formed bony trabeculae may be present and the cartilage may be on the surface, simulating osteochondroma. However, the radiographic appearance of the two tumors is so different that differentiating them is not usually a practical problem. Conventional osteosarcoma may be chondroblastic and indistinguishable from periosteal osteosarcoma. Only the involvement of the medullary cavity differentiates conventional osteosarcoma from periosteal osteosarcoma. The radiographic features of periosteal osteosarcoma overlap those of high-grade surface osteosarcoma. Although high-grade surface osteosarcomas are predominantly osteoblastic, they may be chondroblastic. High-grade surface osteosarcoma is considered a grade 3 or 4 osteosarcoma, whereas periosteal osteosarcoma is grade 2 or 3. The histologic features of the two tumors also overlap, and occasionally the distinction is arbitrary.

Because of its chondroblastic nature, periosteal osteosarcoma may be mistaken for chondrosarcoma. Indeed, one study has used the term "juxtacortical chondrosarcoma" (220), but several studies have favored the concept of osteosarcoma over chondrosarcoma (217). Periosteal

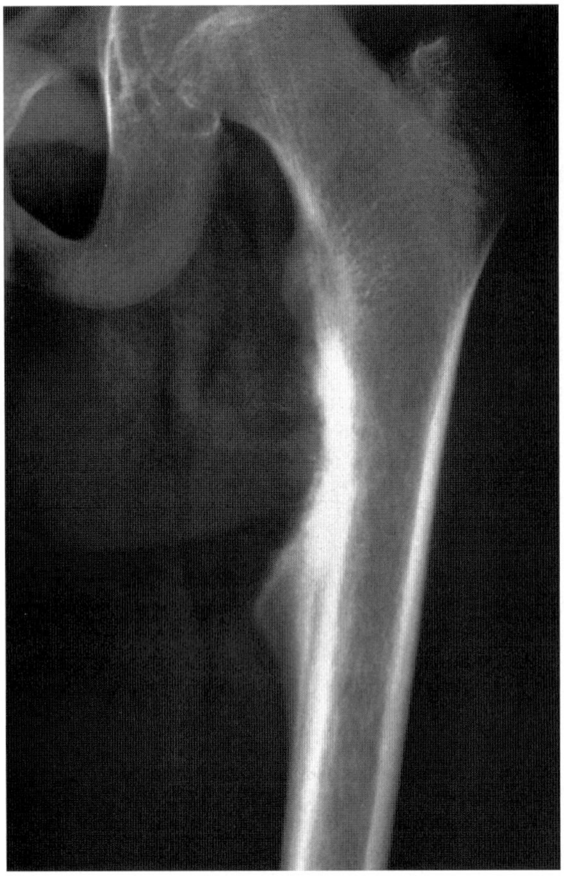

Figure 5-127

PERIOSTEAL OSTEOSARCOMA

The saucer-shaped depression in the proximal femur is strongly suggestive of periosteal osteosarcoma.

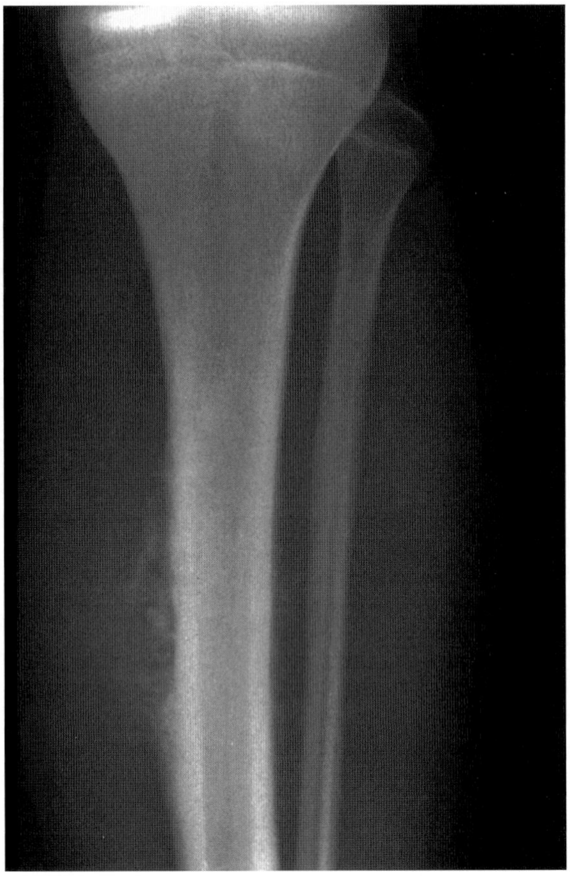

Figure 5-128

PERIOSTEAL OSTEOSARCOMA

The tumor involves the cortex but not the medullary canal, and merges into soft tissue. Note the partial ossification.

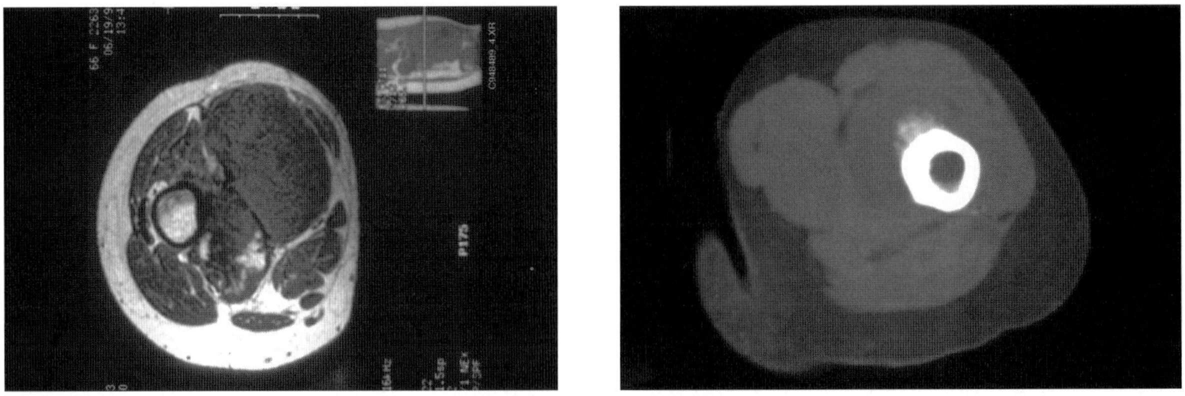

Figure 5-129

PERIOSTEAL OSTEOSARCOMA

MRI (left) and CT (right) do not demonstrate medullary involvement by these two examples of periosteal osteosarcoma.

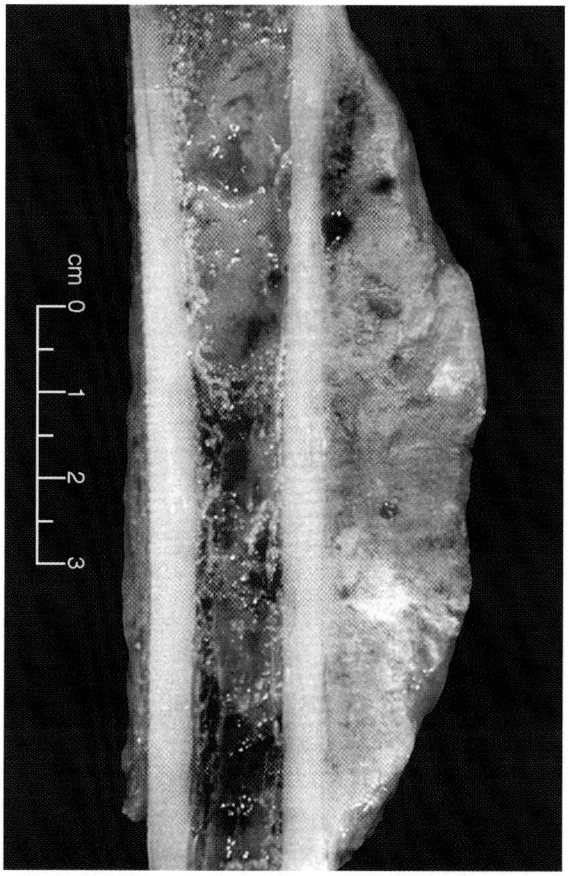

Figure 5-130

PERIOSTEAL OSTEOSARCOMA

The tumor, a firm gray-white mass, is attached to the periosteal surface and does not involve the medulla.

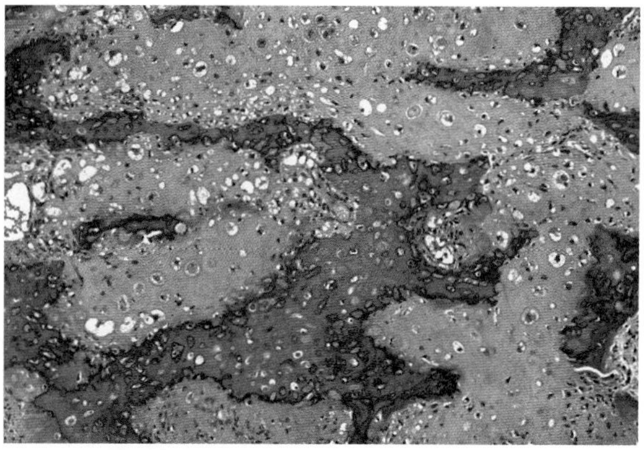

Figure 5-131

PERIOSTEAL OSTEOSARCOMA

Chondroblastic osteosarcoma shows irregular spicules of bone in the center of the cartilaginous nodules.

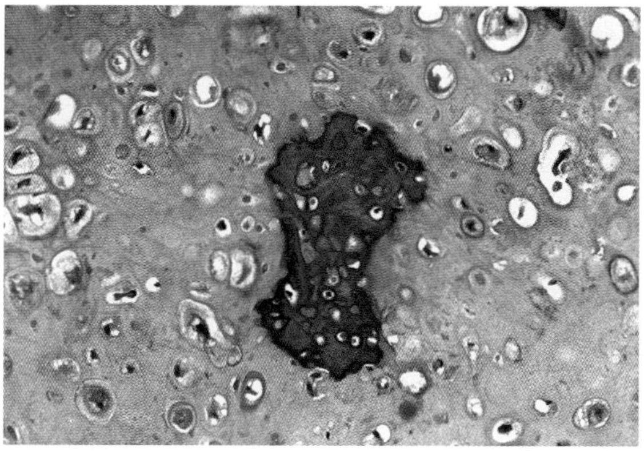

Figure 5-132

PERIOSTEAL OSTEOSARCOMA

The tumor contains cartilaginous differentiation with moderate cytologic atypia.

chondrosarcomas tend to be large, poorly marginated lesions on the surface of bone. The peripheral condensation of nuclei and spindling typical of periosteal osteosarcoma is not present in chondrosarcoma.

Treatment and Prognosis. Prognosis is excellent. Bertoni et al. (217) reported a 15 percent metastatic rate and Ritts et al. (219), an 18 percent rate. Although this rate is higher than that of parosteal osteosarcoma, it is considerably less than that of conventional osteosarcoma. Because of the rarity of the tumor, experience with chemotherapy is limited. Most periosteal osteosarcomas are treated with surgical resection, and orthopedic oncologists are reluctant to perform resection without preoperative chemotherapy.

High-Grade Surface Osteosarcoma

Definition. High-grade surface osteosarcoma is a malignant bone-forming neoplasm with high-grade cytologic features; it is situated predominantly on the surface of bone (223).

General Features. High-grade surface osteosarcoma is the least common type of surface osteosarcoma. Until the year 2000, the Mayo Clinic files contained only 12 cases (fig. 5-134).

Clinical Features. Patients present with swelling, with or without pain. There is a definite male predominance. Patients generally are

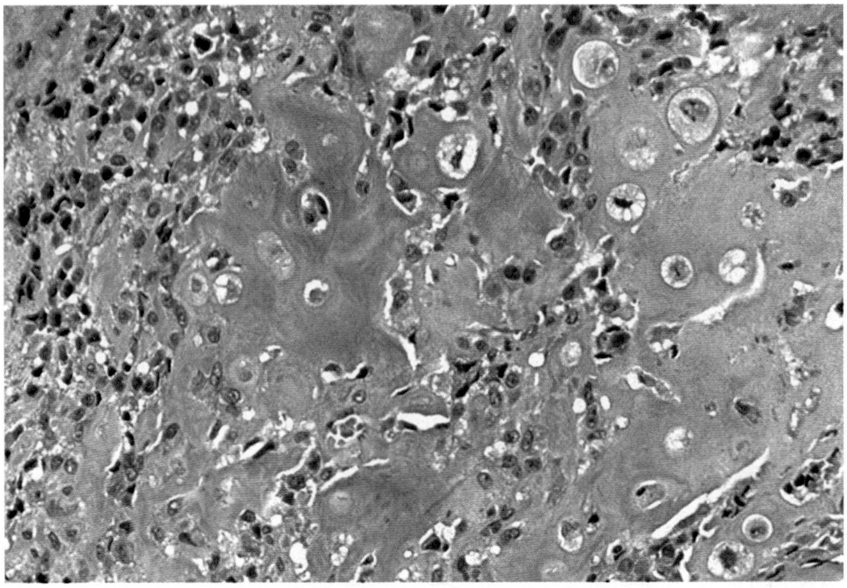

Figure 5-133

PERIOSTEAL OSTEOSARCOMA

This chondroblastic osteosarcoma contains cellular areas of hyperchromatic spindle-shaped cells associated with matrix production.

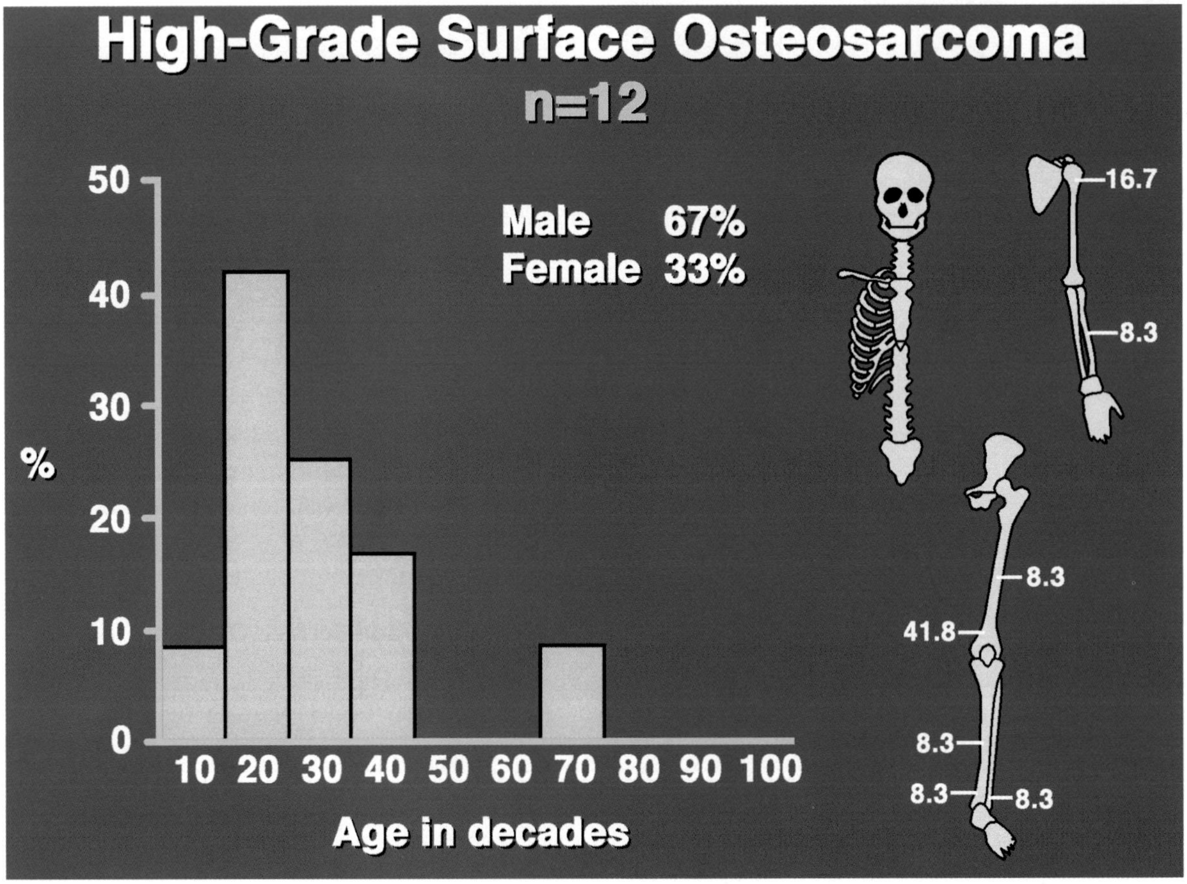

Figure 5-134

HIGH-GRADE SURFACE OSTEOSARCOMAS

Distribution of high-grade osteosarcoma according to the age and sex of the patient and the site of the lesion.

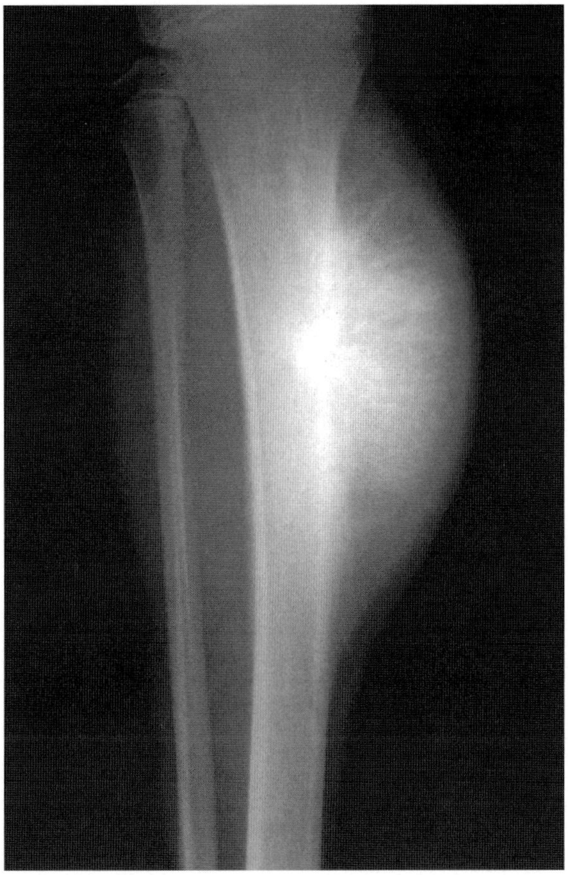

Figure 5-135

HIGH-GRADE SURFACE OSTEOSARCOMA

This mineralized mass involves the surface of the proximal tibia and has a sunburst appearance.

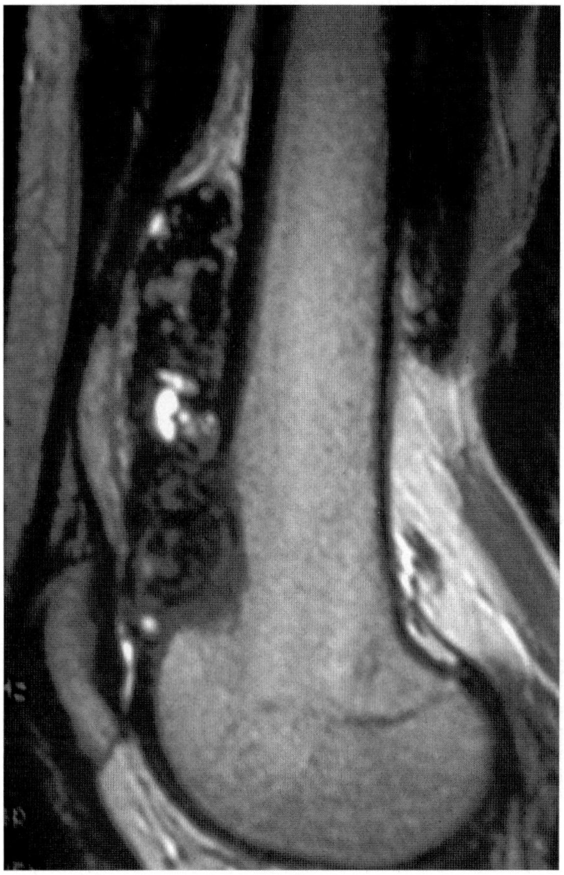

Figure 5-136

HIGH-GRADE SURFACE OSTEOSARCOMA

MRI of this high-grade surface osteosarcoma shows only focal medullary involvement.

young adults, with the highest incidence occurring in the second and third decades of life. Long tubular bones are usually involved, and more than half of the tumors are diaphyseal.

Radiographic Findings. Radiographs show a lesion with variable mineralization arising from the surface of bone (fig. 5-135). The margins are indistinct, and the appearance of the majority of lesions suggests a malignancy. Periosteal reaction is uncommon. In up to one third of the tumors, CT and MRI show minimal medullary involvement (fig. 5-136).

Gross Findings. Grossly, the tumors are attached to the cortex and show a mixture of fleshy and hard areas (fig. 5-137).

Microscopic Findings. Histologically, all tumors are considered high grade (grade 3 or 4) (fig. 5-138). In a study of Okada et al. (222), the majority were osteoblastic.

Differential Diagnosis. The differential diagnosis of high-grade surface osteosarcoma includes parosteal osteosarcoma, periosteal osteosarcoma, and conventional osteosarcoma. The radiographic features may suggest either parosteal osteosarcoma or periosteal osteosarcoma. However, the high-grade cytologic features rule out the former. The distinction between high-grade surface osteosarcoma and periosteal osteosarcoma can be considerably more difficult, as indicated in the above discussion on periosteal osteosarcoma. High-grade surface osteosarcoma is differentiated from conventional osteosarcoma purely on the basis of whether the lesion arose from the medullary cavity or the surface of bone.

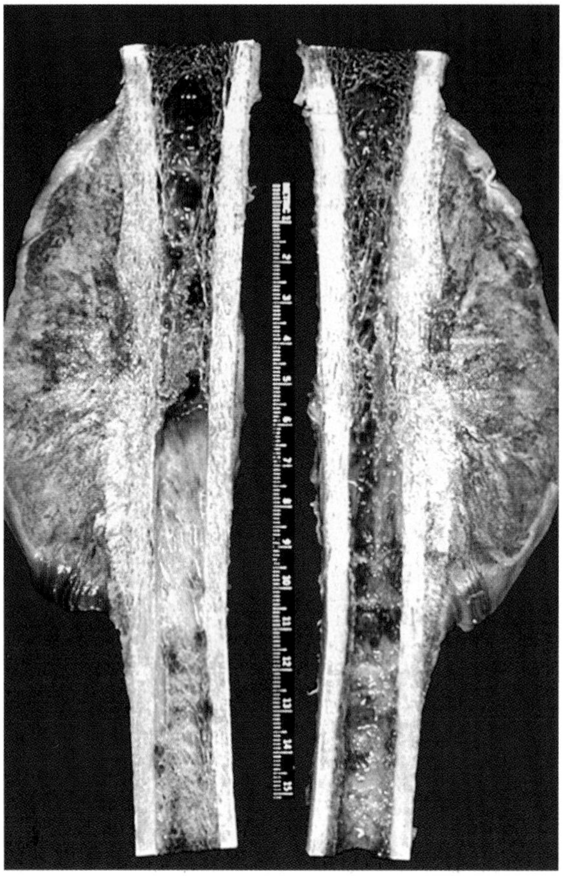

Figure 5-137

HIGH-GRADE SURFACE OSTEOSARCOMA

This osteosarcoma in a 16-year-old girl involves nearly the circumference of the femur.

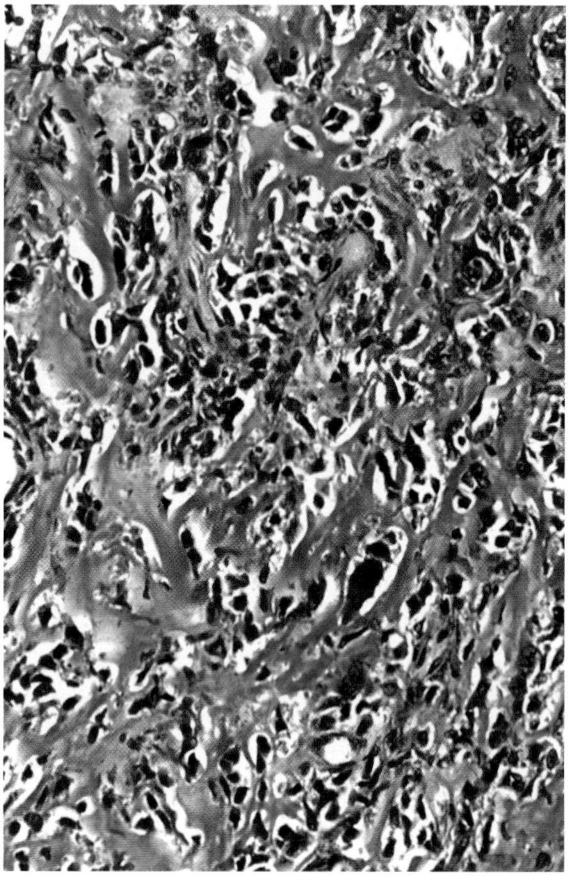

Figure 5-138

HIGH-GRADE SURFACE OSTEOSARCOMA

The entire tumor consisted of grade 4 osteoblastic osteosarcoma.

Treatment and Prognosis. Ideally, the treatment is preoperative chemotherapy followed by surgical resection. In the series reported by Okada et al. (222), the 5-year survival rate was 46 percent. The outcome of patients with grade 3 sarcomas was considerably better than that of those with grade 4 sarcomas. A poor response to chemotherapy is associated with a poor outcome.

REFERENCES

Osteoid Osteoma

1. Ayala AG, Murray JA, Erling MA, Raymond AK. Osteoid-osteoma: intraoperative tetracycline-fluorescence demonstration of the nidus. J Bone Joint Surg Am 1986;68:747–51.
2. Baruffi MR, Volpon JB, Neto JB, Casartelli C. Osteoid osteomas with chromosome alterations involving 22q. Cancer Genet Cytogenet 2001;124:127–31.
3. Dal Cin P, Sciot R, Samson I, De Wever I, Van den Berghe H. Osteoid osteoma and osteoblastoma with clonal chromosome changes. Br J Cancer 1998;78:344–8.
4. Fechner RE, Mills SE. Tumors of the bones and joints. Atlas of Tumor Pathology, 3rd Series, Fascicle 8. Washington, DC: Armed Forces Institute of Pathology; 1993:28–32.
5. Flaherty RA, Pugh DG, Dockerty MB. Osteoid osteoma. Am J Roentgenol Radium Ther Nucl Med 1956;76:1041–51.
6. Franchi A, Calzolari A, Zampi G. Immunohistochemical detection of c-fos and c-jun expression in osseous and cartilaginous tumours of the skeleton. Virchows Arch [B] 1998;432:515–9.
7. Helms CA. Osteoid osteoma. The double density sign. Clin Orthop 1987;222:167–73.
8. Kneisl JS, Simon MA. Medical management compared with operative treatment for osteoid-osteoma. J Bone Joint Surg Am 1992;74:179–85.
9. Makley JT, Dunn MJ. Prostaglandin synthesis by osteoid osteoma [Letter]. Lancet 1982;2:42.
10. McDermott MB, Kyriakos M, McEnery K. Painless osteoid osteoma of the rib in an adult. A case report and a review of the literature. Cancer 1996;77:1442–9.
11. Muscolo DL, Velan O, Pineda Acero G, Ayerza MA, Calabrese ME, Santini Araujo E. Osteoid osteoma of the hip. Percutaneous resection guided by computed tomography. Clin Orthop 1995;310:170–5.
12. Roger B, Bellin MF, Wioland M, Grenier P. Osteoid osteoma: CT-guided percutaneous excision confirmed with immediate follow-up scintigraphy in 16 outpatients. Radiology 1996;201:239–42.
13. Rosenthal DI, Springfield DS, Gebhardt MC, Rosenberg AE, Mankin HJ. Osteoid osteoma: percutaneous radio-frequency ablation. Radiology 1995;197:451–4.
14. Schulman L, Dorfman HD. Nerve fibers in osteoid osteoma. J Bone Joint Surg Am 1970;52:1351–6.
15. Sim FH, Dahlin CD, Beabout JW. Osteoid-osteoma: diagnostic problems. J Bone Joint Surg Am 1975;57:154–9.
16. Swee RG, McLeod RA, Beabout JW. Osteoid osteoma. Detection, diagnosis, and localization. Radiology 1979;130:117–23.
17. Unni KK. Dahlin's bone tumors: general aspects and data on 11,087 cases, 5th ed. Philadelphia: Lippincott-Raven; 1996:121–30.

Osteoblastoma

18. Angervall L, Persson S, Stenman G, Kindblom LG. Large cell, epithelioid, telangiectatic osteoblastoma: a unique pseudosarcomatous variant of osteoblastoma. Hum Pathol 1999;30:1254–9.
19. Belchis DA, Meece CA, Benko FA, Rogan PK, Williams RA, Gocke CD. Loss of heterozygosity and microsatellite instability at the retinoblastoma locus in osteosarcomas. Diagn Mol Pathol 1996;5:214–9.
20. Camitta B, Wells R, Segura A, Unni KK, Murray K, Dunn D. Osteoblastoma response to chemotherapy. Cancer 1991;68:999–1003.
21. Dahlin DC, Johnson EW Jr. Giant osteoid osteoma. J Bone Joint Surg Am 1954;36:559–72.
22. Dal Cin P, Sciot R, Samson I, De Wever I, Van den Berghe H. Osteoid osteoma and osteoblastoma with clonal chromosome changes. Br J Cancer 1998;78:344–8.
23. Dorfman HD, Czerniak B, eds. Bone tumors. St. Louis: Mosby; 1998:103–27.
24. Dorfman HD, Weiss SW. Borderline osteoblastic tumors: problems in the differential diagnosis of aggressive osteoblastoma and low-grade osteosarcoma. Semin Diagn Pathol 1984;1:215–34.
25. Franchi A, Calzolari A, Zampi G. Immunohistochemical detection of c-fos and c-jun expression in osseous and cartilaginous tumours of the skeleton. Virchows Arch [B] 1998;432:515–9.
26. Kroon HM, Schurmans J. Osteoblastoma: clinical and radiologic findings in 98 new cases. Radiology 1990;175:783–90.
27. Lucas DR, Unni KK, McLeod RA, O'Connor MI, Sim FH. Osteoblastoma: clinicopathologic study of 306 cases. Hum Pathol 1994;25:117–34.
28. Mascarello JT, Krous HF, Carpenter PM. Unbalanced translocation resulting in the loss of the chromosome 17 short arm in an osteoblastoma. Cancer Genet Cytogenet 1993;69:65–7.

29. McLeod RA, Dahlin DC, Beabout JW. The spectrum of osteoblastoma. Am J Roentgenol 1976;126:321–5.
30. Mirra JM, Cove K, Theros E, Paladugu R, Smasson J. A case of osteoblastoma associated with severe systemic toxicity. Am J Surg Pathol 1979;3:463–71.
31. Mirra JM, Kendrick RA, Kendrick RE. Pseudomalignant osteoblastoma versus arrested osteosarcoma: a case report. Cancer 1976;37:2005–14.
32. Radig K, Schneider-Stock R, Mittler U, Neumann HW, Roessner A. Genetic instability in osteoblastic tumors of the skeletal system. Pathol Res Pract 1998;194:669–77.
33. Schajowicz F, Lemos C. Malignant osteoblastoma. J Bone Joint Surg Br 1976;58:202–11.
34. Walaas L, Kindblom LG. Light and electron microscopic examination of fine-needle aspirates in the preoperative diagnosis of osteogenic tumors: a study of 21 osteosarcomas and two osteoblastomas. Diagn Cytopathol 1990;6:27–38.
35. Willems JS. Aspiration biopsy cytology of tumors and tumor-suspect lesions of bone. In: Linsk JA, Franzen S, eds. Clinical aspiration cytology. Philadelphia: Lippincott; 1983:356–7.

Osteosarcoma of Bone

36. Age and dose of chemotherapy as major prognostic factors in a trial of adjuvant therapy of osteosarcoma combining two alternating drug combinations and early prophylactic lung irradiation. French Bone Tumor Study Group. Cancer 1988;61:1304–11.
37. Aue G, Muralidhar B, Schwartz HS, Butler MG. Telomerase activity in skeletal sarcomas. Ann Surg Oncol 1998;5:627–34.
38. Bacci G, Picci P, Ferrari S, et al. Primary chemotherapy and delayed surgery for nonmetastatic osteosarcoma of the extremities. Results in 164 patients preoperatively treated with high doses of methotrexate followed by cisplatin and doxorubicin. Cancer 1993;72:3227–38.
39. Baldini N, Scotlandi K, Serra M, et al. P-glycoprotein expression in osteosarcoma: a basis for risk-adapted adjuvant chemotherapy. J Orthop Res 1999;17:629–32.
40. Ballance WA Jr, Mendelsohn G, Carter JR, Abdul-Karim FW, Jacobs G, Makley JT. Osteogenic sarcoma. Malignant fibrous histiocytoma subtype. Cancer 1988;62:763–71.
41. Bathurst N, Sanerkin N, Watt I. Osteoclast-rich osteosarcoma. Br J Radiol 1986;59:667–73.
42. Bayani J, Zielenska M, Pandita A, et al. Spectral karyotyping identifies recurrent complex rearrangements of chromosomes 8, 17, and 20 in osteosarcomas. Genes Chromosomes Cancer 2003;36:7–16.
43. Beedles KE, Sharpe PT, Wagner EF, Grigoriadis AE. A putative role for c-Fos in the pathophysiology of Paget's disease. J Bone Miner Res 1999;14(Suppl 2):21–8.
44. Belchis DA, Meece CA, Benko FA, Rogan PK, Williams RA, Gocke CD. Loss of heterozygosity and microsatellite instability at the retinoblastoma locus in osteosarcomas. Diagn Mol Pathol 1996;5:214–9.
45. Bell DW, Varley JM, Szydlo TE, et al. Heterozygous germ line hCHK2 mutations in Li-Fraumeni syndrome. Science 1999;286:2528–31.
46. Benassi MS, Molendini L, Gamberi G, et al. Alteration of pRb/p16/cdk4 regulation in human osteosarcoma. Int J Cancer 1999;84:489–93.
47. Benassi MS, Molendini L, Gamberi G, et al. Involvement of INK4A gene products in the pathogenesis and development of human osteosarcoma. Cancer 2001;92:3062–7.
48. Bertoni F, Dallera P, Bacchini P, Marchetti C, Campobassi A. The Istituto Rizzoli-Beretta experience with osteosarcoma of the jaw. Cancer 1991;68:1555–63.
49. Bertoni F, Unni KK, McLeod RA, Dahlin DC. Osteosarcoma resembling osteoblastoma. Cancer 1985;55:416–26.
50. Bieling P, Rehan N, Winkler P, et al. Tumor size and prognosis in aggressively treated osteosarcoma. J Clin Oncol 1996;14:848–58.
51. Bjornsson J, Inwards CY, Wold LE, Sim FH, Taylor WF. Prognostic significance of spontaneous tumour necrosis in osteosarcoma. Virchows Arch A Pathol Anat Histopathol 1993;423:195–9.
52. Bodey B, Groger AM, Bodey B Jr, Siegel SE, Kaiser HE. Immunohistochemical detection of p53 protein overexpression in primary human osteosarcomas. Anticancer Res 1997;17:493–8.
53. Boehm AK, Neff JR, Squire JA, Bayani J, Nelson M, Bridge JA. Cytogenetic findings in 36 osteosarcoma specimens and a review of the literature. Pediatr Pathol Mol Med 2000;19:359–76.
54. Bookstein R, Shew JY, Chen PL, Scully P, Lee WH. Suppression of tumorigenicity of human prostate carcinoma cells by replacing a mutated RB gene. Science 1990;247:712–5.
55. Brandwood CP, Hoyland JA, Hillarby MC, et al. Apoptotic gene expression in Paget's disease: a possible role for Bcl-2. J Pathol 2003;201:504–12.
56. Brien WW, Salvati EA, Healey JH, Bansal M, Ghelman B, Betts F. Osteogenic sarcoma arising in the area of a total hip replacement. A case report. J Bone Joint Surg Am 1990;72:1097–9.
57. Campanacci M, Cervellati G. Osteosarcoma: a review of 345 cases. Ital J Orthop Traumatol 1975;1:5–22.

58. Carrasco CH, Charnsangavej C, Raymond AK, et al. Osteosarcoma: angiographic assessment of response to preoperative chemotherapy. Radiology 1989;170:839–42.
59. Chan HS, Grogan TM, Haddad G, DeBoer G, Ling V. P-glycoprotein expression: critical determinant in the response to osteosarcoma chemotherapy. J Natl Cancer Inst 1997;89:1706–15.
60. Chano T, Ikegawa S, Kontani K, Okabe H, Baldini N, Saeki Y. Identification of RB1CC1, a novel human gene that can induce RB1 in various human cells. Oncogene 2002;21:1295-8.
61. Chene P, Bechter E. p53 mutants without a functional tetramerisation domain are not oncogenic. J Mol Biol 1999;286:1269–74.
62. Cheng CL, Ma J, Wu PC, Mason RS, Posen S. Osteomalacia secondary to osteosarcoma. A case report. J Bone Joint Surg Am 1989;71:288–92.
63. Cho Y, Gorina S, Jeffrey PD, Pavletich NP. Crystal structure of a p53 tumor suppressor-DNA complex: understanding tumorigenic mutations. Science 1994;265:346–55.
64. Clark JL, Unni KK, Dahlin DC, Devine KD. Osteosarcoma of the jaw. Cancer 1983;51:2311–6.
65. Collins BT, Cramer HM, Ramos RR. Fine needle aspiration biopsy of recurrent and metastatic osteosarcoma. Acta Cytol 1998;42:357–61.
66. Cordon-Cardo C. Mutations of cell cycle regulators. Biological and clinical implications for human neoplasia. Am J Pathol 1995;147:545–60.
67. Dahlin DC, Coventry MB. Osteogenic sarcoma. A study of six hundred cases. J Bone Joint Surg Am 1967;49:101–10.
68. Davis AM, Bell RS, Goodwin PJ. Prognostic factors in osteosarcoma: a critical review. J Clin Oncol 1994;12:423–31.
69. Dhaini HR, Thomas DG, Giordano TG, et al. Cytochrome p450 CYP3A4/5 expression as a biomarker of outcome in osteosarcoma. J Clin Oncol 2003;21:2481–5.
70. DiBiase SJ, Guan J, Curran WJ Jr, Iliakis G. Repair of DNA double-strand breaks and radiosensitivity to killing in an isogenic group of *p53* mutant cell lines. Int J Radiat Oncol Biol Phys 1999;45:743–51.
71. Dodd LG, Chai C, McAdams HP, Layfield LJ. Fine needle aspiration of osteogenic sarcoma metastatic to the lung. A report of four cases. Acta Cytol 1998;42:754–8.
72. Dorfman HD, Czerniak B. Bone cancers. Cancer 1995;75(Suppl):203–10.
73. Draper GJ, Sanders BM, Kingston JE. Second primary neoplasms in patients with retinoblastoma. Br J Cancer 1986;53:661–71.
74. Dryja TP, Cavenee W, White R, et al. Homozygosity of chromosome 13 in retinoblastoma. N Engl J Med 1984;310:550–3.
75. Eilber F, Giuliano A, Eckardt J, Patterson K, Moseley S, Goodnight J. Adjuvant chemotherapy for osteosarcoma: a randomized prospective trial. J Clin Oncol 1987;5:21–6.
76. el-Naggar AK, Hurr K, Tu ZN, et al. DNA and RNA content analysis by flow cytometry in the pathobiologic assessment of bone tumors. Cytometry 1995;19:256–62.
77. Enneking WF, Kagan A. "Skip" metastases in osteosarcoma. Cancer 1975;36:2192–205.
78. Fan J, Bertino JR. Modulation of cisplatinum cytotoxicity by p53: effect of p53-mediated apoptosis and DNA repair. Mol Pharmacol 1999;56:966–72.
79. Fellenberg J, Krauthoff A, Pollandt K, Delling G, Parsch D. Evaluation of the predictive value of Her-2/neu gene expression on osteosarcoma therapy in laser-microdissected paraffin-embedded tissue. Lab Invest 2004;84:113–21.
80. Ferrari S, Bertoni F, Zanella L, et al. Evaluation of P-glycoprotein, HER-2/ErbB-2, p53, and Bcl-2 in primary tumor and metachronous lung metastases in patients with high-grade osteosarcoma. Cancer 2004;100:1936–42.
81. Feugeas O, Guriec N, Babin-Boilletot A, et al. Loss of heterozygosity of the RB gene is a poor prognostic factor in patients with osteosarcoma. J Clin Oncol 1996;14:467–72.
82. Fitzgerald RH Jr, Dahlin DC, Sim FH. Multiple metachronous osteogenic sarcoma. Report of twelve cases with two long-term survivors. J Bone Joint Surg Am 1973;55:595–605.
83. Franchi A, Calzolari A, Zampi G. Immunohistochemical detection of c-fos and c-jun expression in osseous and cartilaginous tumours of the skeleton. Virchows Arch 1998;432:515–9.
84. Friend SH, Bernards R, Rogelj S, et al. A human DNA segment with properties of the gene that predisposes to retinoblastoma and osteosarcoma. Nature 1986;323:643–6.
85. Gamberi G, Benassi MS, Bohling T, et al. C-myc and c-fos in human osteosarcoma: prognostic value of mRNA and protein expression. Oncology 1998;55:556–63.
86. Garcia-Castellano JM, Villanueva A, Healey JH, et al. Methylthioadenosine phosphorylase gene deletions are common in osteosarcoma. Clin Cancer Res 2002;8:782–7.
87. Gillespy T 3rd, Manfrini M, Ruggieri P, Spanier SS, Pettersson H, Springfield DS. Staging of intraosseous extent of osteosarcoma: correlation of preoperative CT and MR imaging with pathologic macroslides. Radiology 1988;167:765–7.
88. Glasser DB, Lane JM, Huvos AG, Marcove RC, Rosen G. Survival, prognosis, and therapeutic response in osteogenic sarcoma. The Memorial Hospital experience. Cancer 1992;69:698–708.

89. Gokgoz N, Wunder JS, Mousses S, Eskandarian S, Bell RS, Andrulis IL. Comparison of p53 mutations in patients with localized osteosarcoma and metastatic osteosarcoma. Cancer 2001;92:2181–9.
90. Good DA, Busfield F, Fletcher BH, et al. Linkage of Paget disease of bone to a novel region on human chromosome 18q23. Am J Hum Genet 2002;70:517–25.
91. Goorin AM, Abelson HT, Frei E 3rd. Osteosarcoma: fifteen years later. N Engl J Med 1985;313:1637–43.
92. Gorlick R, Anderson P, Andrulis I, et al. Biology of childhood osteogenic sarcoma and potential targets for therapeutic development: meeting summary. Clin Cancer Res 2003; 9:5442–53.
93. Gorlick R, Huvos AG, Heller G, et al. Expression of HER2/erbB-2 correlates with survival in osteosarcoma. J Clin Oncol 1999;17;2781–8.
94. Greenblatt MS, Bennett WP, Hollstein M, Harris CC. Mutations in the p53 tumor suppressor gene: clues to cancer etiology and molecular pathogenesis. Cancer Res 1994;54:4855–78.
95. Gunawardena S, Chintagumpala M, Trautwein L, et al. Multifocal osteosarcoma: an unusual presentation. J Pediatr Hematol Oncol 1999;21:58–62.
96. Hansen MF, Koufos A, Gallie BL, et al. Osteosarcoma and retinoblastoma: a shared chromosomal mechanism revealing recessive predisposition. Proc Natl Acad Sci U S A 1985;82:6216–20.
97. Hansen MF, Nellissery MJ, Bhatia P. Common mechanisms of osteosarcoma and Paget's disease. J Bone Miner Res 1999;14(Suppl 2):39–44.
98. Hasegawa T, Hirose T, Kudo E, Hizawa K, Usui M, Ishii S. Immunophenotypic heterogeneity in osteosarcomas. Hum Pathol 1991;22:583–90.
99. Hawkins MM, Draper GJ, Kingston JE. Incidence of second primary tumours among childhood cancer survivors. Br J Cancer 1987;56:339–47.
100. Hoang BH, Kubo T, Healey JH, et al. Expression of LDL receptor-related protein 5 (LRP5) as a novel marker for disease progression in high-grade osteosarcoma. Int J Cancer 2004;109:106–11.
101. Huang HJ, Yee JK, Shew JY, et al. Suppression of the neoplastic phenotype by replacement of the RB gene in human cancer cells. Science 1988;242:1563–6.
102. Hudson M, Jaffe MR, Jaffe N, et al. Pediatric osteosarcoma: therapeutic strategies, results, and prognostic factors derived from a 10-year experience. J Clin Oncol 1990;8:1988–97.
103. Hulsebos TJ, Bijleveld EH, Oskam NT, et al. Malignant astrocytoma-derived region of common amplification in chromosomal band 17p12 is frequently amplified in high-grade osteosarcomas. Genes Chromosomes Cancer 1997;18:279–85.
104. Huvos AG. Osteogenic sarcoma of bones and soft tissues in older persons. A clinicopathologic analysis of 117 patients older than 60 years. Cancer 1986;57:1442–9.
105. Huvos AG, Butler A, Bretsky SS. Osteogenic sarcoma associated with Paget's disease of bone. A clinicopathologic study of 65 patients. Cancer 1983;52:1489–95.
106. Huvos AG, Rosen G, Bretsky SS, Butler A. Telangiectatic osteogenic sarcoma: a clinicopathologic study of 124 patients. Cancer 1982;49:1679–89.
107. Huvos AG, Sundaresan N, Bretsky SS, Butler A. Osteogenic sarcoma of the skull. A clinicopathologic study of 19 patients. Cancer 1985;56:1214–21.
108. Inoue YZ, Frassica FJ, Sim FH, Unni KK, Petersen IA, McLeod RA. Clinicopathologic features and treatment of postirradiation sarcoma of bone and soft tissue. J Surg Oncol 2000;75:42–50.
109. Kakar S, Mihalov M, Chachlani NA, Ghosh L, Johnstone H. Correlation of c-fos, p53, and PCNA expression with treatment outcome in osteosarcoma. J Surg Oncol 2000;73:125–6.
110. Kamb A. Cyclin-dependent kinase inhibitors and human cancer. Curr Top Microbiol Immunol 1998;227:139–48.
111. Kamijo T, Zindy F, Roussel MF, et al. Tumor suppression of the mouse INK4a locus mediated by the alternative reading frame product p19ARF. Cell 1997;91:649–59.
112. Kanoe H, Nakayama T, Murakami H, et al. Amplification of the CDK4 gene in sarcomas: tumor specificity and relationship with the RB gene mutation. Anticancer Res 1998;18:2317–21.
113. Kloen P, Gebhardt MC, Perez-Atayde A, et al. Expression of transforming growth factor-beta (TGF-beta) isoforms in osteosarcomas: TGF-beta3 is related to disease progression. Cancer 1997;80:2230–9.
114. Knudson AG Jr. Mutation and cancer: statistical study of retinoblastoma. Proc Natl Acad Sci U S A 1971;68:820–3.
115. Kragh LV, Dahlin DC, Erich JB. Osteogenic sarcoma of the jaws and facial bones. Am J Surg 1958;96:496–505.
116. Kramer K, Hicks DG, Palis J, et al. Epithelioid osteosarcoma of bone. Immunocytochemical evidence suggesting divergent epithelial and mesenchymal differentiation in a primary osseous neoplasm. Cancer 1993;71:2977–82.
117. Kreicbergs A. DNA cytometry of musculoskeletal tumors. A review. Acta Orthop Scand 1990; 61:282–97.

118. Kruzelock RP, Murphy EC, Strong LC, Naylor SL, Hansen MF. Localization of a novel tumor suppressor locus on human chromosome 3q important in osteosarcoma tumorigenesis. Cancer Res 1997;57:106–9.
119. Kunisada T, Ozaki T, Kawai A, Sugihara S, Taguchi K, Inoue H. Imaging assessment of the responses of osteosarcoma patients to preoperative chemotherapy: angiography compared with thallium-201 scintigraphy. Cancer 1999;86:949–56.
120. Kurt AM, Unni KK, McLeod RA, Pritchard DJ. Low-grade intraosseous osteosarcoma. Cancer 1990;65:1418–28.
121. Kusuzaki K, Takeshita H, Murata H, et al. Relation between cellular doxorubicin binding ability to nuclear DNA and histologic response to preoperative chemotherapy in patients with osteosarcoma. Cancer 1998;82:2343–9.
122. Kyriakos M. Intracortical osteosarcoma. Cancer 1980;46:2525–33.
123. Lane DP, Crawford LV. T antigen is bound to a host protein in SV40-transformed cells. Nature 1979;278:261–3.
124. Layfield LJ, Glasgow BJ, Anders KH, Mirra JM. Fine needle aspiration cytology of primary bone lesions. Acta Cytol 1987;31:177–84.
125. Levine AJ. p53, the cellular gatekeeper for growth and division. Cell 1997;88:323–31.
126. Li FP, Fraumeni JF Jr. Soft-tissue sarcomas, breast cancer, and other neoplasms. A familial syndrome? Ann Intern Med 1969;71:747–52.
127. Li WW, Fan J, Hochhauser D, Bertino JR. Overexpression of p21waf1 leads to increased inhibition of E2F-1 phosphorylation and sensitivity to anticancer drugs in retinoblastoma-negative human sarcoma cells. Cancer Res 1997;57:2193–9.
128. Lichtenstein L, ed. Bone tumors, 4th ed. Saint Louis: Mosby; 1972:215–43.
129. Link MP, Goorin AM, Miser AW, et al. The effect of adjuvant chemotherapy on relapse-free survival in patients with osteosarcoma of the extremity. N Engl J Med 1986;314:1600–6.
130. Lonardo F, Ueda T, Huvos AG, Healey J, Ladanyi M. p53 and MDM2 alterations in osteosarcomas: correlation with clinicopathologic features and proliferative rate. Cancer 1997;79:1541–7.
131. Look AT, Douglass EC, Meyer WH. Clinical importance of near-diploid tumor stem lines in patients with osteosarcoma of an extremity. N Engl J Med 1988;318:1567–72.
132. Lukas J, Sorensen CS, Lukas C, Santoni-Rugiu E, Bartek J. p16INK4a, but not constitutively active pRb, can impose a sustained G1 arrest: molecular mechanisms and implications for oncogenesis. Oncogene 1999;18:3930–5.
133. Malkin D, Li FP, Strong LC, et al. Germ line p53 mutations in a familial syndrome of breast cancer, sarcomas, and other neoplasms. Science 1990;250:1233–8.
134. Manara MC, Baldini N, Serra M, et al. Reversal of malignant phenotype in human osteosarcoma cells transduced with the alkaline phosphatase gene. Bone 2000;26:215–200.
135. Marcove RC, Mike V, Hajek JV, Levin AG, Hutter RV. Osteogenic sarcoma under the age of twenty-one. A review of one hundred and forty-five operative cases. J Bone Joint Surg Am 1970;52:411–23.
136. Matsuno T, Unni KK, McLeod RA, Dahlin DC. Telangiectatic osteogenic sarcoma. Cancer 1976;38:2538–47.
137. McLeod RA, Berquist TH. Bone tumor imaging: contribution of CT and MRI. Contemp Issues Surg Pathol 1988;11:1–34.
138. Mervak TR, Unni KK, Pritchard DJ, McLeod RA. Telangiectatic osteosarcoma. Clin Orthop 1991;270:135–9.
139. Meyer WH, Schell MJ, Kumar AP, et al. Thoracotomy for pulmonary metastatic osteosarcoma. An analysis of prognostic indicators of survival. Cancer 1987;59:374–9.
140. Miller CW, Ikezoe T, Krug U, et al. Mutations of the CHK2 gene are found in some osteosarcomas, but are rare in breast, lung, and ovarian tumors. Genes Chromosomes Cancer 2002;33:17–21.
141. Mirra JM, Kameda N, Rosen G, Eckardt J. Primary osteosarcoma of toe phalanx: first documented case. Review of osteosarcoma of short tubular bones. Am J Surg Pathol 1988;12:300–7.
142. Mohney BG, Robertson DM, Schomberg PJ, Hodge DO. Second nonocular tumors in survivors of heritable retinoblastoma and prior radiation therapy. Am J Ophthalmol 1998;126:269–77.
143. Nakajima H, Sim FH, Bond JR, Unni KK. Small cell osteosarcoma of bone. Review of 72 cases. Cancer 1997;79:2095–106.
144. Nellissery MJ, Padalecki SS, Brkanac Z, et al. Evidence for a novel osteosarcoma tumor-suppressor gene in the chromosome 18 region genetically linked with Paget disease of bone. Am J Hum Genet 1998;63:817–24.
145. Neuburger M, Xia Y, Herget GW, Huang Y, Adler CP. Prognostic significance of DNA image cytophotometry for osteosarcoma. Anal Quant Cytol Histol 1999;21:461–7.
146. Nicol KK, Ward WG, Savage PD, Kilpatrick SE. Fine-needle aspiration biopsy of skeletal versus extraskeletal osteosarcoma. Cancer 1998;84:176–85.

147. Nielsen GP, Burns KL, Rosenberg AE, Louis DN. CDKN2A gene deletions and loss of p16 expression occur in osteosarcomas that lack RB alterations. Am J Pathol 1998;153:159–63.
148. Nora FE, Unni KK, Pritchard DJ, Dahlin DC. Osteosarcoma of extragnathic craniofacial bones. Mayo Clin Proc 1983;58:268–72.
149. Ochi K, Daigo Y, Katagiri T, et al. Prediction of response to neoadjuvant chemotherapy for osteosarcoma by gene-expression profiles. Int J Oncol 2004;24:647–55.
150. Okada K, Wold LE, Beabout JW, Shives TC. Osteosarcoma of the hand. A clinicopathologic study of 12 cases. Cancer 1993;72:719–25.
151. Oliner JD, Kinzler KW, Meltzer PS, George DL, Vogelstein B. Amplification of a gene encoding a p53-associated protein in human sarcomas [Letter]. Nature 1992;358:80–3.
152. Oliveira P, Nogueira M, Pinto A, Almeida MO. Analysis of p53 expression in osteosarcoma of the jaw: correlation with clinicopathologic and DNA ploidy findings. Hum Pathol 1997;28: 1361–5.
153. Onda M, Matsuda S, Higaki S, et al. ErbB-2 expression is correlated with poor prognosis for patients with osteosarcoma. Cancer 1996;77: 71–8.
154. Onikul E, Fletcher BD, Parham DM, Chen G. Accuracy of MR imaging for estimating intraosseous extent of osteosarcoma. AJR Am J Roentgenol 1996;167:1211–5.
155. Overholtzer M, Rao PH, Favis R, et al. The presence of p53 mutations in human osteosarcomas correlates with high levels of genomic instability. Proc Natl Acad Sci U S A 2003;100: 11547–52.
156. Papachristou DJ, Batistatou A, Sykiotis GP, Varakis I, Papavassilou AG. Activation of the JNK–AP-1 signal transduction pathway is associated with pathogenesis and progression of human osteosarcomas. Bone 2003;32:364–71.
157. Patino-Garcia A, Pineiro ES, Diez MZ, Iturriagagoitia LG, Klussmann FA, Ariznabarreta LS. Genetic and epigenetic alterations of the cell cycle regulators and tumor suppressor genes in pediatric osteosarcomas. J Pediatr Hematol Oncol 2003;25:362–7.
158. Pollock R, Lang A, Ge T, Sun D, Tan M, Yu D. Wild-type p53 and a p53 temperature-sensitive mutant suppress human soft tissue sarcoma by enhancing cell cycle control. Clin Cancer Res 1998;4:1985–94.
159. Pompetti F, Rizzo P, Simon RM, et al. Oncogene alterations in primary, recurrent, and metastatic human bone tumors. J Cell Biochem 1996;63:37–50.
160. Rab GT, Ivins JC, Childs DS Jr, Cupps RE, Pritchard DJ. Elective whole lung irradiation in the treatment of osteogenic sarcoma. Cancer 1976;38:939–42.
161. Radig K, Schneider-Stock R, Haeckel C, Neumann W, Roessner A. p53 gene mutations in osteosarcomas of low-grade malignancy. Hum Pathol 1998;29:1310–6.
162. Radig K, Schneider-Stock R, Mittler U, Neumann HW, Roessner A. Genetic instability in osteoblastic tumors of the skeletal system. Pathol Res Pract 1998;194:669–77.
163. Raymond AK, Ayala AG. Specimen management after osteosarcoma chemotherapy. Contemp Issues Surg Pathol 1988;11:157–81.
164. Redmond OM, Stack JP, Dervan PA, Hurson BJ, Carney DN, Ennis JT. Osteosarcoma: use of MR imaging and MR spectroscopy in clinical decision making. Radiology 1989;172:811–5.
165. Roussel MF. The INK4 family of cell cycle inhibitors in cancer. Oncogene 1999;18:5311–7.
166. Ruggieri P, Sim FH, Bond JR, Unni KK. Malignancies in fibrous dysplasia. Cancer 1994;73: 1411–24.
167. Saeter G, Elomaa I, Wahlqvist Y, et al. Prognostic factors in bone sarcomas. Acta Orthop Scand Suppl 1997;273:156–60.
168. Salvati M, Ciappetta P, Raco A. Osteosarcomas of the skull. Clinical remarks on 19 cases. Cancer 1993;71:2210–6.
169. Sandig V, Brand K, Herwig S, Lukas J, Bartek J, Strauss M. Adenovirally transferred p16INK4/CDKN2 and p53 genes cooperate to induce apoptotic tumor cell death. Nat Med 1997;3:313–9.
170. Sanerkin NG. Definitions of osteosarcoma, chondrosarcoma, and fibrosarcoma of bone. Cancer 1980;46:178–85.
171. Schajowicz F, de Prospero JD, Cosentino E. Case report 641: chondroblastoma-like osteosarcoma. Skeletal Radiol 1990;19:603–6.
172. Scheel C, Schaefer KL, Jauch A, et al. Alternative lengthening of telomeres is associated with chromosomal instability in osteosarcomas. Oncogene 2001;20:3835–44.
173. Schofield D, Triche TJ. cDNA microanalysis of global gene expression in sarcomas. Curr Opin Oncol 2002;14:406–11.
174. Selivanova G, Iotsova V, Okan I, et al. Restoration of the growth suppression function of mutant p53 by a synthetic peptide derived from p53 C-terminal domain. Nat Med 1997;3:632–8.
175. Serra M, Scotlandi K, Reverter-Branchat G, et al. Value of P-glycoprotein and clinicopathologic factors as the basis for new treatment strategies in high-grade osteosarcoma of the extremities. J Clin Oncol 2003;21:536–42.

176. Sherr CJ. The INK4a/ARF network in tumour suppression. Mol Cell Biol 2001;2:731–7.
177. Sherr CJ, Roberts JM. Inhibitors of mammalian G1 cyclin-dependent kinases. Genes Dev 1995;9:1149–63.
178. Shives TC, Dahlin DC, Sim FH, Pritchard DJ, Earle JD. Osteosarcoma of the spine. J Bone Joint Surg Am 1986;68:660–8.
179. Simon MA, Aschliman MA, Thomas N, Mankin HJ. Limb-salvage treatment versus amputation for osteosarcoma of the distal end of the femur. J Bone Joint Surg Am 1986;68:1331–7.
180. Simons A, Janssen IM, Suijkerbuijk RF, et al. Isolation of osteosarcoma-associated amplified DNA sequences using representational difference analysis. Genes Chromosomes Cancer 1997;20:196–200.
181. Simons A, Schepens M, Forus A, et al. A novel chromosomal region of allelic loss, 4q32-q34, in human osteosarcomas revealed by representational difference analysis. Genes Chromosomes Cancer 1999;26:115–24.
182. Squire JA, Pei J, Marrano P, et al. High-resolution mapping of amplifications and deletions in pediatric osteosarcoma by use of CGH analysis of cDNA microarrays. Genes Chromosomes Cancer 2003;38:215–25.
183. Stock C, Kager L, Fink FM, Gadner H, Ambros PF. Chromosomal regions involved in the pathogenesis of osteosarcomas. Genes Chromosomes Cancer 2000;28:329–36.
184. Tarkkanen M, Elomaa I, Blomqvist C, et al. DNA sequence copy number increase at 8q: a potential new prognostic marker in high-grade osteosarcoma. Int J Cancer 1999;84:114–21.
185. Taylor WF, Ivins JC, Dahlin DC, Edmonson JH, Pritchard DJ. Trends and variability in survival from osteosarcoma. Mayo Clin Proc 1978;53:695–700.
186. Taylor WF, Ivins JC, Unni KK, Beabout JW, Golenzer HJ, Black LE. Prognostic variables in osteosarcoma: a multi-institutional study. J Natl Cancer Inst 1989;81:21–30.
187. Thomas DG, Giordano TJ, Sanders D, Biermann JS, Baker L. Absence of HER2/neu gene expression in osteosarcoma and skeletal Ewing's sarcoma. Clin Cancer Res 2002;8:788–93.
188. Tiemann F, Hinds PW. Induction of DNA synthesis and apoptosis by regulated inactivation of a temperature-sensitive retinoblastoma protein. EMBO J 1998;17:1040–52.
189. Toguchida J, Yamaguchi T, Dayton SH, et al. Prevalence and spectrum of germline mutations of the p53 gene among patients with sarcoma. N Engl J Med 1992;326:1301–8.
190. Troup JB, Dahlin DC, Coventry MB. The significance of giant cells in osteogenic sarcoma: do they indicate a relationship between osteogenic sarcoma and giant cell tumor of bone? Proc Staff Meet Mayo Clin 1960;35:179–86.
191. Uozaki H, Horiuchi H, Ishida T, Iijima T, Imamura T, Machinami R. Overexpression of resistance-related proteins (metallothioneins, glutathione-S-transferase pi, heat shock protein 27, and lung resistance-related protein) in osteosarcoma. Relationship with poor prognosis. Cancer 1997;79:2336–44.
192. Ulaner GA, Huang HY, Otero J, et al. Absence of a telomere maintenance mechanism as a favorable prognostic factor in patients with osteosarcoma. Cancer Res 2003;63:1759–63.
193. Uribe-Botero G, Russell WO, Sutow WW, Martin RG. Primary osteosarcoma of bone. Clinicopathologic investigation of 243 cases, with necropsy studies in 54. Am J Clin Pathol 1977; 67:427–35.
194. van Dartel M, Redeker S, Bras J, Kool M, Hulsebos TJ. Overexpression through amplification of genes in chromosome region 17p11.2 approximately p12 in high-grade osteosarcoma. Cancer Genet Cytogenet 2004;152:8–14.
195. Varley JM, Evans DG, Birch JM. Li-Fraumeni syndrome—a molecular and clinical review. Br J Cancer 1997;76:1–14.
196. Walaas L, Kindblom LG. Light and electron microscopic examination of fine-needle aspirates in the preoperative diagnosis of osteogenic tumors: a study of 21 osteosarcomas and two osteoblastomas. Diagn Cytopathol 1990;6:27–38.
197. Wei G, Lonardo F, Ueda T, et al. CDK4 gene amplification in osteosarcoma: reciprocal relationship with INK4A gene alterations and mapping of 12q13 amplicons. Int J Cancer 1999;80:199–204.
198. White VA, Fanning CV, Ayala AG, Raymond AK, Carrasco CH, Murray JA. Osteosarcoma and the role of fine-needle aspiration. A study of 51 cases. Cancer 1988;62:1238–46.
199. Wick MR, Siegal GP, Unni KK, McLeod RA, Greditzer HG 3rd. Sarcomas of bone complicating osteitis deformans (Paget's disease): fifty years' experience. Am J Surg Pathol 1981;5:47–59.
200. Willems JS. Aspiration biopsy cytology of tumors and tumor-suspect lesions of bone. In: Linsk JA, Franzen S, eds. Clinical aspiration cytology. Philadelphia: Lippincott; 1983:356–7.
201. Willen H. Tumor necrosis and prognosis in osteosarcoma. Acta Orthop Scand Suppl 1997;68: 126–9.
202. Wong FL, Boice JD Jr, Abramson DH, et al. Cancer incidence after retinoblastoma. Radiation dose and sarcoma risk. JAMA 1997;278:1262–7.

203. Wunder JS, Czitrom AA, Kandel R, Andrulis IL. Analysis of alterations in the retinoblastoma gene and tumor grade in bone and soft-tissue sarcomas. J Natl Cancer Inst 1991;83:194–200.
204. Zucchini C, Bianchini M, Valvassori L, et al. Identification of candidate genes involved in the reversal of malignant phenotype of osteosarcoma cells transfected with the liver/bone/kidney alkaline phosphatase gene. Bone 2004;672–9.

Parosteal Osteosarcoma

205. Ahuja SC, Villacin AB, Smith J, Bullough PG, Huvos AG, Marcove RC. Juxtacortical (parosteal) osteogenic sarcoma: histological grading and prognosis. J Bone Joint Surg Am 1977;59:632–47.
206. Bertoni F, Present D, Hudson T, Enneking WF. The meaning of radiolucencies in parosteal osteosarcoma. J Bone Joint Surg Am 1985;67:901–10.
207. Geschickter CF, Copeland MM. Parosteal osteoma of bone: a new entity. Ann Surg 1951;133:790–806.
208. Gisselsson D, Palsson E, Hoglund M, et al. Differentially amplified chromosome 12 sequences in low- and high-grade osteosarcoma. Genes Chromosomes Cancer 2002;33:133–40.
209. Nobel-Topham SE, Burrow SR, Eppert K, et al. SAS is amplified predominantly in surface osteosarcoma. J Orthop Res 1996;14:700–5.
210. Okada K, Frassica FJ, Sim FH, Beabout JW, Bond JR, Unni KK. Parosteal osteosarcoma. A clinicopathological study. J Bone Joint Surg Am 1994;76:366–78.
211. Ragazzini P, Gamberi G, Benassi MS, et al. Analysis of SAS gene and CDK4 and MDM2 proteins in low-grade osteosarcoma. Cancer Detect Prev 1999;23:129–36.
212. Sinovic JF, Bridge JA, Neff JR. Ring chromosome in parosteal osteosarcoma. Clinical and diagnostic significance. Cancer Genet Cytogenet 1992;62:50–2.
213. Szymanska J, Mandahl N, Mertens F, Tarkkanen M, Karaharju E, Knuutila S. Ring chromosomes in parosteal osteosarcoma contain sequences from 12q13-15: a combined cytogenetic and comparative genomic hybridization study. Genes Chromosomes Cancer 1996;16:31–4.
214. Tarkkanen M, Bohling T, Gamberi G, et al. Comparative genomic hybridization of low-grade central osteosarcoma. Mod Pathol 1998;11:421–6.
215. Wold LE, Unni KK, Beabout JW, Sim FH, Dahlin DC. Dedifferentiated parosteal osteosarcoma. J Bone Joint Surg Am 1984;66:53–9.
216. Wunder JS, Eppert K, Burrow SR, et al. Co-amplification and overexpression of CDK4, SAS and MDM2 occur frequently in human parosteal osteosarcomas. Oncogene 1999;18:783–8.

Periosteal Osteosarcoma

217. Bertoni F, Boriani S, Laus M, Campanacci M. Periosteal chondrosarcoma and periosteal osteosarcoma. Two distinct entities. J Bone Joint Surg Br 1982;64:370–6.
218. deSantos LA, Murray JA, Finklestein JB, Spjut HJ, Ayala AG. The radiographic spectrum of periosteal osteosarcoma. Radiology 1978;127: 123–9.
219. Ritts GD, Pritchard DJ, Unni KK, Beabout JW, Eckardt JJ. Periosteal osteosarcoma. Clin Orthop 1987;219:299–307.
220. Schajowicz F. Juxtacortical chondrosarcoma. J Bone Joint Surg Br 1977;59:473–80.
221. Unni KK, Dahlin DC, Beabout JW. Periosteal osteogenic sarcoma. Cancer 1976;37:2476–85.

High-Grade Surface Osteosarcoma

222. Okada K, Unni KK, Swee RG, Sim FH. High grade surface osteosarcoma: a clinicopathologic study of 46 cases. Cancer 1999;85:1044–54.
223. Wold LE, Unni KK, Beabout JW, Pritchard DJ. High-grade surface osteosarcomas. Am J Surg Pathol 1984;8:181–6.

6 FIBROGENIC TUMORS

DESMOPLASTIC FIBROMA

Definition. Desmoplastic fibroma is a hypocellular spindle cell tumor of fibroblasts that produces abundant collagen and is identical histologically to the more common desmoid tumor of soft tissues.

General Features. The term desmoplastic fibroma was introduced in 1958 by Jaffe (7) who discussed it in relation to fibrosarcoma of bone, emphasizing the kinship between the two tumors. The true incidence is difficult to evaluate because the cases of desmoplastic fibroma described in the literature undoubtedly include examples of fibrous dysplasia, low-grade osteosarcoma, and low-grade fibrosarcoma. Nevertheless, desmoplastic fibroma is one of the rarest of bone tumors, with only 14 cases reported in the Mayo Clinic files through 1999 (fig. 6-1). The term "periosteal desmoid" is a misnomer, referring to a harmless non-neoplastic condition, that is, cortical avulsive irregularity (5).

Clinical Features. Patients with desmoplastic fibroma are generally in the second or third

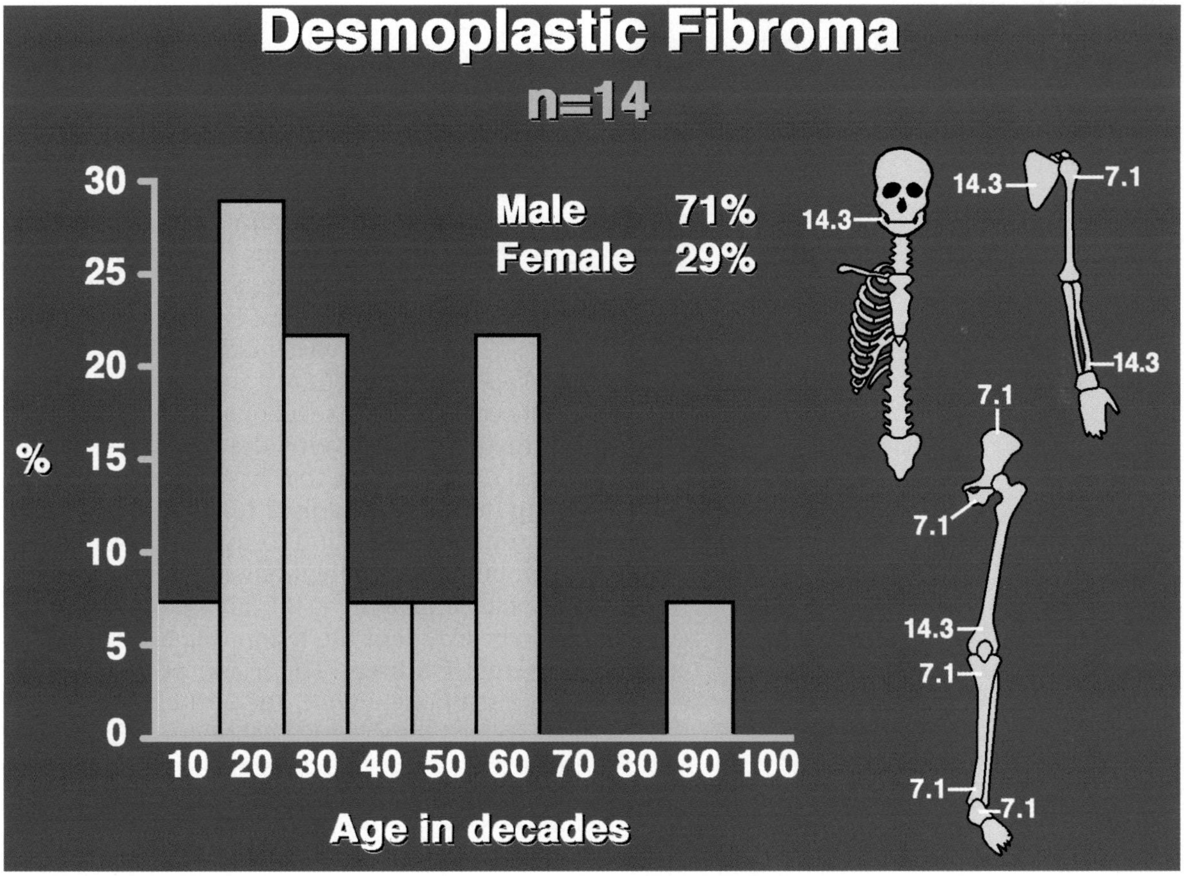

Figure 6-1

DESMOPLASTIC FIBROMA

Distribution of desmoplastic fibroma according to the age and sex of the patient and the site of the lesion.

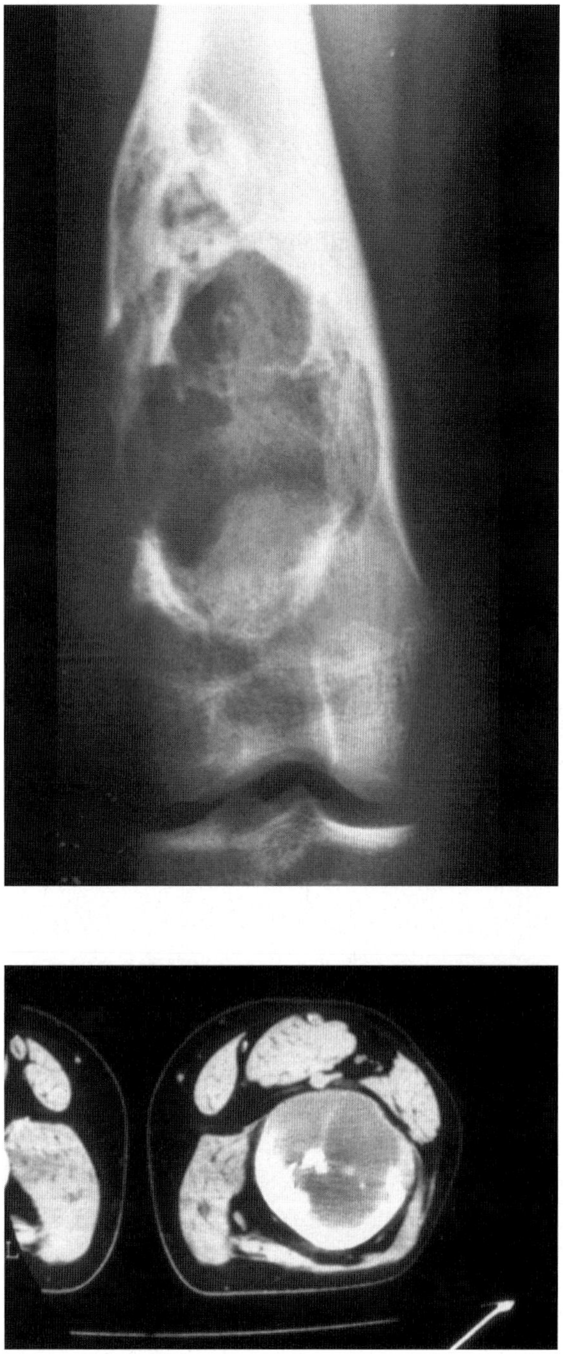

Figure 6-2

DESMOPLASTIC FIBROMA

Top: Large, mixed lytic and sclerotic destructive tumor of the distal femur. The lesion has features suggestive of a benign or low-grade malignant lesion, given the associated osseous expansion and cortical thickening.

Bottom: Corresponding computerized tomography (CT) image shows destruction of the cortex and extension into soft tissue.

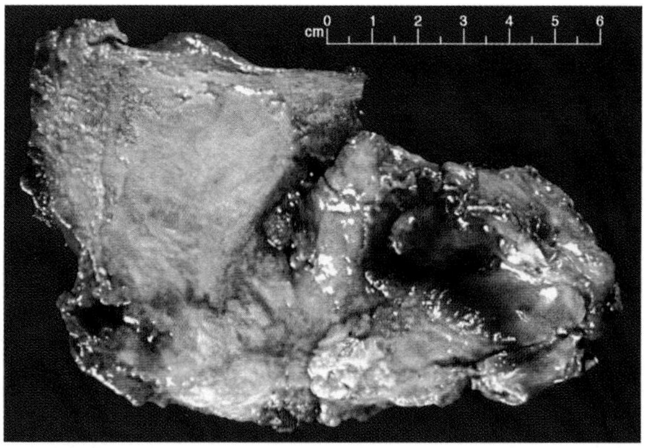

Figure 6-3

DESMOPLASTIC FIBROMA

The tumor appears firm and fibrous.

decade of life (9). Males slightly outnumber females. Pain is the predominant symptom; rarely, the tumor is an incidental radiographic finding (6,9). About 10 percent of patients present with pathologic fracture (4).

Sites. Desmoplastic fibroma has been reported in many skeletal sites. According to two comprehensive reviews of the literature (2,4), the bone involved most commonly is the mandible. The femur and ilium also are involved frequently.

Radiographic Findings. Desmoplastic fibroma presents as an oval lytic defect (fig. 6-2, top). The lesion is well demarcated, but if peripheral sclerosis is present, it is incomplete. No mineral occurs within the lesional tissue. The cortex of the bone is unevenly destroyed, leaving behind ridges of bone that have a trabeculated or soap-bubble appearance (6). The tumor may destroy the cortex and form a soft tissue mass. Computerized tomography (CT) and magnetic resonance imaging (MRI) are helpful in defining the extent of the lesion (fig. 6-2, bottom).

Gross Findings. The lesion peels off easily from the bone; hence, the entire mass usually is received intact in the laboratory. The tumor is white to gray, rubbery, and firm, and has a whorled appearance, similar to that of a desmoid tumor (fig. 6-3). Small cystic areas containing liquid matrix may be noted.

Microscopic Findings. Desmoplastic fibroma is a permeative, hypocellular spindle cell tumor associated with large amounts of collagen (fig. 6-4). The spindle cells have slender nuclei

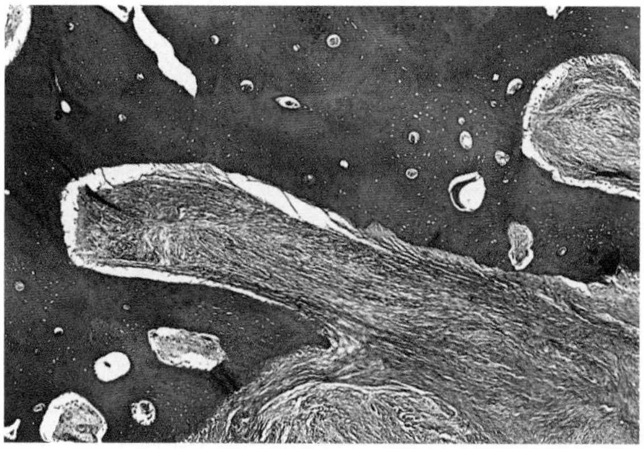

Figure 6-4

DESMOPLASTIC FIBROMA

Desmoplastic fibroma of the mandible infiltrating cortical bone.

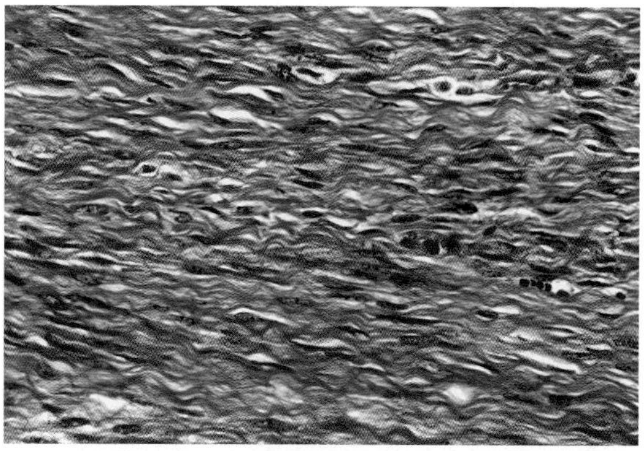

Figure 6-5

DESMOPLASTIC FIBROMA

Cells with slender, tapered nuclei without atypia are surrounded by wavy collagen fibers.

with no cytologic features of malignancy (fig. 6-5). Mitotic figures are sparse. The amount of cellularity varies, and some areas may be relatively hypercellular. However, marked hypercellularity with interlacing fascicles of spindle cells is inconsistent with a diagnosis of desmoplastic fibroma. Large gaping vascular spaces without a muscular wall, as seen in desmoid tumors, are present (fig. 6-6). The collagen is fibrillar or hyalinized; keloid-like collagen is rarely seen.

Electron microscopic studies have demonstrated features typical of fibroblasts (11). One study identified three types of cells: fibroblasts, myofibroblasts, and primitive mesenchymal cells (8).

Genetics and Other Special Techniques. Trisomy 8 and trisomy 20, nonrandom aberrations in desmoid tumors, have been observed in desmoplastic fibroma (3,10). These findings indicate that, analogous to soft tissue fibrous lesions, trisomy 8 and trisomy 20 contribute to aberrant cell proliferation in primary fibrous lesions of bone, supporting a common or related mechanism of pathogenesis.

Differential Diagnosis. Desmoplastic fibroma may be confused, on the one hand, with fibrous dysplasia and, on the other hand, with low-grade fibrosarcoma and osteosarcoma. Fibrous dysplasia has a characteristic radiographic appearance, with a rind of sclerotic bone surrounding a lucency. Microscopically, fibrous dysplasia can have large areas of spindle cell proliferation without bone formation, and biopsy specimens

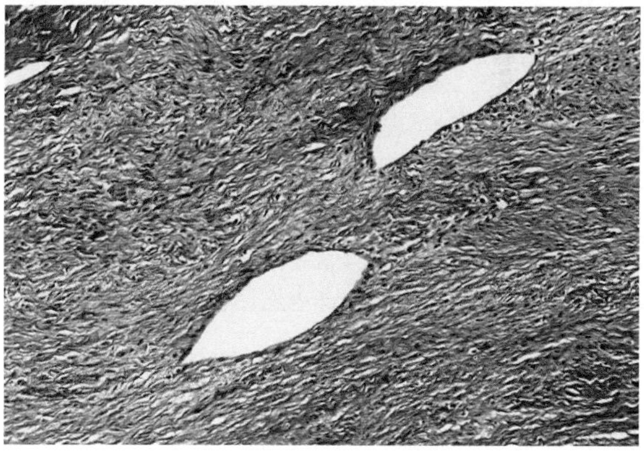

Figure 6-6

DESMOPLASTIC FIBROMA

Sweeping fascicles of spindle-shaped cells and dilated vascular spaces.

from such areas may be mistaken for desmoplastic fibroma. However, adequate sampling obviates this problem. Distinguishing between desmoplastic fibroma and low-grade fibrosarcoma can be difficult and somewhat arbitrary (1). It is best to insist on the amount of cellularity that would be acceptable in a desmoid tumor. Any bone formation by the tumor rules out desmoplastic fibroma and supports the diagnosis of low-grade osteosarcoma.

Treatment and Prognosis. Treatment should be complete surgical removal either by thorough curettage (9) or resection (11). If the resection is

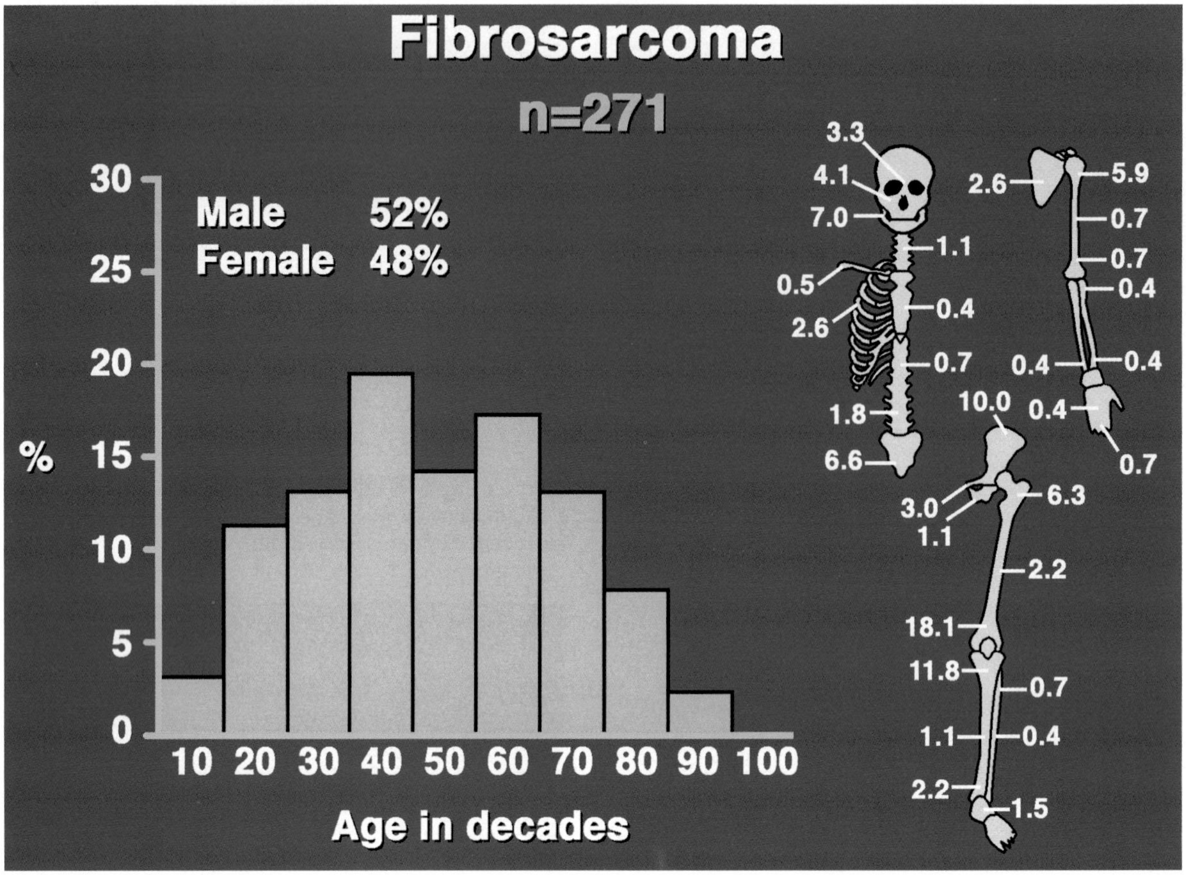

Figure 6-7

FIBROSARCOMA

Distribution of fibrosarcoma according to the age and sex of the patient and the site of the lesion.

inadequate, the tumor may recur (6). There have been no well-documented examples of distant metastasis with desmoplastic fibroma. Two authors (KK Unni, CY Inwards, Mayo Clinic) recently saw a high-grade spindle cell sarcoma that occurred about 15 years after removal of a desmoplastic fibroma from the same site.

FIBROSARCOMA

Definition. Fibrosarcoma is a malignant tumor composed of spindle cells that often are arranged in fascicles. A variable amount of collagen is produced, but there is no deposition of osteoid or cartilage.

General Features. Fibrosarcoma tends to be a diagnosis of exclusion, and differentiating it from fibroblastic osteosarcoma is often arbitrary. Of the cases reported at Mayo Clinic, 30 percent were secondary, arising in Paget's disease or other conditions (13). Ducatman et al. (14) described three spindle cell sarcomas in patients with Recklinghausen's disease: one fibrosarcoma and two malignant fibrous histiocytomas. These tumors did not have the features of malignant peripheral nerve sheath tumors. In the Swedish registry, fibrosarcomas account for 3.5 percent of all sarcomas of bone (17). Dahlin and Ivins (13) reported that osteosarcoma is seven times as common as fibrosarcoma. The Mayo Clinic files contain the records of 271 fibrosarcomas (fig. 6-7).

Clinical Features. Patients present with pain, sometimes associated with swelling. Males and females are affected about equally, and all age groups are involved. Very few patients are in the first 5 years of life. The lack of a pronounced

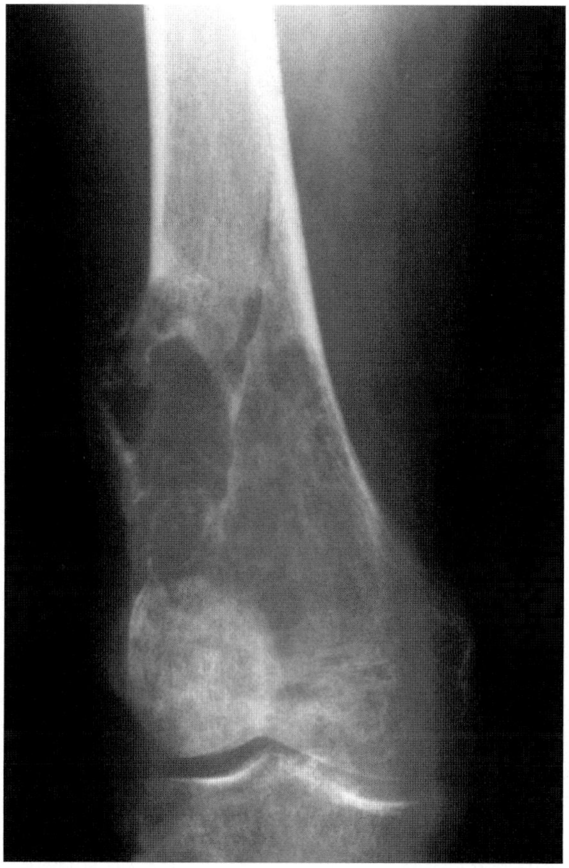

Figure 6-8

FIBROSARCOMA

A purely lytic tumor of the distal femur is seen. There is destruction of the cortex and a pathologic fracture.

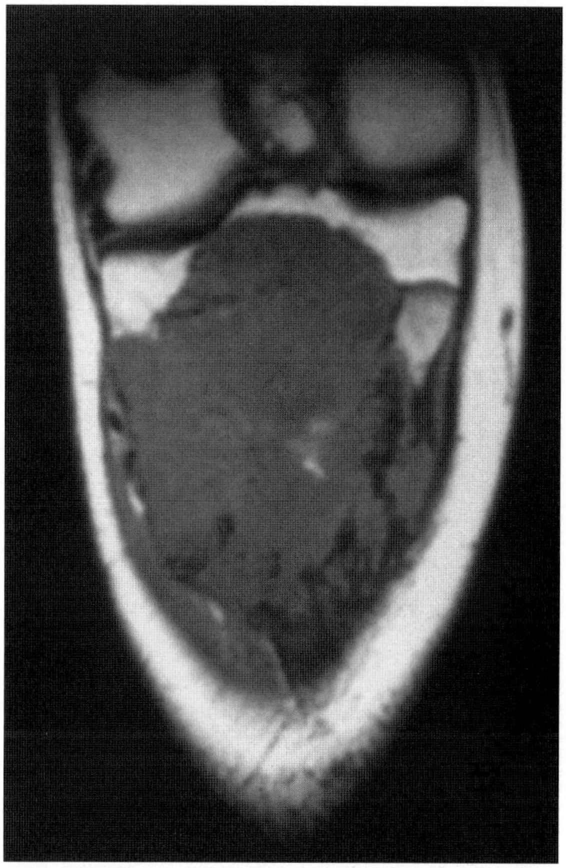

Figure 6-9

FIBROSARCOMA

Coronal T_1-weighted magnetic resonance image (MRI) shows a large destructive fibrosarcoma of the proximal tibial metaphysis with an associated soft tissue mass. The tumor crosses the open growth plate to involve a portion of the epiphysis.

tendency to affect children and adolescents is in sharp contrast to the incidence of osteosarcoma and is more similar to that of malignant fibrous histiocytoma.

Sites. Most of the tumors occur around the knee joint, with the distal femur and proximal tibia being the most common sites. Multicentric skeletal involvement has been described (16).

Radiographic Findings. Fibrosarcoma presents as a purely lytic destructive process, usually involving the metaphysis of a long bone (fig. 6-8). The margins generally are indistinct, and the lesion may destroy the cortex to extend into soft tissues (fig. 6-9). CT and MRI are helpful in defining the extent of the tumor.

Gross Findings. The gross appearance reflects the histologic grade of the tumor. Low-grade tumors tend to be firm and fibrous, and they may have a whorled appearance. High-grade tumors tend to be soft and fleshy and more obviously permeative (fig. 6-10). Rarely, the tumor has a distinctly gelatinous appearance.

Microscopic Findings. Fibrosarcomas consist of spindle cells arranged in fascicles that generally intersect to create a herringbone pattern (fig. 6-11). The nuclei are long and slender and have tapered ends. The cytoplasm is usually indistinct. The amount of collagen produced varies, ranging from abundant to slight. By definition, no mineralized matrix is found.

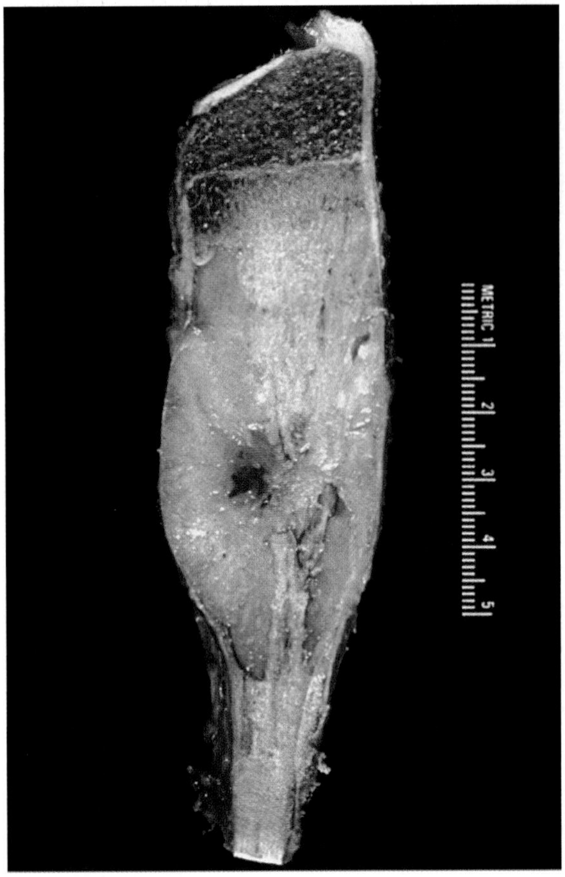

Figure 6-10

FIBROSARCOMA

A fleshy white tumor of the proximal fibula fills the bone marrow cavity, destroys the cortex, and extends into soft tissue.

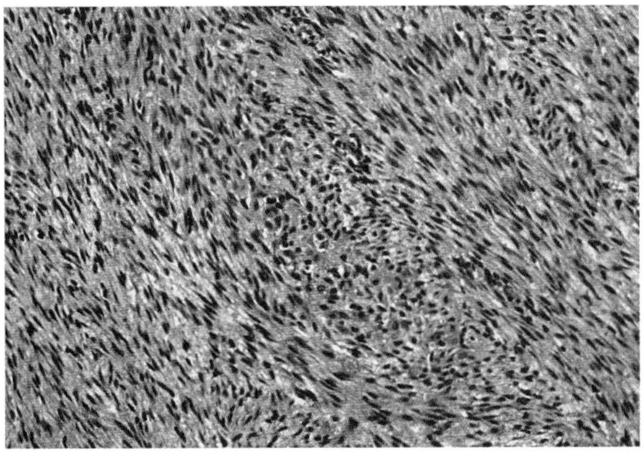

Figure 6-11

FIBROSARCOMA

A hypercellular high-grade fibrosarcoma contains spindle-shaped cells arranged in a herringbone pattern.

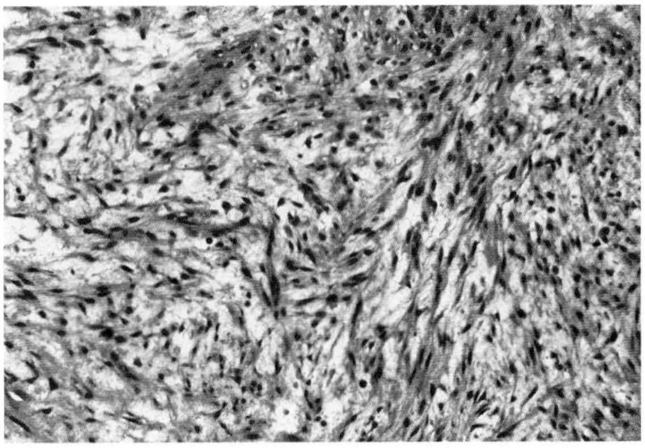

Figure 6-12

FIBROSARCOMA

Myxoid change within a fibrosarcoma.

The matrix may become myxoid and the term *myxoid fibrosarcoma* may be used (fig. 6-12). Rarely, a fibrosarcoma has cells with very small nuclei and the term *small cell fibrosarcoma* may be applied (fig. 6-13).

Grading. Fibrosarcomas are graded on the basis of the cellularity of the tumor and the cytologic features of the tumor cells. Grade 1 fibrosarcomas show abundant collagen production; the tumor cells have nuclei that are regular and have little hyperchromasia. Grade 2 fibrosarcomas have less collagen production and more spindle cells, which are somewhat enlarged and hyperchromatic (fig. 6-14). Grade 3 fibrosarcomas are extremely cellular and have little collagen formation. The cell nuclei are packed closely together and are very hyperchromatic. Grade 4 fibrosarcomas have little or no collagen formation, and the spindle cell nuclei are extremely dense and hyperchromatic. Pleomorphism, as in other high-grade sarcomas (such as osteosarcoma), is not a feature of fibrosarcoma. Mitotic figures and foci of necrosis are more common in high-grade tumors.

This grading system is subjective, as evidenced by the differences in the relative numbers of the different grades in reported series. Whereas Dahlin and Ivins (13) found only one grade 1 fibrosarcoma in a series of 114 tumors, Taconis and van Rijssel (18) found 14 of 114 tumors to be grade 1. Nevertheless, all studies have confirmed that the grade of the tumor correlates with prognosis (12,13,18).

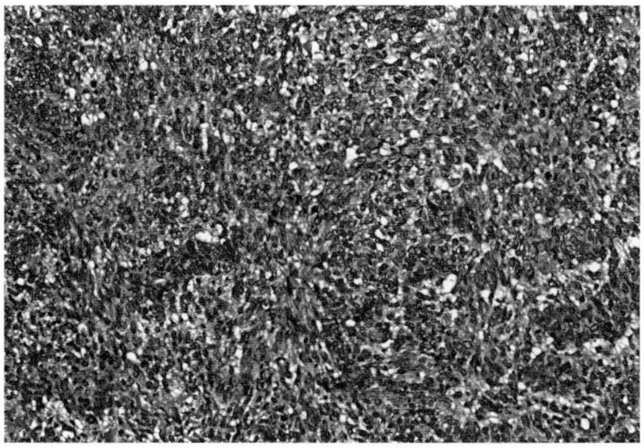

Figure 6-13

FIBROSARCOMA

A high-grade tumor with relatively small cells imparts a "small cell" appearance.

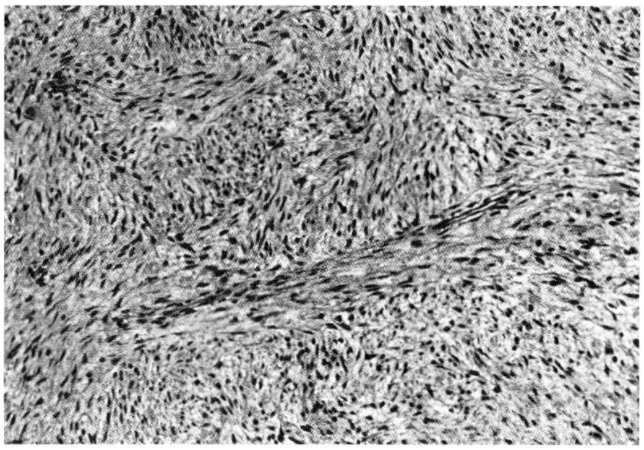

Figure 6-14

FIBROSARCOMA

This grade 2 (of 4) fibrosarcoma is only moderately cellular, and the tumor cells are less plump than those seen in high-grade fibrosarcoma.

Differential Diagnosis. Low-grade fibrosarcoma has to be differentiated from fibrous dysplasia and desmoplastic fibroma. The cells of fibrous dysplasia tend to be plump, whereas those of fibrosarcoma tend to be slender and tapered. The finding of typical areas of metaplastic bone formation confirms the diagnosis of fibrous dysplasia. The distinction between fibrosarcoma and desmoplastic fibroma may be arbitrary (see above).

High-grade fibrosarcomas have to be differentiated from fibroblastic osteosarcoma. This differentiation is based solely on identifying osteoid matrix in the latter. The spindle cells of malignant fibrous histiocytoma are more pleomorphic than those of fibrosarcoma. Taconis and van Rijssel (18) found no difference in prognosis between patients with fibrosarcoma and those with malignant fibrous histiocytoma.

Sarcomatoid metastatic carcinoma can simulate fibrosarcoma. Spindled carcinoma cells usually have plump nuclei, whereas those of fibrosarcoma are slender. A good clinical history and immunoperoxidase studies for epithelial markers are useful in making the diagnosis.

Treatment and Prognosis. Treatment is surgical ablation. Patients with low-grade tumors do not require adjunctive treatment, but those with high-grade fibrosarcomas probably require preoperative chemotherapy. One study has suggested that the prognosis for patients with fibrosarcoma is worse than for those with osteosarcoma (17). In the series of Jeffree and Price (15), the 5-year survival rate was 16 percent. Patients with low-grade tumors fared better than those with high-grade tumors. Dahlin and Ivins (13) also confirmed better survival with low-grade tumors, but their overall survival (28.7 percent) was better than for osteosarcoma at that time. Bertoni et al. (12) reported an even better survival rate of 42 percent; the 5-year survival rate was 83 percent for patients with low-grade fibrosarcomas but only 34 percent for those with high-grade tumors.

REFERENCES

Desmoplastic Fibroma

1. Bertoni F, Calderoni P, Bacchini P, Campanacci M. Desmoplastic fibroma of bone. A report of six cases. J Bone Joint Surg Br 1984;66:265–8.
2. Bohm P, Krober S, Greschniok A, Laniado M, Kaiserling E. Desmoplastic fibroma of the bone. A report of two patients, review of the literature, and therapeutic implications. Cancer 1996;78:1011–23.
3. Bridge JA, Swarts SJ, Buresh C, et al. Trisomies 8 and 20 characterize a subgroup of benign fibrous lesions arising in both soft tissue and bone. Am J Pathol 1999;154:729–33.
4. Crim JR, Gold RH, Mirra JM, Eckardt JJ, Bassett LW. Desmoplastic fibroma of bone: radiographic analysis. Radiology 1989;172:827–32.
5. Fechner RE, Mills SE. Tumors of the bones and joints. Atlas of Tumor Pathology, 3rd Series, Fascicle 8.Washington, DC: Armed Forces Institute of Pathology; 1993:154–6.
6. Inwards CY, Unni KK, Beabout JW, Sim FH. Desmoplastic fibroma of bone. Cancer 1991;68:1978–83.
7. Jaffe HL. Tumors and tumorous conditions of the bones and joints. Philadelphia: Lea & Febiger; 1958:298–304.
8. Lagace R, Delage C, Bouchard HL, Seemayer TA. Desmoplastic fibroma of bone. An ultrastructural study. Am J Surg Pathol 1979;3:423–30.
9. Nishida J, Tajima K, Abe M, et al. Desmoplastic fibroma. Aggressive curettage as a surgical alternative for treatment. Clin Orthop 1995;320:142–8.
10. Qi H, Dal Cin P, Hernandez JM, et al. Trisomies 8 and 20 in desmoid tumors. Cancer Genet Cytogenet 1996;92:147–9.
11. Sugiura I. Desmoplastic fibroma. Case report and review of the literature. J Bone Joint Surg Am 1976;58:126–30.

Fibrosarcoma

12. Bertoni F, Capanna R, Calderoni P, Patrizia B, Campanacci M. Primary central (medullary) fibrosarcoma of bone. Semin Diagn Pathol 1984;1:185–98.
13. Dahlin DC, Ivins JC. Fibrosarcoma of bone. A study of 114 cases. Cancer 1969;23:35–41.
14. Ducatman BS, Scheithauer BW, Dahlin DC. Malignant bone tumors associated with neurofibromatosis. Mayo Clin Proc 1983;58:578–82.
15. Jeffree GM, Price CH. Metastatic spread of fibrosarcoma of bone. A report on forty-nine cases, and a comparison with osteosarcoma. J Bone Joint Surg Br 1976;58:418–25.
16. Kabukcuoglu Y, Kabukcuoglu F, Carter S, Ozturk I, Erseven G, Kuzgun U. Multiple diffuse fibrosarcoma of bone. Am J Orthop 1999;28:715–7.
17. Larsson SE, Lorentzon R, Boquist L. Fibrosarcoma of bone. A demographic, clinical and histopathological study of all cases recorded in the Swedish cancer registry from 1958 to 1968. J Bone Joint Surg Br 1976;58:412–7.
18. Taconis WK, van Rijssel TG. Fibrosarcoma of long bones. A study of the significance of areas of malignant fibrous histiocytoma. J Bone Joint Surg Br 1985;67:111–6.

7 "HISTIOCYTIC" TUMORS

BENIGN FIBROUS HISTIOCYTOMA

Definition. Benign fibrous histiocytoma is a primary neoplasm of bone that is composed of fibroblasts and histiocytes whose cytologic features do not suggest a malignant neoplasm.

General Features. The term fibrous histiocytoma was used originally to denote a soft tissue tumor considered to be composed of fibroblasts and histiocytes. Although the terms *benign fibrous histiocytoma* and *atypical fibrous histiocytoma* were in vogue many years ago, they are less common today. Benign fibrous histiocytoma of skin is probably not a true neoplasm. The presence of a pronounced storiform pattern of spindle cells and lipid-laden histiocytes led to the term *fibroxanthoma,* or *fibrous histiocytoma,* for the common metaphyseal fibrous defect (nonossifying fibroma). This concept has not received support because metaphyseal fibrous defect is probably not a true neoplasm but a developmental defect. The term benign fibrous histiocytoma of bone is now applied to a lesion that has the histologic features of a metaphyseal fibrous defect but differs from the latter in: 1) causing symptoms; 2) occurring in a wider age group; and 3) having an unusual location (4).

Some of the benign fibrous histiocytomas that have been reported occurred at the ends of long bones. Giant cell tumors may have a prominent fibrohistiocytic component, and at least some of these reported examples are probably giant cell tumors. The diagnosis of atypical fibrous histiocytoma is even more of a problem. Saito and Caines (6) reported one case of atypical fibrous histiocytoma of bone. The tumor had features generally associated with a fibrohistiocytic tumor; although it had cellular pleomorphism, there were no atypical mitotic figures. The patient was well 5 years after radical surgery. The diagnostic criteria for atypical fibrous histiocytoma are so tenuous that it hardly can be considered a diagnostic entity. The Mayo Clinic files contain the records of only nine cases of fibrous histiocytoma (fig. 7-1).

Clinical Features. Patients range in age from 5 to 75 years (4). There is a slight male predominance. Pain is the usual symptom.

Sites. The iliac wing is the most common site, followed by the femur.

Radiographic Findings. The tumor presents as a well-defined lytic defect. When a long bone is affected, the diaphysis or metaphyseal regions are involved.

Gross Findings. The gross appearance varies from fleshy to fibrous, and the tumor is gray or yellow.

Microscopic Findings. The microscopic appearance suggests a metaphyseal fibrous defect. Spindle cells with plump or slender nuclei are arranged in a loose storiform pattern (fig. 7-2). Some of the cells have vesicular nuclei and pink or foamy cytoplasm, which suggest a histiocytic origin. The nuclei lack atypical features. Mitotic figures may be present, but are not atypical. There are usually clusters of foam cells and multinucleated giant cells (fig. 7-3).

Differential Diagnosis. The microscopic features of benign fibrous histiocytoma are identical to those of metaphyseal fibrous defects, and the distinction between the two is based on the characteristic location in the metaphysis and the lack of symptoms caused by a metaphyseal defect. Some benign fibrous histiocytomas are reported to occur in the epiphysis (1,2,5). In these instances, the differentiation from a giant cell tumor with prominent fibrohistiocytic features is necessarily arbitrary. The distinction between benign and malignant fibrous histiocytomas depends entirely on the cytologic features of malignancy in the latter.

Treatment and Prognosis. Treatment consists of thorough curettage. In the series of eight cases reported by Clarke et al. (3), there were three recurrences. There have not been any reports of distant metastasis.

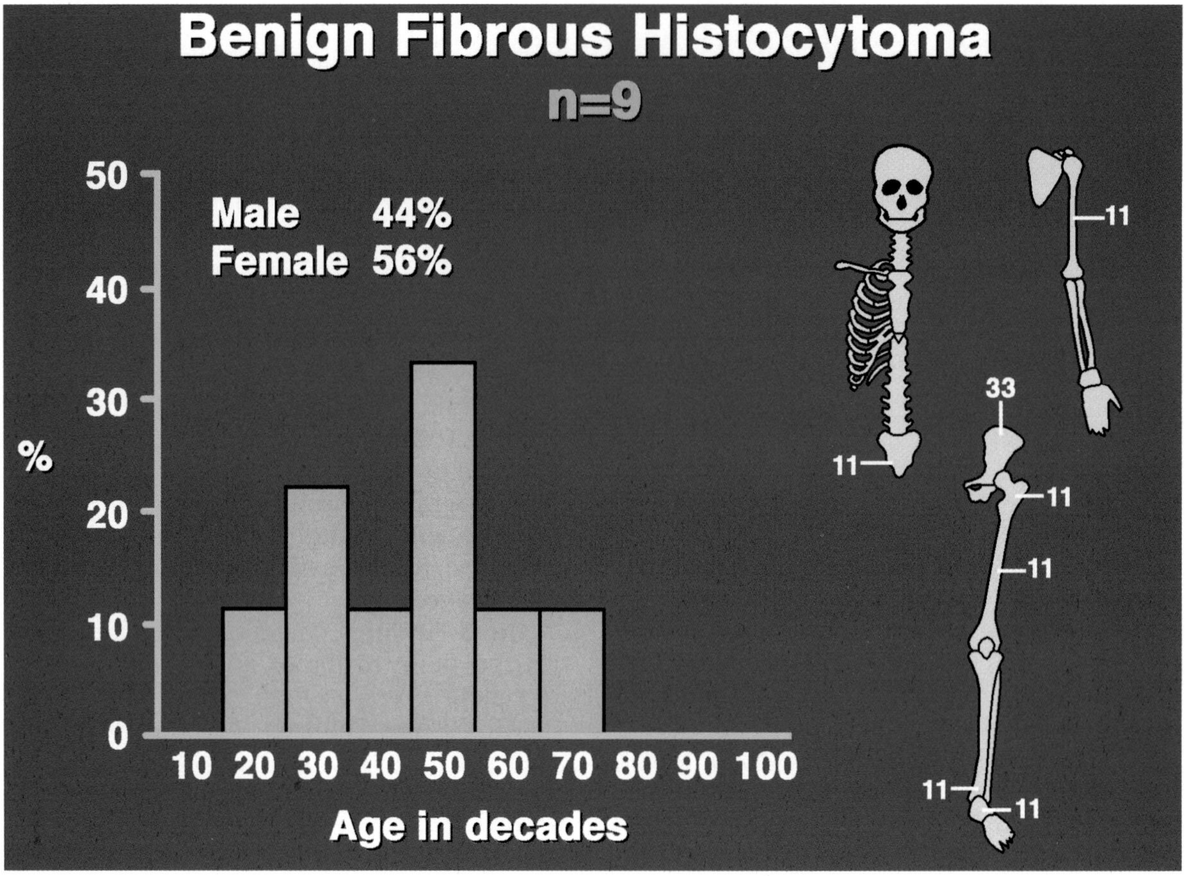

Figure 7-1

BENIGN FIBROUS HISTIOCYTOMA

Distribution of benign fibrous histiocytoma according to the age and sex of the patient and the site of the lesion.

MALIGNANT FIBROUS HISTIOCYTOMA

Definition. Malignant fibrous histiocytoma is a primary pleomorphic sarcoma of bone with a variable morphology in which the tumor cells do not produce osteoid or cartilage matrix.

General Features. The term *malignant fibrous histiocytoma* was introduced to describe a tumor of soft tissues because tissue culture studies had shown that the tumor cells could have fibroblastic and histiocytic properties (20). The results of immunohistochemical studies have been conflicting: some have confirmed that the tumor cells show monocyte-macrophage differentiation (22); others have not (25). Fletcher (11) has suggested that malignant fibrous histiocytoma is a reproducible histologic pattern, but this does not imply that the tumor cells have a histiocytic derivation. Even if the histogenesis is unclear, malignant fibrous histiocytoma of bone appears well accepted as a clinicopathologic entity.

It is difficult to evaluate the incidence of malignant fibrous histiocytoma because most of the reported series have been culled by reexamining cases of osteosarcoma and fibrosarcoma (9, 10,15). The Mayo Clinic files contain the records of 90 cases of malignant fibrous histiocytoma compared with 271 cases of fibrosarcoma and 1,941 cases of osteosarcoma. It appears that about one fourth of all cases are secondary. Tumors have been described secondary to bone infarcts (12,17) in the setting of previous radiation (15) and Paget's disease. There have been single case reports of malignant fibrous histiocytoma of bone arising at the site of a previous arthroplasty (14, 23) and a previous shrapnel wound (16).

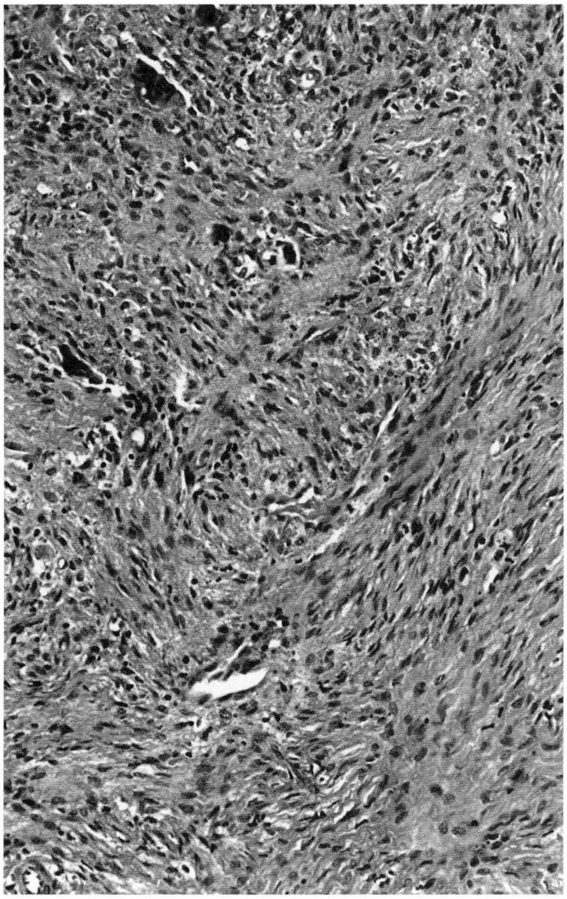

Figure 7-2

BENIGN FIBROUS HISTIOCYTOMA

Plump spindle cells arranged in a storiform pattern suggest the diagnosis of metaphyseal fibrous defect. However, this tumor was located in the clavicle.

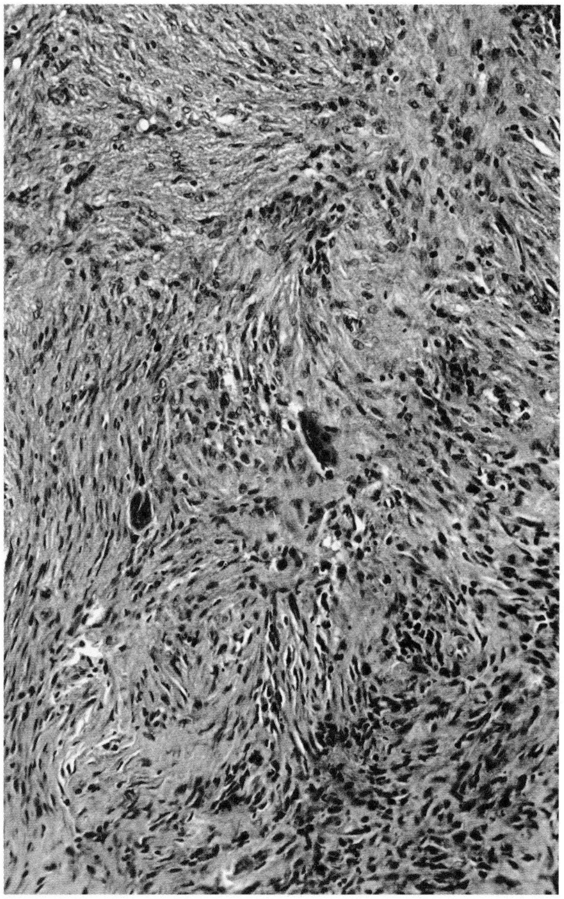

Figure 7-3

BENIGN FIBROUS HISTIOCYTOMA

The tumor contains multinucleated giant cells, hemosiderin-laden macrophages, and scattered lymphocytes.

Clinical Features. There is a modest male predominance. In most reported large series, the age distribution is even among the decades. In the Mayo Clinic files, the youngest patient was 6 years of age and the oldest was 81 (fig. 7-4). Pain is the predominant symptom; rarely, a patient presents with a pathologic fracture.

Sites. Any portion of the skeleton may be involved, but the majority of tumors affect the metaphysis of long bones, especially around the knee joint. Rarely, the tumor is diaphyseal. Multicentric skeletal disease is unusual and, if present, the diagnosis of malignant lymphoma should be excluded.

Radiographic Findings. The most common appearance is that of a purely lytic destructive process involving the metaphysis of long bones (fig. 7-5). The margins are poorly defined, and the tumor frequently breaks through the cortex to involve the soft tissues. Periosteal reaction is uncommon (9). The radiographic features are nonspecific but usually suggest a malignancy (fig. 7-6).

Gross Findings. The gross appearance is quite variable (figs. 7-7, 7-8). The tumor is soft, poorly demarcated, and fleshy white. Areas of yellow discoloration may be present, reflecting foci of foam cells. Areas of necrosis are common.

Microscopic Findings. The microscopic appearance of malignant fibrous histiocytoma is similar to that of the soft tissue counterpart. The tumor consists predominantly of two cell

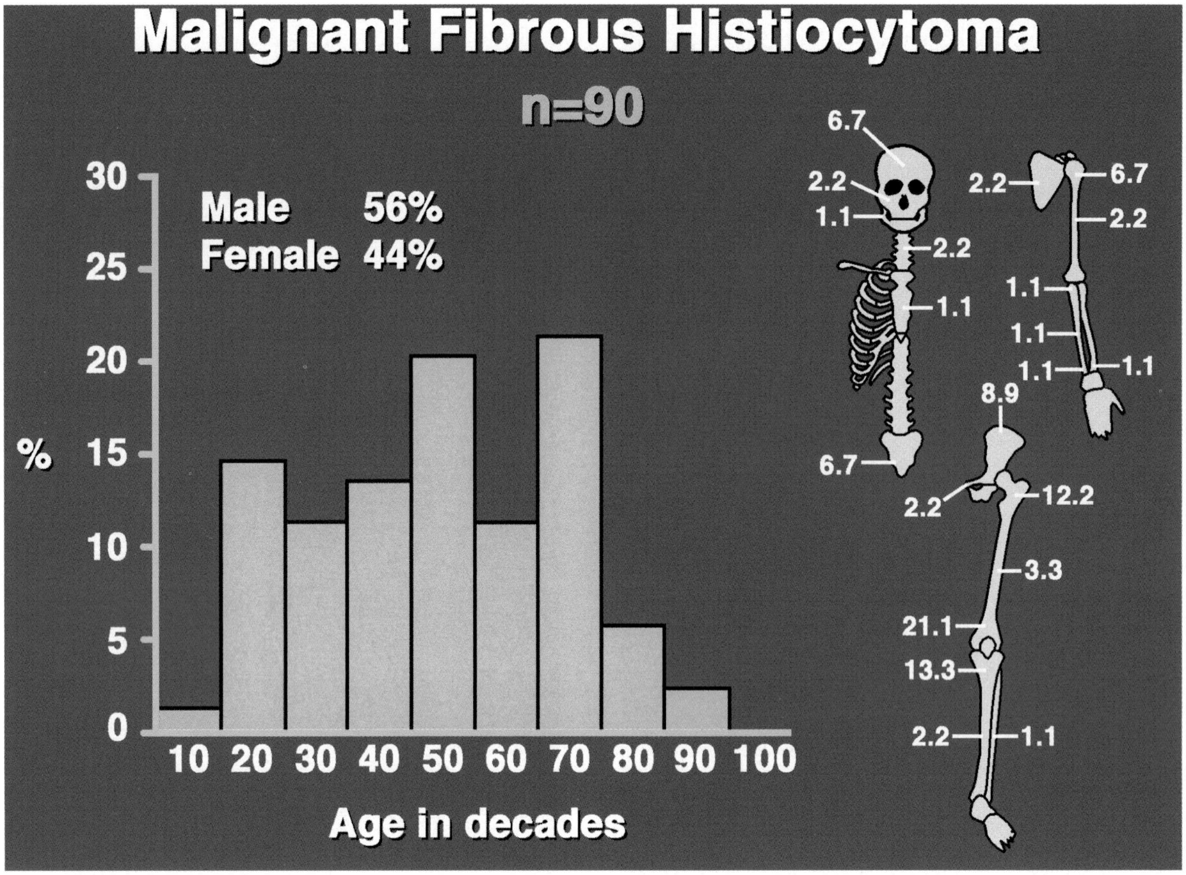

Figure 7-4

MALIGNANT FIBROUS HISTIOCYTOMA

Distribution of malignant fibrous histiocytoma according to the age and sex of the patient and the site of the lesion.

types: fibroblasts and histiocytes. In addition, benign and malignant multinucleated giant cells are always present, but their number varies from few to many. When giant cells dominate the histologic features, the diagnosis of giant cell tumor may be suggested.

The relative amounts of spindle cells and histiocytes vary greatly, which is the basis for attempts to subclassify these tumors into storiform-pleomorphic and histiocytic types. However, because the variation in the histologic appearance of any given tumor is so great, it does not seem reasonable to subclassify malignant fibrous histiocytomas of bone.

The spindle cells have enlarged hyperchromatic nuclei and tend to be arranged in a storiform or cartwheel pattern (fig. 7-9). The spindle cell areas may have variable amounts of collagen. Fine filamentous collagen is common between tumor cells. Differentiating this matrix from osteoid is necessarily arbitrary. Occasionally, large amounts of collagen are laid down and the spindle cell areas are hypocellular. Even in these areas, a storiform pattern is maintained. Myxoid change in the matrix is unusual.

The histiocytic cells have irregular or round nuclei that are hyperchromatic and may have grooves (fig. 7-10). The cytoplasm is pink and abundant, and may be granular or foamy. Clusters of foam cells may be prominent. These foam cells may be multinucleated, and Touton giant cells may be present.

Infiltration with lymphocytes is not unusual; polymorphonuclear leukocytes and eosinophils are less common. It generally is accepted that

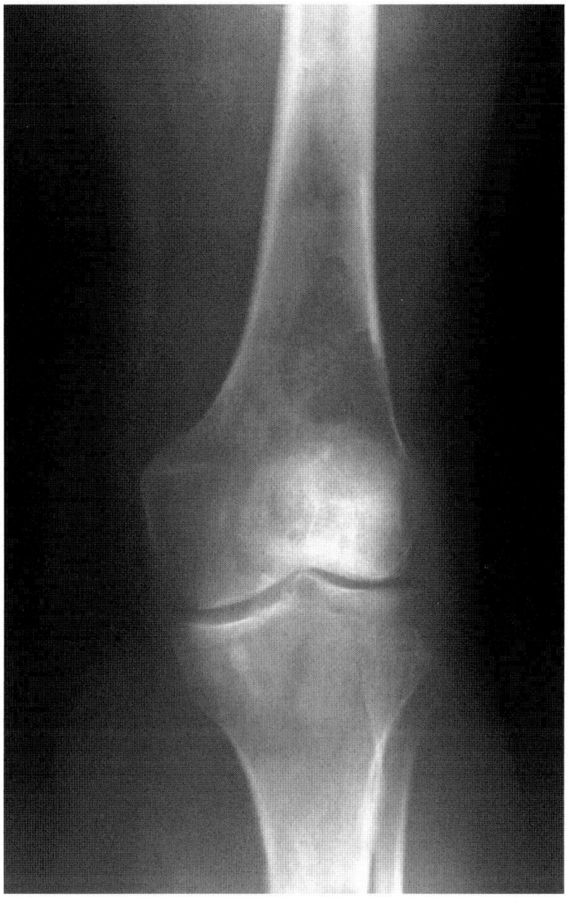

Figure 7-5

MALIGNANT FIBROUS HISTIOCYTOMA

Large destructive tumor of the distal femur. Although not apparent on plain films, at the time of amputation the tumor had a large soft tissue component.

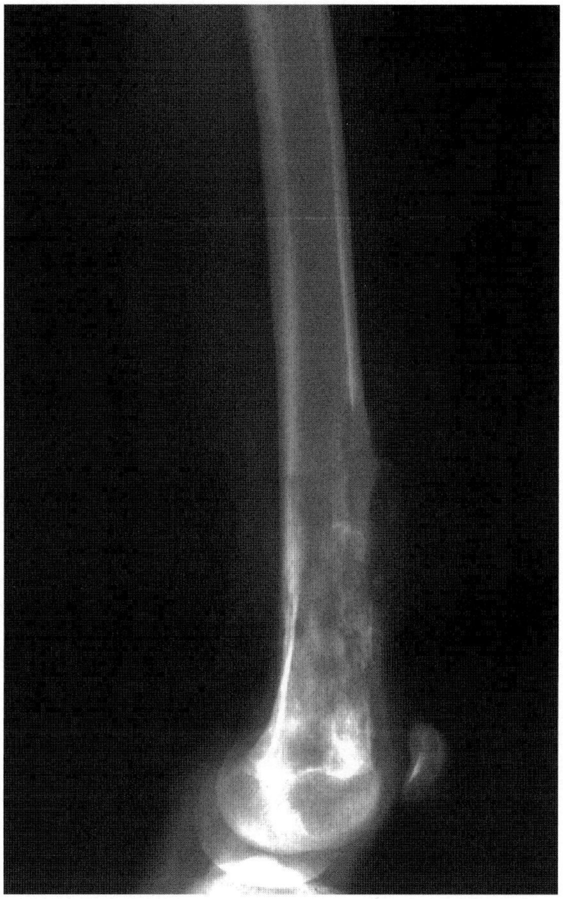

Figure 7-6

MALIGNANT FIBROUS HISTIOCYTOMA

This tumor of the distal femur had a permeative appearance.

malignant fibrous histiocytoma is largely a high-grade sarcoma. Rarely, well-differentiated sarcomas have been reported (15).

The results of immunohistochemical studies have varied. Some have suggested a more macrophage differentiation of the tumors, but others have not (22,25). Several electron microscopic studies have shown histiocytic and fibroblastic differentiation (13,19,21). Ghandur-Mnaymneh et al. (13) demonstrated cells that had both fibroblastic and histiocytic differentiation, and Shapiro (21) was able to demonstrate cells that had myofibroblastic differentiation.

Cytologic Findings. The cytologic features of a fine-needle aspiration (FNA) biopsy specimen of primary malignant fibrous histiocytoma of bone closely parallel those seen in soft tissue (8,24). Most tumors are high grade, with smears containing an admixture of atypical polygonal and spindled fibroblastic cells with a single, dense nucleus and large binucleated or multinucleated bizarre giant cells (fig. 7-11). The giant cells have abundant foamy or vacuolated cytoplasm that may contain phagocytosed cell debris or pigment. Tumor cell nuclei are highly variable in size and shape, and have a coarse chromatin pattern and prominent nucleoli. Mitotic figures, including atypical ones, are frequent. There may be a prominent component of benign-appearing osteoclasts. Because malignant

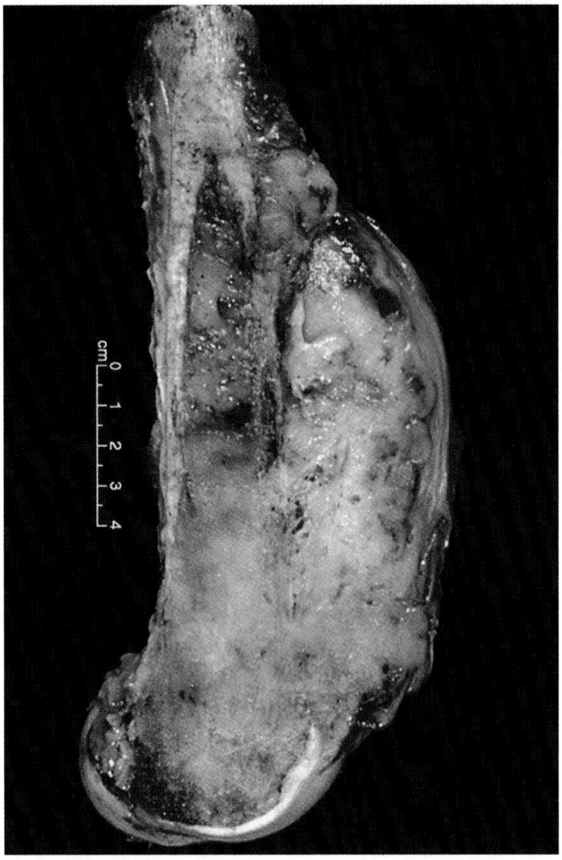

Figure 7-7

MALIGNANT FIBROUS HISTIOCYTOMA

This fleshy tumor extends to the end of the bone, with extensive cortical destruction. The tumor has yellow areas which represent foam cells.

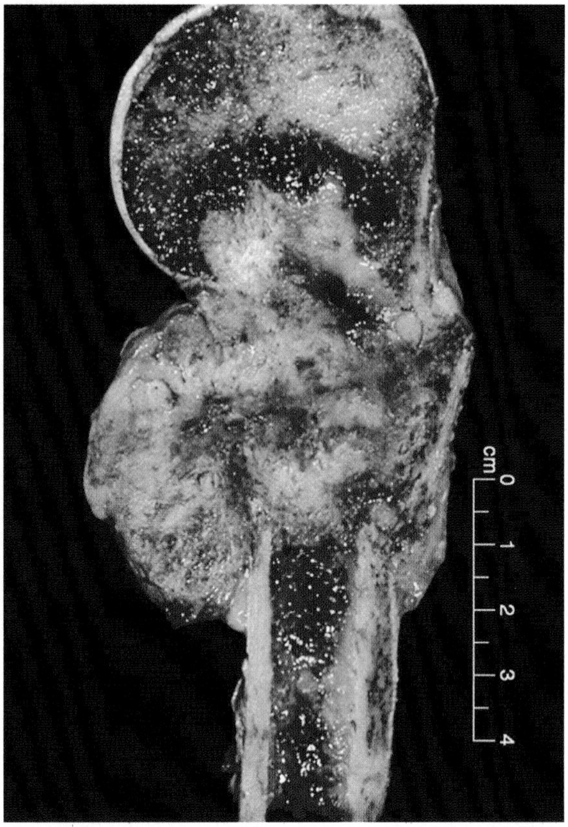

Figure 7-8

MALIGNANT FIBROUS HISTIOCYTOMA

This patient received preoperative chemotherapy, followed by surgery. Grossly and microscopically, the tumor was almost entirely viable.

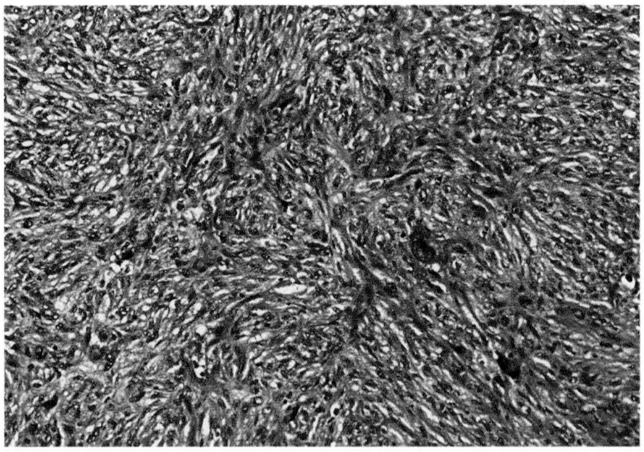

Figure 7-9

MALIGNANT FIBROUS HISTIOCYTOMA

Cytologically malignant spindle cells are arranged in a storiform growth pattern.

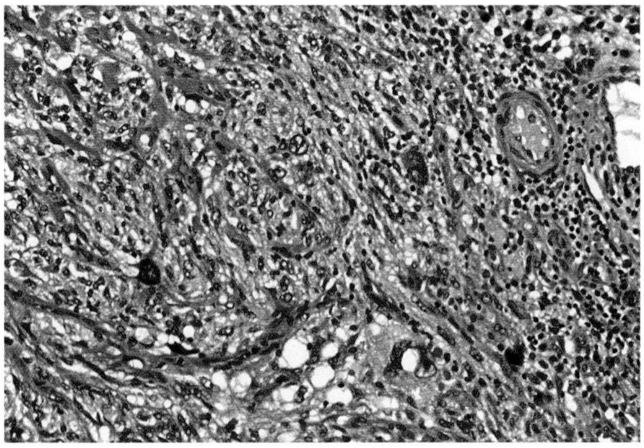

Figure 7-10

MALIGNANT FIBROUS HISTIOCYTOMA

Pleomorphic histiocytic cells with vesicular nuclei, hemosiderin, and a cluster of lymphocytes are within a malignant fibrous histiocytoma arising in the tibia of a 55-year-old woman.

fibrous histiocytoma is a diagnosis of exclusion, a descriptive FNA diagnosis of high-grade spindled and pleomorphic sarcoma is preferred.

Differential Diagnosis. Because of the pleomorphism of the nuclei, the diagnosis of malignancy is usually straightforward. In older patients, metastatic sarcomatoid carcinoma has to be ruled out. Careful clinical examination and the results of immunostaining are helpful in this regard. The distinction between malignant fibrous histiocytoma and fibroblastic osteosarcoma may be arbitrary. Fibrosarcomas do not have the pronounced pleomorphism seen in malignant fibrous histiocytomas. A malignant lymphoma with spindled cells may be mistaken for malignant fibrous histiocytoma. Diffuse permeation of the bone marrow, with intact bony trabeculae, favors the diagnosis of malignant lymphoma. When multicentric malignant fibrous histiocytoma is suspected, malignant lymphoma should be excluded with appropriate immunoperoxidase stains.

Treatment and Prognosis. Malignant fibrous histiocytoma behaves like a high-grade sarcoma. The reported 5-year survival rates have ranged from 34 percent (9) to 53 percent (15). Modern chemotherapy has reportedly improved prognosis, and a 7-year survival rate of 69 percent has been reported (7). In the series of Bacci et al. (7), patients with tumors that had necrosis after chemotherapy fared better than those whose tumors responded poorly. The response to chemotherapy is not as good as with osteosarcoma. According to Naka et al. (18), the difference in prognosis between malignant fibrous histiocytoma and malignant fibrous histiocytoma-like osteosarcoma is not statistically significant. Patients with malignant fibrous histiocytoma of bone are now treated as if they had osteosarcoma.

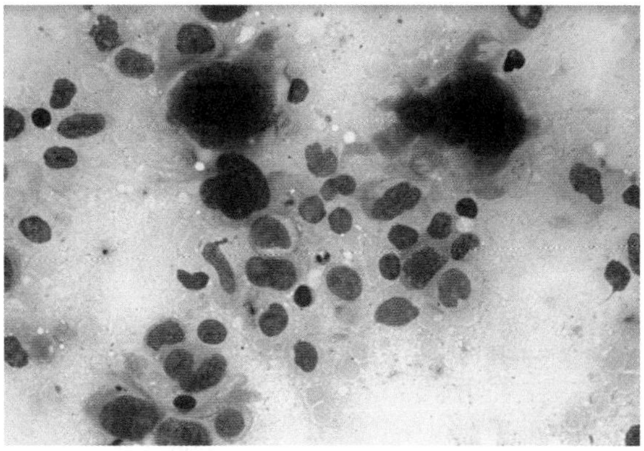

Figure 7-11

MALIGNANT FIBROUS HISTIOCYTOMA

Cellular aspirate with markedly pleomorphic nuclei.

REFERENCES

Benign Fibrous Histiocytoma

1. Bertoni F, Calderoni P, Bacchini P, et al. Benign fibrous histiocytoma of bone. J Bone Joint Surg Am 1986;68:1225–30.
2. Bertoni F, Capanna R, Calderoni P, Bacchini P. Case report 223. Benign fibrous histiocytoma. Skeletal Radiol 1983;9:215–7.
3. Clarke BE, Xipell JM, Thomas DP. Benign fibrous histiocytoma of bone. Am J Surg Pathol 1985;9:806–15.
4. Fechner RE, Mills SE. Tumors of the bones and joints. Atlas of Tumor Pathology, 3rd Series, Fascicle 8. Washington, DC: Armed Forces Institute of Pathology; 1993:161–73.
5. Matsuno T. Benign fibrous histiocytoma involving the ends of long bone. Skeletal Radiol 1990;19:561–6.
6. Saito R, Caines MJ. Atypical fibrous histiocytoma of the humerus: a light and electron microscopic study. Am J Clin Pathol 1977;68:409–15.

Malignant Fibrous Histiocytoma

7. Bacci G, Picci P, Mercuri M, Bertoni F, Ferrari S. Neoadjuvant chemotherapy for high grade malignant fibrous histiocytoma of bone. Clin Orthop 1998;346:178–89.
8. Berardo MD, Powers CN, Wakely PE Jr, Almeida MO, Frable WJ. Fine-needle aspiration cytopathology of malignant fibrous histiocytoma. Cancer 1997;81:228–37.

9. Capanna R, Bertoni F, Bacchini P, Bacci G, Guerra A, Campanacci M. Malignant fibrous histiocytoma of bone. The experience at the Rizzoli Institute: report of 90 cases. Cancer 1984;54:177–87.
10. Dahlin DC, Unni KK, Matsuno T. Malignant (fibrous) histiocytoma of bone—fact or fancy? Cancer 1977;39:1508–16.
11. Fletcher CD. Malignant fibrous histiocytoma? Histopathology 1987;11:433–7.
12. Frierson HF Jr, Fechner RE, Stallings RG, Wang GJ. Malignant fibrous histiocytoma in bone infarct. Association with sickle cell trait and alcohol abuse. Cancer 1987;59:496–500.
13. Ghandur-Mnaymneh L, Zych G, Mnaymneh W. Primary malignant fibrous histiocytoma of bone: report of six cases with ultrastructural study and analysis of the literature. Cancer 1982;49:698–707.
14. Haag M, Adler CP. Malignant fibrous histiocytoma in association with hip replacement. J Bone Joint Surg Br 1989;71:701.
15. Huvos AG, Heilweil M, Bretsky SS. The pathology of malignant fibrous histiocytoma of bone. A study of 130 patients. Am J Surg Pathol 1985;9:853–71.
16. Lindeman G, McKay MJ, Taubman KL, Bilous AM. Malignant fibrous histiocytoma developing in bone 44 years after shrapnel trauma. Cancer 1990;66:2229–32.
17. Mirra JM, Bullough PG, Marcove RC, Jacobs B, Huvos AG. Malignant fibrous histiocytoma and osteosarcoma in association with bone infarcts; report of four cases, two in caisson workers. J Bone Joint Surg Am 1974;56:932–40.
18. Naka T, Fukuda T, Shinohara N, Iwamoto Y, Sugioka Y, Tsuneyoshi M. Osteosarcoma versus malignant fibrous histiocytoma of bone in patients older than 40 years. A clinicopathologic and immunohistochemical analysis with special reference to malignant fibrous histiocytoma-like osteosarcoma. Cancer 1995;76:972–84.
19. Nakashima Y, Morishita S, Kotoura Y, et al. Malignant fibrous histiocytoma of bone. A review of 13 cases and an ultrastructural study. Cancer 1985;55:2804–11.
20. Ozzello L, Stout AP, Murray MR. Cultural characteristics of malignant histiocytomas and fibrous xanthomas. Cancer 1963;16:331-44.
21. Shapiro F. Malignant fibrous histiocytoma of bone: an ultrastructural study. Ultrastruct Pathol 1981;2:33–42.
22. Strauchen JA, Dimitriu-Bona A. Malignant fibrous histiocytoma. Expression of monocyte/macrophage differentiation antigens detected with monoclonal antibodies. Am J Pathol 1986;124:303–9.
23. Troop JK, Mallory TH, Fisher DA, Vaughn BK. Malignant fibrous histiocytoma after total hip arthroplasty. A case report. Clin Orthop 1990;253:297–300.
24. Walaas L, Angervall L, Hagmar B, Save-Soderbergh J. A correlative cytologic and histologic study of malignant fibrous histiocytoma: an analysis of 40 cases examined by fine-needle aspiration cytology. Diagn Cytopathol 1986;2:46–54.
25. Wood GS, Beckstead JH, Turner RR, Hendrickson MR, Kempson RL, Warnke RA. Malignant fibrous histiocytoma tumor cells resemble fibroblasts. Am J Surg Pathol 1986;10:323–35.

8 SMALL CELL MALIGNANCIES

EWING'S SARCOMA

Definition. Ewing's sarcoma is a highly malignant neoplasm composed of small, round, rather uniform cells that do not form matrix.

General Features. In 1921, Ewing (24) described the small cell sarcoma of bone that now bears his name. Since his description of a diffuse endothelioma, the histogenesis of this highly lethal neoplasm has been debated. Because of the undifferentiated appearance of the tumor cells, it seems reasonable to consider that the cell of origin is an undifferentiated mesenchymal cell. Immunohistochemical studies and, more importantly, cytogenetic studies have established that the so-called primitive neuroectodermal tumor (PNET) is within the spectrum of Ewing's sarcoma and Ewing's sarcoma cells are of neuroectodermal derivation. It is now well recognized that Ewing's sarcoma may occur as a primary tumor in soft tissues (1).

Ewing's sarcoma is the fourth most common primary neoplasm of bone, exceeded in incidence only by myeloma, osteosarcoma, and chondrosarcoma. The Mayo Clinic series includes 578 cases (8.6 percent of all malignant tumors) (fig. 8-1).

Clinical Features. There is a definite male predilection. Children and adolescents are usually affected, a younger population than with any other primary bone tumor. About 75 percent of the patients with Ewing's sarcoma are in the first two decades of life. Of the cases included in the Mayo Clinic files, only 8 patients were in the sixth decade of life. In the Intergroup Ewing's Sarcoma Study group, the youngest patient was 5 months old and about 9 percent were in the first 5 years of life (43). Maygarden et al. (58) found 19 patients younger than 3 years; they constituted 2.6 percent of all cases in the Intergroup Study.

Patients present with pain, with or without swelling. Pathologic fracture is rare. Some patients present with fever associated with laboratory findings of anemia, leukocytosis, and increased erythrocyte sedimentation rate, all of which suggest infection.

Sites. Any portion of the skeleton may be involved. However, it is unusual for Ewing's sarcoma to occur in the small bones of the hands and feet. About 60 percent of the tumors are in the pelvic girdle and lower extremities. Kissane et al. (43) found that the femur was the most common site, followed by the ilium and fibula.

Any portion of a long tubular bone may be affected. Although the metaphysis is involved most commonly, Ewing's sarcoma involves the shaft more often than do most other primary neoplasms. At presentation, multiple skeletal sites may be involved. This is considered a manifestation of metastases.

Radiographic Findings. Ewing's sarcoma tends to involve a large portion of the bone. In long bones, the metaphysis and diaphysis are involved preferentially. The tumor presents as a permeative destructive process with poorly defined margins. As the tumor permeates the cortex, it incites periosteal new bone formation. This new bone usually forms as concentric layers, producing an onionskin appearance (fig. 8-2). However, spiculated bone, as seen in osteosarcoma, may also be present. Although Ewing's sarcoma does not produce a matrix, reactive new bone formation may be present within the lesion. This appearance of a mixture of lysis and sclerosis, especially in conjunction with spiculated periosteal new bone, makes it virtually impossible to distinguish between Ewing's sarcoma and osteosarcoma (fig. 8-3).

Radiographically, there may be a relatively well-demarcated geographic area of destruction, with little or no periosteal new bone formation, suggesting a benign lesion (fig. 8-4), or the cortex may appear thickened because of the periosteal new bone. Occasionally, medullary involvement is slight, and much of the tumor is in the soft tissues. This soft tissue mass may appear to invade the cortex, producing the rather typical appearance of saucerization (fig. 8-5).

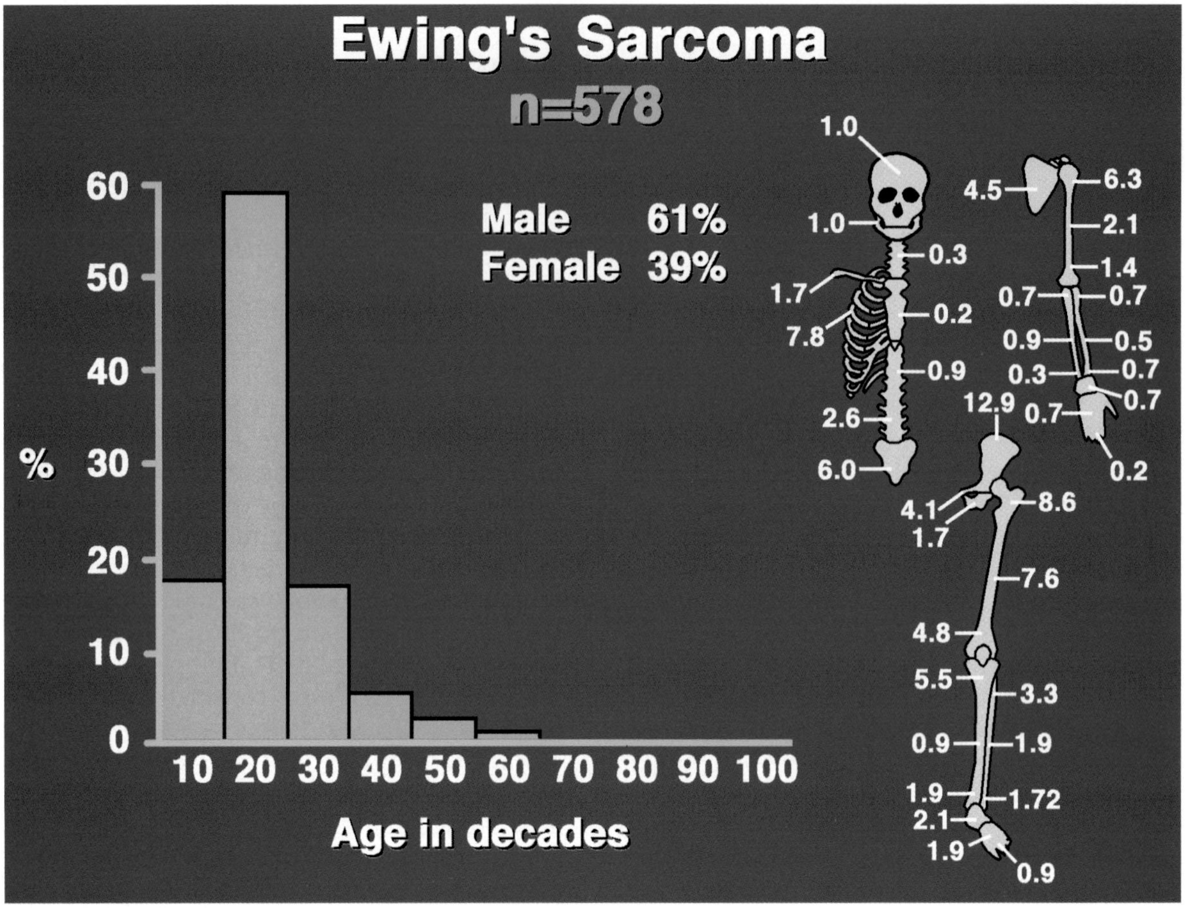

Figure 8-1

EWING'S SARCOMA

Distribution of Ewing's sarcoma by the age and sex of the patient and the site of the lesion.

Computerized tomography (CT) helps define the extent of the lesion, especially the soft tissue involvement. With magnetic resonance imaging (MRI), Ewing's sarcoma tends to have low signal intensity on T_1-weighted images, which is in contrast with the high signal intensity of bone marrow (fig. 8-6). On T_2-weighted images, the tumor is hyperintense in comparison to skeletal muscle (23). Sites involved by Ewing's sarcoma tend to be hot on radionuclide bone scans, an excellent technique for ruling out skeletal metastasis.

Gross Findings. Ewing's tumor is a soft, white (fish-flesh) mass of almost liquid consistency (fig. 8-7). When the tumor is sectioned, the contents may run like pus, and this may lead to a mistaken diagnosis of osteomyelitis. Geographic or punctate areas of necrosis may be prominent. The cortex is often thickened, and fleshy tumor is seen between layers of thickened periosteum. In the modern era, almost all patients receive preoperative chemotherapy, radiotherapy, or both before surgical resection. In a resected specimen, the area of the tumor may be fibrotic or scarred (fig. 8-8). Occasionally, the area is cystic, containing liquid necrotic debris.

Microscopic Findings. The essential microscopic finding is a proliferation of small, round, uniform cells and no matrix production. The Intergroup Ewing's Sarcoma Study divided the growth pattern of this tumor into three types based on histologic findings: 1) diffuse: broad fields of tumor without topographic features; 2) lobular: islands of tumor cells separated by

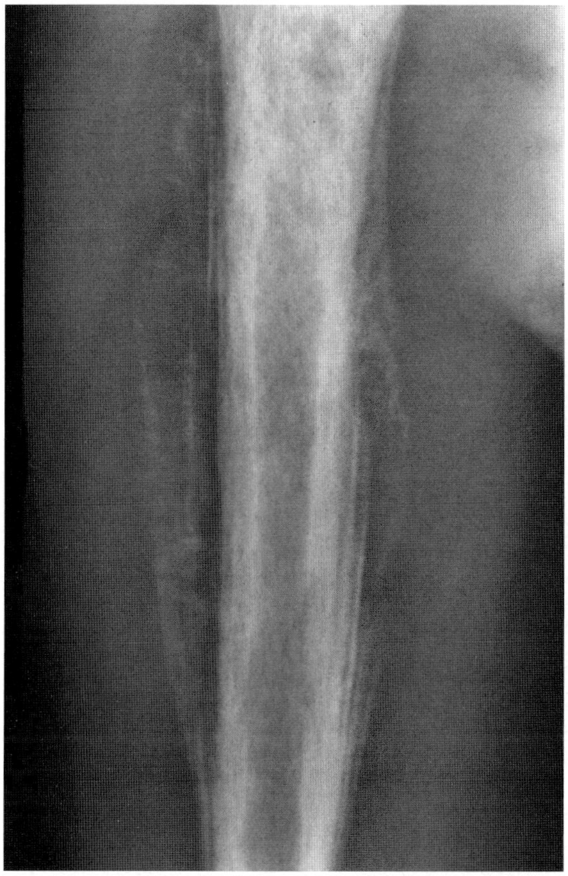

Figure 8-2

EWING'S SARCOMA

Ewing's sarcoma involving the proximal humerus of a 15-year-old boy. Pronounced periosteal new bone formation produces an onionskin appearance. (Fig. 18-3 from Unni KK. Dahlin's bone tumors: general aspects and data on 11,087 cases, 5th ed. Philadelphia: Lippincott-Raven; 1996:251. By permission of Mayo Foundation.)

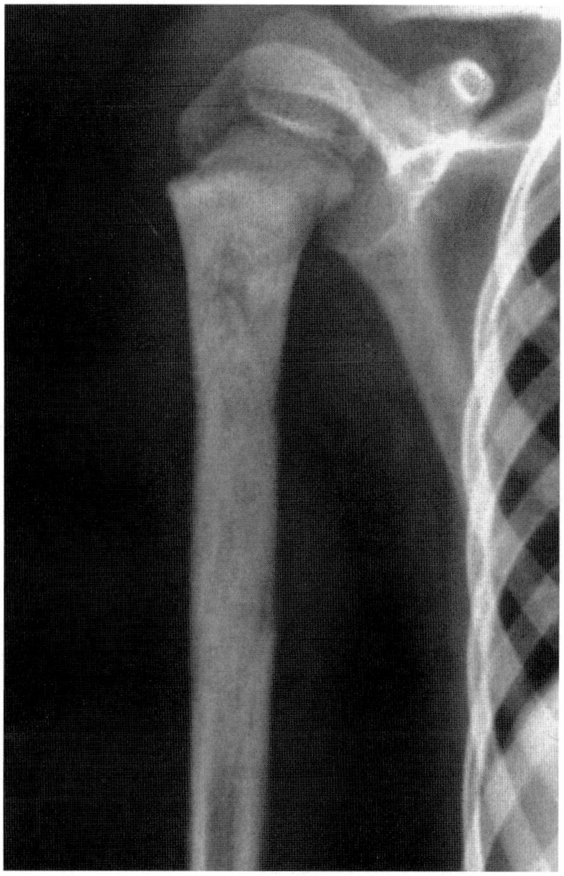

Figure 8-3

EWING'S SARCOMA

Occasionally, Ewing's sarcoma has a sclerotic appearance, as in this tumor involving the proximal humerus of a 7-year-old boy. Almost all of the proximal humerus is involved by extensive sclerosis. (Fig. 18-6 from Unni KK. Dahlin's bone tumors: general aspects and data on 11,087 cases, 5th ed. Philadelphia: Lippincott-Raven; 1996:252. By permission of Mayo Foundation.)

fibrous septa; and 3) filagree: delicate bicellular anastomosing strands separated by fibrovascular stroma (43).

In our experience, Ewing's sarcoma most often grows in a diffuse or sheet-like pattern in the bone marrow and may assume lobular and filagree patterns when it invades soft tissues (fig. 8-9). The tumor cells have clear cytoplasm without well-defined cytoplasmic boundaries, creating the impression of a sea of cytoplasm peppered with almost uniformly placed nuclei. The nuclei are round or slightly oval, but clear-cut spindling (not caused by crushing during biopsy) is unacceptable for Ewing's sarcoma. The nuclei have finely dispersed chromatin and one or two indistinct nucleoli (fig. 8-10). Mitotic activity is variable (fig. 8-11). Llombart-Bosch et al. (50) pointed out the presence of very dense nuclei in a small proportion of cells, which they considered to be degenerated.

Necrosis may be slight or extensive; viable tumor may be arranged in a perivascular pattern. Nuclear dust may encrust vessels, producing the Azzopardi phenomenon, best known with small cell carcinoma of the lung.

Dahlin et al. (13) reported that just over 10 percent of Ewing's sarcomas had larger, more pleomorphic cells (fig. 8-12). The nuclei are more

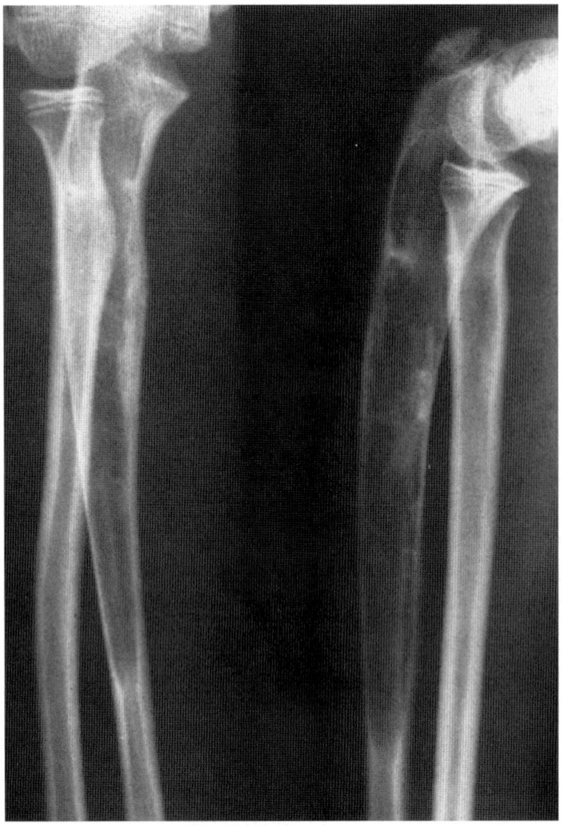

Figure 8-4

EWING'S SARCOMA

This is an unusual radiographic appearance of Ewing's sarcoma because the neoplasm involves almost half of the length of the ulna, commences at the joint margin, and does not breach the cortex. These features are reminiscent of fibrous dysplasia.

irregular than those seen in the classic lesion, and mitotic activity is more pronounced as well. In all other respects, this large cell or atypical form of Ewing's sarcoma) is similar to typical Ewing's sarcoma (62).

Since the original description by Ewing, it has been recognized that the tumor may contain rosettes, which is a feature considered typical of primitive neural tumors. Indeed, a small subset of Ewing's sarcoma has a lobulated growth pattern, prominent rosettes, and even a fibrillary background, features that strongly suggest neural differentiation (fig. 8-13). The term *primitive neuroectodermal tumor (PNET)* has been applied to this lesion. Immunohistochemical and cytogenetic studies have confirmed that Ewing's sarcoma may be derived from neuroectoderm and that classic Ewing's sarcoma, large cell Ewing's sarcoma, and PNET (including the so-called Askin's tumor [6]) all belong to the same family but have different degrees of differentiation.

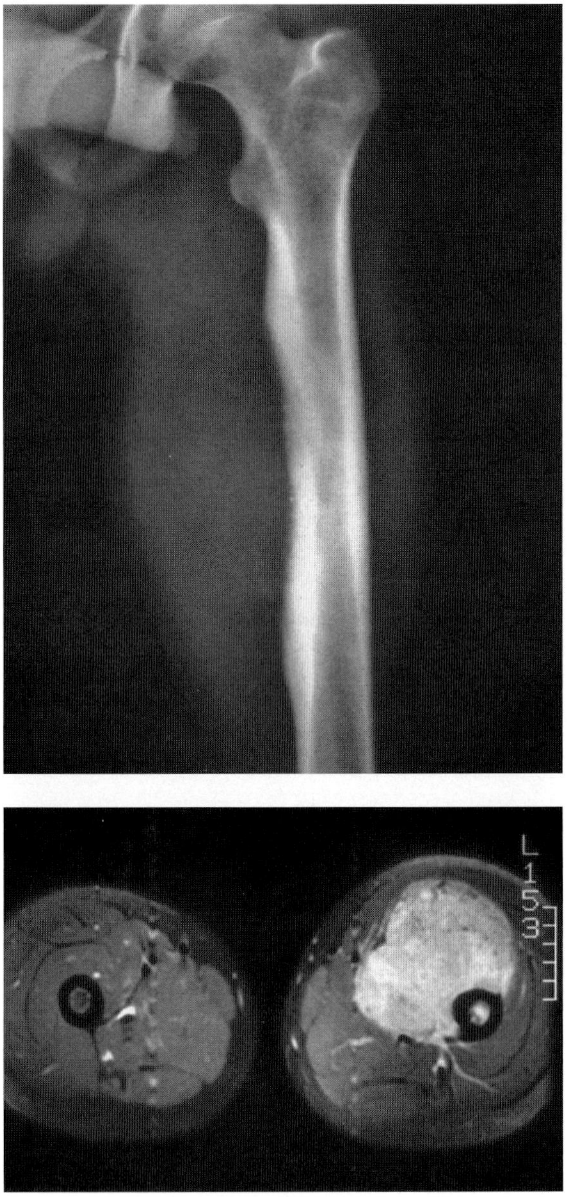

Figure 8-5

EWING'S SARCOMA

Top: Radiograph of the left femur showing a diaphyseal lesion. Saucerization of the medial cortex is associated with cortical thickening proximally and distally.

Bottom: Magnetic resonance image (MRI) demonstrates the true extent of the soft tissue mass, which cannot be appreciated on the radiograph. (Courtesy of Dr. R. Shishido, San Diego, CA.)

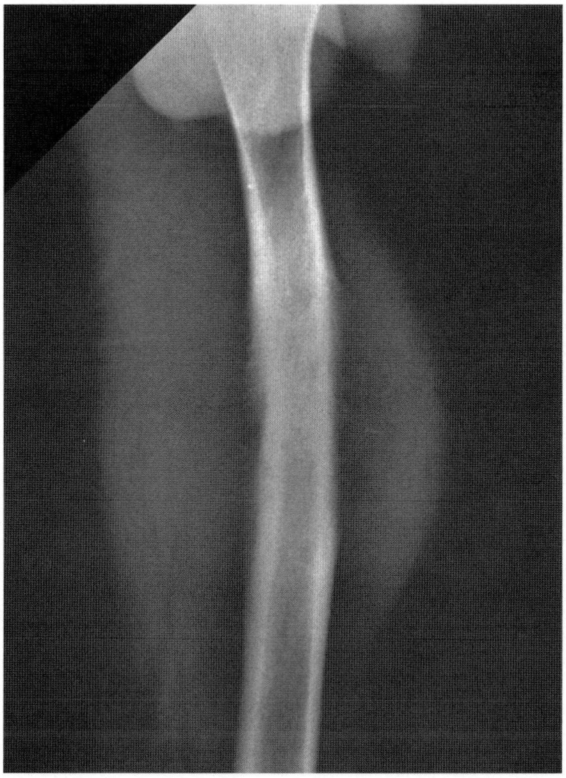

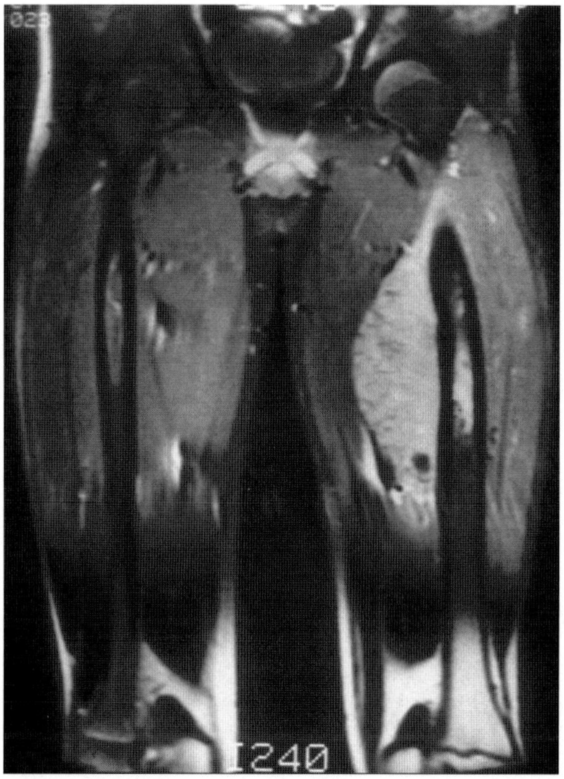

Figure 8-6

EWING'S SARCOMA

Left: Radiograph of a lesion involving the mid-shaft of the left femur in a 15-year-old girl. It shows cortical destruction and periosteal reaction.

Right: Gadolinium-enhanced T_1-weighted MRI highlights the extent of intraosseous involvement and also clearly demonstrates a large soft tissue mass.

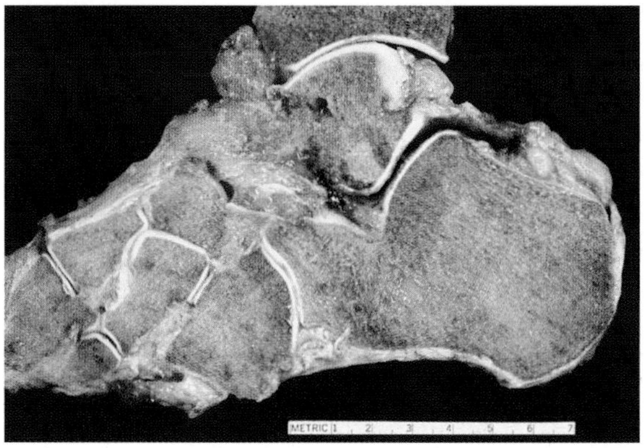

Figure 8-7

EWING'S SARCOMA

This tan-gray tumor extensively involves the foot of a 16-year-old boy. It occupies the entire talus and has invaded all the surrounding joint spaces and navicular bone.

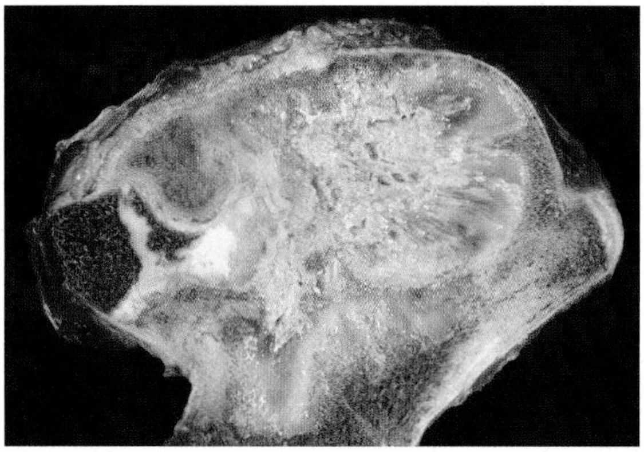

Figure 8-8

EWING'S SARCOMA

The patient received chemotherapy before resection of this tumor involving the left ilium. The yellow-gray mass contained no histologic evidence of viable tumor.

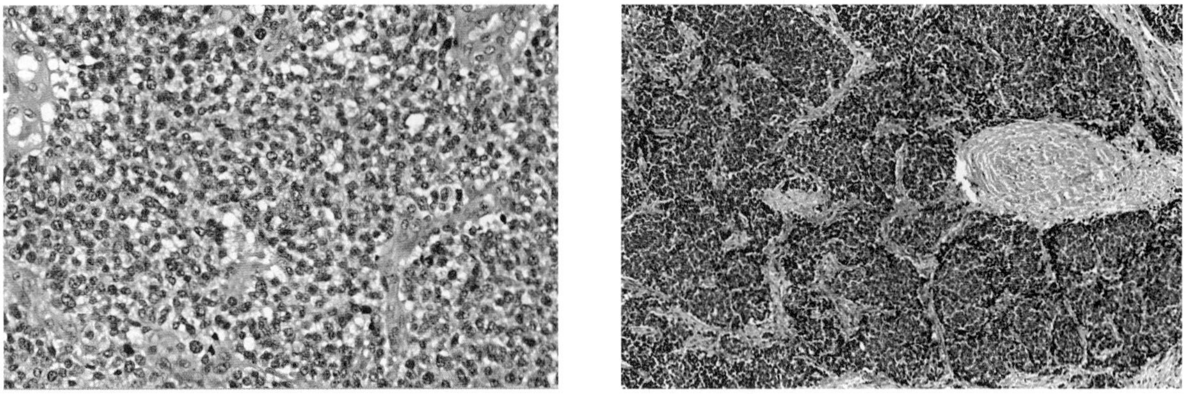

Figure 8-9

EWING'S SARCOMA

Left: Diffuse sheets of uniform small round cells.
Right: A lobulated growth pattern in a tumor invading surrounding soft tissue.

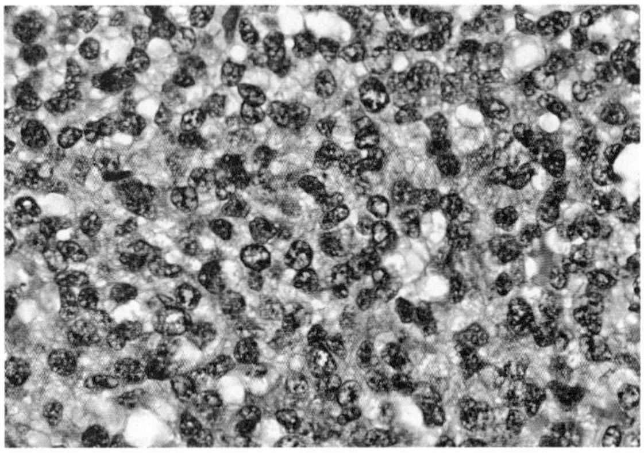

Figure 8-10

EWING'S SARCOMA

This typical histologic specimen shows round to oval nuclei, finely dispersed nuclear chromatin, and indistinct eosinophilic cytoplasm.

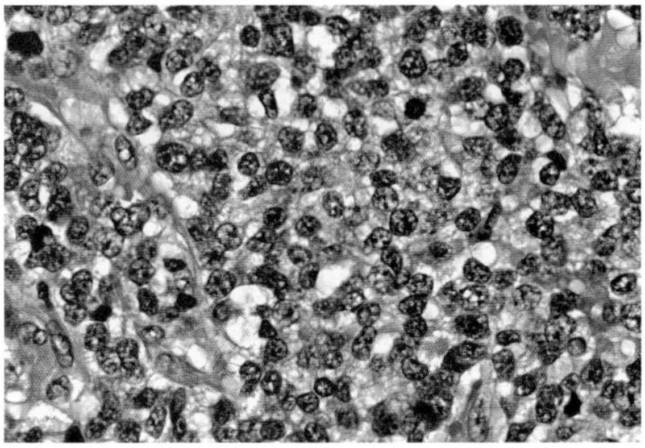

Figure 8-11

EWING'S SARCOMA

Although scattered mitotic figures are seen, mitotic activity generally is low to moderate.

Histologic grading is not practical because of the uniform appearance from tumor to tumor. All small cell sarcomas are high-grade tumors (grade 4 of 4).

Open biopsies are rarely necessary to confirm the diagnosis of Ewing's sarcoma. If the findings on fine-needle aspiration cytology are not diagnostic, open biopsy is performed and a frozen section must be examined to confirm the presence of viable tumor and to allocate material for all special studies.

Immunohistochemical Findings. Since Schajowicz (76) showed that the periodic acid–Schiff (PAS) stain was useful in differentiating Ewing's sarcoma from malignant lymphoma, special stains have been important in the work-up of small round cell tumors of bone. The PAS stain is positive in Ewing's sarcoma but usually negative in malignant lymphoma, whereas a reticulin stain shows a network of fibers in malignant lymphoma but not in Ewing's sarcoma.

The characteristic 11;22 translocation of Ewing's sarcoma produces a protein (MIC-2) that can be identified with immunoperoxidase stains (fig. 8-14). Initially, several commercially available antibodies were considered specific and

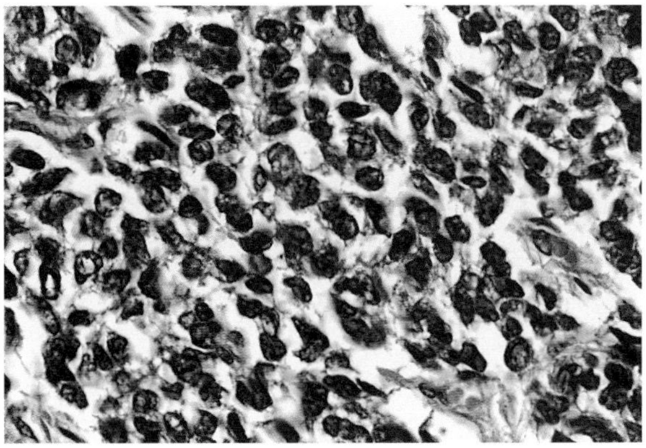

Figure 8-12

EWING'S SARCOMA

Atypical (large cell) Ewing's sarcoma contains larger, more irregularly shaped nuclei than those of typical Ewing's sarcoma.

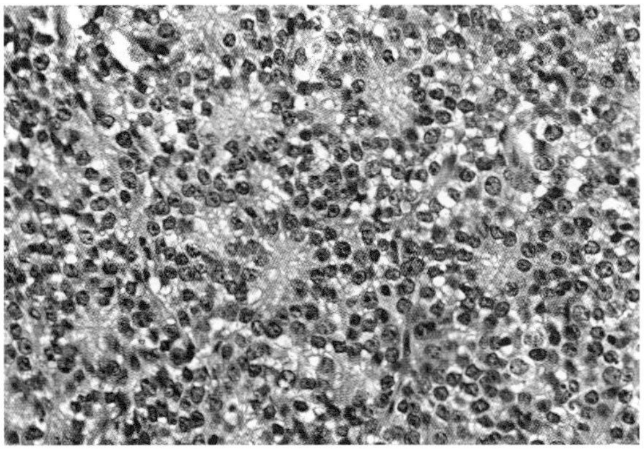

Figure 8-13

EWING'S SARCOMA

Prominent rosette formation occurs throughout the tumor.

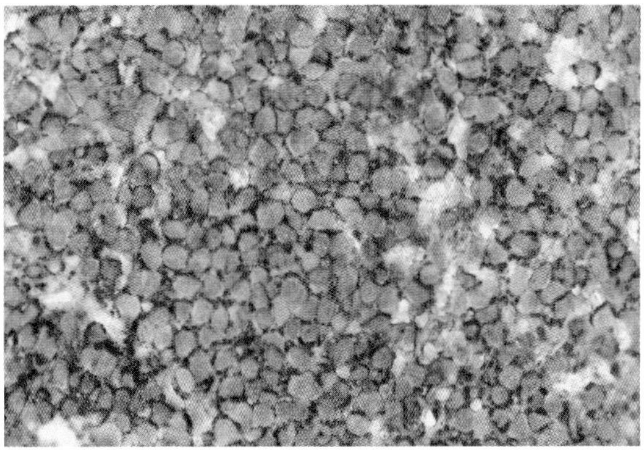

Figure 8-14

EWING'S SARCOMA

The tumor cells show diffuse immunoreactivity for CD99.

sensitive for diagnosing Ewing's sarcoma. However, further studies have shown that although MIC-2 staining is quite sensitive (a small cell malignancy in which MIC-2 is negative is likely not Ewing's tumor), it is not specific (51). Hence, it is important to use a panel of immunoperoxidase stains, especially to rule out lymphoma (51). Several studies have reported positive results with epithelial markers in Ewing's sarcoma (32,94).

Ultrastructural Findings. Ultrastructural findings are notable for lack of differentiation. Many tumors have large amounts of glycogen in the cytoplasm (26). Intermediate filaments may be seen. Occasionally, they are organized as tonofilaments.

Cytologic Findings. Fine-needle aspiration (FNA) biopsy specimens of primary Ewing's sarcoma/pPNET of bone are typically highly cellular. Two main cell types can be recognized in classic cases of Ewing's sarcoma. The predominant population consists of relatively uniform cells with sparse, poorly defined cytoplasm and rounded, uniform nuclei containing finely dispersed chromatin and inconspicuous nucleoli. Less frequent are scattered, smaller cells with hyperchromatic, dense nuclei (fig. 8-15) (12,28,73,101). In addition, occasional cells with abundant glycogen and finely vacuolated cytoplasm are seen.

Atypical variants of Ewing's sarcoma/pPNET have a uniform population of somewhat larger cells with more well-developed cytoplasm, enlarged nuclei with more irregular chromatin, and clearly discernable nucleoli. In these cases, mitotic figures are often seen. Although rosette-like arrangements of tumor cells have been described in aspirates of PNET, its distinction from classic Ewing's sarcoma is usually impossible with FNA cytology.

Immunocytochemistry is useful in confirming the diagnosis of Ewing's sarcoma and particularly helpful in differentiating it from lymphoma. The limited diagnostic value of MIC-2 antigen immunoreactivity must be noted because it may occur in other small cell malignancies besides Ewing's sarcoma (11).

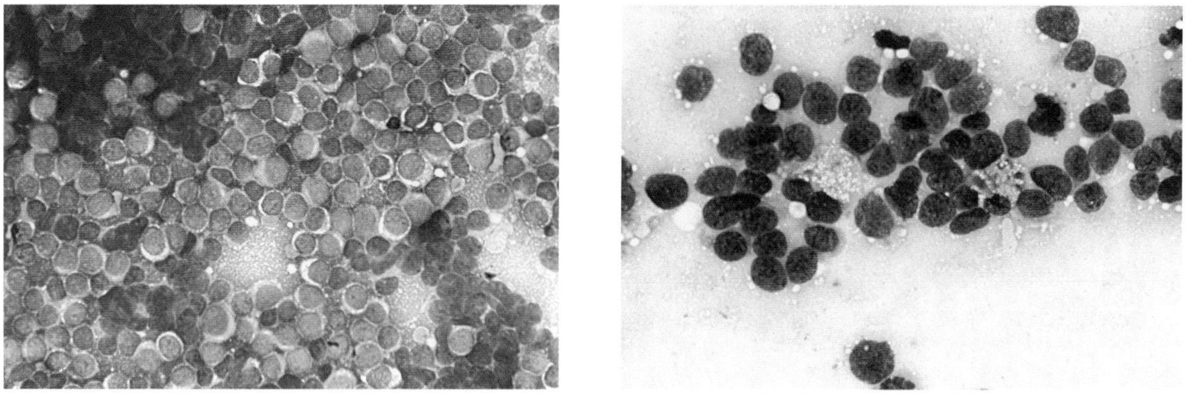

Figure 8-15

EWING'S SARCOMA

Highly cellular aspirates from two bone tumors of the Ewing's sarcoma/primitive neuroectodermal tumor (PNET) family. The tumor cells are characterized by relatively uniform nuclei with finely dispersed chromatin and inconspicuous nucleoli. Occasional cells have more abundant, vacuolated cytoplasm. Scattered, smaller, hyperchromatic nuclei are also typically seen.

Genetics and Other Special Techniques. Cytogenetic analysis has provided insight into the histopathogenesis of several bone and soft tissue tumors for which the derivation was previously unknown. Translocations, or exchange of chromosomal material between two or more homologous chromosomes, are frequently encountered as tumor-specific anomalies in mesenchymal neoplasms. These translocations are often present as the sole cytogenetic abnormality and are therefore likely to be etiologic. Ewing's sarcoma was the first sarcoma to be defined by a specific chromosomal translocation, t(11;22)(q24;q12) (7,91).

Ewing's sarcoma most often arises within the bones of children or adolescents. Primary soft tissue Ewing's sarcoma is much less frequent and appears more closely related pathologically to peripheral (p)PNET. The latter demonstrates more definite neural features, and although it may arise in bone, it is located most often in deep soft tissues. Ewing's sarcoma (a tumor of unknown histopathogenesis) shares a functionally identical chromosomal rearrangement, t(11;22)(q24;q12) (fig. 8-16), with pPNET, indicating a common mechanism of oncogenesis and a similar tissue of origin (neural) for these distinct clinicopathologic entities (99).

The 11;22 translocation, or variants thereof, is detectable cytogenetically or by molecular approaches in more than 95 percent of Ewing's sarcomas and pPNETs (10). As a consequence of the 11;22 translocation, the 5' portion of the *EWS* gene from 22q12 is fused to the 3' portion of the *FLI1* gene (a member of the E-twenty-six specific [ETS] family of transcription factors) from 11q24. The fusion results in the formation of a tumor-specific chimeric RNA that encodes a novel transcription factor which retains ETS domain-specific DNA binding capability in combination with *EWS* transactivational properties (17,18).

In some cases of Ewing's sarcoma/pPNET, the 11;22 translocation involves a third chromosome ("complex translocation") such as 4q21, 5q31, 6p21, 7q12, 10p11.2, 12q14, 14q11, or 18p23, or even two additional chromosomes (75). In other cases, rearrangement of 22q12 occurs with a chromosomal partner other than 11q24. These are referred to as "cytogenetic variant translocations." An example is the 21;22 translocation [t(11;22)(q22;q12)] that fuses *EWS* with another ETS family member, *ERG* (localized to 21q22), and is seen in approximately 5 percent of Ewing's sarcomas/pPNETs (83,106). At least six variant translocations (including *EWS/ERG*) have been defined cytogenetically and molecularly (Table 8-1) (39,54,83).

Less commonly, the 11;22 translocation and known variant translocations of Ewing's sarcoma and pPNET are cryptic or masked, requiring other technical approaches such as fluorescence in situ hybridization (FISH) or reverse transcriptase polymerase chain reaction (RT-PCR) analysis for detection. FISH analysis, a highly sensitive and

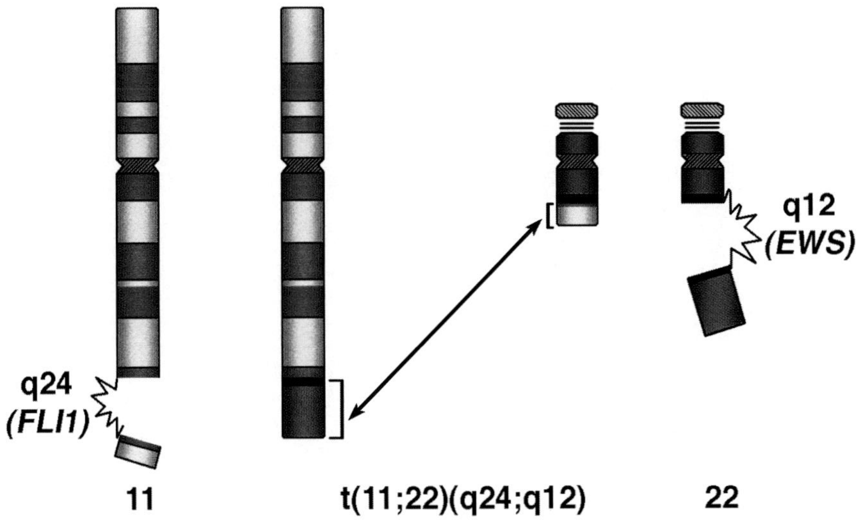

Figure 8-16

11;22 TRANSLOCATION IN EWING'S SARCOMA/pPNET

Schematic illustration of the 11;22 translocation [t(11;22)(q24;q12)].

Table 8-1

CHARACTERISTIC AND VARIANT CYTOGENETIC TRANSLOCATIONS AND ASSOCIATED FUSION GENES, AND THE RELATIVE FREQUENCY IN EWING'S SARCOMA/pPNET[a]

Translocation	Fusion Gene	Estimated Prevalence (%)	Original References
t(11;22)(q24;q12)	*EWS/FLI1*	95	18
t(21;22)(q22;q12)	*EWS/ERG*	5	83,106
t(7;22)(p22;q12)	*EWS/ETV1*	<1	39
t(17;22)(q21;q12)	*EWS/EIAF*	<1	41,92
t(2;22)(q33;q12)	*EWS/FEV*	<1	70
inv(22)	*EWS/ZSG*	<1	54
t(16;21)(p11;q22)	*FUS/ERG*	<1	80

[a]pPNET = peripheral primitive neuroectodermal tumor.

reliable technique, may be performed on chromosomal metaphase cells or interphase cells (fig. 8-17). Interphase FISH, optimally performed on cell suspensions or cytologic touch preparations of fresh or frozen tumor but also adaptable to paraffin-embedded tissue, is a rapid and effective alternative to RT-PCR (46). The 11;22 translocation or variant translocations can be visualized in interphase cells by the use of site-specific probes labeled with fluorescent dyes. Typically, different colored dyes linked with translocation breakpoint "flanking" or translocation breakpoint "spanning" cosmid probes, or larger human genomic DNA fragments propagated as yeast artificial chromosomes (YACs) or bacterial artificial chromosomes (BACs), are used to assess the presence of the translocation (20,21, 45,59–61,88). Some investigators, however, have used whole chromosome "painting" probes that bind to sequences along the length of chromosomes 11 and 22 to detect a rearrangement (84).

An unbalanced translocation, der(16)t(1;16), with variable breaks on both chromosomes, is considered the most common secondary structural abnormality in Ewing's sarcoma/pPNET (fig. 8-18) (22). The result of the unbalanced 1;16 translocation is the generation of one or two der(16), leading to either partial trisomy 1q or

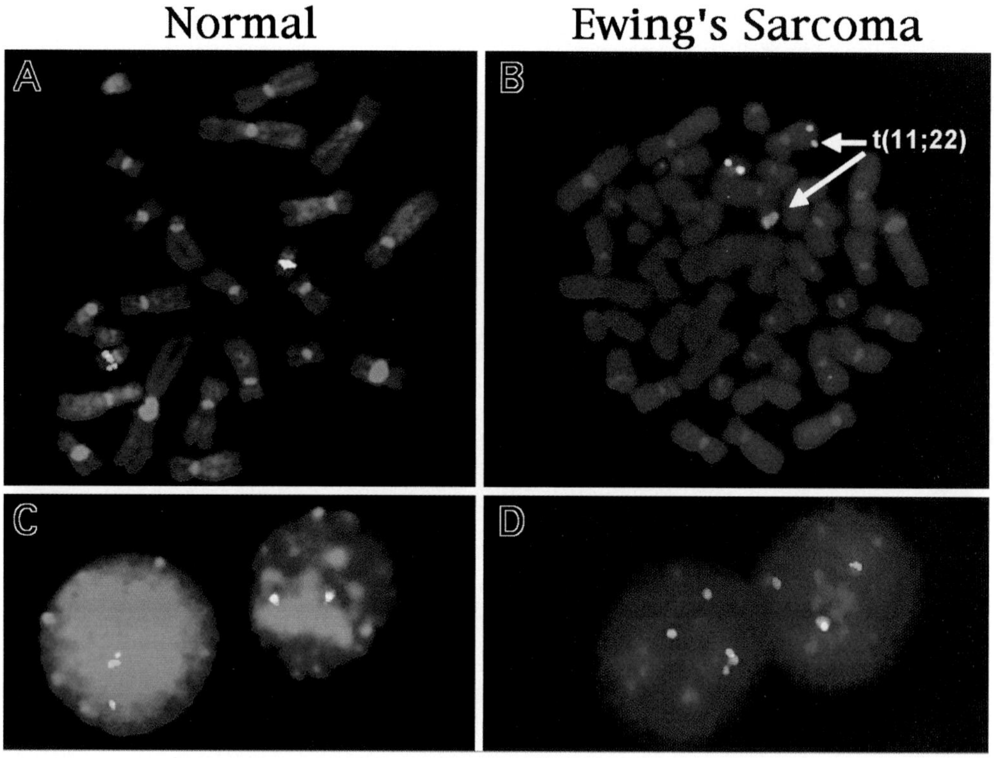

Figure 8-17

FLUORESCENCE IN SITU HYBRIDIZATION (FISH) IN EWING'S SARCOMA

A: Bicolor FISH studies performed on normal control metaphase cells with chromosomal probes proximal and distal to the 22q12 translocation breakpoint (red and green signals, respectively) show localization of the two probes to the normal chromosome 22 homologues.

B: FISH performed on Ewing's sarcoma metaphase cells with the 22q12 translocation breakpoint-flanking probe set, described in A, confirms the presence of an 11;22 translocation [one green signal has now translocated to the der(11)].

C: FISH performed on normal control interphase cells with the 22q12 breakpoint-flanking probe set shows two fused red and green signals as expected in normal cells.

D: FISH performed on a Ewing's sarcoma cytologic touch preparation with the 22q12 breakpoint-flanking probe set shows a splitting of one of the fused signal sets, indicating a rearrangement.

partial tetrasomy 1q and monosomy 16 in all cases. Cytogenetic detection of the der(16) has also been described in other malignancies such as leukemia, Wilms' tumor, alveolar rhabdomyosarcoma, and extraskeletal myxoid chondrosarcoma. In Ewing's sarcoma/pPNET, the der(16) is most often present with t(11;22)(q24;q12) (86). A der(16) may also be detected by double-target FISH in interphase nuclei of Ewing's sarcoma (35).

Certain numerical changes are frequent in Ewing's sarcomas/pPNETs. Conventional cytogenetic analysis, FISH, or comparative genomic hybridization studies have revealed extra copies of chromosome 8 in 35 to 55 percent of the tumors examined and extra copies of chromosome 12 in 24 to 33 percent (75). These aneuploidies appear to be independent events acquired in a flexible order during Ewing's sarcoma/pPNET genetic progression (55). Of possible prognostic significance is the observation of a higher frequency of trisomy 8 and trisomy 12 in relapsed tumors than in primary tumors (4,36,55,87); others have suggested that trisomy 8 is not a predictive factor for outcome (34). Deletions or loss of 1p or gain of 1q material (or both), or other secondary structural abnormalities such as loss of 16q, may also have a prognostic effect (associated with an unfavorable outcome in patients with localized disease) (34,36,74,85,87,103).

Ewing's sarcoma/pPNET–specific chromosomal translocations fuse the *EWS* gene (22q12) to a subset of the ETS transcription factor family members, most commonly the *FLI1* gene (11q24) and less frequently genes *ERG* (21q22), *ETV1* (7p22), *E1A-F* (17q21), *FEV* (2q33), or *ZSG* (22q12); in rare cases, the *FUS* gene (16p11) has been shown to be fused to *ERG* (21q22) (see Table 8-1). These highly specific gene fusions encode aberrant chimeric transcription factors thought to be responsible for cell transformation in Ewing's sarcoma/pPNET. The molecular analyses of the 11;22 translocation and its variants have had an important effect on the clinical management of patients with Ewing's sarcoma/pPNET (fig. 8-19). These patients can now be identified by the presence of an abnormal fusion product that is inextricably linked to the biology of these tumors (19). Genetic analysis is especially helpful when morphology is not conclusive or when tumors present in unusual clinical settings or anatomic locations (46). In the event of unexpected or discrepant results, it is advisable to have more than one diagnostic modality available.

The nature of the novel chimeric transcription factor encoded by *EWS/FLI1* and its downstream targets are being investigated. Transfection with *EWS/FLI1* or *EWS/ERG* can transform mouse NIH3T3 fibroblasts so that they acquire tumor-like properties, such as growth in soft agar and immunodeficient mice (56). Compared with native FLI1, the EWS/FLI1 fusion protein is more efficient at inducing neoplastic transformation of fibroblasts in vitro and is a stronger transcriptional activator of promoters responsive to native FLI1 (57). One study has implicated the transforming growth factor-beta (TGF-β) type II receptor (RII) as a target of the oncoproteins of the various fusion genes in Ewing's sarcoma/pPNET (33). *TGF-β* is a putative tumor suppressor gene. Levels of TGF-β are decreased when *EWS/FLI1* is introduced into embryonic stem cells. TGF-β sensitivity is restored and tumorigenicity in cell lines containing the fusion gene is blocked with antisense oligonucleotides to *EWS/FLI1* (38).

Other examples of genes or genetic pathways that appear to have a role in the development or progression of Ewing's sarcoma include *BARO1* (with *BRCA1* breast cancer susceptibility gene

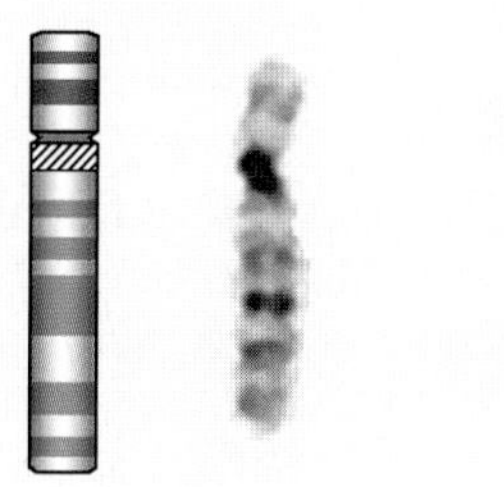

Figure 8-18

SECONDARY STRUCTURAL ANOMALY IN EWING'S SARCOMA

The der(16)t(1;16)(q12;q11.2) is the most common secondary structural anomaly in Ewing's sarcoma.

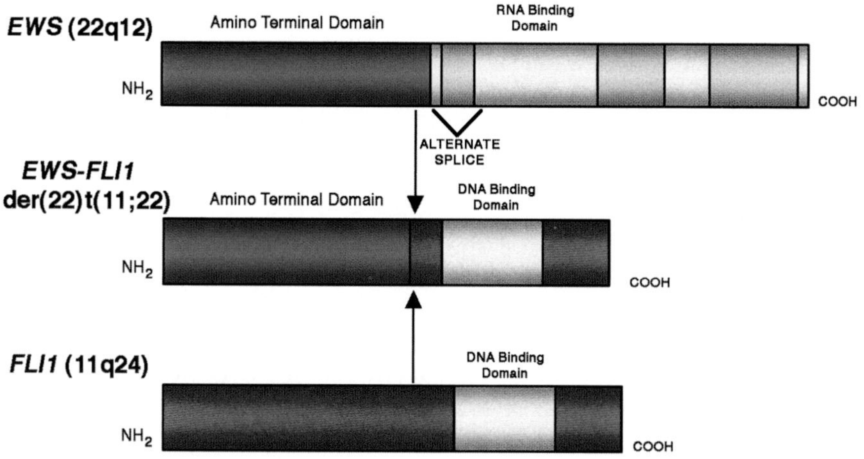

Figure 8-19

EWS/FLI1 CHIMERIC PROTEIN PRODUCT

(Modified from fig. 2 from de Alava E, Gerald WL. Molecular biology of the Ewing's sarcoma/primitive neuroectodermal tumor family. J Clin Oncol 2000;18: 204-13.)

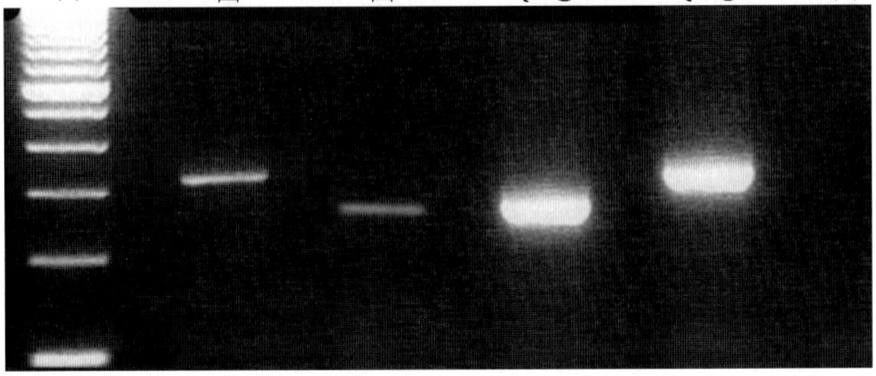

Figure 8-20

REVERSE TRANSCRIPTASE POLYMERASE CHAIN REACTION ANALYSIS OF EWING'S SARCOMA

Lane 1, 100-bp ladder; lane 4, positive type 1 *EWS/FLI1* cell line control; lane 5, positive type 2 *EWS/FLI1* cell line control; lane 6, negative control, no RNA.)

interaction), pRB pathway (with loss of cell cycle inhibitor p16^{INK4a}), *PI3K-AKT* pathway, insulin-like growth factor pathway (particularly *IGF-IR* and *IGFBP-3*), poly(ADP-ribose) polymerase (*PARP*), platelet-derived growth factor pathway (PDGF-C, β-PDGFR), MAP kinase pathway (upregulation of cyclin D1 [*CCND1*]), *Id2* (inhibitor of DNA binding 2), *c-myc, p57^{KIP2}, VEGF* (vascular endothelial growth factor), *TNC* (Tenascin-C), *CCN* (cysteine-rich *CYR61*, connective tissue growth factor [*CTGF*], nephroblastoma overexpressed gene [*Nov*]), and the p53/p14^{ARF} tumor suppressor gene pathway (5,14,29,30,37,42,44,47,48, 52,53,64,65,72,79,82,85,90,93,95–97,107,108).

RT-PCR is the archetype for the molecular detection of Ewing's sarcoma/pPNET–specific chimeric RNA transcripts (fig. 8-20). The PCR technique uses specific synthetic oligonucleotides to amplify a section of a given gene in vitro. With the additional step of reverse transcription (RNA⇒DNA), PCR can be performed on RNA. Consensus primers capable of detecting *EWS/FLI1* or *EWS/ERG* transcripts have been designed, providing diagnostic utility in more than 95 percent of cases. Good quality snap-frozen tissue is the ideal starting material for RNA extraction, but archival (paraffin-embedded) tissue may be acceptable in some cases (provided RNA degradation is not extensive). The high sensitivity of RT-PCR allows for the detection of as little as one tumor cell among 1 million normal cells. Consequently, several groups have demonstrated that, with this approach, minimal disease (occult tumor cells) can be detected in peripheral blood and bone marrow (16,25,98,105). Molecular detection of occult tumor cells in peripheral blood or bone marrow will likely contribute to patient management. Schleiermacher et al. (77) reported that patients with localized Ewing's sarcoma and occult tumor cells in peripheral blood, bone marrow, or both, as detected by RT-PCR analysis, are comparable to patients with metastases in terms of the localization of the primary tumor, outcome, and relapse pattern. Telomerase activity, alone or in combination with RT-PCR, appears to be a significant prognostic marker for Ewing's sarcoma patients during therapy and follow-up (67).

In addition to the variably involved chromosomes in the Ewing's sarcoma/pPNET rearrangements listed in Table 8-1, considerable heterogeneity also exists with respect to specific *EWS/FLI1* molecular breakpoints. "Molecular variants" in this text refer to alternative forms of a given fusion product, reflecting differences in exon composition. To date, all *EWS/FLI1* chimeric transcripts have consistently included exons 1–7 of *EWS* and exons 8 and 9 of *FLI1*. All have shown an intact *FLI1* DNA-binding domain, suggesting that this function is necessary for biologic activity (17,106). Approximately 85 to 90 percent of *EWS/FLI1* fusion transcripts are characterized by the fusion of exon 7 of *EWS* to exon 6 of *FLI1* (referred to as a "type 1 *EWS/FLI1* chimeric transcript") or fusion of exon 7 of *EWS* to exon 5 of *FLI1* (referred to as a "type 2 *EWS/FLI1* chimeric transcript") (106).

Identification of the 11;22 translocation or *EWS/FLI1* fusion transcript is not only useful diagnostically in Ewing's sarcoma/pPNET, but distinguishing type 1 and type 2 *EWS/FLI1* transcripts may also be important prognostically. Specifically, two large clinical studies have shown that the most common type of *EWS/FLI1* fusion (type 1), seen in approximately two thirds of cases, is associated with significantly better survival (15,104). The better clinical behavior of Ewing's sarcoma/pPNETs with the *EWS/FLI1* type 1 fusion is correlated with functional differences between the type 1 fusion protein and other alternative forms of *EWS/FLI1* (49).

Differential Diagnosis. Small cell malignancies of all kinds have to be considered in the differential diagnosis. Purely on a cytologic basis, small cell carcinoma of the lung may be impossible to differentiate from Ewing's sarcoma. However, the clinical features are so different that it is hardly a practical consideration.

Metastatic neuroblastoma has always been considered in the differential diagnosis of Ewing's sarcoma. Most patients with metastatic neuroblastoma are younger than 2 years. Neuroblastomas tend to produce marked crush artifact. The presence of rosettes and neurofilaments should suggest the diagnosis of neuroblastoma. Most patients with metastatic neuroblastoma have clinically obvious primary and serum markers.

Other small cell sarcomas of childhood, especially embryonal and alveolar rhabdomyosarcoma, may present with bone involvement. Embryonal rhabdomyosarcoma is essentially a spindle cell sarcoma, and spindling is not a feature of Ewing's sarcoma. The cells of alveolar rhabdomyosarcoma are more pleomorphic and have more prominent nucleoli than those of Ewing's sarcoma. Rhabdomyosarcoma cells stain with desmin and MyoD1, but Ewing's sarcoma cells do not.

Malignant lymphoma of bone usually affects adults, although children are not exempt. Most malignant lymphomas have nuclei that vary in size and shape and do not have the uniform appearance typical of those of Ewing's sarcoma. Immunoperoxidase staining for CD45 is positive in lymphoma cells but not Ewing's sarcoma cells. The cells of lymphoblastic lymphoma can be difficult to differentiate from Ewing's sarcoma; they may also be stained with stains against MIC-2. However, they also stain with terminal deoxytransferase (TdT) (51).

As indicated above, Ewing's sarcoma can simulate osteomyelitis clinically, radiographically, and even grossly. It is important not to mistake areas of necrosis in Ewing's sarcoma for osteomyelitis. Insistence on finding an inflammatory infiltrate and granulation tissue before making the diagnosis of osteomyelitis avoids this problem.

Small cell osteosarcoma can be very difficult to distinguish from Ewing's sarcoma. It is appropriate to identify clear-cut matrix production, preferably calcified, before diagnosing osteosarcoma. It is our practice to err on the side of diagnosing Ewing's sarcoma in questionable cases.

Although mesenchymal chondrosarcoma may be considered in the differential diagnosis, these cells are cytologically quite different from those in Ewing's sarcoma. The tumor cells are not as hyperchromatic as in Ewing's sarcoma and show a hemangiopericytomatous vascular proliferation, which is never seen in Ewing's sarcoma. The identification of chondroid matrix is the ultimate criterion in confirming the diagnosis of mesenchymal chondrosarcoma.

Treatment and Prognosis. Modern multiagent chemotherapy and radiotherapy have significantly improved the prognosis for patients with Ewing's sarcoma, although limited surgical treatment is undergoing a resurgence. In 1961, Dahlin et al. (13) reported a 5-year survival rate of 15 percent for patients with Ewing's sarcoma and a 10-year rate of 10.7 percent. The treatment regimens used were varied and included radiotherapy and surgery. In 2001, Paulussen et al. (69) reported a 10-year event-free survival rate of 52 percent after intensive chemotherapy, followed by surgery, radiotherapy, or both.

In addition to the administration of chemotherapy, many other factors have been reported to be correlated with prognosis.

Site. Many studies have confirmed the poor prognosis associated with pelvic tumors (9,27, 63,66,100). However, a few have reported no correlation with the site of involvement (2,102). Reporting on the results from the Intergroup Ewing's Sarcoma Study group, Siegal et al. (81) found that the patients with tumors in the skeleton of the head and neck had a considerably better prognosis.

Tumor Volume. Several studies have suggested that large primary tumors are associated with a poor prognosis (2,31,40,102). However, others did not find any correlation between tumor volume and prognosis (8,40,71).

Microscopic Features. Several studies have shown that histologic classification into typical Ewing's sarcoma, atypical Ewing's sarcoma, and PNET did not affect prognosis (13,50,68,89). Only one study has suggested that the diagnosis of PNET is associated with a significantly worse prognosis (78). The presence of a filagree pattern has been reported to be associated with a worse prognosis (43). Also, the presence of dark cells has been reported to be an unfavorable prognostic sign (89).

Response to Chemotherapy. Several studies have shown a correlation between histologic response to chemotherapy and prognosis (3,40,71,102). Some groups use the same technique to evaluate tumor necrosis in Ewing's sarcoma that they use to evaluate osteosarcoma, that is, mapping the surgical specimen and calculating the residual viable tumor as a percentage of the entire neoplasm (102). However, Picci et al. (71) pointed out that there is a difference in response to chemotherapy between osteosarcoma and Ewing's sarcoma. In osteosarcoma, necrotic tumor is replaced with fibrous tissue and reactive new bone formation so that the size of the original tumor can still be evaluated. In Ewing's sarcoma, there is no such replacement of necrotic tumor; hence, the tumor shrinks. They suggested that the viable tumor be evaluated, and they devised the following grading system: grade 1, at least one nodule of viable tumor covers one low-power microscopic field; grade 2, isolated nodules of viable tumor but not covering more than one low-power field; and grade 3, no viable tumor is identified. This grading system correlated very well with prognosis.

Cytogenetics. See above section on Genetics and Other Special Techniques.

MYELOMA

Myeloma is divided into three groups: multiple myeloma, solitary plasmacytoma, and osteosclerotic myeloma. Each is discussed separately.

Multiple Myeloma

Definition. Multiple myeloma is a disorder in which malignant plasma cells accumulate in the bone marrow and produce an immunoglobulin, usually monoclonal IgG or IgA (113).

General Features. Multiple myeloma is the most common primary neoplasm of bone, accounting for about 44 percent of all malignant tumors. Most are diagnosed on the basis of bone marrow aspirate findings. About 15 percent are diagnosed on the basis of surgical biopsy findings, with the biopsy performed because the patient presents with either a destructive lesion or a pathologic fracture.

The etiology of multiple myeloma is unknown. Up to 16 percent of patients with monoclonal gammopathy of undetermined significance eventually develop multiple myeloma, but it may take up to 30 years (113). It is not known how often multiple myeloma progresses from monoclonal gammopathy. Rarely, multiple myeloma develops in chronic osteomyelitis (142); there is one example of this in the Mayo Clinic files. In one patient whose case is in the Mayo Clinic files, an anaplastic myeloma developed in association with systemic mastocytosis. The Mayo Clinic files contain the records of 986 cases of multiple myeloma (fig. 8-21). In all of them, the diagnosis was confirmed with biopsy (cases diagnosed with a bone marrow aspirate are not included).

Clinical Features. Multiple myeloma is a disease of older adults. Only about 6.5 percent of patients are in the first three decades of life; in the Mayo Clinic series, the youngest patient was 16 years old. The largest concentration of patients is in the sixth and seventh decades of life. There is a definite male predominance, with a male to female ratio of 16 to 10 (137). Bone pain, usually of the back, is the most common symptom. The pain generally is of less than 6 months' duration, although some patients have symptoms for many years. Weakness and weight loss are common complaints. Sudden pain may herald a pathologic fracture, which is especially common in the spine. Spinal cord compression caused by pathologic fracture or tumor can produce neurologic symptoms.

Laboratory findings are of critical importance in the diagnosis of multiple myeloma. Anemia, usually normocytic and normochromic, is common. The peripheral blood smear frequently shows rouleau formation. Renal insufficiency occurs in most patients and is associated with hypercalcemia, hyperuricemia, and obstruction

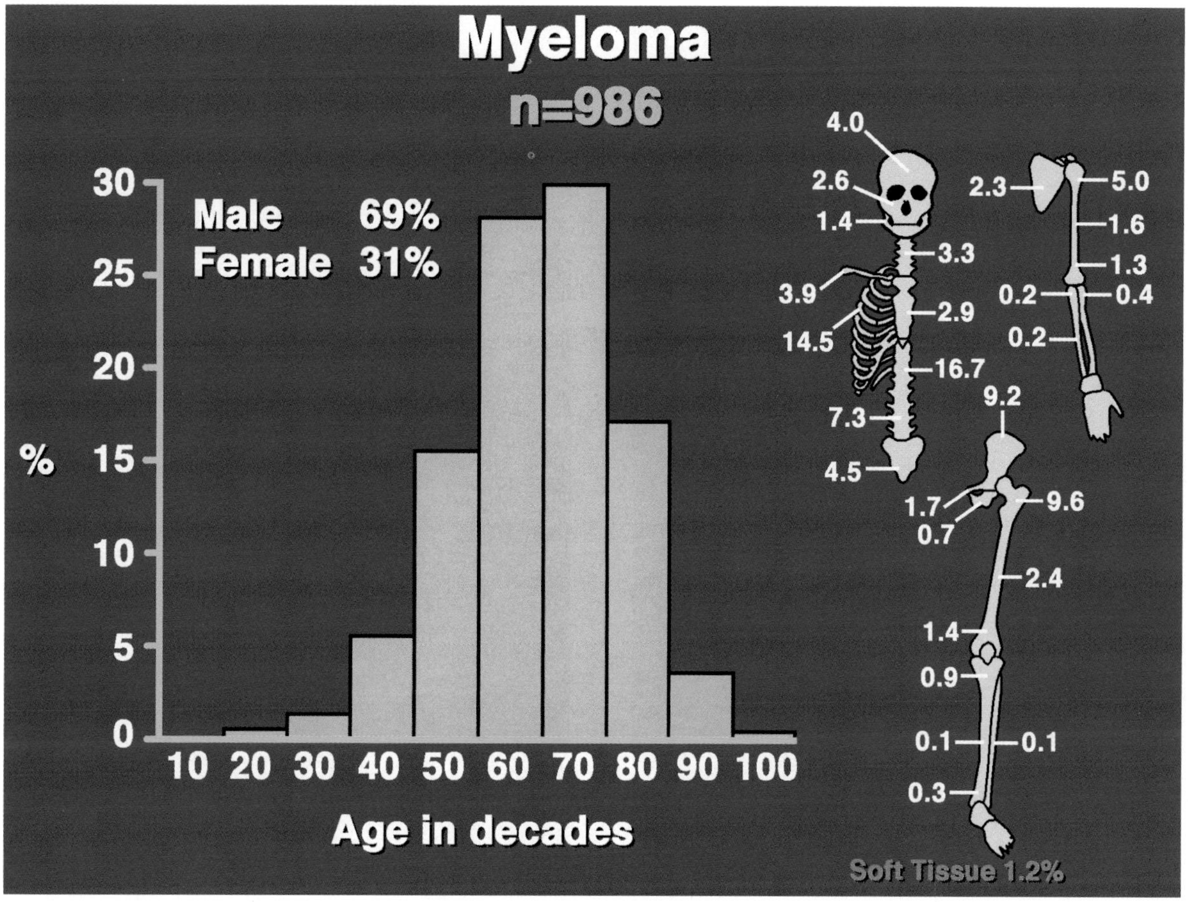

Figure 8-21

MYELOMA

Distribution of myeloma according to the age and sex of the patient and the site of the lesion.

of the renal tubules by protein casts. Serum and urine studies demonstrate monoclonal protein in the majority of patients.

Sites. Multiple myeloma tends to occur in bones that contain hematopoietic marrow: the thoracic cage, skull, pelvic bones, and proximal portions of the femur and humerus are the most common sites. The small bones of the hands and feet are rarely involved.

Radiographic Findings. Classically, multiple myeloma presents as punched-out areas of bone destruction without surrounding sclerosis (figs. 8-22, 8-23). Expansion of the bone may produce a ballooned-out appearance. Variable osteoporosis is common, often resulting in pathologic fracture (fig. 8-24), especially in vertebrae. In up to 25 percent of patients, lesions are not apparent

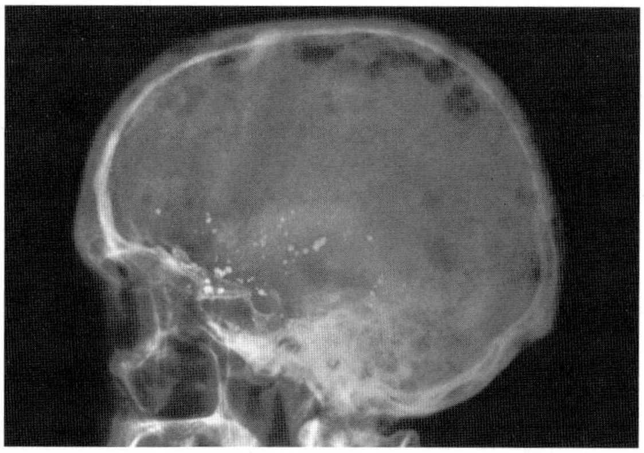

Figure 8-22

MULTIPLE MYELOMA

Multiple lytic, well-circumscribed lesions involve the calvarium. In addition to multiple myeloma, the radiographic differential diagnosis includes metastatic carcinoma.

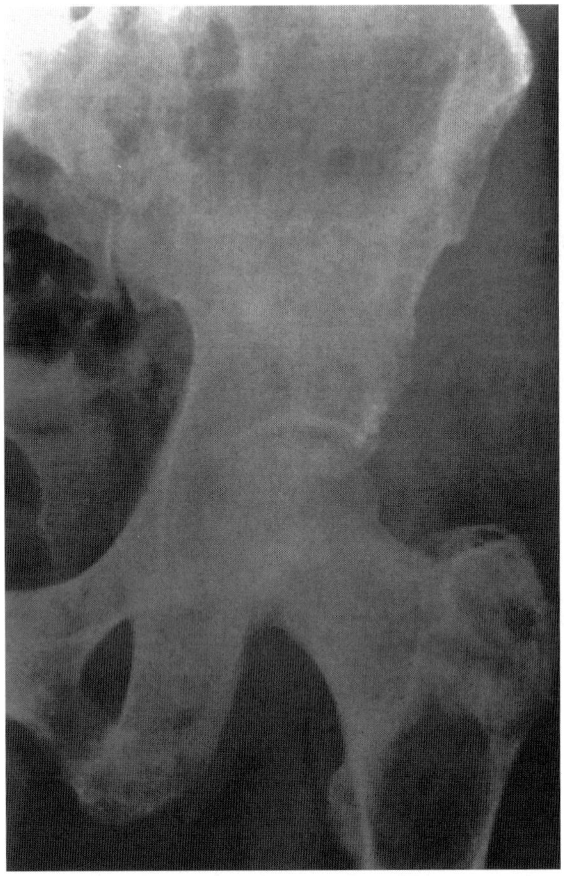

Figure 8-23

MYELOMA

A purely lytic and discrete lesion with endosteal erosion and cortical thinning involves the proximal femur.

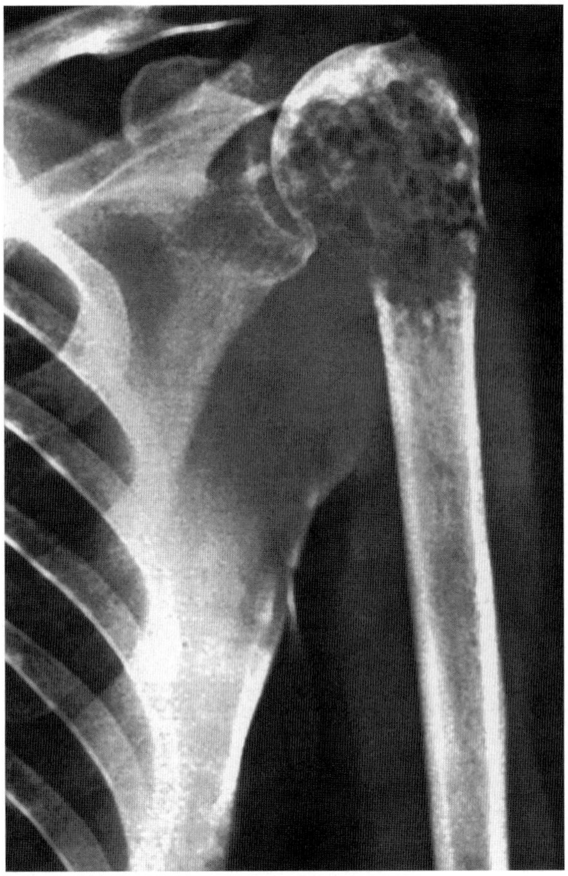

Figure 8-24

MYELOMA

The patient presented with a pathologic fracture through a destructive lytic lesion involving the proximal humerus.

on plain radiographs. There is a diffuse demineralization not apparent on plain X rays. CT and MRI may reveal small discrete lesions. The appearance on MRI varies because the disease does not involve the bone marrow in a homogeneous fashion. Calcification of amyloid deposits may suggest chondrosarcoma (141).

Gross Findings. Multiple myeloma is soft and has a typical currant-jelly appearance (fig. 8-25). Occasionally, the tumor is white and fleshy, similar to the appearance of malignant lymphoma. If large deposits of amyloid are present, the lesion appears dark brown and glassy.

Microscopic Findings. Under low-power magnification, multiple myeloma shows small, round cells arranged in sheets. The cells have abundant light blue or pink cytoplasm. The nuclei are round and eccentric and have a characteristic pattern of chromatin, which is arranged in clumps at the periphery, producing a clock-face appearance (fig. 8-26). Mitotic figures are uncommon. Double and multinucleated cells are common (fig. 8-27).

The histologic features vary. The tumor may be quite vascular. In some tumors, the vessels are small and capillary-like with thick walls; in others, the vessels are large and dilated, and create a stag-horn appearance, simulating the appearance of hemangiopericytoma (fig. 8-28).

The nuclear features vary from those of normal plasma cells to nuclei that are very pleomorphic, with prominent nucleoli (fig. 8-29). In the latter, it may not be obvious that the cell is a plasma cell. The nuclei may be sufficiently pleomorphic to suggest sarcoma. The cells may be discohesive or clustered, suggesting an epithelial neoplasm. Occasionally, the immunoglobulins crystalize and fill the cytoplasm of the plasma cells; histiocytes containing crystalline material may also be present (133).

Deposits of amyloid are found in about 10 to 15 percent of tumors. The amount varies and may be associated with a giant cell reaction (fig. 8-30). Proliferating plasma cells are usually found among amyloid deposits. Rarely, the deposits are so heavy that no plasma cells remain. Any deposit of amyloid in bone is considered multiple myeloma unless proved otherwise.

The neoplastic cells of multiple myeloma produce a monoclonal cytoplasmic immunoglobulin; hence, they stain for either kappa or lambda light chains. The cells usually are negative for CD45 and CD20, but frequently express CD56. Although keratin stains are negative, myeloma cells often are positive for epithelial membrane antigen. Positivity for CD138 is considered specific for plasma cells.

Cytologic Findings. FNA cytology is useful in rapidly establishing the diagnosis of multiple myeloma, particularly when it occurs as a solitary bone lesion that radiographically includes a wide spectrum of differential diagnoses. In smears of well-differentiated myeloma, the plasma cell differentiation is obvious. The tumor cells are uniform, with abundant, well-delineated cytoplasm that often has perinuclear clearing; the eccentric rounded nuclei have dense, coarse chromatin (153). In less well-differentiated tumors, the

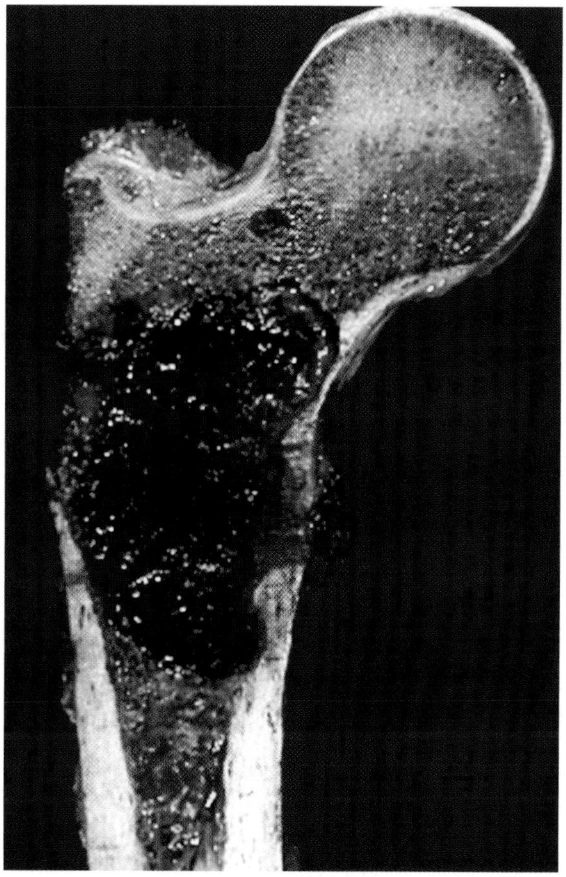

Figure 8-25

MYELOMA

This tumor in the proximal femur has a glistening cut surface and a dark red-brown color typical of myeloma.

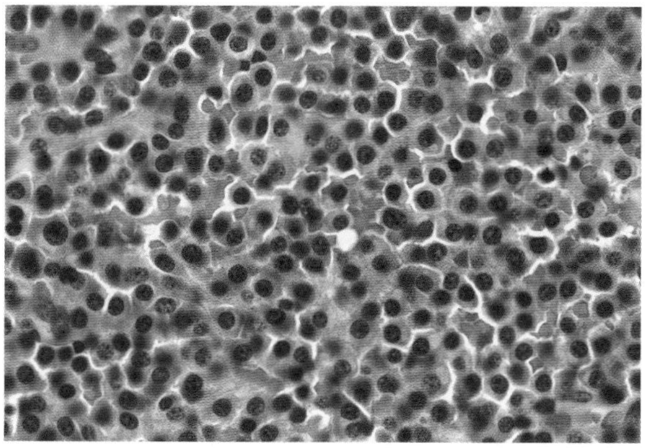

Figure 8-26

MYELOMA

Mature plasma cell myeloma with small round nuclei, clumped nuclear chromatin, and abundant cytoplasm.

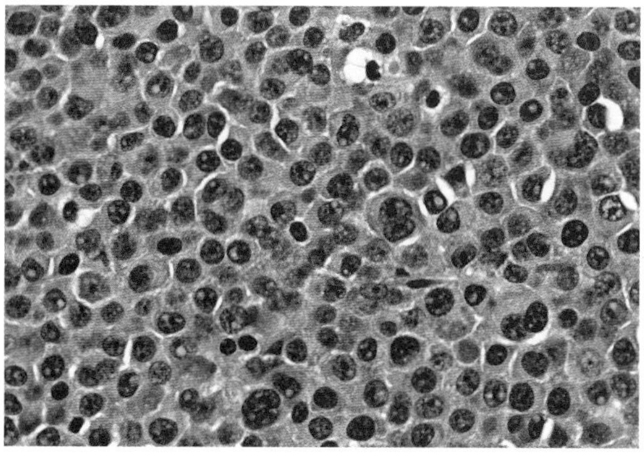

Figure 8-27

MYELOMA

Binucleated plasma cells are common in this tumor.

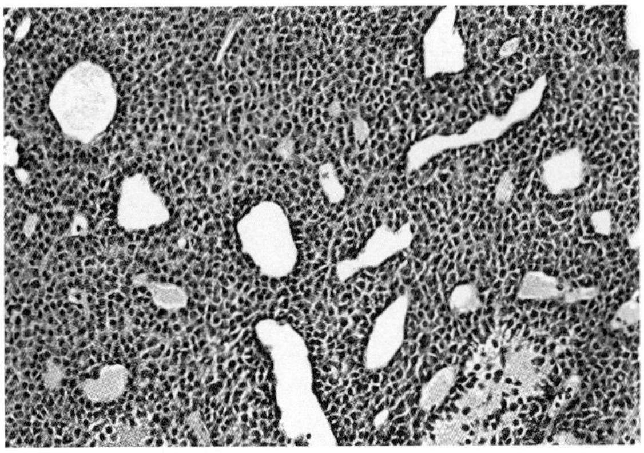

Figure 8-28

MYELOMA

The distended vascular spaces impart a hemangiopericytoma-like pattern. When the tumor cells cluster in small nests, they may resemble a neuroendocrine carcinoma.

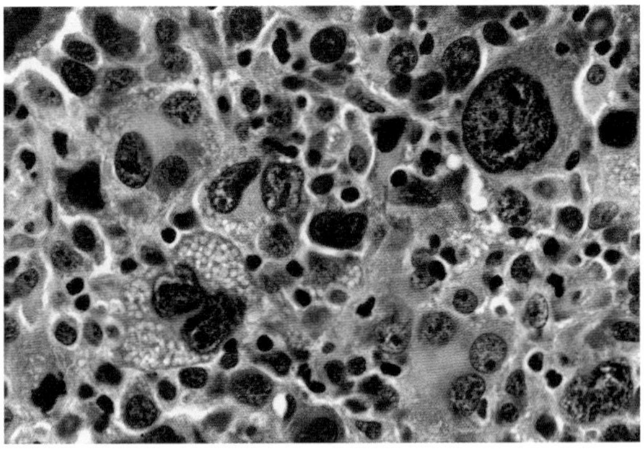

Figure 8-29

ANAPLASTIC MYELOMA

Pleomorphic plasma cells show marked variation in nuclear size and shape. Several prominent nucleoli are present. The smaller background cells provide more recognizable evidence of plasmacytic differentiation.

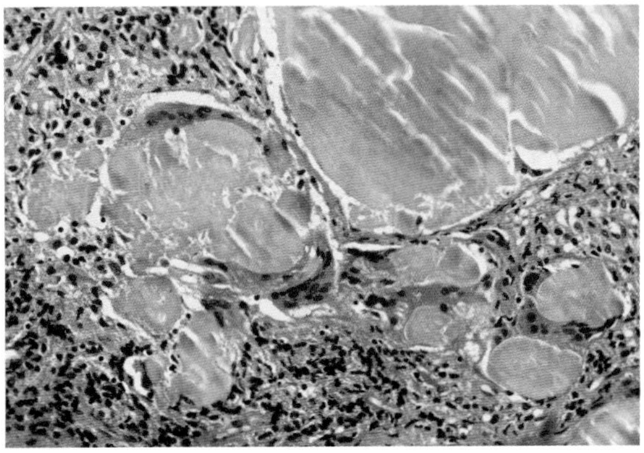

Figure 8-30

MYELOMA

Nodular eosinophilic masses of amyloid are associated with foreign body multinucleated giant cells. Neoplastic plasma cells fill the spaces between the amyloid deposits.

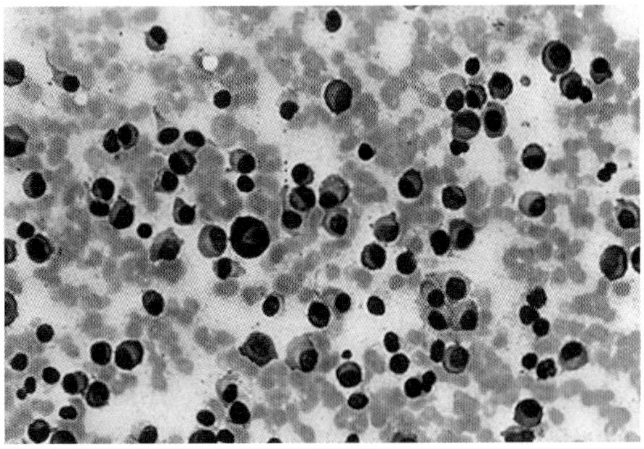

Figure 8-31

MYELOMA

Fine-needle aspiration (FNA) smear shows a high degree of plasma cell differentiation despite variability in cell size and multinucleated forms.

variation in cell size is more prominent, and binucleated and multinucleated cell forms occur. Even in these cases, however, plasma cell differentiation is usually easily recognized (fig. 8-31). Poorly differentiated multiple myeloma may be extremely difficult to differentiate from both lymphoma and metastatic carcinoma. Immunocytochemistry is helpful in these cases. However, immunoreactivity for epithelial membrane antigen is notably of no use in the differential diagnosis between multiple myeloma and carcinoma.

Genetics and Other Special Techniques. Clinically, cytogenetic analysis has been invaluable in the diagnosis, prognosis, and management of hematologic malignancies. However, for multiple myeloma, cytogenetic information is limited because this malignancy is composed mainly of terminally differentiated B cells and it is difficult to obtain analyzable metaphases in this hypoproliferative entity. Clonal chromosomal abnormalities are observed in only 30 to 45 percent of cases (most often in cases of previously

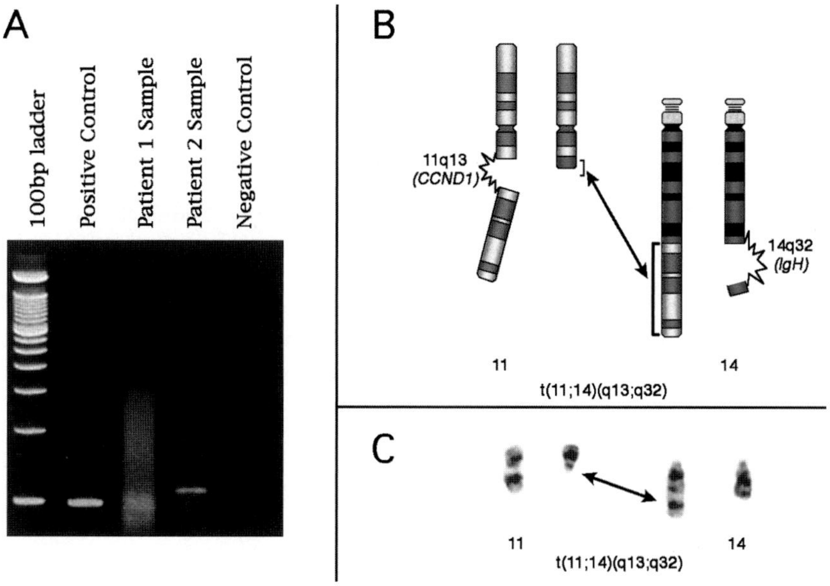

Figure 8-32

MOLECULAR TECHNIQUES IN MULTIPLE MYELOMA

A: Polymerase chain reaction analysis for *IgH* rearrangements uses consensus primers for the *IgH* framework III and joins region genes detected on an 8 percent nondenaturing polyacrylamide gel. Staining with ethidium bromide shows that patient 2 with multiple myeloma exhibits a monoclonal *IgH* rearrangement, whereas patient 1 is negative for this rearrangement.

B,C: Schematic illustration and partial G-banded karyotype, respectively, of the 11;14 translocation [t(11;14)(q13;q32)] commonly seen in multiple myeloma. This translocation leads to overexpression of cyclin D1.

treated and relapsed disease) in contrast to flow cytometric analysis of nuclear DNA content of $G_{I/O}$ cells, which has demonstrated aneuploidy in 50 to 80 percent of patients (112,130,144).

Multiple myeloma karyotypes are complex and characterized by multiple numerical and structural aberrations (123,149). Hypodiploidy is associated with shortened survival. The most consistent structural abnormality is rearrangement of 14q32, the locus for the immunoglobulin heavy chain (*IgH*) gene, found in more than one fourth of cytogenetically abnormal patients (114,134). Over the last decade, modern molecular techniques have revealed an even higher percentage (70 to 90 percent) of 14q32 rearrangements (117,127). Reciprocal chromosomal translocations, which are mediated by errors in *IgH* switch recombination or somatic hypermutation as plasma cells are generated in germinal centers, are present (fig. 8-32A) (150). These translocations dysregulate known or candidate proto-oncogenes that are juxtaposed to a strong *IgH* enhancer.

In the majority of cases, the abnormal 14q32 is the result of a t(11;14)(q13.3;q32.3), leading to overexpression of cyclin D1 (fig. 8-32B,C) (115, 127). Other recurrent translocations in multiple myeloma include t(4;14)(p16.3;q32.3), t(14;16)(q32.3;q23.1), t(6;14)(p25;q32.3), t(6;14)(p21.1;q32.3), t(8;14)(q24.1;q32.3), t(9;14)(p13;q32.3), t(14;18)(q32.3;q21.3), t(14;19)(q32.3;q13), t(14;20)(q32.3;q11), t(14;22)(q32.3;q11), t(1;14)(p34;q32.3), t(11;22)(q13;q13), t(6;8)(p10;q10), der(8;18)(q10;q10), and der(8;20)(q10;q10) (Table 8-2) (115,118,128,129,131,147,148,150,152). Several of these abnormalities are similar to those found in other B-cell disorders involving the *IgH* locus (14q32). The nearly universal presence of *IgH* rearrangements in multiple myeloma supports the concept that Ig sequence alterations play a critical role in the pathogenesis of this neoplasm.

The 4;14 chromosomal translocation observed in 10 to 20 percent of patients with multiple myeloma results in the dysregulation of two genes localized to 4p16.3: fibroblast growth factor receptor 3 (*FGFR3*) and the putative transcription factor multiple myeloma SET domain (*MMSET*) (119,143). A subset of multiple myelomas harboring the 4;14 chromosomal translocation lack expression of *FGFR3*, yet express *MMSET* and have an *IgH/MMSET* fusion transcript, suggesting that activation of *MMSET*, not *FGFR3*, may be the critical transforming event of this recurrent translocation (146). Mutated *FGFR3* has been shown to confer resistance to caspase 3-related apoptosis (119), and patients with a 4;14 translocation have a poor outcome (short event-free and short overall survival periods) (138). Molecular analysis of the 14;16 translocation has demonstrated that the 16q23.1 breakpoints are distributed 500 kb centromeric to the c-*maf* proto-oncogene and that this translocation leads to increased c-*maf* transcription

Table 8-2

CHROMOSOMAL ABNORMALITIES IN MULTIPLE MYELOMA[a]

Chromosomal Lesion	Gene(s) Involved	Estimated Prevalence (%)
add(14)(q32)	*IgH*	45-90
t(11;14)(q13.3;q32.3)	*CCND1*	30-40 of 14q+ cases
t(4;14)(p16.3;q32.3)	*FGFR3/MMSET*	20-35 of 14q+ cases
t(14;16)(p32.3;q23.1)	*c-maf*	1-25 of 14q+ cases
t(6;14)(p21.1;q32.3)	*CCND3*	<20 of 14q+ cases
t(8;14)(q24.1;q32.3)	*c-myc*	<10 of 14q+ cases
t(6;14)(p25;q32.3)	*IRF4*	NA[b]
t(9;14)(p13;q32.3)	*PAX5*	NA
t(14;18)(q32.3;q21.3)	*BCL2*	NA
t(14;19)(q32.3;q13)	*BCL3*	NA
t(14;20)(q32.3;q11)	*mafb*	NA
t(1;14)(p34;q32.3)	*E3/LAPTm5*	NA
Monosomy 13, del(13)(q14)	*RB1*	20-80
Abnormalities of 1q[c]	-	40

[a]From references 114 and 134.
[b]NA = not assessed because of limited number of studies.
[c]Multiple translocation partners (50 percent), deletions of 1p (30 percent), rarely observed as sole change.

(116). Cyclin D3 is dysregulated as a consequence of the 6;14 translocation [t(6;14)(p21;q32)] (150). Three D-type cyclin genes encode proteins, each of which can interact with the CDK4 or the CDK6 cyclin D-dependent kinases that phosphorylate RB (retinoblastoma), thus regulating a process that promotes the G_1/S cell cycle transition. As mentioned above, the 11;14 translocation [t(11;14) (q13;q32)] results in ectopic expression of cyclin D1, in contrast to the absence of cyclin D1 expression in normal B cells.

The detection of partial or complete loss of chromosome 13 is an independent prognostic factor associated with a poor prognosis for patients with multiple myeloma and suggests the presence of a putative tumor suppressor gene (fig. 8-33) (123,124,135,140,156,158). Loss of 13q14, the locus for the *RB* gene, appears to be the common minimal deletion region; however, most chromosome 13 abnormalities as identified by FISH analysis represent monosomy 13 or large q arm deletions (110,126). Routine assessment of chromosome 13 abnormalities by FISH or other technical approaches has been strongly recommended for patients with multiple myeloma considered for high-dose chemotherapy (fig. 8-33) (124,125). CT-guided biopsy of MRI-detected focal lesions is a safe technique that can provide important cytogenetic information in a substantial number of patients with multiple myeloma not identified during random bone marrow sampling (111).

Interleukin (IL)-6 cytokine and insulin-like growth factor-1 are essential growth and survival factors for myeloma cell lines and primary cells, protecting them from apoptosis induced by chemotherapeutic agents. Binding of IL-6 to its receptor (IL-6R) triggers myeloma cell immortalization or proliferation through utilization of the Jak-STAT or *ras* signal transduction pathways (or both) (134). Serum IL-6 levels or C-reactive protein levels, an indirect measurement of IL-6 activity, correlate with the extent of disease and survival (134,139).

High levels of expression of the antiapoptotic gene *BCL2* have been detected in the majority of myeloma patients. A significant correlation between *BCL2* expression and resistance to therapy with interferon has been described (145). $BCLX_L$, another antiapoptotic gene of the same family, has been linked to multidrug resistance (157). Phosphatase and tensin homolog deleted on chromosome 10 *(PTEN)* suppresses the *P13K/Akt* pathway and induces apoptosis of myeloma cells (120). Preliminary studies suggest that *PTEN*-deficient myeloma cells are remarkably sensitive to mTOR inhibitors (151). Abnormalities of other genes that may confer a poor prognosis include some of the following: *p53*, fibroblast growth factor receptor genes (*FGFR*), and *N-* and *K-ras* (134).

Microarray technology and gene expression studies have recently contributed to the identification of large numbers of genes that may have a role in multiple myeloma (125). De Vos et al. (122) reported 250 genes as significantly upregulated and 159 downregulated in malignant plasma cell samples compared with normal plasma cell samples. The results of Inoue et al. (132) indicate that upregulation of *PDZK1* (the PDZ domain containing 1) is likely a target for 1q12-22 amplification in multiple myeloma and

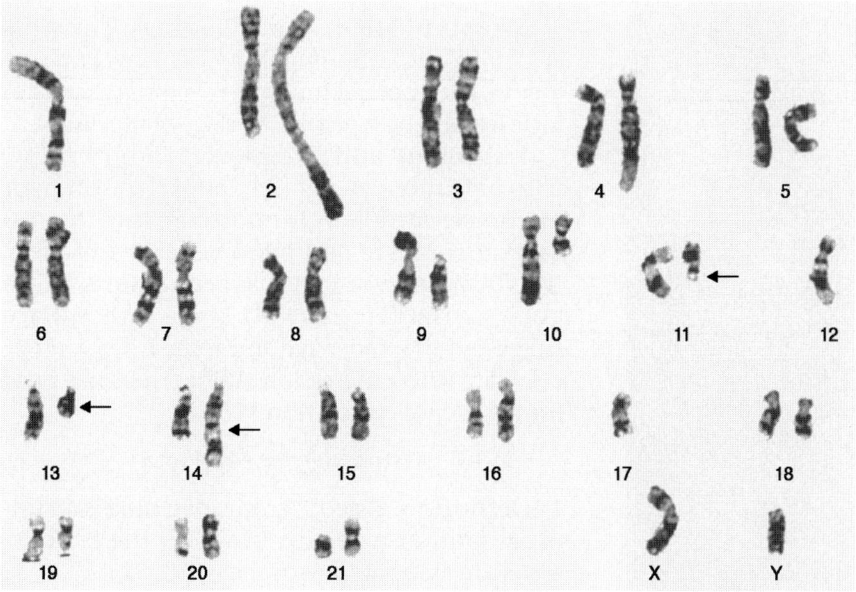

Figure 8-33

PARTIAL LOSS OF CHROMOSOME 13 IN MULTIPLE MYELOMA

Representative G-banded karyotype from a case of multiple myeloma exhibits complex rearrangements including an interstitial deletion of the long arm of chromosome 13 as well as a t(11;14)(q13;q32) (arrows).

may be associated with a drug resistance phenotype in this neoplasm.

Claudio et al. (121) created a molecular resource of genes expressed in primary malignant plasma cells with the identification of 9,732 nonredundant expressed genes. Examples of highly expressed genes identified by sequencing include a novel putative disulfide isomerase (MGC3178), a tumor rejection enzyme (*TRA1*), a heat shock 70-kD protein 5, and an annexin (A2).

Microarray studies are leading to the identification of novel genes of potential biologic significance, genes that are differentially expressed between multiple myeloma and B-cell lymphoma, and genes encoding enzymes that could be therapeutic targets.

Differential Diagnosis. Reactive plasmacytosis associated with infection can be difficult to differentiate from multiple myeloma. Osteomyelitis shows fibrosis, capillary proliferation, and a mixed infiltrate even if plasma cells are dominant. A polyclonal pattern of immunostains for light chains confirms the diagnosis of osteomyelitis. Plasmacytoid lymphoma or immunoblastic lymphoma can also present problems; positive staining for CD45 and CD20 strongly supports the diagnosis of lymphoma.

Treatment and Prognosis. Systemic chemotherapy is of value, and some patients have remission. The long-term prognosis continues to be bleak. Radiotherapy is useful for localized problems, such as spinal cord compression. Surgical intervention may be necessary. Fewer than 10 percent of patients survive longer than 10 years. Cytologic atypia and mitotic activity reportedly are associated with a worse prognosis (154,155). Performance status, anemia, renal failure, and hypercalcemia are also associated with a worse prognosis (109,113). Kyle (136) reported on 19 long-term survivors (of a total of 870 patients with multiple myeloma) and found that response to chemotherapy was the most important factor for long-term survival.

Solitary Myeloma (Plasmacytoma)

Definition. Solitary myeloma is a neoplasm of plasma cells that produces a single osseous lesion. *Solitary plasmacytoma* is a synonymous term.

General Features. The diagnosis of solitary myeloma requires careful staging to rule out disseminated disease and should include: 1) skeletal survey; 2) complete blood count; 3) chemistry panel; 4) bone marrow aspirate and biopsy; and 5) serum and urine protein studies (161).

Bataille and Sany (159) suggested the following diagnostic criteria: 1) solitary lesion on a radiograph; 2) histologic evidence of tumor; 3) negative bone marrow findings; 4) absence of anemia, hypercalcemia, or renal involvement; 5) absence of monoclonal protein or lower levels detected only with immunoelectrophoresis; and 6) normal or low levels of immunoglobulins

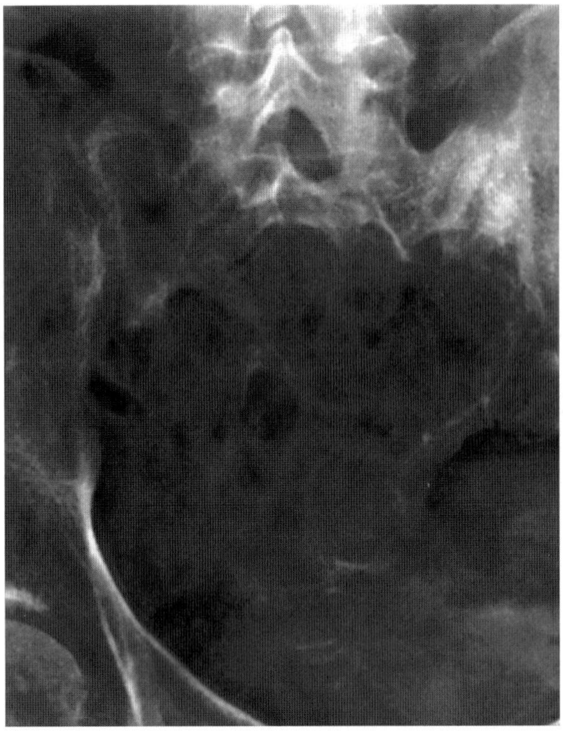

Figure 8-34

SOLITARY MYELOMA

A 33-year-old woman had a large lytic lesion that involved the entire mid and lower sacrum, with cortical destruction on the right. There was no radiographic evidence of other osseous lesions. She had no evidence of disease progression 4 years after treatment for this solitary myeloma.

that return to normal after therapy. Frassica et al. (161) thought that criterion 6 was not reasonable because it is impossible to know at the time of diagnosis; they believed that bone marrow plasmocytosis of 10 percent or less was compatible with the diagnosis of solitary myeloma. About 5 percent of myelomas are solitary (160).

Clinical Features. The majority of patients present with bone pain. Neurologic symptoms and pathologic fracture are other presenting features. Occasionally, the lesion is an incidental radiographic finding (161). Males outnumber females about 2 to 1, and most patients are older than 50 years.

Sites. The spine is the site involved most commonly (159–161). The pelvic girdle and ribs are other common sites.

Radiographic Findings. Radiographs show a solitary, purely lytic lesion that may destroy the cortex and extend into soft tissue (fig. 8-34).

Gross and Microscopic Findings. The gross and microscopic findings in solitary myeloma are identical to those of multiple myeloma. No histologic features help predict the stage of the disease.

Treatment and Prognosis. Radiotherapy, with or without chemotherapy, is the treatment of choice. Although in most patients the disease progresses to multiple myeloma (159–161), the 10-year survival rate has been reported to be as high as 68 percent (159). Some authors have suggested that older age and spine involvement correlate with progression (159); others have not found such a correlation (161).

Osteosclerotic Myeloma

Definition. Osteosclerotic myeloma is an unusual form of myeloma in which the bone lesions are associated with sclerosis.

General Features. Osteosclerotic myeloma accounts for fewer than 3 percent of all myelomas (162). The tumor may be solitary or polyostotic. In the series reported by Kelly et al. (162), just over 50 percent of patients had multiple lesions.

Clinical Features. Patients with osteosclerotic myeloma are younger than those with classic multiple myeloma. They do not present with bone pain or other systemic problems such as fatigue and renal failure. About 50 percent of patients present with peripheral neuropathy. The cause of the neuropathy is obscure, but it is not associated with amyloid deposition in the nerves (162). Some patients present with other paraneoplastic symptoms such as skin pigmentation, organomegaly, and endocrine dysfunction (164). The acronym POEMS (polyneuropathy, organomegaly, endocrinopathy, M-protein, and skin changes) describes the constellation of findings. For patients with polyneuropathy, the correct diagnosis may not be made for a long time. Polyneuropathy occurs in only 5 percent of the patients with conventional myeloma, but in 50 percent of those with osteosclerotic myeloma (162). In a 1971 review of the literature, Mangalik and Veliath (163) found 36 patients with osteosclerotic myeloma, of which 13 had peripheral neuropathy.

Sites. Osteosclerotic myeloma involves the spine, ribs, and pelvic girdle; lesions in the appendicular skeleton or skull are unusual.

Radiographic Features. The lesion may be completely sclerotic, have a mixture of lysis and

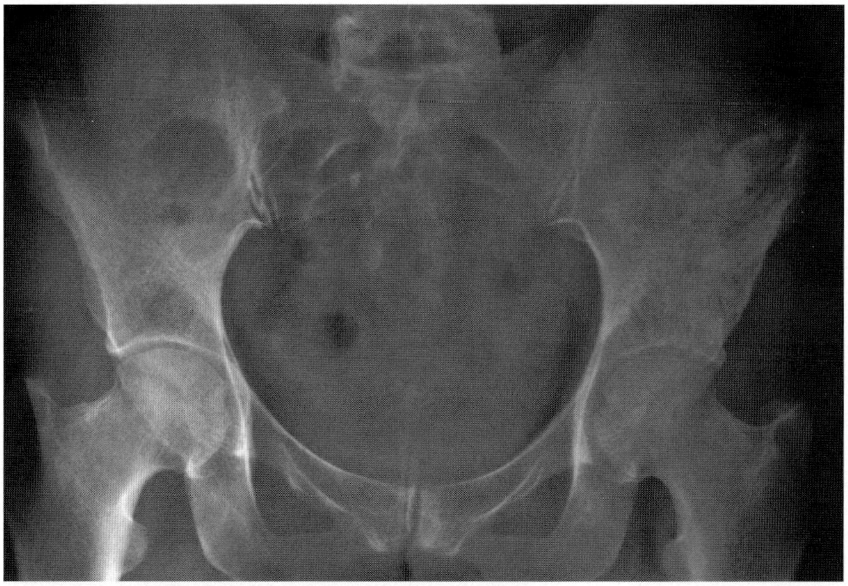

Figure 8-35

OSTEOSCLEROTIC MYELOMA

Plain radiographs of the spine and pelvis show multiple sclerotic lesions involving several bones throughout the pelvis and spine.

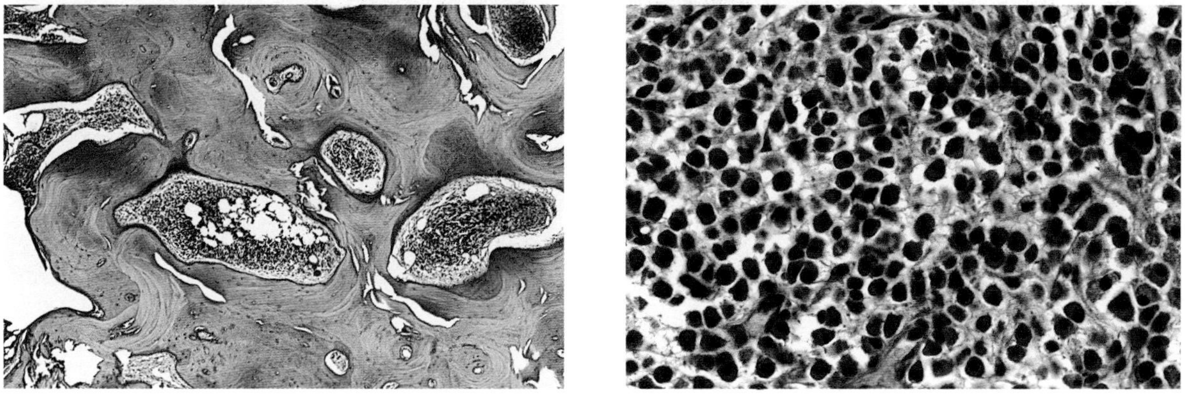

Figure 8-36

OSTEOSCLEROTIC MYELOMA

Left: In small biopsy specimens, it can be particularly difficult to find nests of neoplastic plasma cells because of the dense sclerosis of the surrounding bone.

Right: Higher-power view shows the tumor cells.

sclerosis, or have areas of lysis surrounded by a rim of sclerosis (fig. 8-35).

Microscopic Findings. A needle or open biopsy may be performed to confirm the diagnosis. The bone present in the specimen is usually quite hard and much decalcification may be required to allow sectioning; consequently, the cytologic features are not preserved. Medullary bone is thickened and irregular, and the diagnosis is made by finding an increased number of plasma cells in the bone marrow (fig. 8-36). Amyloid deposits have been reported in association with osteosclerotic myeloma (165).

Treatment and Prognosis. Treatment is often delayed because the disease is not diagnosed. Radiotherapy is useful for solitary lesions. The efficacy of chemotherapy in multiple lesions is not clear.

MALIGNANT LYMPHOMA

Definition. Malignant lymphoma is a malignant neoplasm that is composed of lymphoid cells and produces a tumefactive process within bone.

General Features. Malignant lymphoma of bone was described first by Parker and Jackson in 1939 (185) when they differentiated it from Ewing's sarcoma. The term *reticulum cell sarcoma*

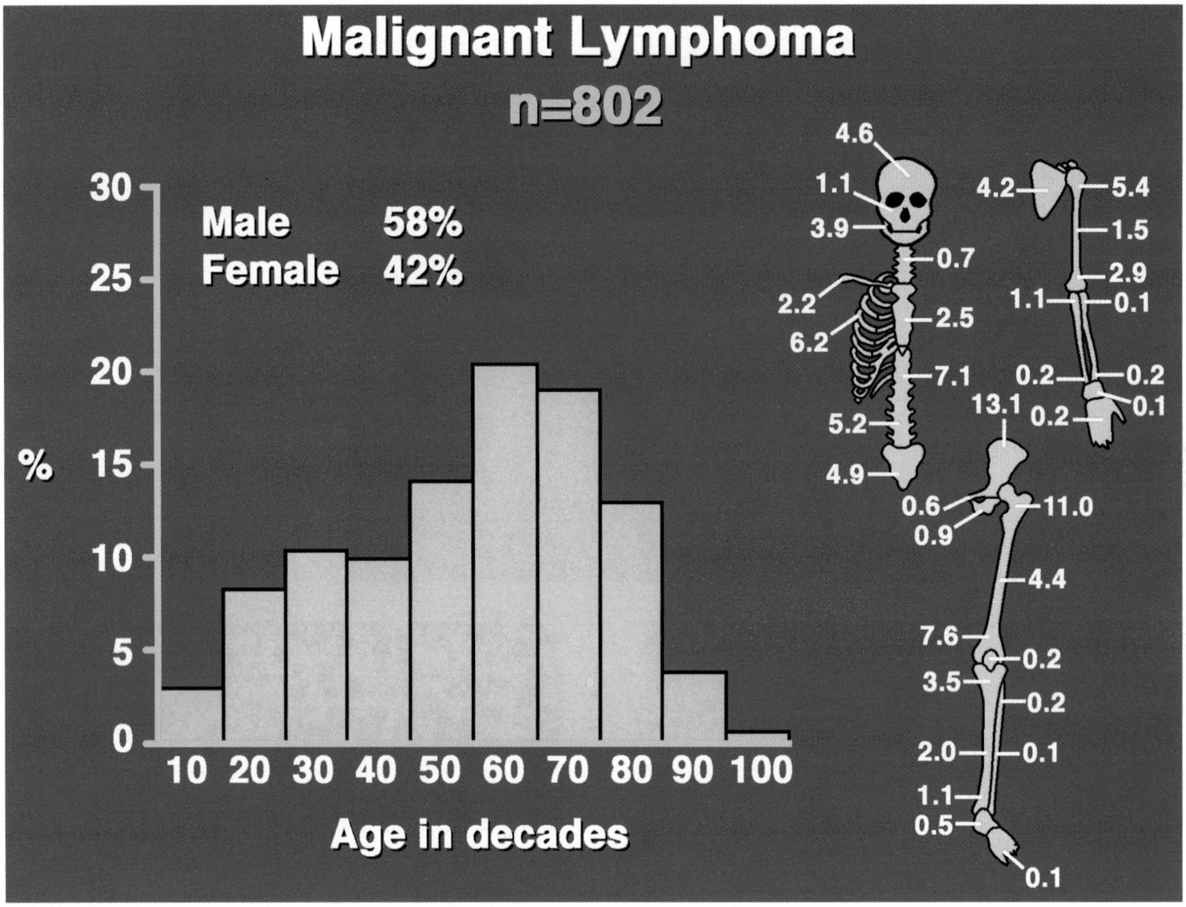

Figure 8-37

MALIGNANT LYMPHOMA

was used because of the fine reticulin network present within the tumor. It is now recognized that this neoplasm is similar to the much more common lymph node counterpart, although histologic peculiarities do exist. Leukemias and Hodgkin's disease can also present as neoplasms of the skeleton.

Malignant lymphoma constitutes about 7 percent of all bone sarcomas, and lymphomas of bone account for 5 percent of extranodal lymphomas (166). The Pediatric Oncology Study Group reported that 5.5 percent of children with lymphoma have primary skeletal disease. In a radiographic study, Braunstein (169) found that 16 percent of patients with lymphoma had evidence of bone involvement. The Mayo Clinic files contain 802 biopsy-confirmed examples of skeletal lymphoma, accounting for 12 percent of malignant neoplasms (fig. 8-37).

Clinical Features. Most patients with lymphoma present with bone pain. A mass lesion may be palpated. Neurologic symptoms are common when the vertebral column is affected. Patients with primary lymphoma of bone rarely present with systemic or B symptoms such as fever and night sweats. Occasionally, symptoms associated with hypercalcemia, such as constipation, lethargy, and somnolence, may be present (180). There is a slight male predominance. Any age group may be affected, although the highest incidence is in the fourth and fifth decades of life.

Sites. Lymphomas tend to affect the portions of the skeleton containing red marrow. In the Mayo Clinic files, the femur is the bone most

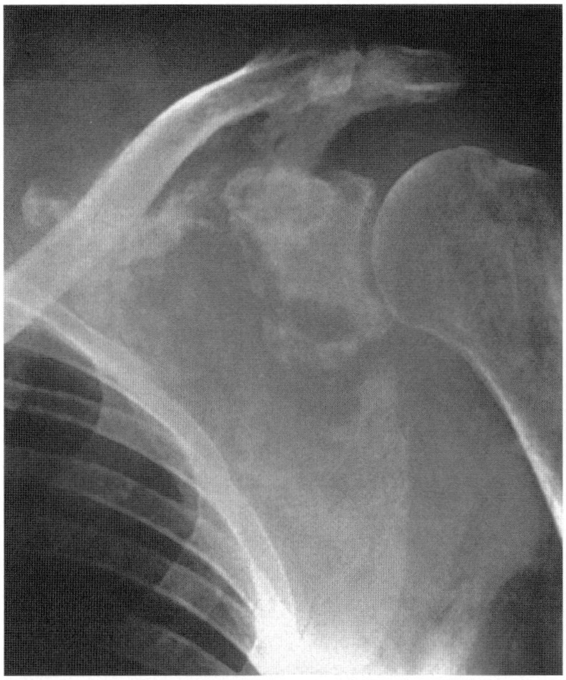

Figure 8-38

MALIGNANT LYMPHOMA

A mixed lytic and sclerotic lesion involves the scapula. There is a pathologic fracture through the body of the scapula.

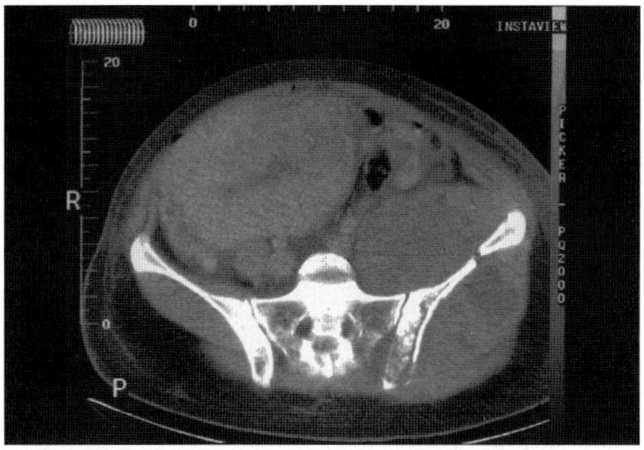

Figure 8-39

MALIGNANT LYMPHOMA

Computerized tomography (CT) shows a destructive lesion involving the left ilium, with a soft tissue mass extending posteriorly and anteriorly from the bone.

commonly involved; the spine and pelvic bones are other common sites. It is extremely unusual to find involvement of the small bones of the hands and feet. When lymphoma presents in the spine or the maxillary antrum, it is often impossible to be sure of the site of origin.

Radiographic Findings. The radiographic findings are quite variable and not specific. In long bones, the diaphysis is preferentially involved. The tumor tends to involve large portions of the bone. It is not unusual to see destruction of 25 to 50 percent of the bone; occasionally, the entire bone is destroyed. The process is poorly defined and has a wide area of transition. The lesion shows variable sclerosis; rarely, the tumor is entirely sclerotic or lytic. The typical pattern is a mixture of lysis and sclerosis, producing a moth-eaten appearance (fig. 8-38). The cortex is usually destroyed, and a soft tissue mass is commonly present. In a flat bone such as the ilium, large areas of destruction with soft tissue extension on both sides of the bone suggest the diagnosis of lymphoma (fig. 8-39). In spite of cortical destruction and soft tissue extension, periosteal new bone formation is uncommon. A purely sclerotic appearance may be mistaken for Paget's disease or osteoblastic metastasis.

Radionuclide bone scan is a sensitive modality for identifying lymphomatous involvement of bone. It may show extensive bone marrow disease that was invisible on plain radiographs. In the proper clinical circumstances, negative results on plain radiography and positive findings on a radionuclide bone scan are suggestive of malignant lymphoma.

MRI is also sensitive for identifying lymphoma of bone (fig. 8-40). Although some studies have suggested that low signal intensity on T_2-weighted images is typical of lymphoma, White et al. (192) did not find this to be a reliable sign. MRI signal changes in the bone marrow, without obvious changes on plain radiographs, are suggestive of malignant lymphoma (fig. 8-41).

Gross Findings. Because most patients with lymphoma are treated with radiotherapy, chemotherapy, or both, gross specimens are uncommon. A portion of bone may be resected if the tumor is associated with a pathologic fracture. Grossly, a large portion of the bone is involved, the cortex is destroyed, the margins are indistinct, and a soft tissue mass is present. The tumor has the fish-flesh appearance usually associated with lymphoma (fig. 8-42).

Although many lymphomas of bone are now diagnosed on the basis of FNA cytology, open

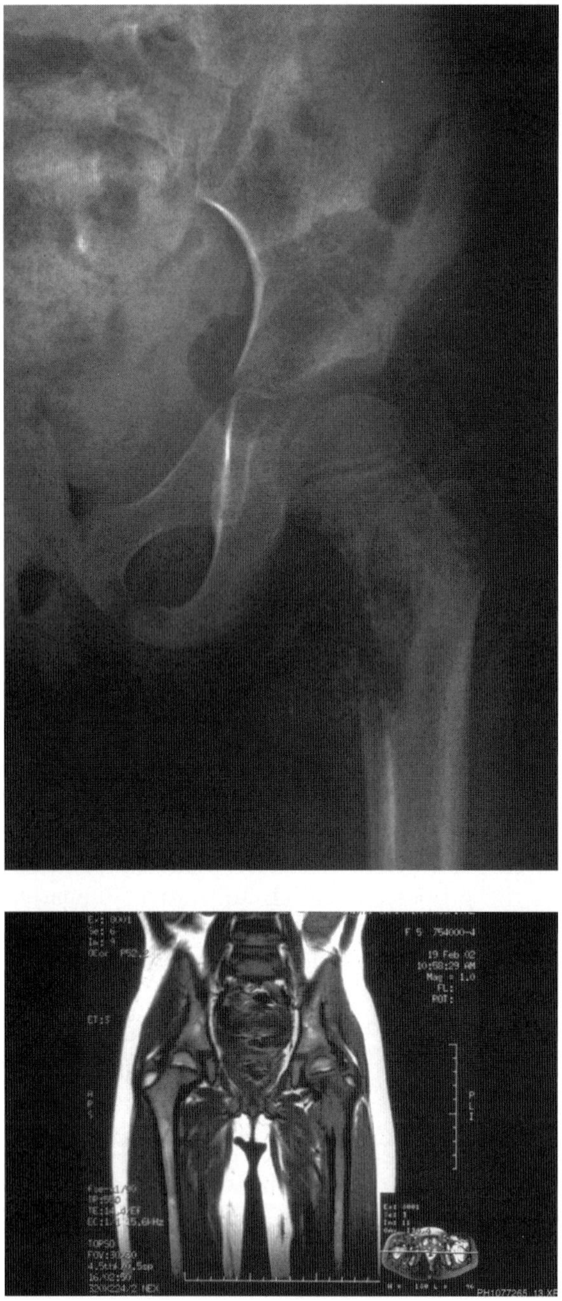

Figure 8-40

MALIGNANT LYMPHOMA

Top: An anteroposterior radiograph shows a large lesion involving the medial aspect of the proximal femur of a 5-year-old boy. There is destruction of the lesser trochanter and periosteal reaction.

Bottom: Coronal T_1-weighted MRI shows replacement of the high signal intensity of bone marrow by tumor, which extends into the medial soft tissues. Biopsy tissue showed anaplastic large cell lymphoma. (Courtesy of Dr. W. Chen, Taipei, Taiwan.)

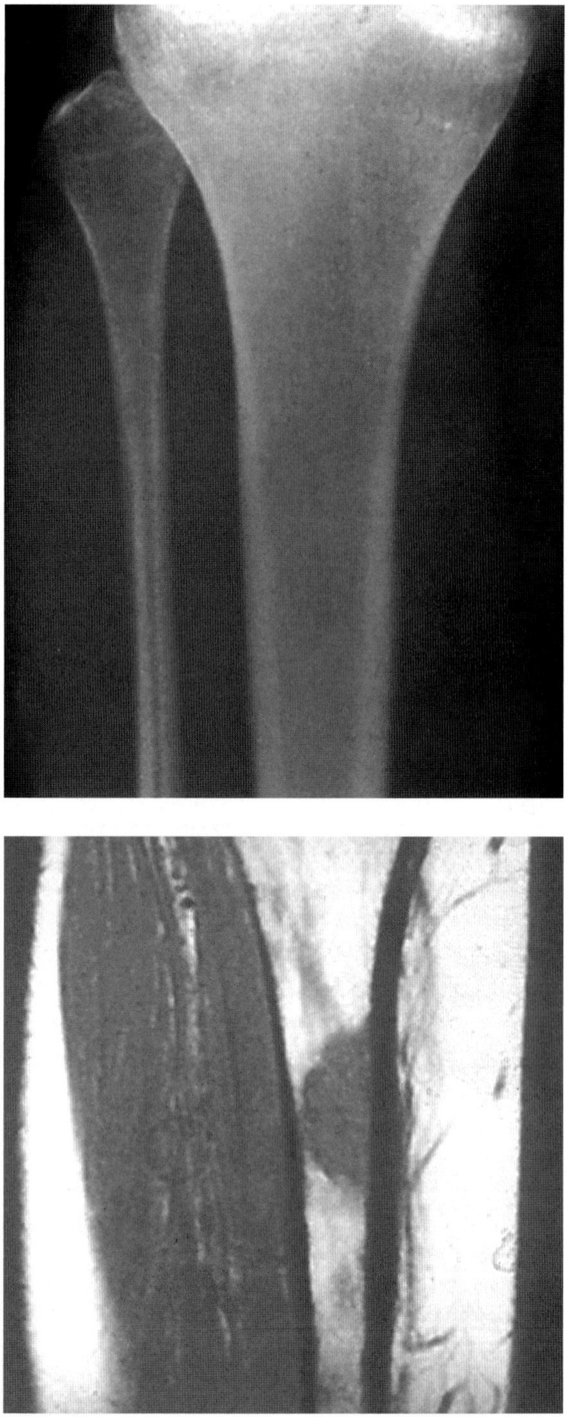

Figure 8-41

MALIGNANT LYMPHOMA

Top: A plain radiograph shows an intact tibia without recognizable evidence of a neoplastic process.

Bottom: The corresponding MRI study, however, shows a lesion in the proximal tibial shaft that is confined to the medullary compartment.

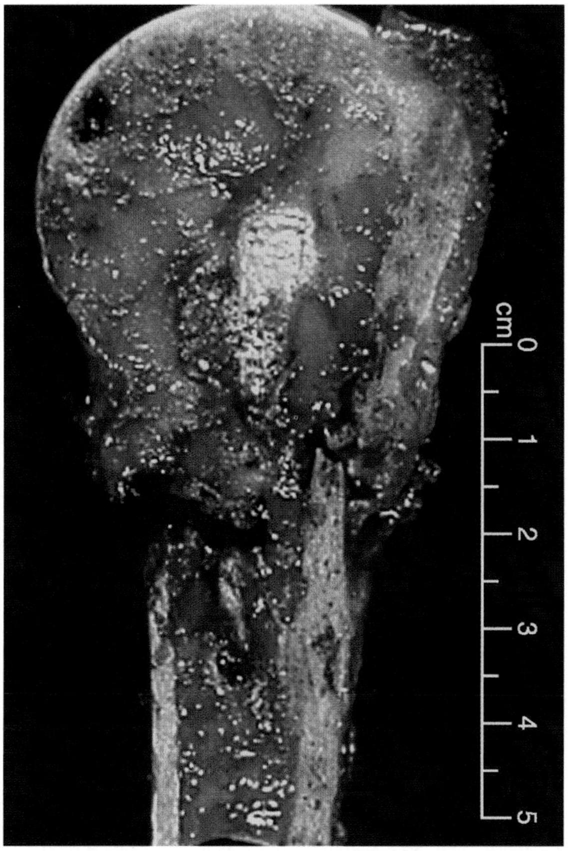

Figure 8-42

MALIGNANT LYMPHOMA

This tumor forms a destructive mass associated with a pathologic fracture in the proximal humerus of a 52-year-old woman. It has the tan-gray, fish-flesh appearance typically seen in lymphomas arising elsewhere.

biopsy may be necessary in some cases. The tumor may be extensively permeative within normal or even thickened medullary bone. Thus, the gross specimen may be quite hard. It is important not to decalcify the entire specimen. If the specimen is sclerotic, decalcification may be prolonged and unnecessarily delay diagnosis. Moreover, decalcification procedures may affect the cytologic features and interfere with immunohistochemical studies. Fleshy tumor tissue can be teased out from between the bony trabeculae; this tissue is amenable to frozen section immunostaining and to rapidly preparing permanent sections.

Microscopic Findings. The majority of lymphomas of the skeleton have a diffuse growth pattern. Although bone marrow involvement is

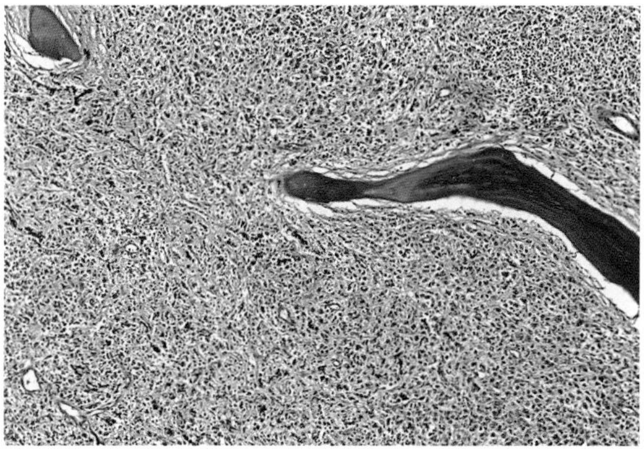

Figure 8-43

MALIGNANT LYMPHOMA

The tumor diffusely involves the marrow spaces, where it permeates between preexisting trabecular bone.

not uncommon in follicular small cleaved cell lymphomas, it is distinctly unusual for them to produce a bone tumor. Similarly, small lymphocytic lymphomas and chronic lymphocytic leukemias are rarely diagnosed in bone biopsy specimens. Consequently, most lymphomas of bone are the diffuse large cell type.

Under low-power magnification, lymphoma of bone has the permeative pattern typical of the disease in other organs. The tumor fills up bone marrow spaces, leaving behind preexisting bony trabeculae (fig. 8-43). Similarly, the tumor cells invade marrow fat and leave fat cells intact. The bony trabeculae may appear normal or thickened and irregular; they may even appear pagetoid.

Fine reticulin fibers occur between individual tumor cells. Occasionally, this produces fibrous bands or even dense, hyalinized collagen (fig. 8-44).

Although most lymphomas may be classified as large cell, the cells vary considerably in size and shape. Frequently, there is a mixture of small, medium, and large cells. Indeed, this polymorphism is typical of lymphoma (fig. 8-45). The nuclei may have irregular outlines and be cleaved. The nucleoli may be prominent. The cytoplasm is not abundant and may be amphophilic.

Rarely, a lymphoma is so fibrotic that the tumor cells spindle, suggesting a sarcoma (fig. 8-46) (178). There may even be formation of a storiform pattern. Other confusing features are clustering of the tumor cells and clearing of the cytoplasm. Lymphomas tend to be crushed during the biopsy procedure. Hence, the biopsy

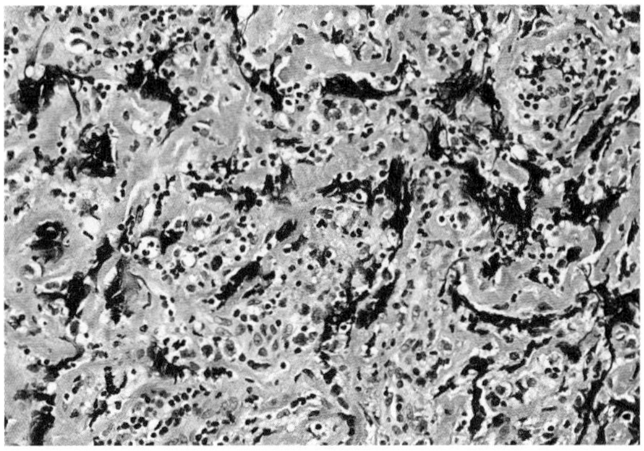

Figure 8-44

MALIGNANT LYMPHOMA

Sclerotic bands of fibrous tissue weave between the tumor cells. The cytologic features of many cells are obscured by crush artifact.

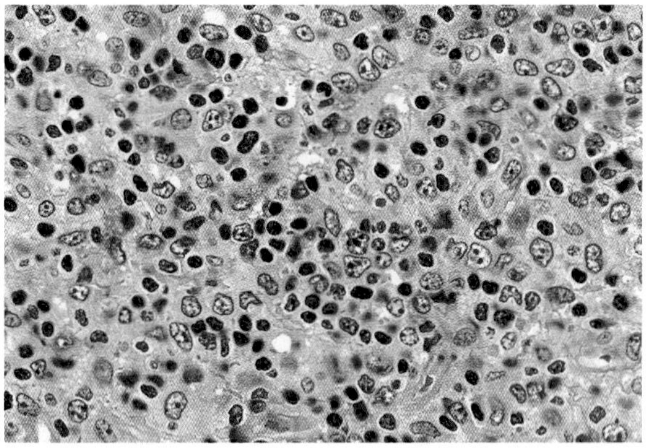

Figure 8-45

MALIGNANT LYMPHOMA

This diffuse large B-cell lymphoma is composed of cells that have a polymorphic appearance and express CD20.

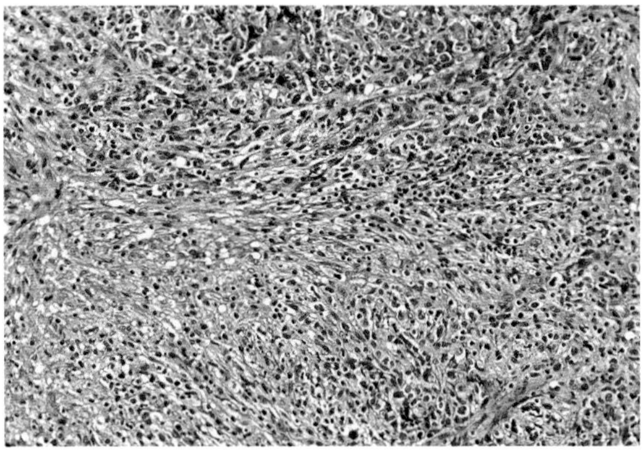

Figure 8-46

MALIGNANT LYMPHOMA

Marked fibrosis in the tumor gives the cells a spindled appearance. This could lead to a mistaken diagnosis of sarcoma.

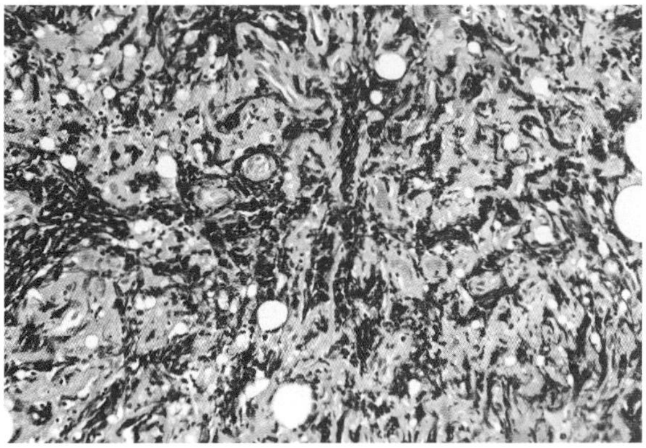

Figure 8-47

MALIGNANT LYMPHOMA

The diagnosis of lymphoma should always be considered when crush artifact is seen in a bone biopsy. This lymphoma contained a large amount of crush artifact. Cells were better preserved in other areas.

specimen may appear as if dense DNA material filled the bone marrow space (fig. 8-47). Such an appearance suggests the diagnosis of malignant lymphoma. Although normal bone marrow cells can be crushed, it is unusual to find extensive crush artifact, similar to that seen in small cell carcinoma of the lung, except in lymphomas and metastatic neuroblastomas in bone. Lymphoblastic lymphomas are especially vulnerable to crush artifact (fig. 8-48).

Hodgkin's disease can involve bone as a secondary phenomenon; rarely is bone disease the initial manifestation. Of 175 patients with Hodgkin's disease reported by Braunstein and White (170), 21 percent had evidence of bone destruction. However, only 7 of 36 patients presented with bone findings. Newcomer et al. (182) found that 15 percent of patients with Hodgkin's disease had bone involvement. Ostrowski et al. (183) reported on 25 patients with biopsy-confirmed Hodgkin's disease of bone, 17 of whom presented with bone lesions. However, the evaluation of 12 of these patients demonstrated lymph node disease. Vertebrae and pelvic bones are involved most

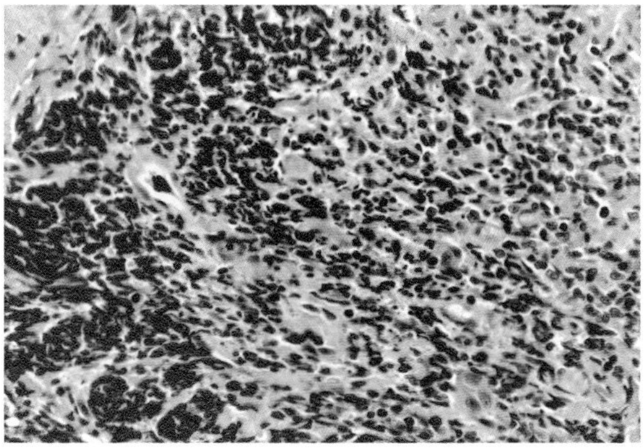

Figure 8-48

MALIGNANT LYMPHOMA

Lymphoblastic lymphoma involving the proximal femur of a 14-year-boy. It is particularly common to see crush artifact in this type of lymphoma. The disease also involved the mediastinum.

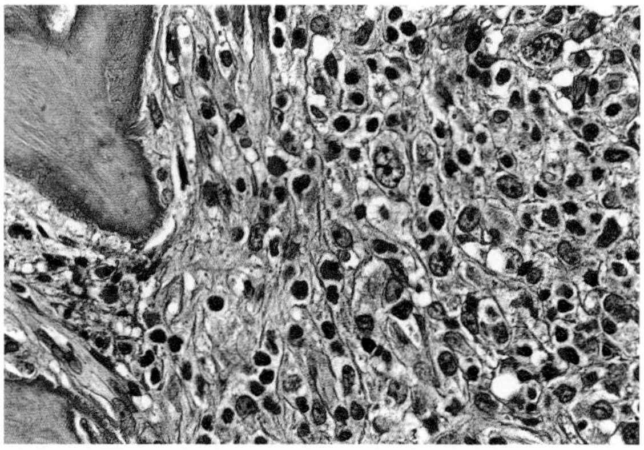

Figure 8-49

HODGKIN'S LYMPHOMA

A binucleated Reed-Sternberg cell is seen in a mixed cellular infiltrate of lymphocytes, macrophages, and eosinophils.

commonly, and the lymph node involvement is usually in the para-aortic areas. Nodular sclerosis and mixed cellularity are the usual types. The presence of bone marrow fibrosis and mixed infiltrate containing eosinophils with occasional large cells with prominent nucleoli should alert one to the possibility of Hodgkin's disease (fig. 8-49). Some tumors have a prominent polymorphonuclear infiltrate. Characteristic Reed-Sternberg cells may be hard to identify.

Leukemic infiltrates can involve bones; this is associated most commonly with a granulocytic tumor (fig. 8-50). In a series of 61 cases of granulocytic sarcoma, Neiman et al. (181) reported that bone, soft tissue, skin, and lymph nodes were involved most often. Granulocytic sarcoma may occur in association with chronic myeloproliferative syndrome or acute granulocytic leukemia or in the absence of bone marrow disease. In some patients with granulocytic sarcoma, leukemic manifestations may not develop for many years (179) and the clinical course may be indolent (191). Neiman et al. (181) described three distinct histologic types of granulocytic sarcoma: well-differentiated (i.e., containing eosinophilic myelocytes), poorly differentiated (rare myelocytes), and blastic (with no granulocytic differentiation and containing large cells with prominent nuclei and nucleoli).

Immunoperoxidase stains have become invaluable in recognizing and subclassifying malignant lymphomas. Lymphomas of bone should be worked up in the same way that the lymph node counterparts are. Nearly all lymphomas of bone are B-cell neoplasms and stain with CD20, although rare T-cell and even Ki-1 lymphomas occur. CD15 and CD30 recognize Reed-Sternberg cells, and myeloperoxidase stain and CD43 help to pinpoint granulocytic differentiation (fig. 8-51).

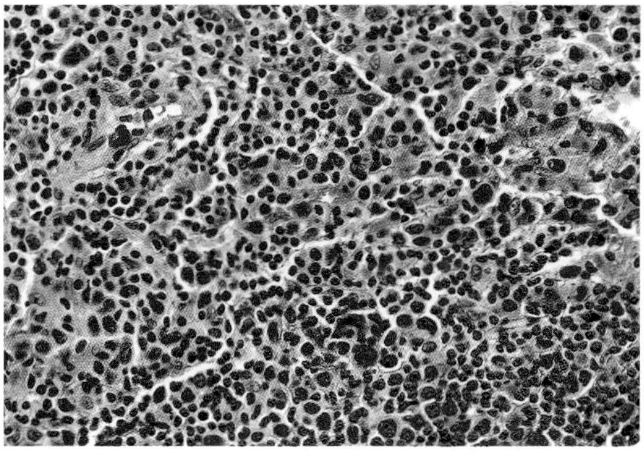

Figure 8-50

GRANULOCYTIC SARCOMA

Without immunohistochemical markers, it would not be possible to distinguish this granulocytic sarcoma from other types of lymphoma. The cells in this tumor expressed myeloperoxidase, but they were negative for other B-cell (CD20) and T-cell (CD3) markers.

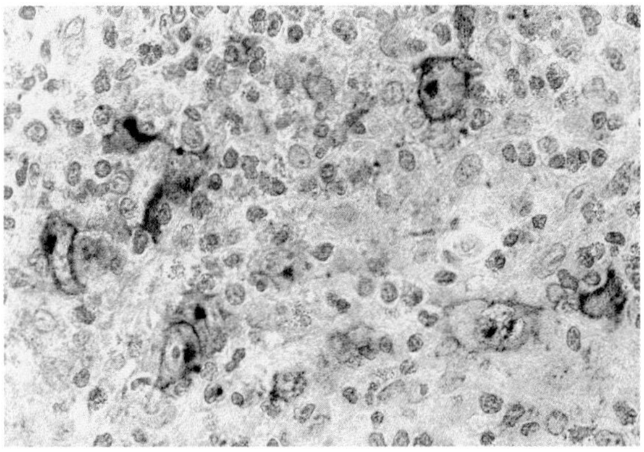

Figure 8-51

HODGKIN'S DISEASE

The Reed-Sternberg cells in this example of Hodgkin's disease (see fig. 8-49) are positive for CD30.

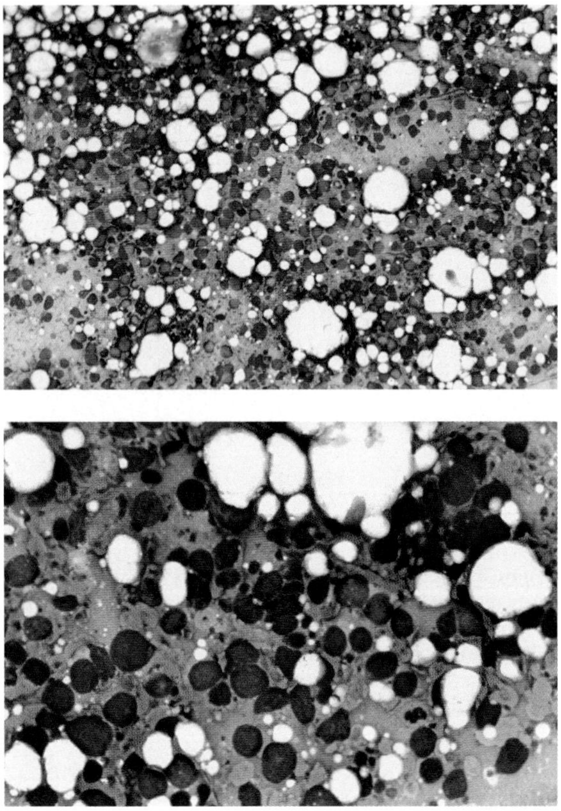

Figure 8-52

LYMPHOMA

Cellular aspirates of a large cell lymphoma of bone. The tumor cells, appearing predominately as naked nuclei, are larger than those of normal lymphocytes and display a condensed chromatin pattern. Small, so-called lymphoglandular bodies are seen in the background.

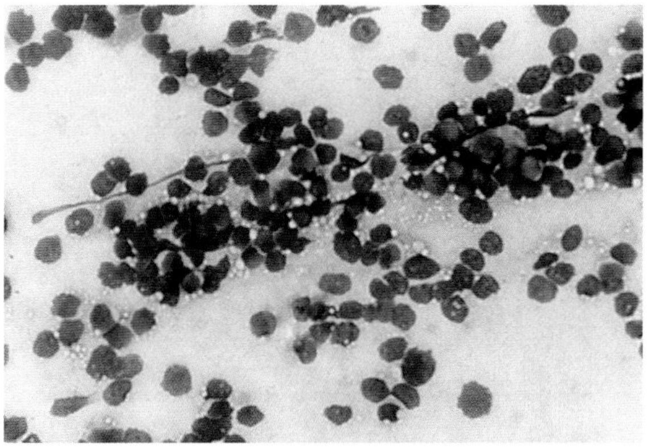

Figure 8-53

LYMPHOMA

FNA of a pre-B-cell acute lymphoblastic leukemia that presented as a solitary bone lesion in the tibia of a 3-year-old boy. The smear shows sheets of small, uniform primitive cells with fine, evenly dispersed chromatin and inconspicuous nucleoli.

Cytologic Findings. FNA cytology is useful in the diagnosis of malignant lymphoma that presents as a primary bone lesion, particularly in quickly differentiating it from other primary bone malignancies and metastatic carcinoma. Large cell lymphomas are characterized by highly cellular aspirates composed of fairly uniform tumor cells that occur primarily as naked, dense nuclei clearly larger than those of normal lymphocytes (fig. 8-52). Distinct nucleoli, scattered mitotic figures, and so-called lymphogranular cytoplasmic bodies are other distinguishing features (177,189). With FNA, large cell, anaplastic lymphoma is occasionally difficult to differentiate from poorly differentiated metastatic carcinomas and from some poorly differentiated primary bone sarcomas. Immunocytochemistry must be performed on the aspirates to diagnose lymphoma, particularly the large cell, anaplastic type. Leukemic infiltrates may also simulate primary bone lesions, particularly in pediatric patients (fig. 8-53), and thus must be considered in the FNA differential diagnosis of small cell malignancies.

Genetics and Other Special Techniques. More than 80 percent of patients with non-Hodgkin's lymphoma (NHL) have clonal chromosomal abnormalities (168,186,188). In contrast to many of the leukemias and sarcomas, single clonal aberrations in NHL are rare; complex numerical and structural changes are observed in most

Table 8-3

"PRIMARY" ACQUIRED CHROMOSOMAL ABNORMALITIES IN LYMPHOMA[a]

Chromosome Lesion	Genes Involved	Cell Lineage	Histology or Disease
Multiple numerical and structural abnormalities (often pseudo-tetraploid state)	?	Reed-Sternberg	Hodgkin's lymphoma
t(8;14)(q24;q32)	*IgH* (14q32)	B cell	Small noncleaved (Burkitt's)
Variants: t(2;8)(p12;q24) or t(8;22)(q24;q11)	*IgK* (2p12) *IgL* (22q11) *myc* (8q24)		
t(14;18)(q32;q21)	*IgH* (14q32) *BCL2* (18q21)	B cell	Follicular (70-90%), high grade (20-40%)
t(3;14)(q27;q32)	*BCL6* (3q27) *IgH* (14q32)	B cell	Diffuse with large cell component
t(11;14)(q13;q32)	*BCL1* (11q13) *IgH* (14q32)	B cell	Mantle cell (centrocytic)
t(9;14)(p13;q32); del(7)(q32)	*PAX5* (9p13) *IgH* (14q32)	B cell	Small cell lymphocytic lymphoma of the plasmacytoid subtype
t(11;18)(q21;q21)	*API2* (11q21) *MALT1* (18q21)	B cell	Low-grade mucosa-associated lymphoid tissue (MALT) type lymphoma
t(2;5)(p23;q35) inv(2)(p23q35)	*ALK* (2p23) *ATIC* (2q35) *NPM* (5q35)	T cell	Anaplastic large cell lymphoma
14q11 rearrangements[b]	*TCRA* (14q11) *TCRD* (14q11)	T cell	T-cell lymphoma

[a]Additional less common variant translocations have been detected in nearly all of the lymphoma subtypes listed below.
[b]Most common rearrangements are inv(14)(q11q32) and t(14;14)(q11;q32).

cases. Although no genetic abnormality is specific for any subtype, each has a nonrandom association with individual classifications of NHL, suggesting a correlation between the altered gene(s) and the histologic, phenotypic, and clinical features of the lymphoma (Tables 8-3, 8-4). Genetic analysis of lesions is used in the clinical management of lymphoma to 1) aid in morphologic diagnosis, 2) provide a prognostic indicator in some cases, and 3) evaluate residual disease by highly specific and sensitive methods (172,173,190). Although microarray gene expression technology has identified many new genes that contribute to accurate classification and prognostication in lymphoma, it is not clear whether this technology will become routine (176). A specific and sensitive cytogenetic or molecular diagnostic marker for the differential diagnosis and clinical monitoring of Hodgkin's lymphoma has not been identified.

Chromosomal translocations of lymphomas of B-cell lineage frequently result in rearrangements of the immunoglobulin heavy and light chain genes, and chromosomal translocations of T-cell lymphomas often produce rearrangements of the beta and gamma/delta chain T-cell receptor genes. Molecular studies show that these types of translocations result in deregulated expression of cellular proto-oncogenes following their juxtaposition with antigen receptor genes. Chromosomal translocations of anaplastic large cell and low-grade mucosa-associated lymphoid tissue type lymphomas often result in the fusion of two genes (nonantigen receptor genes) that result in chimeric mRNA and a novel protein.

There are no genetic aberrations specific for lymphomas involving bone (primary or secondary).

Differential Diagnosis. Malignant lymphoma of bone has to be differentiated from other small cell malignancies such as Ewing's

Table 8-4

PROBABLE "SECONDARY" ACQUIRED CHROMOSOME ABNORMALITIES IN LYMPHOMA AND POSSIBLE CLINICAL SIGNIFICANCE[a]

Chromosomal Lesion	Cinical or Prognostic Significance
1p22	Large cell diffuse lymphoma
1q21-22	Poor survival in intermediate/high-grade lymphoma
2p	Skin infiltration
+3	High-grade lymphoma
+5, +6, +18	Shorter survival
Rearranged 5	Shorter survival
6q13-16	B-cell disease and short survival
+7 with t(14;18)	Diffuse histology
10q22-24	Shorter survival
+12	Large cell diffuse lymphoma
13q21-24	Bulky disease
+17 or i(7q)	Diffuse histology and shorter survival
+der(18)t(14;18)(q32;q21)	Disease progression
Many abnormalities and no normal cells	Rapid progression and short survival
Normal cells present with abnormal clone	Better prognosis than cases without normal cells

[a]Data from reference 188.

sarcoma and metastatic small cell carcinoma. Ewing's sarcoma is almost exclusively a disease of childhood. The tumor cells in Ewing's sarcoma are more uniform than those in malignant lymphoma. Positive staining for CD99 and lack of staining for leukocyte markers help to distinguish the two. Lymphoblastic lymphoma is CD99 positive but also TdT positive. Small cell carcinoma frequently affects the bone marrow but rarely produces a destructive mass lesion.

Polymorphonuclear leukocytes may be prominent, especially in Ki-1 lymphoma and Hodgkin's disease. The neoplastic nature of the background cells must be recognized to avoid a mistaken diagnosis.

Some lymphomas show spindling of tumor cells, suggesting a sarcoma. Diffuse permeation of bone marrow spaces and multicentric involvement of the skeleton should suggest lymphoma and the appropriate stains performed.

Staging. Malignant lymphoma of bone can present with the following four clinical scenarios: 1) one skeletal site is involved; 2) multiple bones are involved but no other organ is involved; 3) a patient presents with a bone tumor, but the work-up shows that other organs are affected; 4) a patient is known to have lymphoma, and a bone biopsy is performed to confirm bone involvement.

Treatment and Prognosis. The appropriate treatment for bone lymphoma is still debated. Some authors have argued that systemic chemotherapy is the sole therapy (167), whereas others have suggested that radiotherapy is the primary modality with additional chemotherapy in cases of systemic disease (175).

Prognosis depends mainly on the stage of the disease (184). Fifty-eight percent of patients with true primary lymphoma of bone survive for 5 years. Unexpectedly, patients with multifocal skeletal disease have a 5-year survival rate of 42 percent. For patients with visceral involvement, the prognosis is poor (5-year survival rate, 22 percent). Dosoretz et al. (174) reported a significantly better prognosis in patients with lymphomas with cleaved cells. Clayton et al. (171) found both stage and histologic type to be important. Reimer et al. (187) found that most patients had disseminated disease at work-up but still achieved remission with chemotherapy.

REFERENCES

Ewing's Sarcoma

1. Ahmad R, Mayol BR, Davis M, Rougraff BT. Extraskeletal Ewing's sarcoma. Cancer 1999;85:725–31.
2. Ahrens S, Hoffmann C, Jabar S, et al. Evaluation of prognostic factors in a tumor volume-adapted treatment strategy for localized Ewing sarcoma of bone: the CESS 86 experience. Cooperative Ewing Sarcoma Study. Med Pediatr Oncol 1999;32:186–95.
3. Akerman M. Tumour necrosis and prognosis in Ewing's sarcoma. Acta Orthop Scand Suppl 1997;273:130–2.
4. Amiel A, Ohali A, Fejgin M, et al. Molecular cytogenetic parameters in Ewing sarcoma. Cancer Genet Cytogenet 2003;140:107–12.
5. Amir G, Issakov J, Meller I, et al. Expression of p53 gene product and cell proliferation marker Ki-67 in Ewing's sarcoma: correlation with clinical outcome. Hum Pathol 2002;33:170–4.
6. Askin FB, Rosai J, Sibley RK, Dehner LP, McAlister WH. Malignant small cell tumor of the thoracopulmonary region in childhood: a distinctive clinicopathologic entity of uncertain histogenesis. Cancer 1979;43:2438–51.
7. Aurias A, Rimbaut C, Buffe D, Dubousset J, Mazabraud A. Chromosomal translocations in Ewing's sarcoma [Letter]. N Engl J Med 1983;309: 496–7.
8. Bacci G, Ferrari S, Bertoni F, et al. Prognostic factors in nonmetastatic Ewing's sarcoma of bone treated with adjuvant chemotherapy: analysis of 359 patients at the Istituto Ortopedico Rizzoli. J Clin Oncol 2000;18:4–11.
9. Bacci G, Toni A, Avella M, et al. Long-term results in 144 localized Ewing's sarcoma patients treated with combined therapy. Cancer 1989;63:1477–86.
10. Bridge JA, Sandberg AA. Cytogenetic and molecular genetic techniques as adjunctive approaches in the diagnosis of bone and soft tissue tumors. Skeletal Radiol 2000;29:249–58.
11. Collins BT, Cramer HM, Frain BE, Davis MM. Fine-needle aspiration biopsy of metastatic Ewing's sarcoma with MIC2 (CD99) immunocytochemistry. Diagn Cytopathol 1998;19:382–4.
12. Dahl I, Akerman M, Angervall L. Ewing's sarcoma of bone. A correlative cytological and histological study of 14 cases. Acta Pathol Microbiol Immunol Scand [A] 1986;94:363–9.
13. Dahlin DC, Coventry MB, Scanlon PW. Ewing's sarcoma: a critical analysis of 165 cases. J Bone Joint Surg Am 1961;43:185–92.
14. Dauphinot L, De Oliveira C, Melot T, et al. Analysis of the expression of cell cycle regulators in Ewing cell lines: EWS-FLI-1 modulates p57KIP2 and c-Myc expression. Oncogene 2001;20:3258–65.
15. de Alava E, Kawai A, Healey JH, et al. EWS-FLI1 fusion transcript structure is an independent determinant of prognosis in Ewing's sarcoma. J Clin Oncol 1998;16:1248–55.
16. de Alava E, Lozano MD, Patino A, Sierrasesumaga L, Pardo-Mindan FJ. Ewing family tumors: potential prognostic value of reverse-transcriptase polymerase chain reaction detection of minimal residual disease in peripheral blood samples. Diagn Mol Pathol 1998;7:152–7.
17. Delattre O, Zucman J, Melot T, et al. The Ewing family of tumors—a subgroup of small-round tumors defined by specific chimeric transcripts. N Engl J Med 1994;331:294–9.
18. Delattre O, Zucman J, Plougastel B, et al. Gene fusion with an ETS DNA-binding domain caused by chromosome translocation in human tumours. Nature 1992;359:162–5.
19. Denny CT. Gene rearrangements in Ewing's sarcoma. Cancer Invest 1996;14:83–8.
20. Desmaze C, Brizard F, Turc-Carel C, et al. Multiple chromosomal mechanisms generate an EWS/FLI1 or an EWS/ERG fusion gene in Ewing tumors. Cancer Genet Cytogenet 1997;97:12–9.
21. Desmaze C, Zucman J, Delattre O, Melot T, Thomas G, Aurias A. Interphase molecular cytogenetics of Ewing's sarcoma and peripheral neuroepithelioma t(11;22) with flanking and overlapping cosmid probes. Cancer Genet Cytogenet 1994;74:13–8.
22. Douglass EC, Rowe ST, Valentine M, Parham D, Meyer WH, Thompson EI. A second nonrandom translocation, der(16)t(1;16)(q21;q13), in Ewing sarcoma and peripheral neuroectodermal tumor. Cytogenet Cell Genet 1990;53:87–90.
23. Eggli KD, Quiogue T, Moser RP Jr. Ewing's sarcoma. Radiol Clin North Am 1993;31:325–37.
24. Ewing J. Diffuse endothelioma of bone. Proc N Y Pathol Soc 1921;21:17–24.
25. Fagnou C, Michon J, Peter M, et al. Presence of tumor cells in bone marrow but not in blood is associated with adverse prognosis in patients with Ewing's tumor: Societe Francaise d'Oncologie Pediatrique. J Clin Oncol 1998;16:1707–11.
26. Fechner RE, Mills SE. Tumors of the bones and joints. Atlas of Tumor Pathology, 3rd Series, Fascicle 8. Washington, DC: Armed Forces Institute of Pathology; 1993.
27. Fizazi K, Dohollou N, Blay JY, et al. Ewing's family of tumors in adults: multivariate analysis of survival and long-term results of multimodality therapy in 182 patients. J Clin Oncol 1998;16:3736–43.

28. Frostad B, Tani E, Brosjo O, Skoog L, Kogner P. Fine needle aspiration cytology in the diagnosis and management of children and adolescents with Ewing sarcoma and peripheral primitive neuroectodermal tumor. Med Pediatr Oncol 2002;38:33–40.
29. Fuchs B, Inwards CY, Janknecht R. Vascular endothelial growth factor expression is up-regulated by EWS-ETS oncoproteins and Sp1 and may represent an independent predictor of survival in Ewing's sarcoma. Clin Cancer Res 2004;10:1344–53.
30. Fukuma M, Okita H, Hata J, Umezawa A. Upregulation of Id2, an oncogenic helix-loop-helix protein, is mediated by the chimeric EWS/ets protein in Ewing sarcoma. Oncogene 2003;22:1–9.
31. Gobel V, Jurgens H, Etspuler G, et al. Prognostic significance of tumor volume in localized Ewing's sarcoma of bone in children and adolescents. J Cancer Res Clin Oncol 1987;113:187–91.
32. Greco MA, Steiner GC, Fazzini E. Ewing's sarcoma with epithelial differentiation: fine structural and immunocytochemical study. Ultrastruct Pathol 1988;12:317–25.
33. Hahm KB, Cho K, Lee C, et al. Repression of the gene encoding the TGF-beta type II receptor is a major target of the EWS-FLI1 oncoprotein. Nat Genet 1999;23:222–7.
34. Hattinger CM, Potschger U, Tarkkanen M, et al. Prognostic impact of chromosomal aberrations in Ewing tumours. Br J Cancer 2002;86:1763–9.
35. Hattinger CM, Rumpler S, Ambros IM, et al. Demonstrations of the translocation der(16)t(1;16)(q12;q11.2) in interphase nuclei of Ewing tumors. Genes Chromosomes Cancer 1996;17:141–50.
36. Hattinger CM, Rumpler S, Strehl S, et al. Prognostic impact of deletions at 1p36 and numerical aberrations in Ewing tumors. Genes Chromosomes Cancer 1999;24:243–54.
37. Hu S, Zhang J, Triche TJ. Characterization of the molecular targets of the Ewing's EWS/FLI-1 fusion gene with a tetracycline regulated inducible expression system. In American Association for Cancer Research. Frontiers in cancer prevention research: genetics, risk modeling, molecular targets for chemoprevention, behavioral prevention research, clinical prevention trials, science, and public policy: proceedings. Philadelphia: 2002:45.
38. Im YH, Kim HT, Lee C, et al. EWS-FLI1, EWS-ERG, and EWS-ETV1 oncoproteins of Ewing tumor family all suppress transcription of transforming growth factor beta type II receptor gene. Cancer Res 2000;60:1536–40.
39. Jeon IS, Davis JN, Braun BS, et al. A variant Ewing's sarcoma translocation (7;22) fuses the EWS gene to the ETS gene ETV1. Oncogene 1995;10:1229–34.
40. Jurgens H, Exner U, Gadner H, et al. Multidisciplinary treatment of primary Ewing's sarcoma of bone. A 6-year experience of a European Cooperative Trial. Cancer 1988;61:23–32.
41. Kaneko Y, Yoshida K, Handa M, et al. Fusion of an ETS-family gene, EIAF, to EWS by t(17;22)(q12;q12) chromosome translocation in an undifferentiated sarcoma of infancy. Genes Chromosomes Cancer 1996;15:115–21.
42. Khan J, Wei JS, Ringner M, et al. Classification and diagnostic prediction of cancers using gene expression profiling and artificial neural networks. Nat Med 2001;7:673–9.
43. Kissane JM, Askin FB, Foulkes M, Stratton LB, Shirley SF. Ewing's sarcoma of bone: clinicopathologic aspects of 303 cases from the Intergroup Ewing's Sarcoma Study. Hum Pathol 1983;14:773–9.
44. Kovar H, Jug G, Aryee DN, et al. Among genes involved in the RB dependent cell cycle regulatory cascade, the p16 tumor suppressor gene is frequently lost in the Ewing family of tumors. Oncogene 1997;15:2225–32.
45. Kumar S, Pack S, Kumar D, et al. Detection of EWS-FLI-1 fusion in Ewing's sarcoma/peripheral primitive neuroectodermal tumor by fluorescence in situ hybridization using formalin-fixed paraffin-embedded tissue. Hum Pathol 1999;30:324–30.
46. Ladanyi M, Bridge JA. Contribution of molecular genetic data to the classification of sarcomas. Hum Pathol 2000;31:532–8.
47. Lawlor ER, Scheel C, Irving J, Sorensen PH. Anchorage-independent multi-cellular spheroids as an in vitro model of growth signaling in Ewing tumors. Oncogene 2002;21:307–18.
48. Lessnick SL, Dacwag CS, Golub TR. The Ewing's sarcoma oncoprotein EWS/FLI induces a p53-dependent growth arrest in primary human fibroblasts. Cancer Cell 2002;1:393–401.
49. Lin PP, Brody RI, Hamelin AC, Bradner JE, Healey JH, Ladanyi M. Differential transactivation by alternative EWS-FLI1 fusion proteins correlates with clinical heterogeneity in Ewing's sarcoma. Cancer Res 1999;59:1428–32.
50. Llombart-Bosch A, Contesso G, Henry-Amar M, et al. Histopathological predictive factors in Ewing's sarcoma of bone and clinicopathological correlations. A retrospective study of 261 cases. Virchows Arch A Pathol Anat Histopathol 1986;409:627–40.
51. Lucas DR, Bentley G, Dan ME, Tabaczka P, Poulik JM, Mott MP. Ewing sarcoma vs lymphoblastic lymphoma. A comparative immunohistochemical study. Am J Clin Pathol 2001;115:11–7.

52. Maitra A, Roberts H, Weinberg AG, Geradts J. Aberrant expression of tumor suppressor proteins in the Ewing family of tumors. Arch Pathol Lab Med 2001;125:1207–12.
53. Manara MC, Perbal B, Benini S, et al. The expression of ccn3(nov) gene in musculoskeletal tumors. Am J Pathol 2002;160:849–59.
54. Mastrangelo T, Modena P, Tornielli S, et al. A novel zinc finger gene is fused to EWS in small round cell tumor. Oncogene 2000;19:3799–804.
55. Maurici D, Perez-Atayde A, Grier HE, Baldini N, Serra M, Fletcher JA. Frequency and implications of chromosomes 8 and 12 gains in Ewing sarcoma. Cancer Genet Cytogenet 1998;100:106–10.
56. May WA, Gishizky ML, Lessnick SL, et al. Ewing sarcoma 11;22 translocation produces a chimeric transcription factor that requires the DNA-binding domain encoded by FLI1 for transformation. Proc Natl Acad Sci U S A 1993;90:5752–6.
57. May WA, Lessnick SL, Braun BS, et al. The Ewing's sarcoma EWS/FLI-1 fusion gene encodes a more potent transcriptional activator and is a more powerful transforming gene than FLI-1. Mol Cell Biol 1993;13:7393–8.
58. Maygarden SJ, Askin FB, Siegal GP, et al. Ewing sarcoma of bone in infants and toddlers. A clinicopathologic report from the Intergroup Ewing's Study. Cancer 1993;71:2109–18.
59. McManus AP, Gusterson BA, Pinkerton CR, Shipley JM. Diagnosis of Ewing's sarcoma and related tumours by detection of chromosome 22q12 translocations using fluorescence in situ hybridization on tumour touch imprints. J Pathol 1995;176:137–42.
60. Monforte-Munoz H, Lopez-Terrada D, Affendie H, Rowland JM, Triche TJ. Documentation of EWS gene rearrangements by fluorescence in-situ hybridization (FISH) in frozen sections of Ewing's sarcoma-peripheral primitive neuroectodermal tumor. Am J Surg Pathol 1999;23:309–15.
61. Nagao K, Ito H, Yoshida H, et al. Chromosomal rearrangement t(11;22) in extraskeletal Ewing's sarcoma and primitive neuroectodermal tumour analysed by fluorescence in situ hybridization using paraffin-embedded tissue. J Pathol 1997; 181:62–6.
62. Nascimento AG, Unni KK, Pritchard DJ, Cooper KL, Dahlin DC. A clinicopathologic study of 20 cases of large-cell (atypical) Ewing's sarcoma of bone. Am J Surg Pathol 1980;4:29–36.
63. Nesbit ME Jr, Gehan EA, Burgert EO Jr, et al. Multimodal therapy for the management of primary, nonmetastatic Ewing's sarcoma of bone: a long-term follow-up of the First Intergroup Study. J Clin Oncol 1990;8:1664–74.
64. Nishimori N, Sasaki Y, Yoshida K, et al. Id2 gene is a novel target of transcriptional activation by EWS-ETS fusion proteins in Ewing family tumors. Oncogene 2002;21:8302–9.
65. Obana K, Yang HW, Piao HY, et al. Aberrations of p16INK4A, p14ARF and p15INK4B genes in pediatric solid tumors. Int J Oncol 2003;23:1151–7.
66. O'Connor MI, Pritchard DJ. Ewing's sarcoma. Prognostic factors, disease control, and the reemerging role of surgical treatment. Clin Orthop 1991;262:78–87.
67. Ohali A, Avigad S, Cohen IJ, et al. High frequency of genomic instability in Ewing family of tumors. Cancer Genet Cytogenet 2004;150:50–6.
68. Parham DM, Hijazi Y, Steinberg SM, et al. Neuroectodermal differentiation in Ewing's sarcoma family of tumors does not predict tumor behavior. Hum Pathol 1999;30:911–8.
69. Paulussen M, Ahrens S, Dunst J, et al. Localized Ewing tumor of bone: final results of the cooperative Ewing's Sarcoma Study CESS 86. J Clin Oncol 2001;19:1818–29.
70. Peter M, Couturier J, Pacquement H, et al. A new member of the ETS family fused to EWS in Ewing tumors. Oncogene 1997;14:1159–64.
71. Picci P, Rougraff BT, Bacci G, et al. Prognostic significance of histopathologic response to chemotherapy in nonmetastatic Ewing's sarcoma of the extremities. J Clin Oncol 1993;11:1763–9.
72. Prieur A, Tirode F, Cohen P, Delattre O. EWS/FLI-1 silencing and gene profiling of Ewing cells reveal downstream oncogenic pathways and a crucial role for repression of insulin-like growth factor binding protein 3. Mol Cell Biol 2004;24: 7275–83.
73. Sahu K, Pai RR, Khadilkar UN. Fine needle aspiration cytology of the Ewing's sarcoma family of tumors. Acta Cytol 2000;44:332–6.
74. Sainati L, Leszl A, Montaldi A, Ninfo V, Basso G. Is the deletion of the short arm of chromosome 1 a prognostic factor in pediatric peripheral primitive neuroepithelioma (PNET)? Med Pediatr Oncol 1996;26:143–4.
75. Sandberg AA, Bridge JA. Updates on cytogenetics and molecular genetics of bone and soft tissue tumors: Ewing sarcoma and peripheral primitive neuroectodermal tumors. Cancer Genet Cytogenet 2000;123:1–26.
76. Schajowicz F. Ewing's sarcoma and reticulum-cell sarcoma of bone; with special reference to the histochemical demonstration of glycogen as an aid to differential diagnosis. J Bone Joint Surg Am 1959;41:349–56.
77. Schleiermacher G, Peter M, Oberlin O, et al. Increased risk of systemic relapses associated with bone marrow micrometastasis and circulating tumor cells in localized ewing tumor. J Clin Oncol 2003;21:85–91.

78. Schmidt D, Herrmann C, Jurgens H, Harms D. Malignant peripheral neuroectodermal tumor and its necessary distinction from Ewing's sarcoma. A report from the Kiel Pediatric Tumor Registry. Cancer 1991;68:2251–9.
79. Scotlandi K, Avnet S, Benini S, et al. Expression of an IGF-I receptor dominant negative mutant induces apoptosis, inhibits tumorigenesis and enhances chemosensitivity in Ewing's sarcoma cells. Int J Cancer 2002;101:11–6.
80. Shing DC, McMullan DJ, Roberts P, et al. FUS/ERG gene fusions in Ewing's tumors. Cancer Res 2003;63:4568–76.
81. Siegal GP, Oliver WR, Reinus WR, et al. Primary Ewing's sarcoma involving the bones of the head and neck. Cancer 1987;60:2829–40.
82. Soldatenkov VA, Trofimova IN, Rouzaut A, McDermott F, Dritschilo A, Notario V. Differential regulation of the response to DNA damage in Ewing's sarcoma cells by ETS1 and EWS/FLI-1. Oncogene 2002;21:2890–5.
83. Sorensen PH, Lessnick SL, Lopez-Terrada D, Liu XF, Triche TJ, Denny CT. A second Ewing's sarcoma translocation, t(21;22), fuses the EWS gene to another ETS-family transcription factor, ERG. Nat Genet 1994;6:146–51.
84. Sozzi G, Minoletti F, Miozzo M, et al. Relevance of cytogenetic and fluorescent in situ hybridization analyses in the clinical assessment of soft tissue sarcoma. Hum Pathol 1997;28:134–42.
85. Spahn L, Petermann R, Siligan C, Schmid JA, Aryee DN, Kovar H. Interaction of the EWS NH2 terminus with BARD1 links the Ewing's sarcoma gene to a common tumor suppressor pathway. Cancer Res 2002;62:4583–7.
86. Stark B, Mor C, Jeison M, et al. Additional chromosome 1q aberrations and der(16)t(1;16), correlation to the phenotypic expression and clinical behavior of the Ewing family of tumors. J Neurooncol 1997;31:3–8.
87. Tarkkanen M, Kiuru-Kuhlefelt S, Blomqvist C, et al. Clinical correlations of genetic changes by comparative genomic hybridization in Ewing sarcoma and related tumors. Cancer Genet Cytogenet 1999;114:35–41.
88. Taylor C, Patel K, Jones T, Kiely F, De Stavola BL, Sheer D. Diagnosis of Ewing's sarcoma and peripheral neuroectodermal tumour based on the detection of t(11;22) using fluorescence in situ hybridisation. Br J Cancer 1993;67:128–33.
89. Terrier P, Henry-Amar M, Triche TJ, et al. Is neuroectodermal differentiation of Ewing's sarcoma of bone associated with an unfavourable prognosis? Eur J Cancer 1995;3:307–14.
90. Tsuchiya T, Sekine K, Hinohara S, Namiki T, Nobori T, Kaneko Y. Analysis of the p16INK4, p14ARF, p15, TP53, and MDM2 genes and their prognostic implications in osteosarcoma and Ewing sarcoma. Cancer Genet Cytogenet 2000;120:91–8.
91. Turc-Carel C, Philip I, Berger MP, Philip T, Lenoir GM. Chromosomal translocations in Ewing's sarcoma [Letter]. N Engl J Med 1983;309:497–8.
92. Urano F, Umezawa A, Hong W, Kikuchi H, Hata J. A novel chimera gene between EWS and E1A-F, encoding the adenovirus E1A enhancer-binding protein, in extraosseous Ewing's sarcoma. Biochem Biophys Res Commun 1996;219:608–12.
93. Uren A, Merchant MS, Sun CJ, et al. Beta-platelet-derived growth factor receptor mediates motility and growth of Ewing's sarcoma cells. Oncogene 2003;22:2334–42.
94. Vakar-Lopez F, Ayala AG, Raymond AK, Czerniak B. Epithelial phenotype in Ewing's sarcoma/primitive neuroectodermal tumor. Int J Surg Pathol 2000;8:59–65.
95. Wai DH, Schaefer KL, Schramm A, et al. Expression analysis of pediatric solid tumor cell lines using oligonucleotide microarrays. Int J Oncol 2002;20:441–56.
96. Watanabe G, Nishimori H, Irefune H, et al. Induction of Tenascin-C by tumor-specific EWS-ETS fusion genes. Genes Chromosomes Cancer 2003;36:224–32.
97. Wei G, Antonescu CR, de Alava E, et al. Prognostic impact of INK4A deletion in Ewing sarcoma. Cancer 2000;89:793–9.
98. West DC, Grier HE, Swallow MM, Demetri GD, Granowetter L, Sklar J. Detection of circulating tumor cells in patients with Ewing's sarcoma and peripheral primitive neuroectodermal tumor. J Clin Oncol 1997;15:583–8.
99. Whang-Peng J, Triche TJ, Knutsen T, Miser J, Douglass EC, Israel MA. Chromosome translocation in peripheral neuroepithelioma. N Engl J Med 1984;311:584–5.
100. Wilkins RM, Pritchard DJ, Burgert EO Jr, Unni KK. Ewing's sarcoma of bone. Experience with 140 patients. Cancer 1986;58:2551–5.
101. Willen H. Fine needle aspiration in the diagnosis of bone tumors. Acta Orthop Scand Suppl 1997;273:47-53.
102. Wunder JS, Paulian G, Huvos AG, Heller G, Meyers PA, Healey JH. The histological response to chemotherapy as a predictor of the oncological outcome of operative treatment of Ewing sarcoma. J Bone Joint Surg Am 1998;80:1020–33.
103. Zielenska M, Zhang ZM, Ng K, et al. Acquisition of secondary structural chromosomal changes in pediatric Ewing sarcoma is a probable prognostic factor for tumor response and clinical outcome. Cancer 2001;91:2156–64.

104. Zoubek A, Dockhorn-Dworniczak B, Delattre O, et al. Does expression of different EWS chimeric transcripts define clinically distinct risk groups of Ewing tumor patients? J Clin Oncol 1996;14:1245–51.
105. Zoubek A, Ladenstein R, Windhager R, et al. Predictive potential of testing for bone marrow involvement in Ewing tumor patients by RT-PCR: a preliminary evaluation. Int J Cancer 1998;79: 56–60.
106. Zucman J, Melot T, Desmaze C, et al. Combinatorial generation of variable fusion proteins in the Ewing family of tumours. EMBO J 1993;12:4481–7.
107. Zwerner JP, Guimbellot J, May WA. EWS/FLI function varies in different cellular backgrounds. Exp Cell Res 2003;290:414–9.
108. Zwerner JP, May WA. Dominant negative PDGF-C inhibits growth of Ewing family tumor cell lines. Oncogene 2002;21:3847–54.

Multiple Myeloma

109. Alexanian R, Balcerzak S, Bonnet JD, et al. Prognostic factors in multiple myeloma. Cancer 1975;36:1192–201.
110. Avet-Loiseau H, Daviet A, Sauner S, Bataille R. Chromosome 13 abnormalities in multiple myeloma are mostly monosomy 13. Br J Haematol 2000;111:1116–7.
111. Avva R, Vanhemert RL, Barlogie B, Munshi N, Angtuaco EJ. CT-guided biopsy of focal lesions in patients with multiple myeloma may reveal new and more aggressive cytogenetic abnormalities. AJNR Am J Neuroradiol 2001;22:781–5.
112. Barlogie B, Epstein J, Selvanayagam P, Alexanian R. Plasma cell myeloma—new biological insights and advances in therapy. Blood 1989;73: 865–79.
113. Bataille R, Harousseau JL. Multiple myeloma. N Engl J Med 1997;336:1657–64.
114. Block AM. Cancer cytogenetics. In: Gersen SL, Keagle MB, eds. The principles of clinical cytogenetics. Totowa, NJ: Humana Press; 1999:345–420.
115. Chesi M, Bergsagel PL, Brents LA, Smith CM, Gerhard DS, Kuehl WM. Dysregulation of cyclin D1 by translocation into an IgH gamma switch region in two multiple myeloma cell lines. Blood 1996;88:674–81.
116. Chesi M, Bergsagel PL, Shonukan OO, et al. Frequent dysregulation of the c-maf proto-oncogene at 16q23 by translocation to an Ig locus in multiple myeloma. Blood 1998;91:4457–63.
117. Chesi M, Kuehl WM, Bergsagel PL. Recurrent immunoglobulin gene translocations identify distinct molecular subtypes of myeloma. Ann Oncol 2000;11(Suppl 1):131–5.
118. Chesi M, Nardini E, Brents LA, et al. Frequent translocation t(4;14)(p16.3;q32.3) in multiple myeloma is associated with increased expression and activating mutations of fibroblast growth factor receptor 3. Nat Genet 1997;16:260–4.
119. Chesi M, Nardini E, Lim RS, Smith KD, Kuehl WM, Bergsagel PL. The t(4;14) translocation in myeloma dysregulates both FGFR3 and a novel gene, MMSET, resulting in IgH/MMSET hybrid transcripts. Blood 1998;92:3025–34.
120. Choi Y, Zhang J, Murga C, et al. PTEN, but not SHIP and SHIP2, suppresses the PI3K/Akt pathway and induces growth inhibition and apoptosis of myeloma cells. Oncogene 2002; 21:5289–300.
121. Claudio JO, Masih-Khan E, Tang H, et al. A molecular compendium of genes expressed in multiple myeloma. Blood 2002;100:2175–86.
122. De Vos J, Thykjaer T, Tarte K, et al. Comparison of gene expression profiling between malignant and normal plasma cells with oligonucleotide arrays. Oncogene 2002;21:6848–57.
123. Dewald GW, Kyle RA, Hicks GA, Greipp PR. The clinical significance of cytogenetic studies in 100 patients with multiple myeloma, plasma cell leukemia, or amyloidosis. Blood 1985;66:380–90.
124. Facon T, Avet-Loiseau H, Guillerm G, et al. Chromosome 13 abnormalities identified by FISH analysis and serum beta2-microglobulin produce a powerful myeloma staging system for patients receiving high-dose therapy. Blood 2001;97:1 566–71.
125. Fonseca R, Barlogie B, Bataille R, et al. Genetics and cytogenetics of multiple myeloma: a workshop report. Cancer Res 2004;64:1546–58.
126. Fonseca R, Oken MM, Harrington D, et al. Deletions of chromosome 13 in multiple myeloma identified by interphase FISH usually denote large deletions of the q arm or monosomy. Leukemia 2001;15:981–6.
127. Hallek M, Bergsagel PL, Anderson KC. Multiple myeloma: increasing evidence for a multistep transformation process. Blood 1998;91:3–21.
128. Hanamura I, Iida S, Akano Y, et al. Ectopic expression of MAFB gene in human myeloma cells carrying (14;20)(q32;q11) chromosomal translocations. Jpn J Cancer Res 2001;92:638–44.
129. Hayami Y, Iida S, Nakazawa N, et al. Inactivation of the E3/LAPTm5 gene by chromosomal rearrangement and DNA methylation in human multiple myeloma. Leukemia 2003;17:1650–7.
130. Heim S, Mitelman F. Cancer cytogenetics, 2nd ed. New York: Wiley-Liss; 1995:237.
131. Iida S, Rao PH, Butler M, et al. Deregulation of MUM1/IRF4 by chromosomal translocation in multiple myeloma. Nat Genet 1997;17:226–30.

132. Inoue J, Otsuki T, Hirasawa A, et al. Overexpression of PDZK1 within the 1q12-q22 amplicon is likely to be associated with drug-resistance phenotype in multiple myeloma. Am J Pathol 2004;165:71–81.
133. Jones D, Bhatia VK, Krausz T, Pinkus GS. Crystal-storing histiocytosis: a disorder occurring in plasmacytic tumors expressing immunoglobulin kappa light chain. Hum Pathol 1999;30:1441–8.
134. Kastrinakis NG, Gorgoulis VG, Foukas PG, Dimopoulos MA, Kittas C. Molecular aspects of multiple myeloma. Ann Oncol 2000;11:1217–28.
135. Kramer A, Schultheis B, Bergmann J, et al. Alterations of the cyclin D1/pRb/p16(INK4A) pathway in multiple myeloma. Leukemia 2002;16:1844–51.
136. Kyle RA. Long-term survival in multiple myeloma. N Engl J Med 1983;308:314–6.
137. Larson RS, Sukpanichnant S, Greer JP, Cousar JB, Collins RD. The spectrum of multiple myeloma: diagnostic and biological implications. Hum Pathol 1997;28:1336–47.
138. Moreau P, Facon T, Leleu X, et al. Recurrent 14q32 translocations determine the prognosis of multiple myeloma, especially in patients receiving intensive chemotherapy. Blood 2002;100:1579–83.
139. Papadaki H, Kyriakou D, Foudoulakis A, Markidou F, Alexandrakis M, Eliopoulos GD. Serum levels of soluble IL-6 receptor in multiple myeloma as indicator of disease activity. Acta Haematol 1997;97:191–5.
140. Perez-Simon JA, Garcia-Sanz R, Tabernero MD, et al. Prognostic value of numerical chromosome aberrations in multiple myeloma: a FISH analysis of 15 different chromosomes. Blood 1998;91:3366–71.
141. Reinus WR, Kyriakos M, Gilula LA, Brower AC, Merkel K. Plasma cell tumors with calcified amyloid deposition mistaken for chondrosarcoma. Radiology 1993;189:505–9.
142. Roger DJ, Bono JV, Singh JK. Plasmacytoma arising from a focus of chronic osteomyelitis. A case report. J Bone Joint Surg Am 1992;74:619–23.
143. Ronchetti D, Greco A, Compasso S, et al. Deregulated FGFR3 mutants in multiple myeloma cell lines with t(14;14): comparative analysis of Y373C, K650E and the novel G384D mutations. Oncogene 2001;20:3553–62.
144. Sandberg AA. The chromosomes in human cancer and leukemia, 2nd ed. New York: Elsevier; 1990:649.
145. Sangfelt O, Osterborg A, Grander D, et al. Response to interferon therapy in patients with multiple myeloma correlates with expression of the Bcl-2 oncoprotein. Int J Cancer 1995;63:190–2.
146. Santra M, Zhan F, Tian E, Barlogie B, Shaughnessy J Jr. A subset of multiple myeloma harboring the t(4;14)(p16;q32) translocation lacks FGFR3 expression but maintains an IGH/MMSET fusion transcript. Blood 2003;101:2374–6.
147. Sawyer JR, Lukacs JL, Munshi N, et al. Identification of new nonrandom translocations in multiple myeloma with multicolor spectral karyotyping. Blood 1998;92:4269–78.
148. Sawyer JR, Lukacs JL, Thomas EL, et al. Multicolour spectral karyotyping identifies new translocations and a recurring pathway for chromosome loss in multiple myeloma. Br J Haematol 2001;112:167–74.
149. Sawyer JR, Waldron JA, Jagannath S, Barlogie B. Cytogenetic findings in 200 patients with multiple myeloma. Cancer Genet Cytogenet 1995;82:41–9.
150. Shaughnessy J Jr, Gabrea A, Qi Y, et al. Cyclin D3 at 6p21 is dysregulated by recurrent chromosomal translocations to immunoglobulin loci in multiple myeloma. Blood 2001;98:217–23.
151. Shi Y, Gera J, Hu L, et al. Enhanced sensitivity of multiple myeloma cells containing PTEN mutations to CCI-779. Cancer Res 2002;62:5027–34.
152. Shou Y, Martelli ML, Gabrea A, et al. Diverse karyotypic abnormalities of the c-myc locus associated with c-myc dysregulation and tumor progression in multiple myeloma. Proc Natl Acad Sci U S A 2000;97:228–33.
153. Soderlund V, Tani E, Skoog L, Bauer HC, Kreicbergs A. Diagnosis of skeletal lymphoma and myeloma by radiology and fine needle aspiration cytology. Cytopathology 2001;12:157–67.
154. Strand WR, Banks PM, Kyle RA. Anaplastic plasma cell myeloma and immunoblastic lymphoma. Clinical, pathologic, and immunologic comparison. Am J Med 1984;76:861–7.
155. Sukpanichnant S, Cousar JB, Leelasiri A, Graber SE, Greer JP, Collins RD. Diagnostic criteria and histologic grading in multiple myeloma: histologic and immunohistologic analysis of 176 cases with clinical correlation. Hum Pathol 1994;25:308–18.
156. Tricot G, Barlogie B, Jagannath S, et al. Poor prognosis in multiple myeloma is associated only with partial or complete deletions of chromosome 13 or abnormalities involving 11q and not with other karyotype abnormalities. Blood 1995;86:4250–6.
157. Tu Y, Renner S, Xu F, et al. BCL-X expression in multiple myeloma: possible indicator of chemoresistance. Cancer Res 1998;58:256–62.
158. Zojer N, Konigsberg R, Ackermann J, et al. Deletion of 13q14 remains an independent adverse prognostic variable in multiple myeloma despite its frequent detection by interphase fluorescence in situ hybridization. Blood 2000;95:1925–30.

Solitary Myeloma (Plasmacytoma)

159. Bataille R, Sany J. Solitary myeloma: clinical and prognostic features of a review of 114 cases. Cancer 1981;48:845–51.
160. Dimopoulos MA, Goldstein J, Fuller L, Delasalle K, Alexanian R. Curability of solitary bone plasmacytoma. J Clin Oncol 1992;10:587–90.
161. Frassica DA, Frassica FJ, Schray MF, Sim FH, Kyle RA. Solitary plasmacytoma of bone: Mayo Clinic experience. Int J Radiat Oncol Biol Phys 1989;16:43–8.

Osteosclerotic Myeloma

162. Kelly JJ Jr, Kyle RA, Miles JM, Dyck PJ. Osteosclerotic myeloma and peripheral neuropathy. Neurology 1983;33:202–10.
163. Mangalik A, Veliath AJ. Osteosclerotic myeloma and peripheral neuropathy. A case report. Cancer 1971;28:1040–5.
164. Resnick D, Greenway GD, Bardwick PA, Zvaifler NJ, Gill GN, Newman DR. Plasma-cell dyscrasia with polyneuropathy, organomegaly, endocrinopathy, M-protein, and skin changes: the POEMS syndrome. Distinctive radiographic abnormalities. Radiology 1981;140:17–22.
165. Voss SD, Murphey MD, Hall FM. Solitary osteosclerotic plasmacytoma: association with demyelinating polyneuropathy and amyloid deposition. Skeletal Radiol 2001;30:527–9.

Malignant Lymphoma

166. Baar J, Burkes RL, Bell R, Blackstein ME, Fernandes B, Langer F. Primary non-Hodgkin's lymphoma of bone. A clinicopathologic study. Cancer 1994;73:1194–9.
167. Bacci G, Jaffe N, Emiliani E, et al. Therapy for primary non-Hodgkin's lymphoma of bone and a comparison of results with Ewing's sarcoma. Ten years' experience at the Istituto Ortopedico Rizzoli. Cancer 1986;57:1468–72.
168. Block AW. Cancer cytogenetics. In: Gersen SL, Keagle MB, eds. The principles of clinical cytogenetics. Totowa, NJ: Humana Press; 1999:345–420.
169. Braunstein EM. Hodgkin disease of bone: radiographic correlation with the histological classification. Radiology 1980;137:643–6.
170. Braunstein EM, White SJ. Non-Hodgkin lymphoma of bone. Radiology 1980;135:59–63.
171. Clayton F, Butler JJ, Ayala AG, Ro JY, Zornoza J. Non-Hodgkin's lymphoma in bone. Pathologic and radiologic features with clinical correlates. Cancer 1987;60:2494–501.
172. Cook JR, Shekhter-Levin S, Swerdlow SH. Utility of routine classical cytogenetic studies in the evaluation of suspected lymphomas: results of 279 consecutive lymph node/extranodal tissue biopsies. Am J Clin Pathol 2004;121:826–35.
173. Dalla-Favera R, Gaidano G, Weinstein HJ. Lymphomas. In: DeVita VT Jr, Hellman S, Rosenberg SA, eds. Cancer, principles and practice of oncology, 6th ed. Philadelphia: Lippincott, Williams & Wilkins; 2001:2215–35.
174. Dosoretz DE, Raymond AK, Murphy GF, et al. Primary lymphoma of bone: the relationship of morphologic diversity to clinical behavior. Cancer 1982;50:1009–14.
175. Fairbanks RK, Bonner JA, Inwards CY, et al. Treatment of stage IE primary lymphoma of bone. Int J Radiat Oncol Biol Phys 1994;28:363–72.
176. Gascoyne RD. Emerging prognostic factors in diffuse large B cell lymphoma. Curr Opin Oncol 2004;16:436–41.
177. Htwe WM, Lucas DR, Bedrossian CW, Ryan JR. Fine-needle aspirate of primary lymphoma of bone. Diagn Cytopathol 1996;15:421–6.
178. Kluin PM, Slootweg PJ, Schuurman HJ, et al. Primary B-cell malignant lymphoma of the maxilla with a sarcomatous pattern and multilobulated nuclei. Cancer 1984;54:1598–605.
179. Meis JM, Butler JJ, Osborne BM, Manning JT. Granulocytic sarcoma in nonleukemic patients. Cancer 1986;58:2697–709.
180. Moses AM, Spencer H. Hypercalcemia in patients with malignant lymphoma. Ann Intern Med 1963;59:531–6.
181. Neiman RS, Barcos M, Berard C, et al. Granulocytic sarcoma: a clinicopathologic study of 61 biopsied cases. Cancer 1981;48:1426–37.
182. Newcomer LN, Silverstein MB, Cadman EC, Farber LR, Bertino JR, Prosnitz LR. Bone involvement in Hodgkin's disease. Cancer 1982; 49:338–42.
183. Ostrowski ML, Inwards CY, Strickler JG, Witzig TE, Wenger DE, Unni KK. Osseous Hodgkin disease. Cancer 1999;85:1166–78.
184. Ostrowski ML, Unni KK, Banks PM, et al. Malignant lymphoma of bone. Cancer 1986;58: 2646–55.
185. Parker F Jr, Jackson H Jr. Primary reticulum cell sarcoma of bone. Surg Gynecol Obstet 1939;68: 45–53.
186. Raimondi SC. Cytogenetics of lymphoid neoplasias. In: Mark HFL, ed. Medical cytogenetics. New York: Marcel Dekker; 2000:372–411.
187. Reimer RR, Chabner BA, Young RC, Reddick R, Johnson RE. Lymphoma presenting in bone: results of histopathology, staging, and therapy. Ann Intern Med 1977;87:50–5.
188. Sanger WG, Dave BJ, Bishop MR. Cytogenetics. In: Hancock BW, Selby PJ, MacLennan K, Armitage JO, eds. Malignant lymphoma. London: Arnold; 2000:91–103.

189. Soderlund V, Tani E, Skoog L, Bauer HC, Kreicbergs A. Diagnosis of skeletal lymphoma and myeloma by radiology and fine needle aspiration cytology. Cytopathology 2001;12:157–67.
190. Vega F, Medeiros LJ. Chromosomal translocations involved in non-Hodgkin lymphomas. Arch Pathol Lab Med 2003;127:1148–60.
191. Welch P, Grossi C, Carroll A, et al. Granulocytic sarcoma with an indolent course and destructive skeletal disease. Tumor characterization with immunologic markers, electron microscopy, cytochemistry, and cytogenetic studies. Cancer 1986;57:1005–10.
192. White LM, Schweitzer ME, Khalili K, Howarth DJ, Wunder JS, Bell RS. MR imaging of primary lymphoma of bone: variability of T2-weighted signal intensity. AJR Am J Roentgenol 1998;170:1243–7.

9 NOTOCHORDAL TUMORS

CHORDOMA

Definition. Chordoma is a low-grade malignant tumor that is thought to arise from the remnants of the notochord. It is confined to the spine, especially the proximal and distal portions. Tumors simulating chordoma can occur outside the midline; they probably represent myxoid chondrosarcomas or parachordomas.

General Features. Chordomas account for about 4 percent of malignant bone tumors (51). The Mayo Clinic files contain the records of 411 chordomas, which account for 6 percent of all malignant bone tumors (fig. 9-1). Although chordomas are thought to arise from notochordal remnants, one study has cast doubt on this by noting histochemical differences between fetal notochord and chordoma (5). Although chordomas do not arise from bony elements, their inclusion among bone tumors is justified because of their clinical presentation.

Clinical Features. The clinical features depend on the site of involvement. Patients with

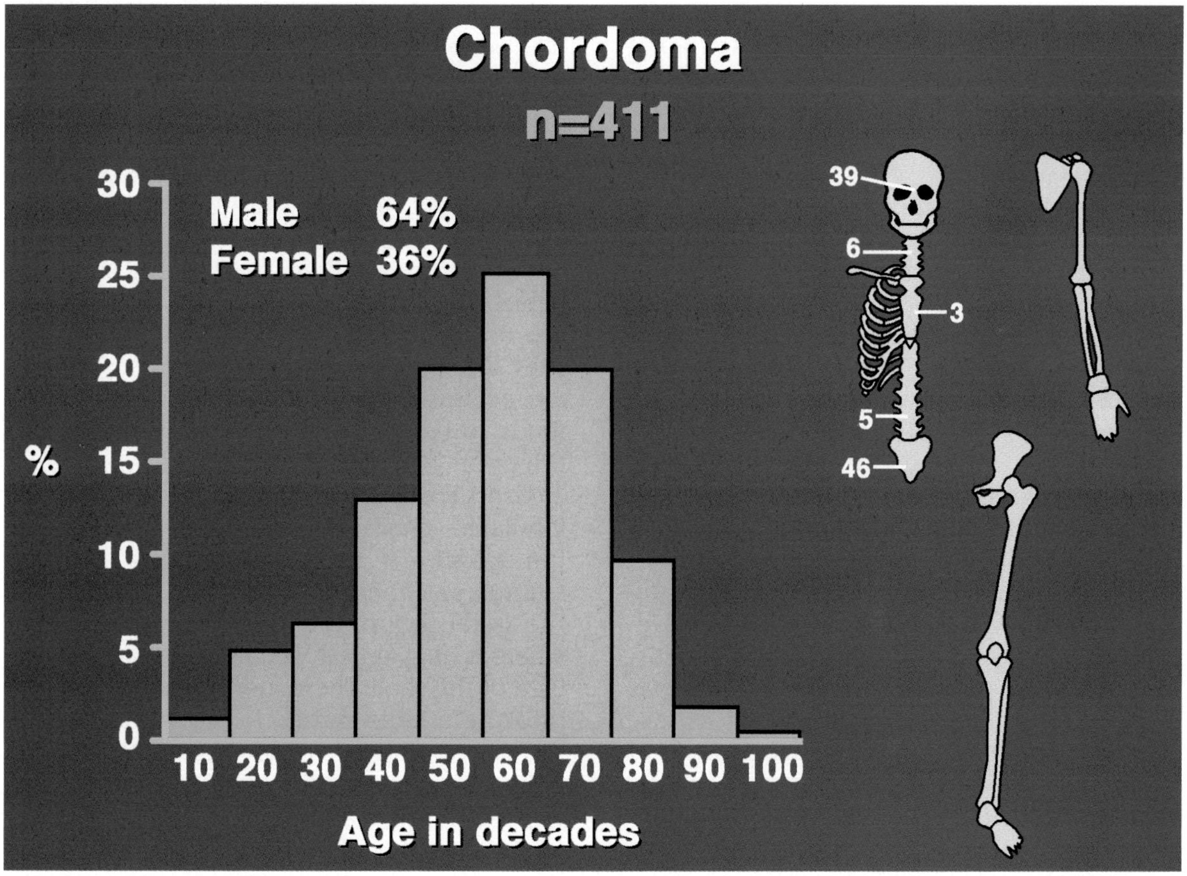

Figure 9-1

CHORDOMA

Distribution of chordoma according to the age and sex of the patient and the site of the lesion.

sacrococcygeal chordomas present with low back pain, frequently of long duration. Constipation and bladder dysfunction may occur by the tumor impinging directly on the bladder or rectum or by involvement of nerves. Chordomas of the spine produce symptoms by impinging on the spinal cord or nerve roots. Patients with spheno-occipital chordomas present with headache and symptoms related to cranial nerve involvement. Although any nerve may be affected, involvement of the sixth cranial nerve is typical, with resultant diplopia. Pressure on the optic nerve may cause blindness. Endocrine dysfunction may result from destruction of the pituitary gland.

Chordoma generally is a disease of adults; most patients are in the fifth to seventh decades of life. Patients with chordomas of the base of the skull generally are a decade younger than those with involvement of the mobile spine and sacrum. In the case records of the Mayo Clinic files, only four of the patients with chordoma were in the first decade of life and all of them had tumors of the spheno-occipital region. The youngest patient with a sacral tumor was a 13-year-old girl.

Males are affected more commonly than females, by a ratio of 2 to 1 (42,53). Some authors have not reported a sex predilection (19).

Sites. The sacrococcygeal region is the site most commonly involved, accounting for about 50 percent of cases (19,51,52). About 37 percent of the tumors involve the basisphenoid, and the rest involve the vertebrae (20). The cervical spine is involved slightly more commonly than the other segments.

Radiographic Findings. Utne and Pugh (52) have described the plain radiographic findings in a series of chordomas. Overall, the plain radiographs showed evidence of bony involvement in 83 percent of the cases and a soft tissue mass in 80 percent. Increased density was found in only 15 percent of cases.

When chordoma involves the sacrococcygeal region, bone involvement is found in 75 percent of cases and a soft tissue mass in 85 percent. Chordoma presents as a lytic destructive process that tends to push into surrounding soft tissues, causing expansion of bone. An increase in radiographic density may be seen in half of the cases and probably represents residual bony trabeculae rather than new bone formation. The soft tissue mass tends to be anterior. Because of the overlying gas shadows, the lesion may be obscured on plain radiographs (fig. 9-2). Kaiser et al. (26) thought in retrospect that the findings on plain radiographs were negative in 17 of 63 cases studied. Computerized tomography (CT) and magnetic resonance imaging (MRI) have made it easier to detect chordomas.

Spinal chordomas start in the body of a vertebra, although de Bruine and Kroon (17) described one tumor that began in the posterior elements. Some studies have suggested that 50 percent (52) or most (22) spinal chordomas involve more than one vertebral body; others have reported a much lower incidence (17). Although the lesions are predominantly lytic, sclerosis may be present in about two thirds of cases (fig. 9-3). Fractures are found only in lower thoracic and lumbar vertebrae affected by tumor, and fracture callus may contribute to the sclerosis seen on plain radiographs.

Cranial chordomas present as destructive lesions that involve the spheno-occipital and hypophyseal area. A portion of the sella turcica is involved in most tumors. Calcification occurs in 30 to 70 percent of cases (fig. 9-4) (22).

All radiographic studies are highly sensitive for detecting chordoma (30). CT is better for detecting calcification (fig. 9-5). MRI is superior for defining the extent of the lesion in all sites, and this has become important for modern aggressive surgical resections. Chordoma tends to be dark on T_1-weighted images and bright on T_2-weighted ones (30,48).

Gross Findings. Chordoma presents as a soft, lobulated, grayish, glistening and translucent tumor and may resemble mucinous adenocarcinoma or chondrosarcoma (figs. 9-6–9-8). In the sacral region, the tumor bulges anteriorly where it may appear well encapsulated. In the base of the skull, the tumor frequently spreads into the middle cranial fossa or into the nasopharynx and even may present as a nasal polyp (10). Recurrent chordoma frequently produces multiple nodules.

Microscopic Findings. Chordomas are lobulated neoplasms, a feature that is always apparent if sufficient tissue is examined. This feature is not helpful in diagnosing spheno-occipital tumors, for which only small amounts

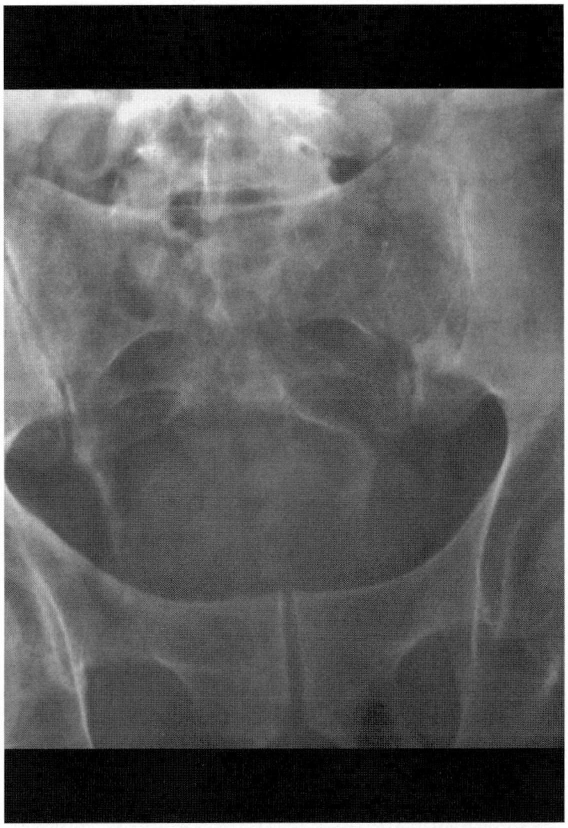

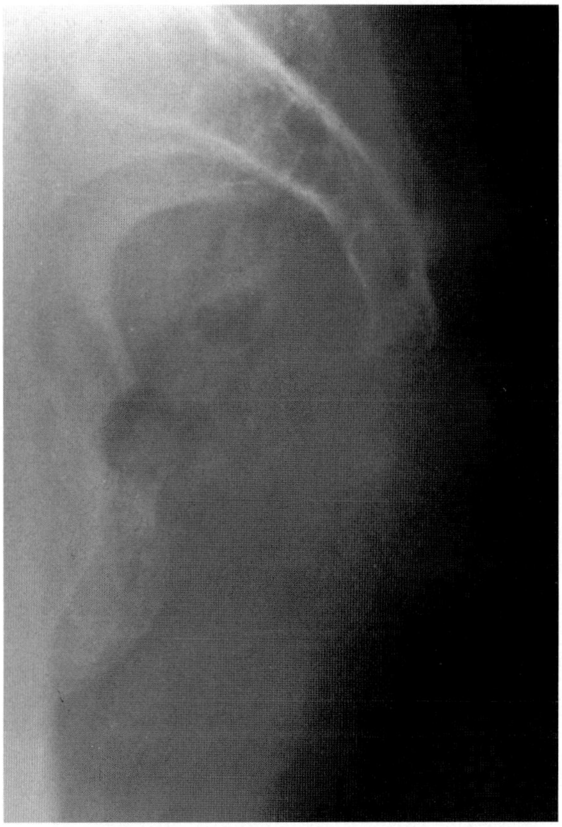

Figure 9-2

CHORDOMA

Left: Plain radiograph shows a tumor characterized by the loss of the usual landmarks. Even large tumors may be difficult to identify because of overlying gas shadows and the complex anatomy.

Right: Lateral radiographs are better for demonstrating the lesion.

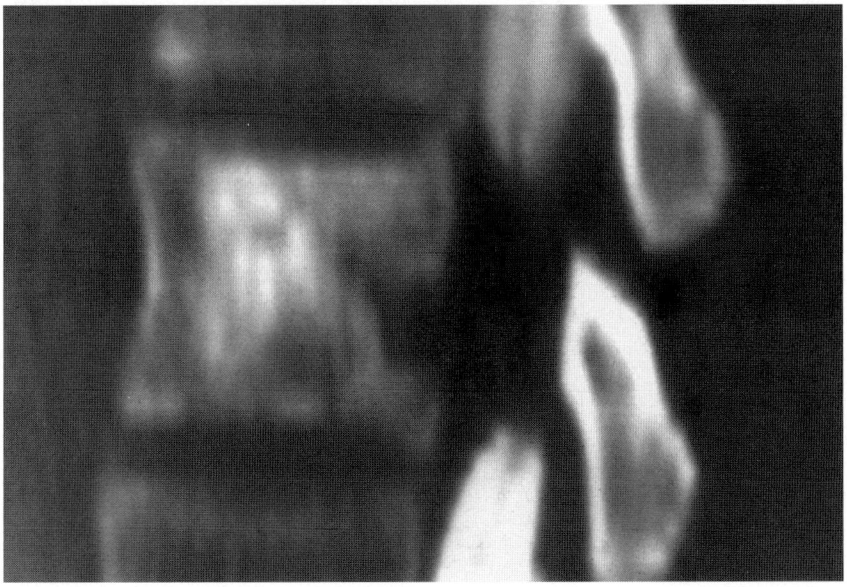

Figure 9-3

CHORDOMA

The tumor involves the lumbar vertebra. There is partial mineralization, and the posterior cortex is destroyed.

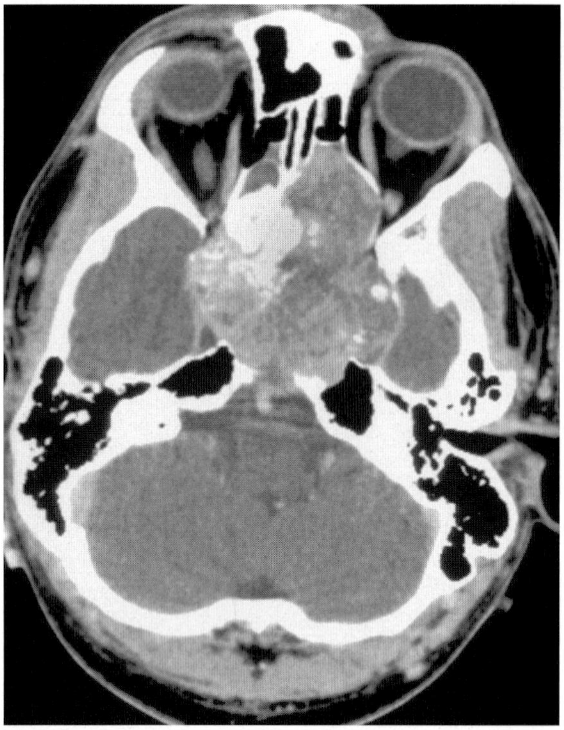

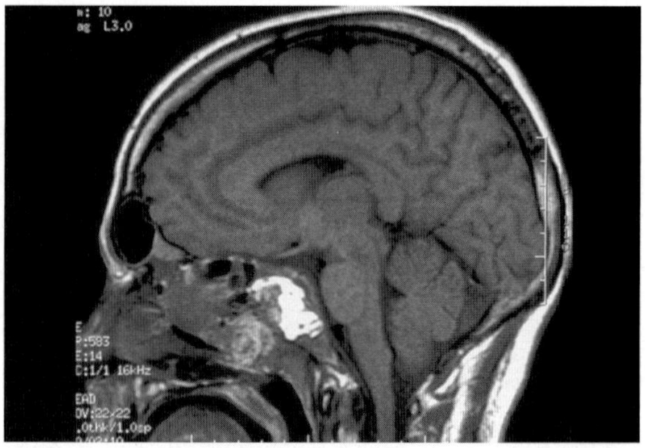

Figure 9-4

CHORDOMA

Chordoma of the base of the skull. Computerized tomography (CT) (left) and magnetic resonance imaging (MRI) (above) both show involvement of the clivus. Mineralization is prominent on CT.

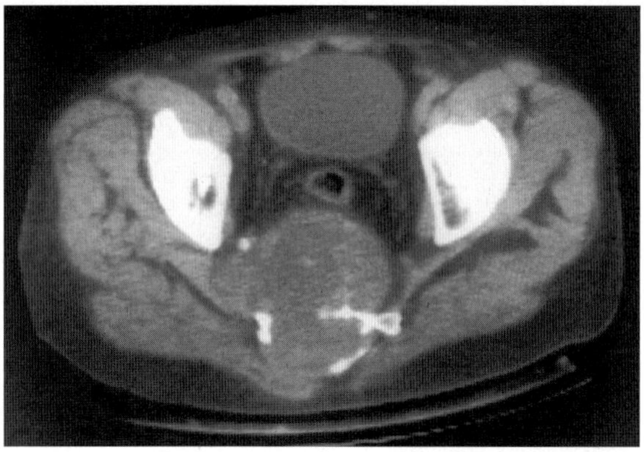

Figure 9-5

CHORDOMA

CT demonstrates destruction of the sacrum, with extensive soft tissue extension. Typically, the tumor forms a presacral mass. The mineralized foci represent fragments of destroyed bone.

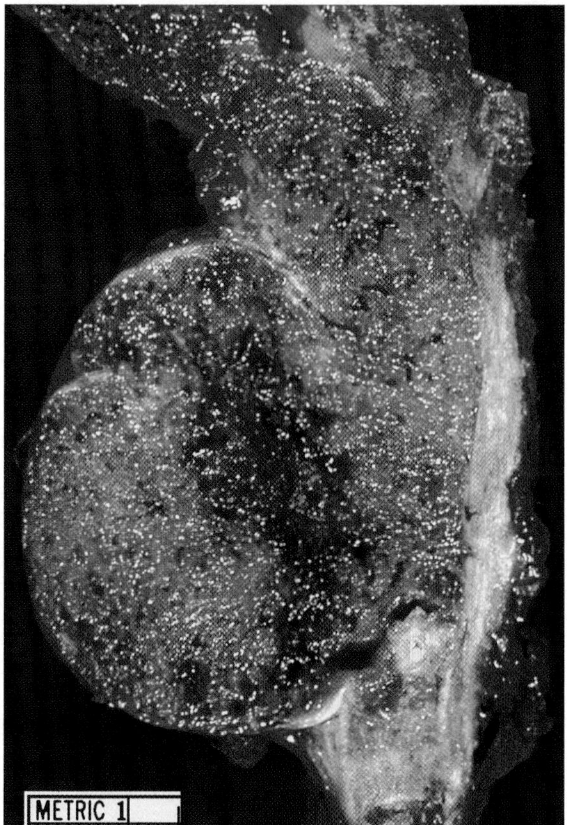

Figure 9-6

CHORDOMA

Resected sacrum. The tumor is glistening and lobulated, and shows a large presacral extension.

of tissue may be available. The tumor is divided into lobules by thin fibrous septa (fig. 9-9). The background is blue, and the cells are arranged in strands and cords against this background (fig. 9-10). The tumor cells have small, round, uniform nuclei and abundant cytoplasm, which

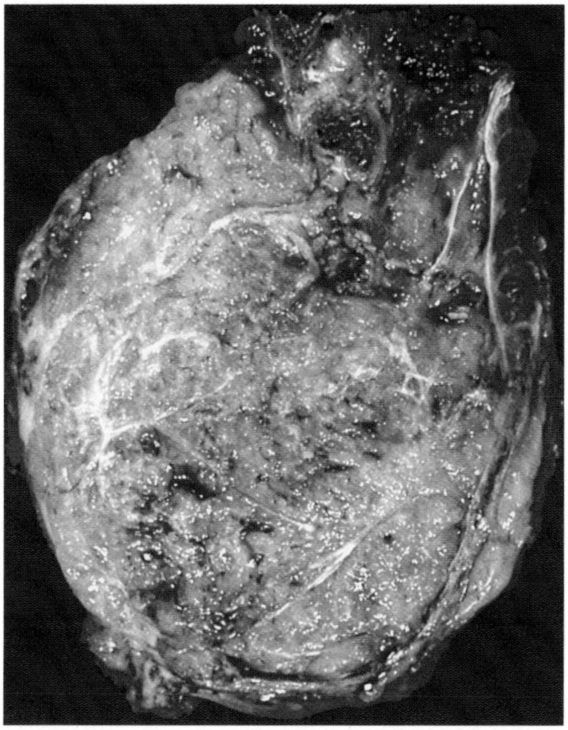

Figure 9-7

CHORDOMA

Such large tumors as this of the sacrum can seldom be completely resected with a wide margin of uninvolved tissue.

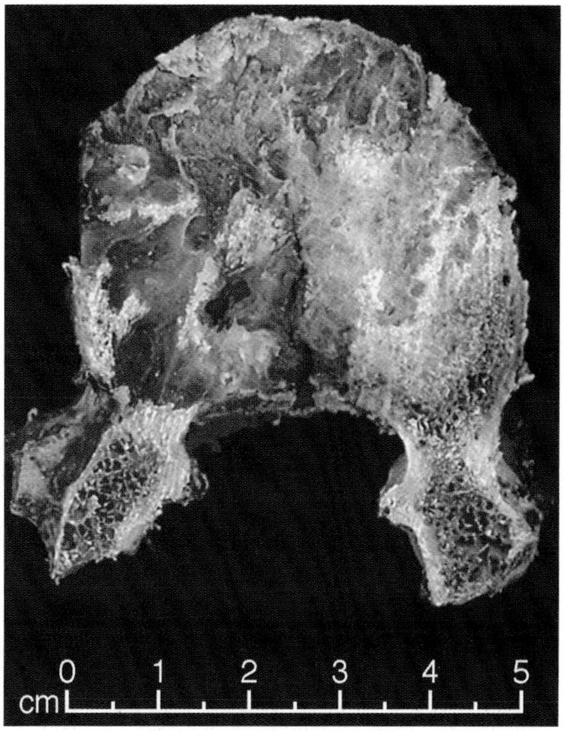

Figure 9-8

CHORDOMA

This blue-gray chordoma filled the entire vertebral body.

usually contains vacuoles, giving rise to physaliferous cells (fig. 9-11). Mitotic activity is generally low. Some chordomas have sheets of tumor cells with eosinophilic cytoplasm, producing an epithelioid appearance (fig. 9-12); some cells are markedly pleomorphic (fig. 9-13). The nuclei are enlarged and hyperchromatic and have a smudged appearance, as in pseudomalignant nuclei. Rarely, a chordoma has spindle cells in or around the lobules (fig. 9-14). These cells do not show marked atypia and do not represent dedifferentiation.

Chordomas stain with the epithelial markers keratin and epithelial membrane antigen (2,7,24,25,34,40,41,55), and less consistently with S-100 protein (fig. 9-15).

Electron microscopy shows such epithelial features as desmosomes, tonofilaments, and intracytoplasmic lumens with microvilli (2).

Cytologic Findings. Chordoma has striking fine-needle aspiration (FNA) cytologic features that closely parallel the histologic features.

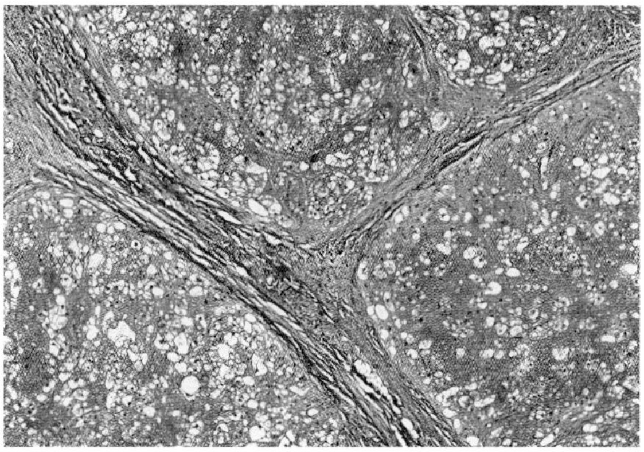

Figure 9-9

CHORDOMA

Typical lobulated appearance of chordoma is seen, with fibrovascular septa separating the lobules.

Three main cell types are embedded in an abundant myxoid matrix (fig. 9-16): large mononucleated or binucleated tumor cells with abundant, bubbly cytoplasm (physaliferous cells);

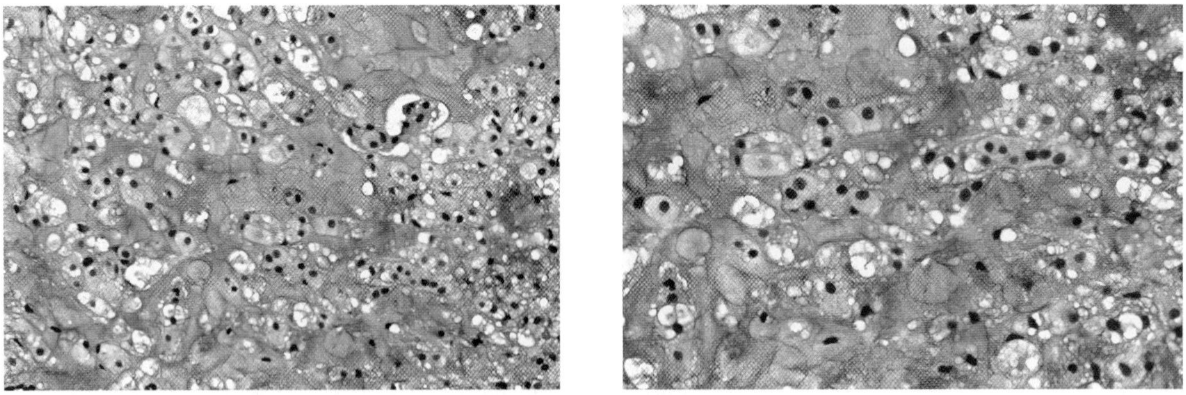

Figure 9-10

CHORDOMA

Left: Cords and small nests of tumor cells are set in a pale blue myxoid background.

Right: Round nuclei with central nucleoli are surrounded by abundant eosinophilic cytoplasm. Numerous intracytoplasmic vacuoles are present.

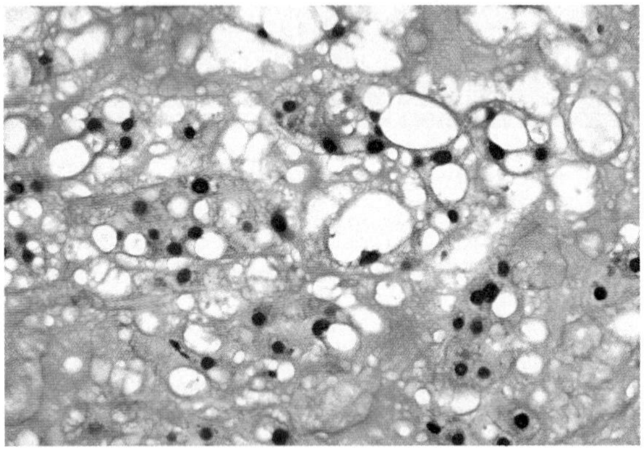

Figure 9-11

CHORDOMA

Prominent intracytoplasmic vacuolization is seen. One or several vacuoles may entrap the nucleus, creating a physaliphorous cell.

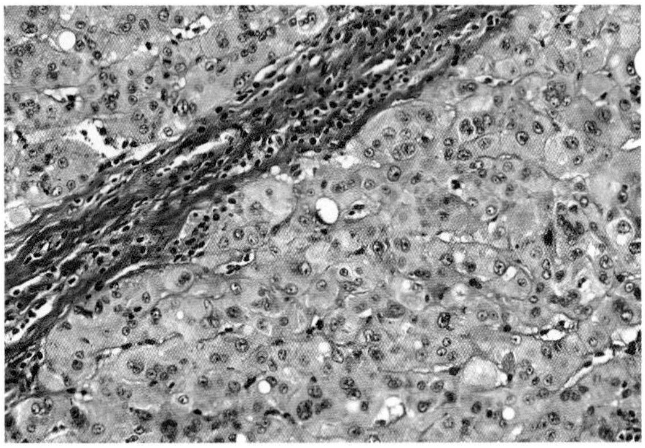

Figure 9-12

CHORDOMA

Solid lobules of tumor cells with abundant eosinophilic cytoplasm produce an epithelioid appearance.

small, rounded uniform cells; and short, plump spindle cells (3,14,21,54). Adjunctive histochemical, immunohistochemical, and ultrastructural techniques, particularly when applied to FNA material, may be particularly useful in distinguishing among chordoma, chondrosarcoma, and carcinoma (21,54).

Genetics and Other Special Techniques. Little is known about the molecular biology of chordoma or the etiologic factors that predispose to it (18,29,35,38). Cytogenetic analyses of nearly 50 sporadic and 2 familial chordomas have documented 28 lesions with a rearranged karyotype (6,8,9,11,15,16,23,31,37,43,46,49). No common tumor-specific rearrangements were found in these analyses; however, certain anomalies were recurrent. Specifically, nearly all cases have been hypodiploid or near diploid, and abnormalities of chromosomes 1 and 3 (most resulting in loss of a portion or all of these chromosomes) were prominent. Lumbosacral and skull base chordomas appear to be cytogenetically similar (43).

Although most chordomas are sporadic, five families with chordoma occurrence have been reported (27). Targeted linkage analysis of one chordoma family and loss of heterozygosity

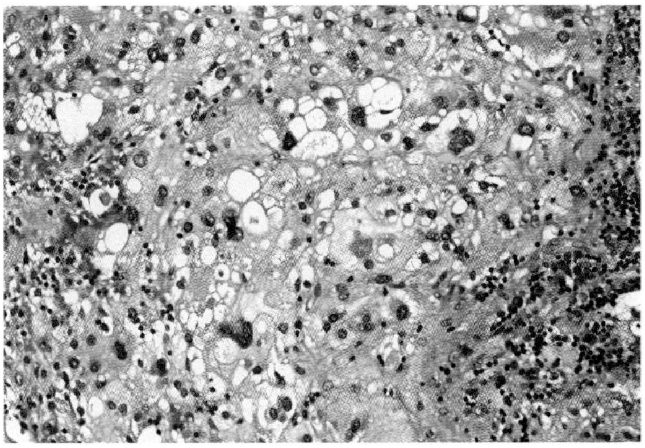

Figure 9-13

CHORDOMA

Occasionally, marked pleomorphism of the tumor cells is present either focally or more diffusely throughout the tumor.

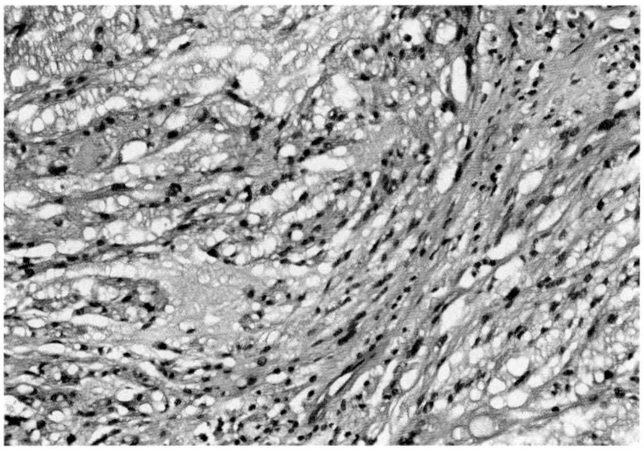

Figure 9-14

CHORDOMA

Elongated nuclei with eosinophilic cytoplasmic extensions create a spindle cell appearance.

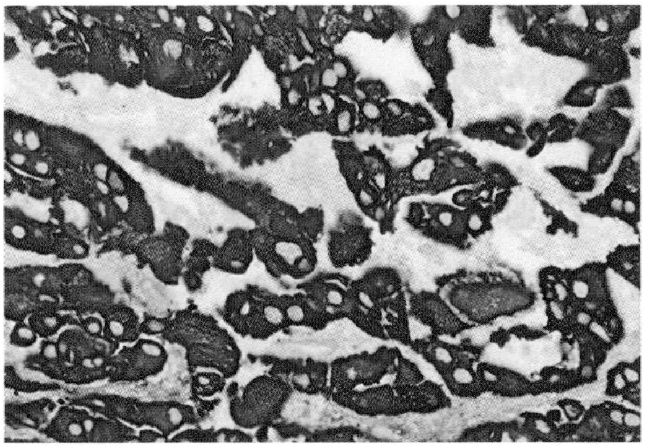

Figure 9-15

CHORDOMA

The tumor cells show strong reactivity with antibodies to keratin.

(LOH) studies of tumor specimens from this family and six additional sporadic chordomas showed a putative tumor suppressor gene locus at 1p36 (32). Specifically, a common molecular lesion at 1p36.13 has been identified with possible loss of function of the *CASP9*, *EPH2A*, and *DVL1* genes (39).

Genome-wide linkage analysis using the extended pedigree of another chordoma family identified chromosomal region 7q33 as a putative locus for familial chordoma (27). DNA sequence analysis of the pleiotrophin gene, *PTN* (localized to 7q33), did not show sequence

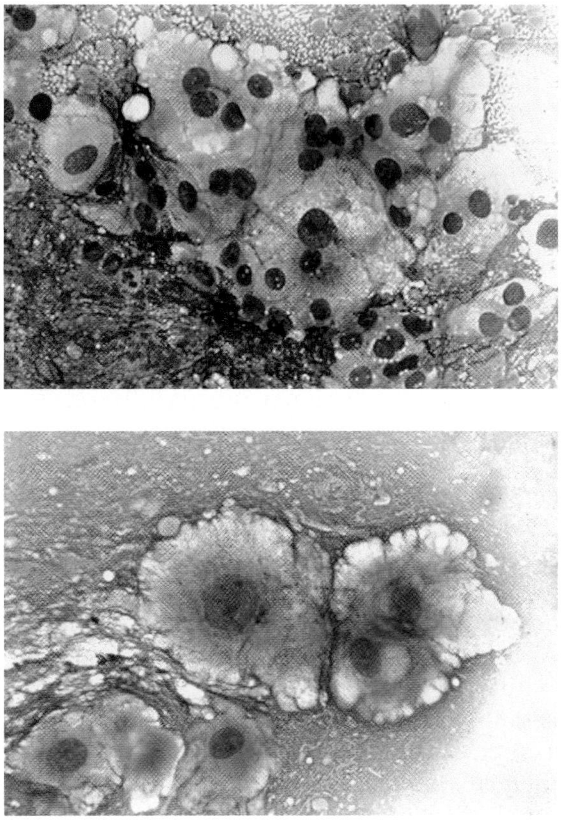

Figure 9-16

CHORDOMA

Top: Clusters of cells have abundant bubbly cytoplasm and a myxoid background.

Bottom: Higher-power view shows the relatively bland cytologic features.

variants, suggesting that *PTN* is not a gene for familial chordoma (27).

Examination for molecular markers of prognostic relevance in a series of 26 chordomas of the skull base revealed reactivation of telomerase as a reliable predictor of outcome for patients with chordoma (36). In contrast, LOH/ microsatellite instability analysis, often instability markers, did not seem to affect the prognosis of patients with skull base chordomas.

Differential Diagnosis. Metastatic carcinoma with intracytoplasmic mucin may present a diagnostic problem, especially if the biopsy sample is limited. Most metastatic carcinomas have more of the cytologic features of malignancy than do chordomas. Myxoid liposarcomas containing signet ring lipoblasts may also simulate the appearance of chordomas. The typical chicken-wire capillary proliferation seen in myxoid liposarcoma is not a feature of chordoma. Chordoma cells stain with keratin, but liposarcoma cells do not. Myxoid chondrosarcoma (chordoid sarcoma) is a sarcoma of soft tissues that resembles chordoma. The occurrence of this tumor in bone is rare. Although both chordomas and chondrosarcomas stain with S-100 protein, myxoid chondrosarcomas do not stain with keratin (56).

Kepes et al. (28) reported a series of unusual meningiomas with a myxoid matrix and coined the term "chordoid meningioma" because of the similarity to chordoma. Some of these tumors had an abundant infiltration of plasma cells and were associated with systemic symptoms. These meningiomas had the cytologic features typical of meningothelial cells. Meningiomas stain with epithelial membrane antigen but not with keratin.

Ecchordosis physalifora are incidental findings at autopsy and typically are seen in the region of the clivus. They are found in about 2 percent of autopsies and have the histologic features of chordoma (57). Ulich and Mirra (50) described a similar case in a vertebral body. It was a microscopic finding in a patient dying of trauma. More cases of this phenomenon are described in the spine. They may be visible on radiographs, are usually sclerotic, and do not destroy bone (33). Microscopically, physaliforous cells are found in the bone marrow but are not arranged in lobules. Longer-term follow-up is necessary before ecchordosis can be accepted as a definite entity in the spine or sacrum.

Treatment and Prognosis. Chordoma is an indolent tumor, and morbidity and mortality are related to local progression of disease rather than to distant metastases. Distant metastases occur in about 20 to 30 percent of cases (2,12, 19,26,53) and usually involve the lungs and, less commonly, other bones and visceral organs. The skin may be involved, usually by direct extension (47).

The prognosis of patients with chordoma has improved considerably since the introduction of radical surgical procedures for tumors of the sacrum and spine (45). Although Eriksson et al. (19) reported only one long-term survivor out of 59 patients, Bergh et al. (2) reported a 59 percent survival rate. Resection of the tumor without contamination at the time of surgery offers the best chance of cure (2,26). Boriani et al. (4) found that resection was the treatment of choice for patients with spinal chordoma and reported a survival rate of 33 percent.

Some reports have suggested that children with chordoma have a worse prognosis than adults (1,13,44); however, some of these cases had atypical histologic features.

CHONDROID CHORDOMA

Definition. Chondroid chordoma is a rare variant of chordoma that contains variable amounts of cartilage; it is found almost exclusively in the base of the skull.

General Features. Chondroid chordoma accounts for 28 percent of all chordomas in the base of the skull reported in the Mayo Clinic files. Rarely, we have seen these tumors in the spine and sacrum.

Chondroid chordoma was delineated as a distinct entity by Heffelfinger et al. (60), who found that prognosis was better for those with chordomas of the base of the skull that contained chondroid areas. This concept has engendered controversy. In some immunoperoxidase studies, chondroid chordomas did not stain with keratin and, hence, were considered to be chondrosarcomas (58,59,67). Jeffrey et al. (61) found that chondroid chordomas and classic chordomas had similar staining patterns. They interpreted their results to suggest that chondroid chordomas do not show true cartilaginous differentiation and, thus, should be classified as hyalinized chordoma. Several other authors have found

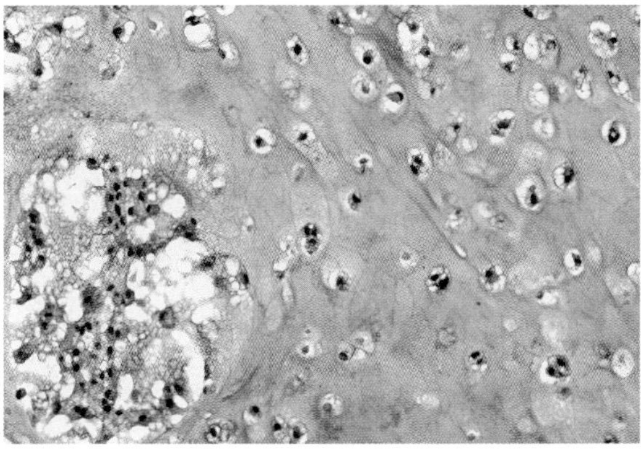

Figure 9-17

CHONDROID CHORDOMA

This tumor involves the clivus and contains areas of hyaline cartilage (right) adjacent to foci showing typical features of chordoma (left).

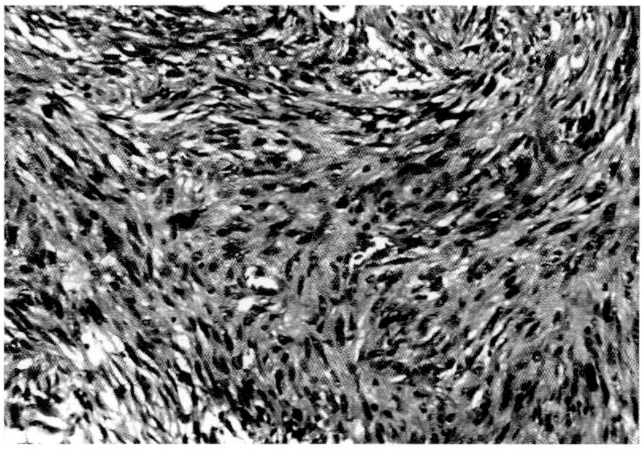

Figure 9-18

DEDIFFERENTIATED CHORDOMA

High-grade spindle cell sarcoma in a chordoma that had been treated previously with irradiation.

that chondroid chordoma stained for keratin, indicating that it is a distinct entity (63–65).

Clinical Features. The clinical features are similar to those of classic chordoma.

Radiographic Findings. The tumor is in the midline, with destruction of the clivus. Calcific densities are more likely to be present than in conventional chordoma (60).

Microscopic Findings. To qualify as chondroid chordoma, foci of cartilaginous differentiation have to be identified juxtaposed to more typical chordoma (fig. 9-17). The amount of cartilage is variable. The chondroid foci show typical hyaline cartilage matrix and cells in lacunae. Cytologic atypia is minimal. Because the amount of tissue obtained from chordomas at the base of the skull is usually minimal, sampling is a problem. If the clinical and radiographic features suggest chordoma, it seems reasonable to diagnose chondroid chordoma even if the biopsy sample shows pure cartilaginous differentiation.

Treatment and Prognosis. Treatment usually consists of debulking the tumor followed by postoperative radiotherapy. Attempts have been made to surgically resect chordomas of the base of the skull (62,66). Heffelfinger et al. (60) found that the survival rate of patients with chondroid chordoma (15.8 years) is considerably better than that for those with conventional chordoma (4.1 years). Mitchell et al. (63) studied 25 patients with chondroid chordomas, compared them with 16 patients with classic chordomas, and found no significant difference in survival. In their series, patients who were younger than 40 years fared better than those older than 40, regardless of the histologic tumor type.

DEDIFFERENTIATED CHORDOMA

Definition. Dedifferentiated chordoma is a high-grade spindle cell sarcoma that occurs in association with or at the site of a previously documented chordoma.

General Features. Conventional chordomas may show some spindle cell proliferation. Dedifferentiated chordomas have the features of a high-grade spindle cell sarcoma. Most are recurrent tumors and the dedifferentiation may be delayed as long as 15 years (72). Most patients have received radiotherapy as part of the treatment for the original chordoma (68,70,71,73). Most dedifferentiated chordomas involve the sacrum, although rare cases in the skull have been described (74).

Microscopic Findings. It is rare to see conventional chordoma juxtaposed to a high-grade sarcoma because most occur after radiotherapy, and the tumor simply shows osteosarcoma, fibrosarcoma, or malignant fibrous histiocytoma (fig. 9-18). The diagnosis can be made on the basis of only the history.

Treatment and Prognosis. Surgical resection, when feasible, is the treatment of choice. Some response to aggressive chemotherapy has been reported (69).

REFERENCES

Chordoma

1. Auger M, Raney B, Callender D, Eifel P, Ordonez NG. Metastatic intracranial chordoma in a child with massive pulmonary tumor emboli. Pediatr Pathol 1994;14:763–70.
2. Bergh P, Gunterberg B, Meis-Kindblom JM, Kindblom LG. Prognostic factors and outcome of pelvic, sacral, and spinal chondrosarcomas: a center-based study of 69 cases. Cancer 2001;91:1201–12.
3. Bergh P, Kindblom LG, Gunterberg B, Remotti F, Ryd W, Meis-Kindblom JM. Prognostic factors in chordoma of the sacrum and mobile spine: a study of 39 patients. Cancer 2000;88:2122–34.
4. Boriani S, Biagini R, De Iure F, et al. [Resection surgery in the treatment of vertebral tumors.] (in Italian.) Chir Organi Mov 1998;83:53–64.
5. Bottles K, Beckstead JH. Enzyme histochemical characterization of chordomas. Am J Surg Pathol 1984;8:443–7.
6. Bridge JA, Pickering D, Neff JR. Cytogenetic and molecular cytogenetic analysis of sacral chordoma. Cancer Genet Cytogenet 1994;75:23–5.
7. Brooks JJ, LiVolsi VA, Trojanowski JQ. Does chondroid chordoma exist? Acta Neuropathol (Berl) 1987;72:229–35.
8. Buonamici L, Roncaroli F, Fioravanti A, et al. Cytogenetic investigation of chordomas of the skull. Cancer Genet Cytogenet 1999;112:49–52.
9. Butler MG, Dahir GA, Hedges LK, Juliao SF, Sciadini MF, Schwartz HS. Cytogenetic, telomere, and telomerase studies in five surgically managed lumbosacral chordomas. Cancer Genet Cytogenet 1995;85:51–7.
10. Campbell WM, McDonald TJ, Unni KK, Laws ER Jr. Nasal and paranasal presentations of chordomas. Laryngoscope 1980;90:612–8.
11. Chadduck WM, Boop FA, Sawyer JR. Cytogenetic studies of pediatric brain and spinal cord tumors. Pediatr Neurosurg 1991;17:57–65.
12. Chambers PW, Schwinn CP. Chordoma. A clinicopathologic study of metastasis. Am J Clin Pathol 1979;72:765–76.
13. Coffin CM, Swanson PE, Wick MR, Dehner LP. Chordoma in childhood and adolescence. A clinicopathologic analysis of 12 cases. Arch Pathol Lab Med 1993;117:927–33.
14. Crapanzano JP, Ali SZ, Ginsberg MS, Zakowski MF. Chordoma: a cytologic study with histologic and radiologic correlation. Cancer 2001;93:40–51.
15. Dalpra L, Malgara R, Miozzo M, et al. First cytogenetic study of a recurrent familial chordoma of the clivus. Int J Cancer 1999;81:24–30.
16. DeBoer JM, Neff JR, Bridge JA. Cytogenetics of sacral chordoma. Cancer Genet Cytogenet 1992;64:95–6.
17. de Bruine FT, Kroon HM. Spinal chordoma: radiologic features in 14 cases. AJR Am J Roentgenol 1988;150:861–3.
18. Eisenberg MB, Woloschak M, Sen C, Wolfe D. Loss of heterozygosity in the retinoblastoma tumor suppressor gene in skull base chordomas and chondrosarcomas. Surg Neurol 1997;47: 156–60.
19. Eriksson B, Gunterberg B, Kindblom LG. Chordoma. A clinicopathologic and prognostic study of a Swedish national series. Acta Orthop Scand 1981;52:49–58.
20. Fechner RE, Mills SE. Tumors of the bones and joints. Atlas of Tumor Pathology, 3rd Series, Fascicle 8. Washington, DC: Armed Forces Institute of Pathology; 1993:239–42.
21. Finley JL, Silverman JF, Dabbs DJ, et al. Chordoma: diagnosis by fine-needle aspiration biopsy with histologic, immunocytochemical, and ultrastructural confirmation. Diagn Cytopathol 1986;2:330–7.
22. Firooznia H, Pinto RS, Lin JP, Baruch HH, Zausner J. Chordoma: radiologic evaluation of 20 cases. Am J Roentgenol 1976;127:797–805.
23. Gibas Z, Miettinen M, Sandberg AA. Chromosomal abnormalities in two chordomas. Cancer Genet Cytogenet 1992;58:169–73.
24. Gottschalk D, Fehn M, Patt S, Saeger W, Kirchner T, Aigner T. Matrix gene expression analysis and cellular phenotyping in chordoma reveals focal differentiation pattern of neoplastic cells mimicking nucleus pulposus development. Am J Pathol 2001;158:1571–8.
25. Jeffrey PB, Biava CG, Davis RL. Chondroid chordoma. A hyalinized chordoma without cartilaginous differentiation. Am J Clin Pathol 1995;103:271–9.
26. Kaiser TE, Pritchard DJ, Unni KK. Clinicopathologic study of sacrococcygeal chordoma. Cancer 1984;53:2574–8.
27. Kelley MJ, Korczak JF, Sheridan E, Yang X, Goldstein AM, Parry DM. Familial chordoma, a tumor of notochordal remnants, is linked to chromosome 7q33. Am J Hum Genet 2001;69:454–60.
28. Kepes JJ, Chen WY, Connors MH, Vogel FS. "Chordoid" meningeal tumors in young individuals with peritumoral lymphoplasmacellular infiltrates causing systemic manifestations of the Castleman syndrome. A report of seven cases. Cancer 1988;62:391–406.

29. Klingler L, Shooks J, Fiedler PN, Marney A, Butler MG, Schwartz HS. Microsatellite instability in sacral chordoma. J Surg Oncol 2000;73:100–3.
30. Larson TC 3rd, Houser OW, Laws ER Jr. Imaging of cranial chordomas. Mayo Clin Proc 1987;62:886–93.
31. Mertens F, Kreicbergs A, Rydholm A, et al. Clonal chromosome aberrations in three sacral chordomas. Cancer Genet Cytogenet 1994;73:147–51.
32. Miozzo M, Dalpra L, Riva P, et al. A tumor suppressor locus in familial and sporadic chordoma maps to 1p36. Int J Cancer 2000;87:68–72.
33. Mirra JM, Brien EW. Giant notochordal hamartoma of intraosseous origin: a newly reported benign entity to be distinguished from chordoma. Report of two cases. Skeletal Radiol 2001;30:698–709.
34. Mitchell A, Scheithauer BW, Unni KK, Forsyth PJ, Wold LE, McGivney DJ. Chordoma and chondroid neoplasms of the spheno-occiput. An immunohistochemical study of 41 cases with prognostic and nosologic implications. Cancer 1993;72:2943–9.
35. Naka T, Iwamoto Y, Shinohara N, Ushijima M, Chuman H, Tsuneyoshi M. Expression of c-met proto-oncogene product (c-MET) in benign and malignant bone tumors. Mod Pathol 1997;10:832–8.
36. Pallini R, Maira G, Pierconti F, et al. Chordoma of the skull base: predictors of tumor recurrence. J Neurosurg 2003;98:812–22.
37. Persons DL, Bridge JA, Neff JR. Cytogenetic analysis of two sacral chordomas. Cancer Genet Cytogenet 1991;56:197–201.
38. Radner H, Katenkamp D, Reifenberger G, Deckert M, Pietsch T, Wiestler OD. New developments in the pathology of skull base tumors. Virchows Arch 2001;438:321–35.
39. Riva P, Crosti F, Orzan F, et al. Mapping of candidate region for chordoma development to 1p36.13 by LOH analysis. Int J Cancer 2003;107:493–7.
40. Rosenberg AE, Brown GA, Bhan AK, Lee JM. Chondroid chordoma—a variant of chordoma. A morphologic and immunohistochemical study. Am J Clin Pathol 1994;101:36–41.
41. Salisbury JR. Demonstration of cytokeratins and an epithelial membrane antigen in chondroid chordoma. J Pathol 1987;153:37–40.
42. Samson IR, Springfield DS, Suit HD, Mankin HJ. Operative treatment of sacrococcygeal chordoma. A review of twenty-one cases. J Bone Joint Surg Am 1993;75:1476–84.
43. Sawyer JR, Husain M, Al-Mefty O. Identification of isochromosome 1q as a recurring chromosome aberration in skull base chordomas: a new marker for aggressive tumors? Neurosurg Focus 2001;10:1–8.
44. Sibley RK, Day DL, Dehner LP, Trueworthy RC. Metastasizing chordoma in early childhood: a pathological and immunohistochemical study with review of the literature. Pediatr Pathol 1987;7:287–301.
45. Stener B, Gunterberg B. High amputation of the sacrum for extirpation of tumors. Principles and technique. Spine 1978;3:351–66.
46. Stepanek J, Cataldo SA, Ebersold MJ, et al. Familial chordoma with probable autosomal dominant inheritance. Am J Med Genet 1998;75:335–6.
47. Su WP, Louback JB, Gagne EJ, Scheithauer BW. Chordoma cutis: a report of nineteen patients with cutaneous involvement of chordoma. J Am Acad Dermatol 1993;29:63–6.
48. Sze G, Uichanco LS 3rd, Brant-Zawadzki MN, et al. Chordomas: MR imaging. Radiology 1988;166:187–91.
49. Tallini G, Dorfman H, Brys P, et al. Correlation between clinicopathological features and karyotype in 100 cartilaginous and chordoid tumours. A report from the Chromosomes and Morphology (CHAMP) Collaborative Study Group. J Pathol 2002;196:194–203.
50. Ulich TR, Mirra JM. Ecchordosis physaliphora vertebralis. Clin Orthop 1982;163:282–9.
51. Unni KK. Dahlin's bone tumors: general aspects and data on 11,087 cases, 5th ed. Philadelphia: Lippincott-Raven; 1996:291–305.
52. Utne JR, Pugh DG. The roentgenologic aspects of chordoma. Am J Roentgenol Radium Ther Nucl Med 1955;74:593–608.
53. Volpe R, Mazabraud A. A clinicopathologic review of 25 cases of chordoma (a pleomorphic and metastasizing neoplasm). Am J Surg Pathol 1983;7:161–70.
54. Walaas L, Kindblom LG. Fine-needle aspiration biopsy in the preoperative diagnosis of chordoma: a study of 17 cases with application of electron microscopic, histochemical, and immunocytochemical examination. Hum Pathol 1991;22:22–8.
55. Walker WP, Landas SK, Bromley CM, Sturm MT. Immunohistochemical distinction of classic and chondroid chordomas. Mod Pathol 1991;4:661–6.
56. Wick MR, Burgess JH, Manivel JC. A reassessment of "chordoid sarcoma." Ultrastructural and immunohistochemical comparison with chordoma and skeletal myxoid chondrosarcoma. Mod Pathol 1988;1:433–43.
57. Wolfe JT 3rd, Scheithauer BW. "Intradural chordoma" or "giant ecchordosis physaliphora"? Report of two cases. Clin Neuropathol 1987;6:98–103.

Chondroid Chordoma

58. Bottles K, Beckstead JH. Enzyme histochemical characterization of chordomas. Am J Surg Pathol 1984;8:443–7.
59. Brooks JJ, LiVolsi VA, Trojanowski JQ. Does chondroid chordoma exist? Acta Neuropathol (Berl) 1987;72:229–35.
60. Heffelfinger MJ, Dahlin DC, MacCarty CS, Beabout JW. Chordomas and cartilaginous tumors at the skull base. Cancer 1973;32:410–20.
61. Jeffrey PB, Biava CG, Davis RL. Chondroid chordoma. A hyalinized chordoma without cartilaginous differentiation. Am J Clin Pathol 1995;103: 271–9.
62. Lanzino G, Sekhar LN, Hirsch WL, Sen CN, Pomonis S, Snyderman CH. Chordomas and chondrosarcomas involving the cavernous sinus: review of surgical treatment and outcome in 31 patients. Surg Neurol 1993;40:359–71.
63. Mitchell A, Scheithauer BW, Unni KK, Forsyth PJ, Wold LE, McGivney DJ. Chordoma and chondroid neoplasms of the spheno-occiput. An immunohistochemical study of 41 cases with prognostic and nosologic implications. Cancer 1993;72:2943–9.
64. Rosenberg AE, Brown GA, Bhan AK, Lee JM. Chondroid chordoma—a variant of chordoma. A morphologic and immunohistochemical study. Am J Clin Pathol 1994;101:36–41.
65. Salisbury JR. Demonstration of cytokeratins and an epithelial membrane antigen in chondroid chordoma. J Pathol 1987;153:37–40.
66. Tai PT, Craighead P, Bagdon F. Optimization of radiotherapy for patients with cranial chordoma. A review of dose-response ratios for photon techniques. Cancer 1995;75:749–56.
67. Walker WP, Landas SK, Bromley CM, Sturm MT. Immunohistochemical distinction of classic and chondroid chordomas. Mod Pathol 1991;4:661–6.

Dedifferentiated Chordoma

68. Belza MG, Urich H. Chordoma and malignant fibrous histiocytoma. Evidence for transformation. Cancer 1986;58:1082–7.
69. Fleming GF, Heimann PS, Stephens JK, et al. Dedifferentiated chordoma. Response to aggressive chemotherapy in two cases. Cancer 1993; 72:714–8.
70. Fukuda T, Aihara T, Ban S, Nakajima T, Machinami R. Sacrococcygeal chordoma with a malignant spindle cell component. A report of two autopsy cases with a review of the literature. Acta Pathol Jpn 1992;42:448–53.
71. Hruban RH, Traganos F, Reuter VE, Huvos AG. Chordomas with malignant spindle cell components. A DNA flow cytometric and immunohistochemical study with histogenetic implications. Am J Pathol 1990;137:435–47.
72. Makek M, Leu HJ. Malignant fibrous histiocytoma arising in a recurrent chordoma. Case report and electron microscopic findings. Virchows Arch A Pathol Anat Histol 1982;397: 241–50.
73. Miettinen M, Lehto VP, Virtanen I. Malignant fibrous histiocytoma within a recurrent chordoma. A light microscopic, electron microscopic, and immunohistochemical study. Am J Clin Pathol 1984;82:738–43.
74. Tomlinson FH, Scheithauer BW, Forsythe PA, Unni KK, Meyer FB. Sarcomatous transformation in cranial chordoma. Neurosurgery 1992; 31:13–8.

10 VASCULAR TUMORS

BENIGN VASCULAR TUMORS

Hemangioma

Definition. A hemangioma is a proliferation of blood vessels lined with a single layer of cytologically bland-appearing endothelial cells. Hemangiomas occur in the medullary cavity and infrequently in the cortex or on the surface of bone.

General Features. Hemangiomas of the spine have been reported in 10 to 12 percent of autopsy cases (6); however, some of these probably represent zones of telangiectasia. Because hemangiomas frequently contain fat, it is unclear whether they are true neoplasms or hamartomas. Occasionally, hemangiomas are multiple. They may involve the bone and soft tissue of an entire extremity and produce consumptive coagulopathy (5). Karlin and Brower (2) suggested that multiple hemangiomas be divided into two types: *diffuse cystic angiomatosis* and *true multiple hemangiomas*. Cystic angiomatosis presents as widespread, multiple cystic areas of bone destruction that are round or oval and sharply circumscribed. It is associated frequently with visceral involvement and patients have a poor prognosis. True multiple hemangiomas consist of multiple lesions, each with the radiographic appearance of a solitary lesion and without visceral involvement.

Hemangiomas are uncommon in surgical series. The Mayo Clinic files contain only 131 cases of hemangioma, accounting for 4.5 percent of all benign tumors (fig. 10-1).

Clinical Features. Hemangiomas may be incidental radiographic findings or they may be painful (3). In the skull, they sometimes produce a palpable mass. Hemangiomas of the spine may cause no symptoms, be painful without spinal cord compression, cause symptoms of spinal cord compression because of extension into the spinal canal, or compress the spinal cord because of pathologic fracture (6).

The peak incidence is the fifth decade of life, and there is a definite female predominance (8).

Sites. The skull and vertebrae are the sites involved most commonly, followed by the jawbones. Long bones are rarely involved. Rare intracortical and periosteal hemangiomas have been described (3).

Radiographic Findings. The radiographic appearance depends on the site of involvement. In long bones, hemangiomas are well-circumscribed lucencies with scattered bony trabeculae coursing through the lesion. Bony contours are often expanded, giving rise to a "soap-bubble" appearance (8). In the skull, hemangiomas produce a well-demarcated zone of rarefaction often associated with outward expansion of the bony profile. This expanded zone frequently shows striations of bone radiating outward, creating a "sunburst" pattern.

In the vertebrae, hemangiomas cause rarefactions with exaggerated vertical striations, producing a "rugger-jersey" appearance. With computerized tomography (CT), the bony trabeculae are seen in cross section, producing a "polka-dot" appearance that is diagnostic of hemangioma (fig. 10-2). Occasionally, the lesion is sclerotic (fig. 10-3). There is increased signal intensity on both T_1- and T_2-weighted magnetic resonance images (MRI) (7), probably because of the fat content of the lesion (figs. 10-4, 10-5).

Gross Findings. Grossly, hemangiomas appear dark blue or red and may have a honeycombed appearance (9). Hemangiomas of the skull have bony trabeculae that extend out and intertrabecular spaces that are soft and dark red (fig. 10-6).

Microscopic Findings. Hemangiomas traditionally have been divided into capillary and cavernous types. As the name suggests, *capillary hemangiomas* are composed of small spaces lined with a single layer of endothelial cells (fig. 10-7). *Cavernous hemangiomas* have larger spaces. A mixture of the two types is often encountered,

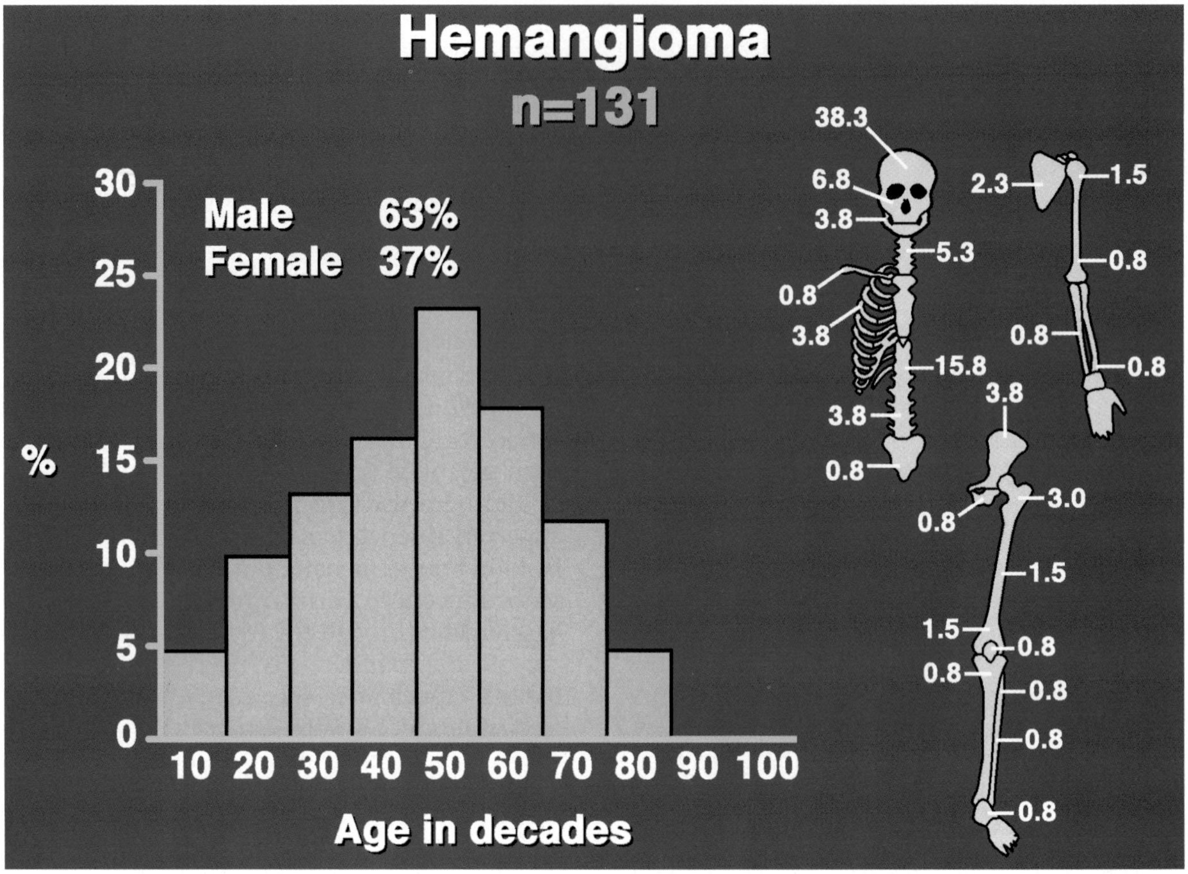

Figure 10-1

HEMANGIOMA

Distribution of hemangioma according to the age and sex of the patient and the site of the lesion.

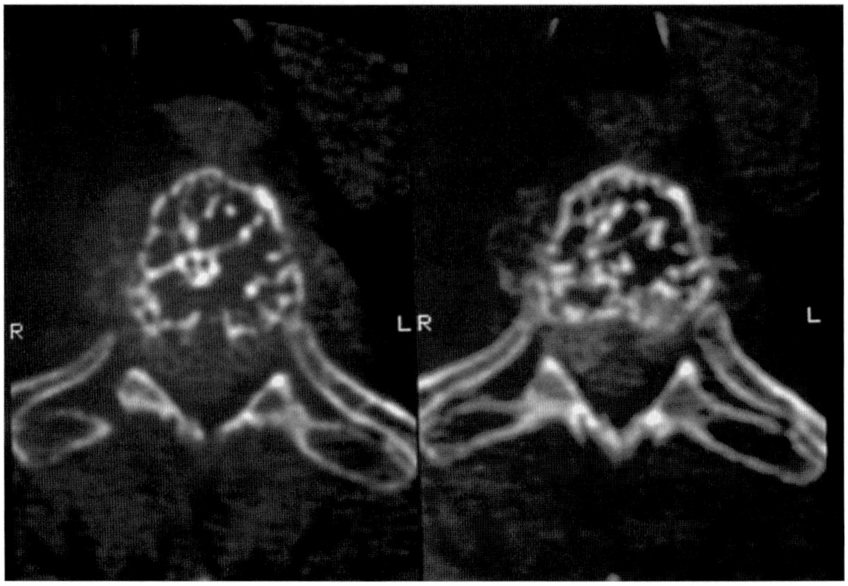

Figure 10-2

HEMANGIOMA

Axial computerized tomography (CT) demonstrating the characteristic polka-dot pattern of a vertebral hemangioma created by thickened vertical trabeculae and intervening low-attenuation fat.

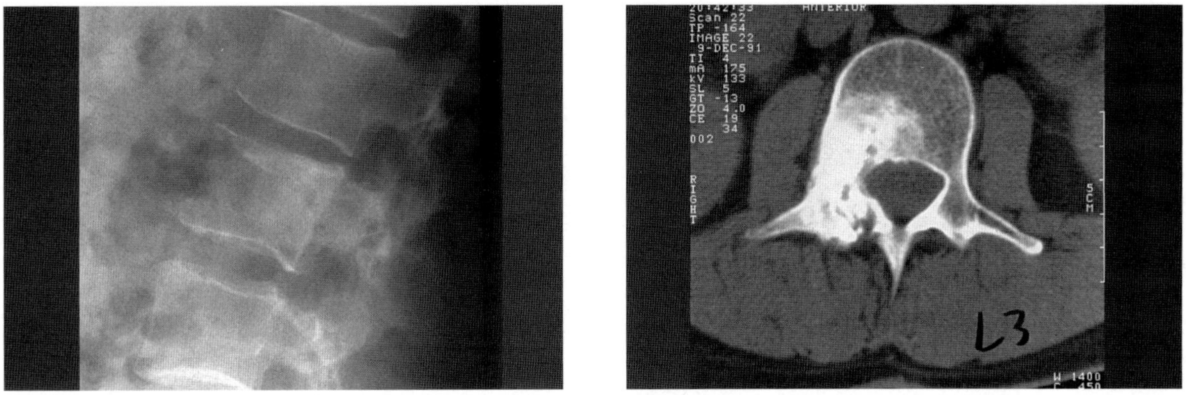

Figure 10-3

HEMANGIOMA

Left: Hemangiomas occasionally are sclerotic. The vertebral pedicle in this radiograph is sclerotic and may be mistaken for metastatic disease.

Right: CT shows involvement of the right pedicle and a portion of the vertebral body.

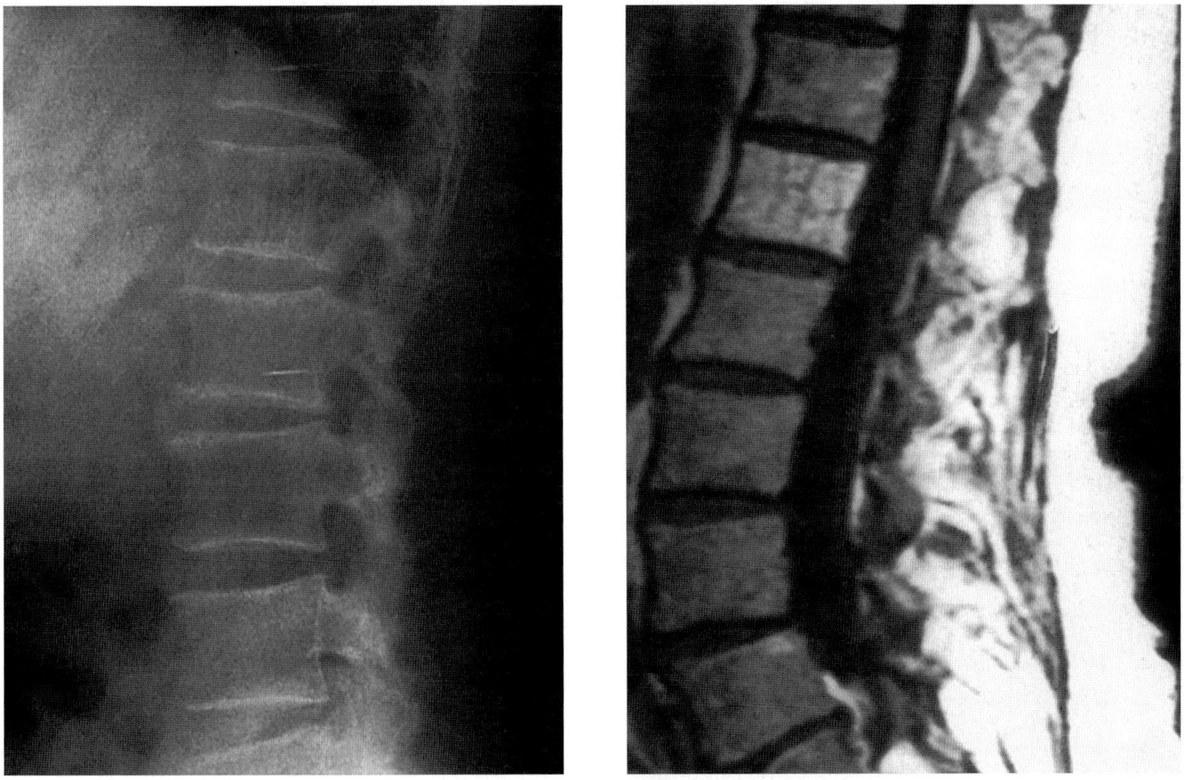

Figure 10-4

HEMANGIOMA

Left: Lateral conventional radiograph of a hemangioma of L1 shows osteopenia. A coarsened vertical trabecular pattern involves the vertebral body and pedicles with a characteristic corduroy pattern.

Right: Sagittal T_1-weighted spin echo magnetic resonance image (MRI) shows the typical features of an asymptomatic vertebral hemangioma of L1. The high signal intensity reflects the presence of intralesional fat. (Figs. 2 and 4a from Wenger DE, Wold LE. Benign vascular lesions of bone: radiologic and pathologic features. Skeletal Radiol 2000;29:63-74.)

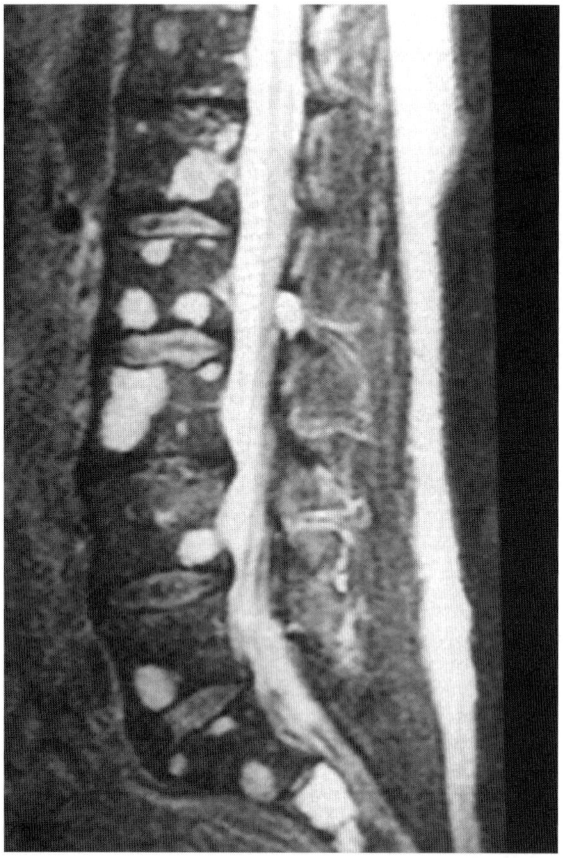

Figure 10-5

HEMANGIOMA

T_2-weighted sagittal MRI of the lumbar spine shows multiple high-signal lesions in all the lumbar vertebrae and in vertebrae S1 and S2.

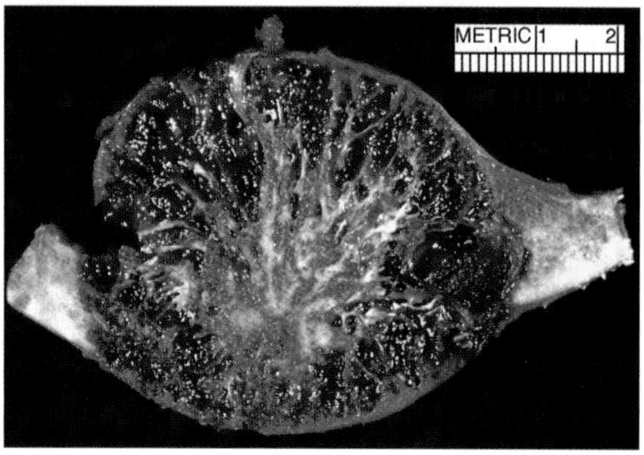

Figure 10-6

HEMANGIOMA

Hemangioma involving the parietal bone of a 48-year-old woman. Sclerotic spicules of bone radiate between red-brown hemorrhagic cavities.

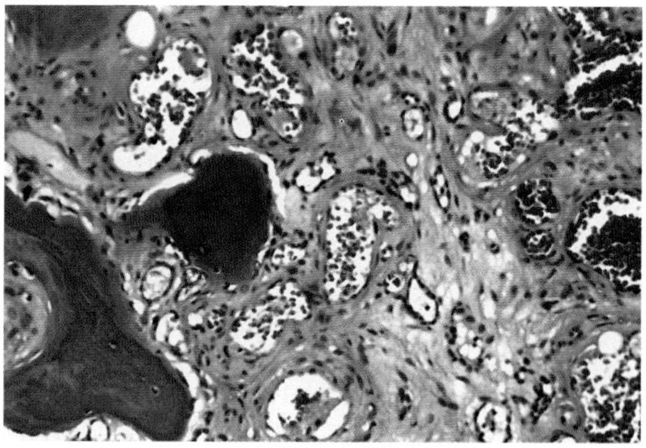

Figure 10-7

HEMANGIOMA

Numerous dilated blood vessels occupy the intertrabecular bone marrow space. The blood vessels are lined by a single layer of flat endothelial cells.

making the subdivision of no practical advantage. Some hemangiomas, especially in the skull, are associated with abundant reactive new bone formation. The bony trabeculae are lined with osteoblasts and the lesion may be mistaken for an osteoblastoma. Some hemangiomas have prominent cubical endothelial cells and may be termed *epithelioid hemangioma (histiocytoid)* (fig. 10-8) (1,4). The histologic features of multiple hemangiomas are the same as those of a solitary lesion. The histologic features are so specific that special stains such as factor VIII, CD31, and CD34 are not necessary.

Differential Diagnosis. It may be difficult to differentiate a hemangioma from a reactive vascular proliferation such as occurs with a fracture. In the reactive process, fibroblasts and inflammatory cells are present in addition to capillaries. The differentiation from low-grade angiosarcoma can be difficult and is based on cytologic features.

Treatment and Prognosis. Most patients with hemangiomas need no treatment. Lesions causing symptoms are treated with intralesional excision. The prognosis is excellent.

Massive Osteolysis

Definition. Massive osteolysis is a rare chronic disorder that begins insidiously and is characterized by progressive regional loss of bone, with resultant deformity (13). *Phantom bone disease, Gorham's disease,* and *disappearing*

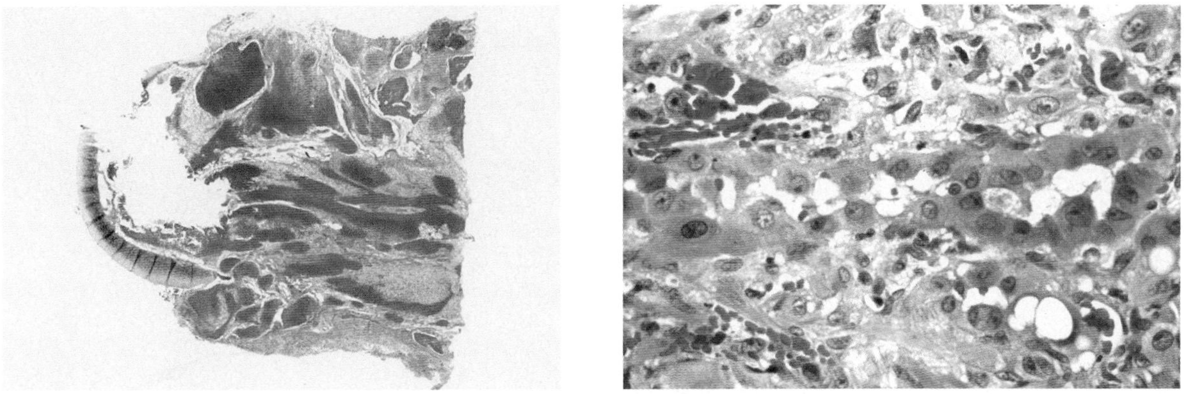

Figure 10-8

EPITHELIOID HEMANGIOMA

Left: A lobular growth pattern is apparent in this epithelioid hemangioma arising in a metatarsal bone. The tumor has grown out of the bone and is at the periphery of the articular surface.

Right: Cuboidal endothelial cells with abundant eosinophilic cytoplasm protrude into well-formed vascular lumens. (Courtesy of Dr. A. Rosenberg, Boston, MA.)

bone disease are other terms used to describe this condition.

General Features. The etiology of massive osteolysis is unknown; trauma has been suggested as a cause. In the series of Shives et al. (14), a definite history of trauma was elicited from only 4 of 11 patients. Lymphangiomatosis and hemangiomatosis have also been reported to cause massive osteolysis (12).

Clinical Features. Most patients are children or young adults, but the disease has been described also in older adults. Pain or pathologic fracture is the presenting symptom.

Sites. Any bone of the skeleton may be involved, but the pelvic and shoulder girdles are involved most frequently. The ribs and vertebrae may also be involved. The pathologic process does not respect the usual boundaries of joints and may spread from one bone to another across a joint space.

Radiographic Findings. The earliest abnormalities may be in the soft tissues, in bone, or in both (14). The disease may start as a soft tissue swelling that involves the cortex with concentric narrowing, an appearance likened to "sucked candy" (fig. 10-9) (10). If the bone is involved initially, lucencies are present in the cortex and medullary cavity. This is followed by concentric shrinkage of the bone, with tapering at the ends. Complete resorption of the bone follows, and the process spreads across joints to contiguous sites.

Gross Findings. The cortex of the involved bone is thinned, and the marrow is replaced with fibrous tissue. The cortex may appear red, suggesting increased vascularity (fig. 10-10).

Microscopic Findings. Most reports have shown vascular proliferation (lymphangiomatous or hemangiomatous) involving bone and surrounding connective tissue (fig. 10-11). Osteoclastic activity is not usually prominent (11). In some cases, the microscopic appearance is unremarkable (14).

Differential Diagnosis. It is impossible to make a diagnosis on the basis of a histologic examination alone. The radiographic features, however, are distinctive.

Treatment and Prognosis. The pathologic process is usually self-limited; however, it is difficult to predict when the disease will arrest. Residual deformities can be a serious problem. Some patients with involvement of the spine or ribs die, usually of infection. One patient received a cortical bone graft with a reportedly good result (15).

Glomus Tumor

Definition. A glomus tumor is a benign, highly vascular tumor composed of small, round, uniform cells arranged around blood vessels.

Clinical Features. Although glomus tumors in cutaneous and soft tissues are common, they are extremely uncommon in bone. Patients present with severe pain.

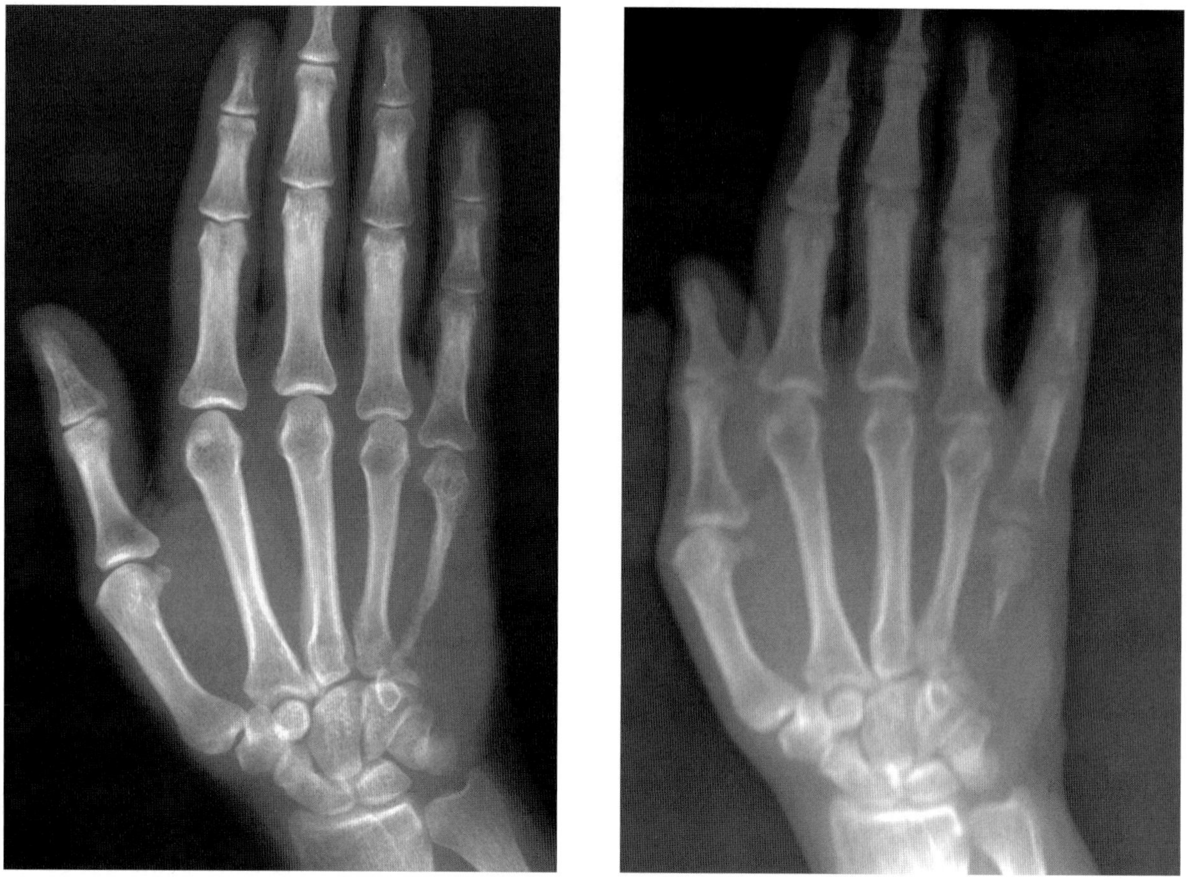

Figure 10-9

MASSIVE OSTEOLYSIS

Left: The fifth metacarpal shows concentric loss of bone. The appearance suggests extrinsic erosion of the bone, a soft tissue process invading the bone.

Right: Ten months later, part of the bone has disappeared.

Sites. The tumors almost always occur in the distal phalanx of a finger, although other bones such as the coccyx and long bones have been reported to be involved (16,17).

Radiographic Findings. The tumor appears as a small, well-circumscribed lucency in the distal phalanx (fig. 10-12).

Gross Findings. The tumor is red, small, and spherical.

Microscopic Findings. Glomus tumors vary in the relative amount of their two components, that is, vessels and small round cells. The lesion may be quite cellular and the spaces occult, or the vessels may be quite prominent and surrounded by a cuff of tumor cells (fig. 10-13).

Treatment and Prognosis. Curettage is curative.

MALIGNANT VASCULAR TUMORS

Angiosarcoma

Definition. Angiosarcoma is a malignant tumor that is composed of anastomosing vascular channels lined with endothelial cells; the cells have cytologic features of malignancy of various degrees.

General Features. Stout (25) defined *hemangioendothelioma* (the term he preferred to angiosarcoma) as a tumor characterized by the formation of atypical endothelial cells in greater numbers than required to line the vessels with a simple endothelial lining, and the formation of vascular tubes with a delicate network of reticulin fibers and a marked tendency for the lu-

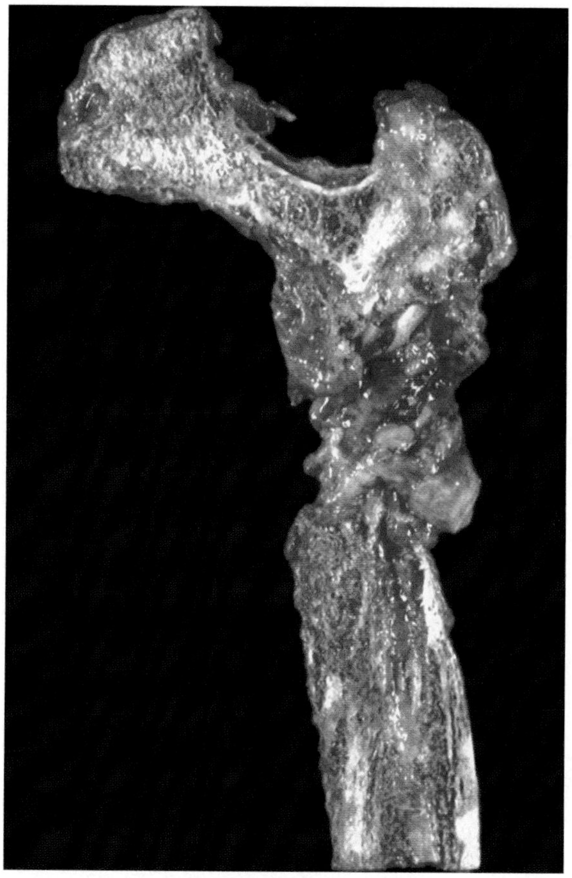

Figure 10-10

MASSIVE OSTEOLYSIS

Extensive bony dissolution, with a patchy red discoloration of the cortical bone corresponding to increased vascularity.

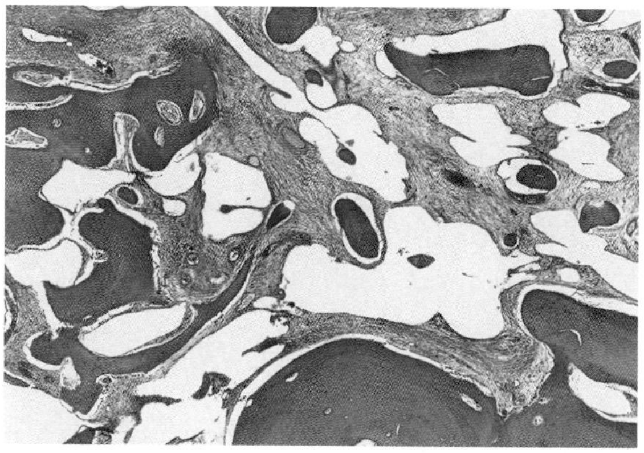

Figure 10-11

MASSIVE OSTEOLYSIS

Cavernous vascular spaces of varying size and shape are surrounded by loose fibrous connective tissue.

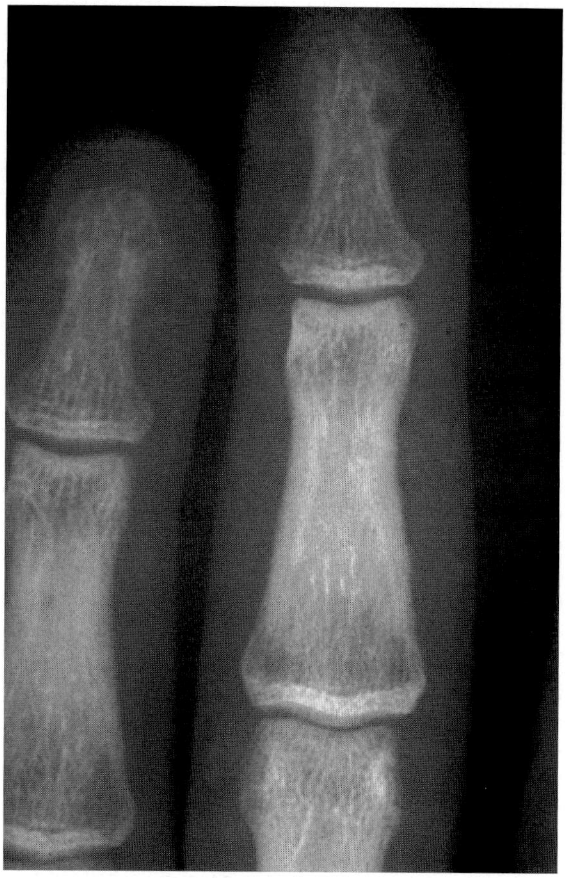

Figure 10-12

GLOMUS TUMOR

A well-circumscribed lesion involves the distal phalanx of the third finger of a 50-year-old man, who complained for 3 years about a burning pain under the nail of this finger.

mens to anastomose. The terminology for malignant vascular tumors has been confusing. *Angiosarcoma, hemangioendothelioma,* and *hemangioendothelial sarcoma* have been used either as synonyms or to refer to different entities. In surgical pathology, the term angiosarcoma has come to mean a high-grade malignancy. Thus, *hemangioendothelioma* has been used for low-grade tumors and *angiosarcoma,* for higher-grade tumors. We prefer to use the term angiosarcoma and to specify grade to suggest prognosis.

Angiosarcoma is extremely uncommon; the Mayo Clinic files contain the records of only 98 cases, accounting for less than 1 percent of all bone tumors (fig. 10-14).

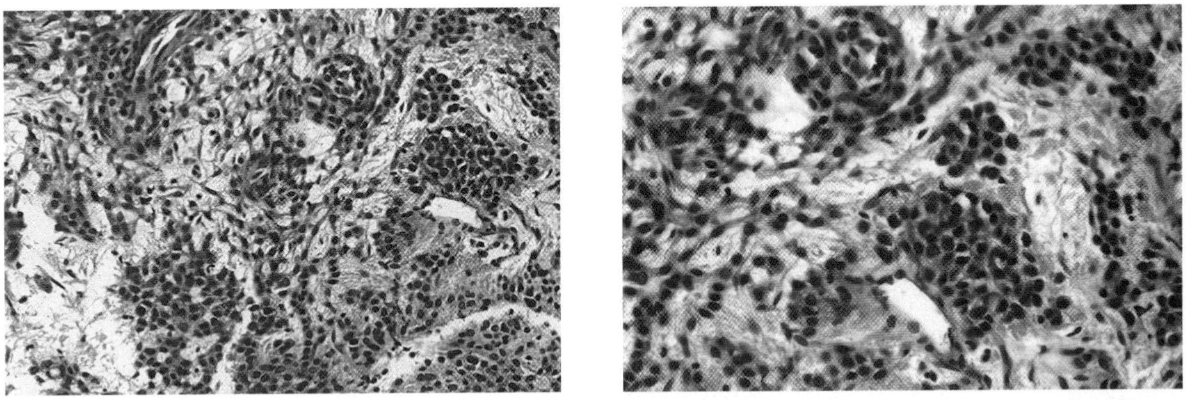

Figure 10-13

GLOMUS TUMOR

Left: Nodular aggregates of cells containing dark round nuclei are surrounded by eosinophilic cytoplasm. Right: The cells tend to cluster around blood vessels. Occasional mitotic figures may be seen.

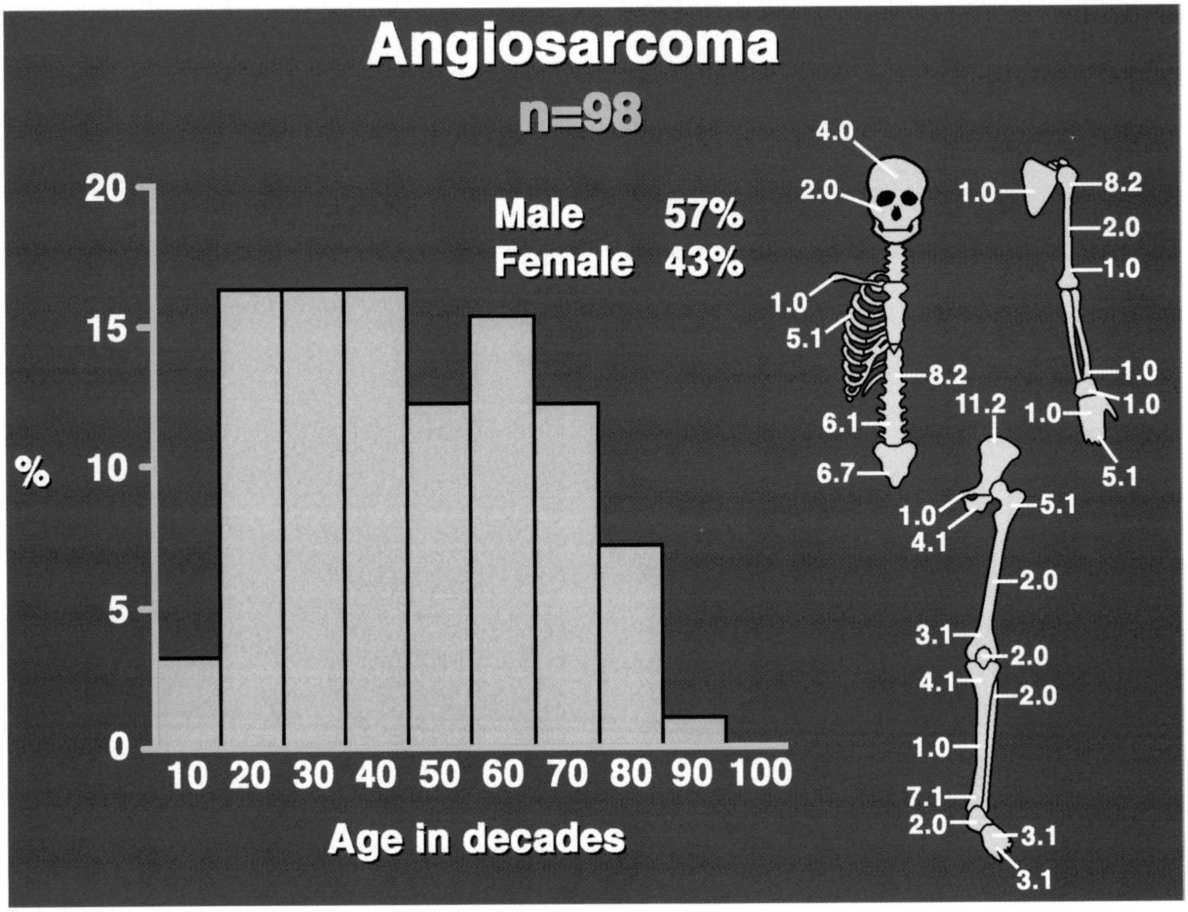

Figure 10-14

ANGIOSARCOMA

Distribution of angiosarcoma according to the age and sex of the patient and the site of the lesion.

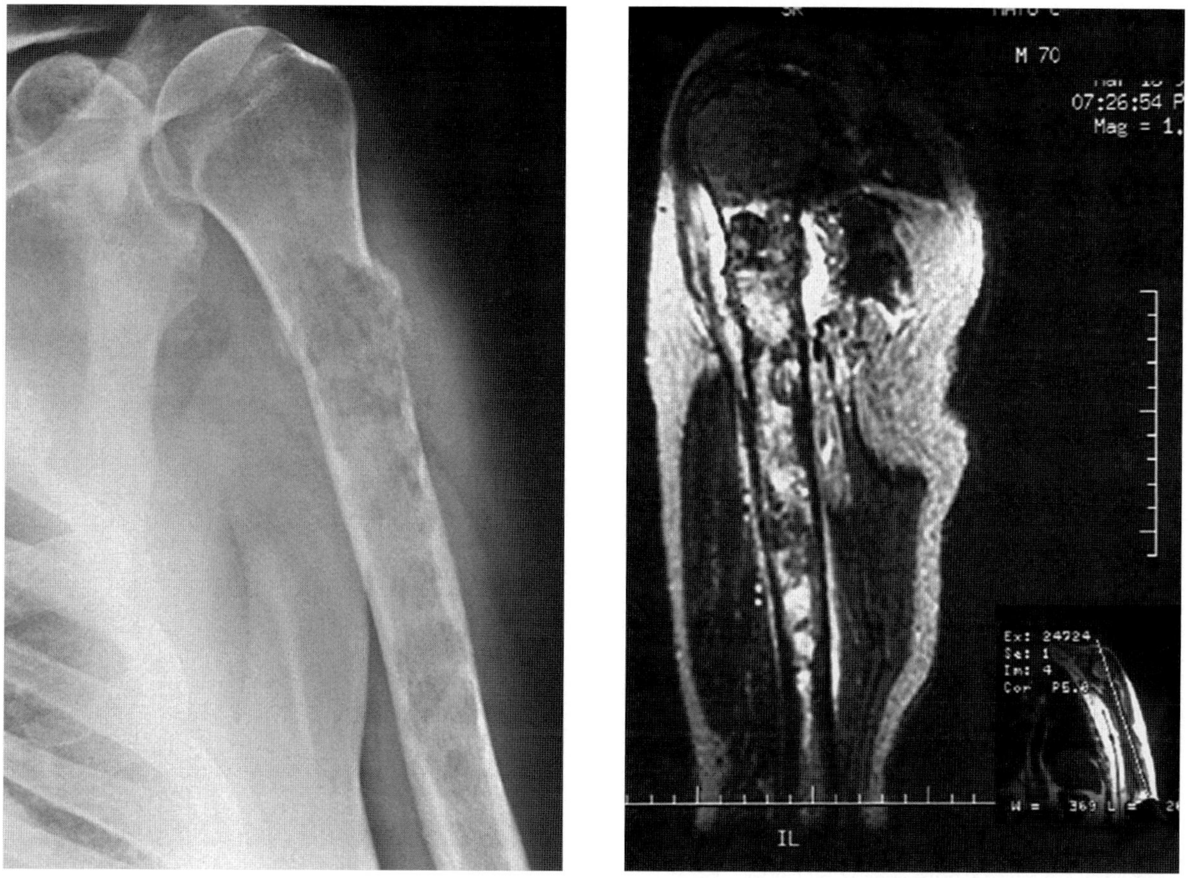

Figure 10-15

ANGIOSARCOMA

Left: Radiograph of the humerus shows a large, aggressive, lytic destructive lesion involving a long segment of the diaphysis with ill-defined margination and endosteal erosion. There is a mildly displaced pathologic fracture near the proximal margin of the tumor.

We have seen one angiosarcoma arise in the sinus tract of a patient with longstanding chronic osteomyelitis, and there has been one convincing case of the tumor arising in a patient with multiple hemangiomas (20).

Clinical Features. Patients present with pain or, occasionally, swelling. Presentation with pathologic fracture is rare, although pathologic fractures are seen slightly more frequently on radiographs (28). Patients with lesions of the spine may present with symptoms of spinal cord compression. There is a slight male predominance (26,27), although one report has suggested a 2 to 1 female predominance (19). Angiosarcoma usually affects young and older adults, with the highest incidence in the fourth decade of life.

Sites. Virtually any portion of the skeleton may be involved, but there is a predilection for the axial skeleton, with involvement of the spine and pelvic bones. From 15 (19) to 33 (26) percent of tumors are multicentric. When the tumor is multicentric, there is a pronounced tendency to involve one anatomic area, such as the bones in one extremity.

Radiographic Findings. Angiosarcomas present mostly as a purely lytic process. In well-differentiated tumors, the lesions tend to be well marginated, whereas higher-grade tumors are poorly demarcated (fig. 10-15) (28). Lesional sclerosis is uncommon, although in some cases sclerosis is in surrounding bone. Periosteal new bone formation is uncommon. Multiple lytic lesions, especially involving contiguous bones,

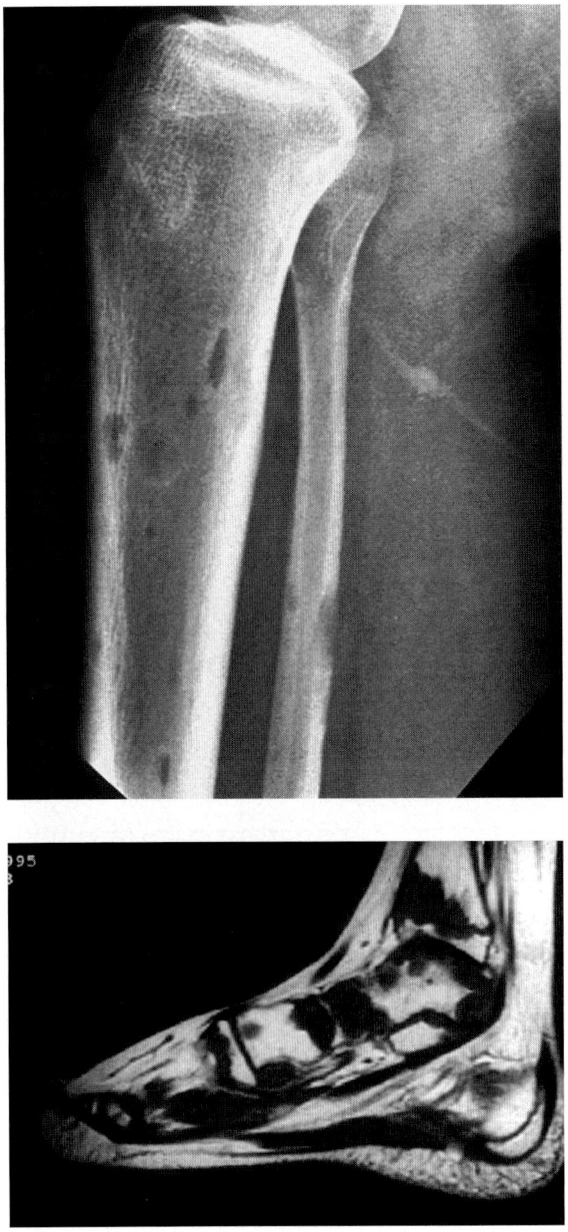

Figure 10-16

ANGIOSARCOMA

Top: Multiple areas of lysis involve the tibia and fibula.

Bottom: Sagittal T_1-weighted MRI shows multiple low-signal lesions in the distal tibia, talus, and navicular and cuneiform bones consistent with a vascular lesion.

are highly suggestive of the diagnosis of angiosarcoma (fig. 10-16).

Gross Findings. Angiosarcoma is characterized by bright red or dark red areas of destruction (figs. 10-17, 10-18). Indeed, the appear-

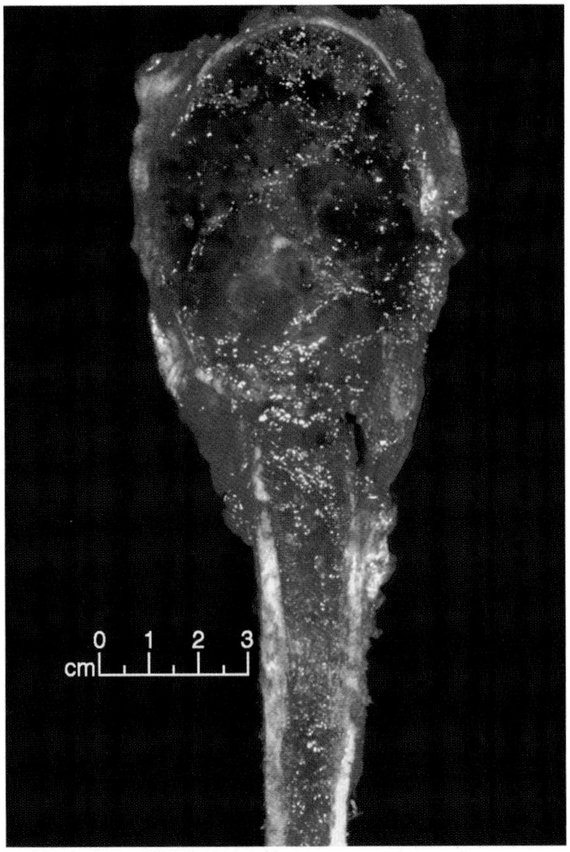

Figure 10-17

ANGIOSARCOMA

A red-brown tumor involving the head, neck, and upper shaft of the humerus is destroying the cortex in a 65-year-old woman, who died 4 months postoperatively with multicentric skeletal disease.

ance may suggest a blood clot. The cortex may be destroyed, and the tumor may extend into soft tissues.

Microscopic Findings. The essential pathologic feature of angiosarcoma is the production of vascular spaces lined with malignant cells. The vascular spaces show a marked tendency for anastomosis. The vessels are packed closely together, and if fibrosis is present, it is focal. Trabeculae or reactive bone may be present (fig. 10-19). Inflammatory cells, especially eosinophils, may be prominent (fig. 10-20). In some angiosarcomas, the endothelial cells are cuboidal and have abundant pink hyaline cytoplasm and vesicular nuclei with a single prominent nucleolus, imparting an epithelioid appearance. This change may be present focally or occur

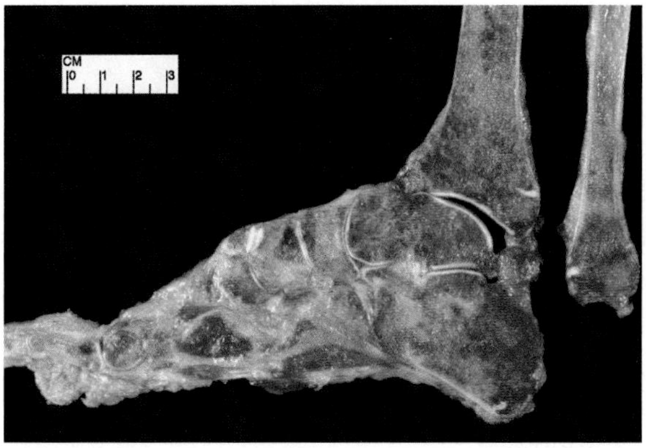

Figure 10-18

ANGIOSARCOMA

A multicentric angiosarcoma forms numerous tan-brown masses involving several bones of the foot, distal tibia, and distal fibula. The patient received radiotherapy preoperatively.

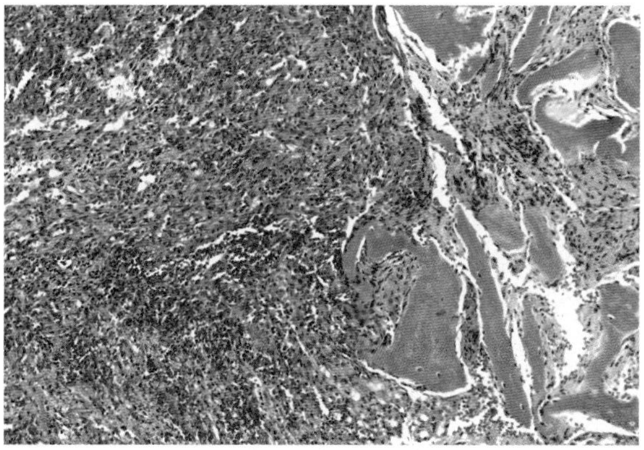

Figure 10-19

ANGIOSARCOMA

Reactive bone formation in angiosarcoma.

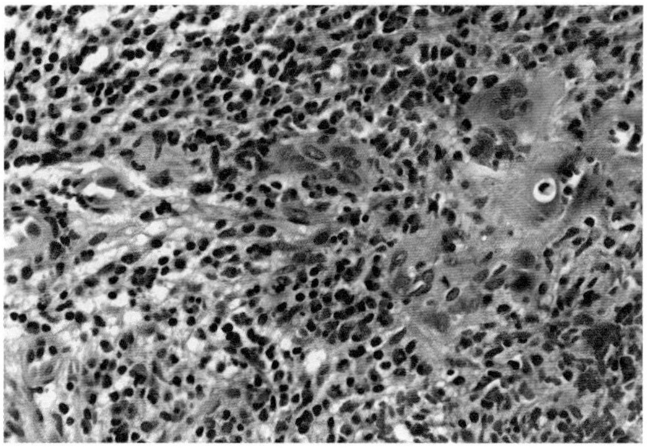

Figure 10-20

ANGIOSARCOMA

This tumor contained numerous eosinophils and a few scattered multinucleated giant cells.

throughout the lesion. If it occurs throughout the lesion, the term *epithelioid angiosarcoma* is used.

Several studies have used a histologic grading system for angiosarcoma (19,26,28). A three-tier grading system seems to work best. In grade 1 angiosarcoma, the vasoformation is obvious and the endothelial cells show minimal atypia (fig. 10-21). In grade 2 lesions, the tumor is still easily recognizable as vasoformative (fig. 10-22). The endothelial cells have moderate atypia, and papillary projections may be present. Grade 3 angiosarcoma is characterized by marked cytologic atypia (fig. 10-23). The tumor cells are

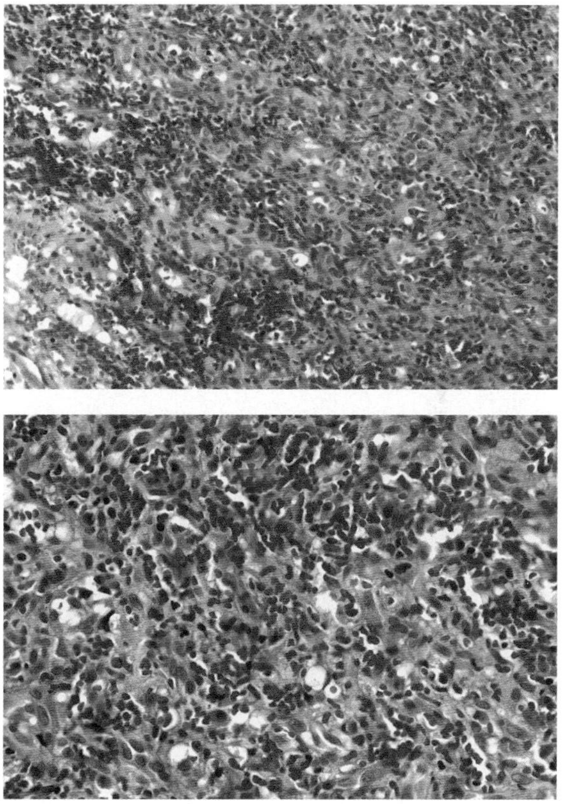

Figure 10-21

GRADE 1 ANGIOSARCOMA

Top: At low power, vasoformation is easy to identify.

Bottom: Higher-power view shows an anastomosing system of irregularly shaped vascular channels. Although not prominent, some degree of cytologic atypia is apparent.

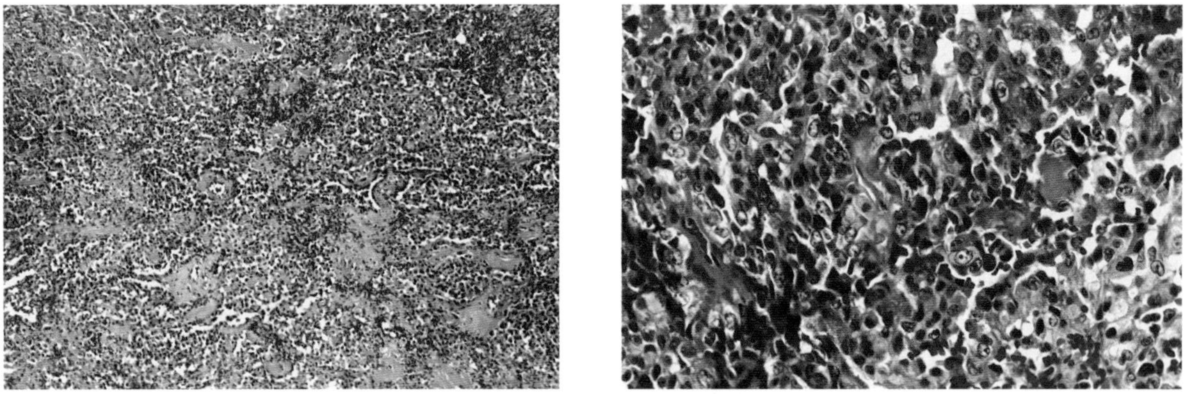

Figure 10-22

GRADE 2 ANGIOSARCOMA

Left: A vasoformative pattern is evident, as is intraluminal budding of endothelial cells.
Right: Higher power shows anaplastic endothelial cells containing enlarged hyperchromatic nuclei with a coarse chromatin pattern.

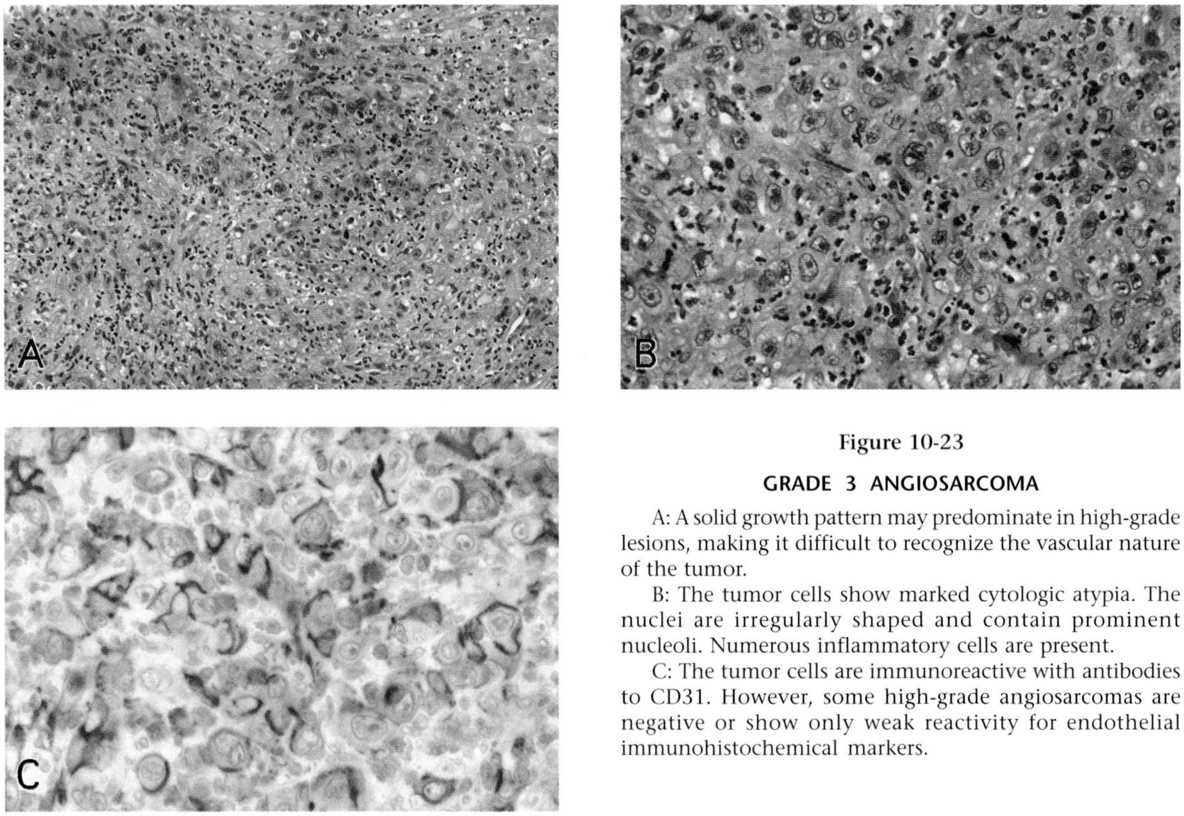

Figure 10-23

GRADE 3 ANGIOSARCOMA

A: A solid growth pattern may predominate in high-grade lesions, making it difficult to recognize the vascular nature of the tumor.

B: The tumor cells show marked cytologic atypia. The nuclei are irregularly shaped and contain prominent nucleoli. Numerous inflammatory cells are present.

C: The tumor cells are immunoreactive with antibodies to CD31. However, some high-grade angiosarcomas are negative or show only weak reactivity for endothelial immunohistochemical markers.

so crowded together that the vasoformative features may not be apparent (fig. 10-24). Epithelioid angiosarcomas are always high grade. Some authors have found so much variation within a given tumor that they do not find grading practical (27).

Weibel-Palade bodies, typical of endothelial cells, are found in the cytoplasm of the tumor cells.

Immunohistochemical Findings. In low-grade tumors, the diagnosis is usually obvious. Reportedly, CD31 antigen is very specific and sensitive for endothelial differentiation (fig. 10-23C)

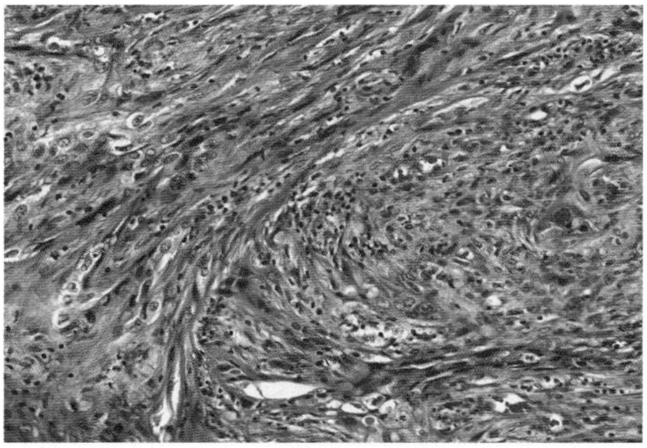

Figure 10-24

GRADE 3 ANGIOSARCOMA

The cells in this high-grade tumor are more spindle-shaped and compactly arranged, with only focal evidence of vascular differentiation.

(21). Epithelioid angiosarcomas usually stain with keratin.

Differential Diagnosis. As with all low-grade tumors, the distinction of grade 1 angiosarcoma from hemangioma can be difficult (24). It has been suggested that some of the grade 1 angiosarcomas reported in the literature are epithelioid hemangiomas that have hobnail-shaped cells lining vascular spaces. In epithelioid hemangioma, the vessels tend not to anastomose and are usually small and lobulated. Grade 1 angiosarcoma has anastomosing channels.

Metastatic carcinoma, especially renal cell carcinoma, can simulate the appearance of angiosarcoma. Recognition of the clear cytoplasm of hypernephroma and the lack of anastomosis are helpful in the diagnosis. Angiosarcomas may stain with keratin, but metastatic carcinomas do not stain with CD31.

Bacillary angiomatosis can produce lytic lesions in the skeleton (18,23). The lesions usually are seen in patients who are immunosuppressed, are caused by a bacillary organism, and are amenable to antibiotic treatment; hence, they are important to recognize. The process is characterized by the proliferation of vessels. The endothelial cells may have epithelioid features and cytologic atypia. However, the vascular proliferation is accompanied by an inflammatory infiltrate, predominantly of neutrophils and clumps of bacteria that stain with the Warthin-Starry silver stain.

Treatment and Prognosis. For solitary lesions, surgical resection is the treatment of choice. Radiotherapy is useful for multicentric disease and if the surgical margins are inadequate.

Some studies have indicated that prognosis is unpredictable and the mortality rate is as high as 50 percent (27). Several other studies have shown a direct correlation with histologic grading. Campanacci et al. (19) reported that no patient with a grade 1 tumor died of disease, but only one patient with a grade 3 tumor survived. Wold et al. (28) reported survival rates of 95, 62, and 20 percent for patients with grade 1, grade 2, and grade 3 tumors, respectively. Dorfman et al. (22) found that 80 percent of patients with well-differentiated tumors survived.

Epithelioid Hemangioendothelioma

Definition. Epithelioid hemangioendothelioma is a low-grade tumor composed of endothelial cells that have epithelial characteristics and in which vasoformation is occult.

General Features. Epithelioid endothelial cells are characterized by a polygonal outline, abundant eosinophilic cytoplasm containing single or multiple vacuoles, and an oval nucleus that may be indented (34). These cells can be seen focally in many vascular tumors, but when they are present throughout the tumor, the lesion can be termed an *epithelioid vascular tumor.* Such tumors can be divided into benign *(epithelioid hemangioma)*, intermediate *(epithelioid hemangioendothelioma)*, and malignant *(epithelioid angiosarcoma)* types.

The concept of epithelioid hemangioendothelioma was first developed in relation to soft tissues (37) to describe a tumor with epithelioid cells in which vasoformation was virtually absent. It had been recognized previously that the so-called intravascular bronchioloalveolar tumor is an epithelioid hemangioendothelioma (29). The lesion described as *myxoid angioblastoma of bone* (32) is the same entity.

Epithelioid hemangioendothelioma is uncommon. Tsuneyoshi et al. (35) classified 14 of 29 hemangioendotheliomas as epithelioid. Of the 18 cases of hemangioendothelioma reported in the Mayo Clinic files, only 4 were classified as epithelioid (36).

Clinical Features. Pain is the most common presentation.

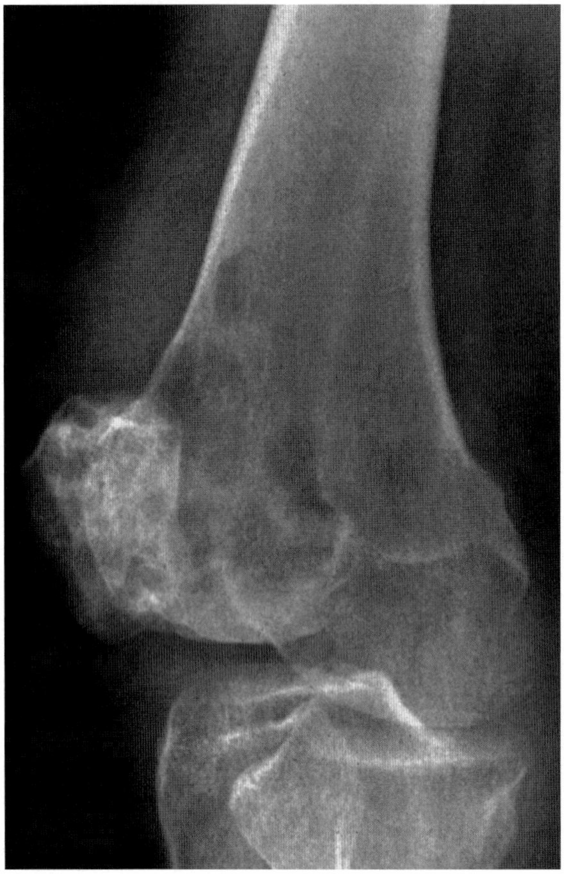

Figure 10-25

EPITHELIOID HEMANGIOENDOTHELIOMA

Oblique view of the right knee shows multiple discrete osteolytic lesions in the distal femur and patella. The patella is an uncommon site for malignant tumors. The patient also had pulmonary metastases. (Courtesy of Dr. J. R. Stange, Tulsa, OK.)

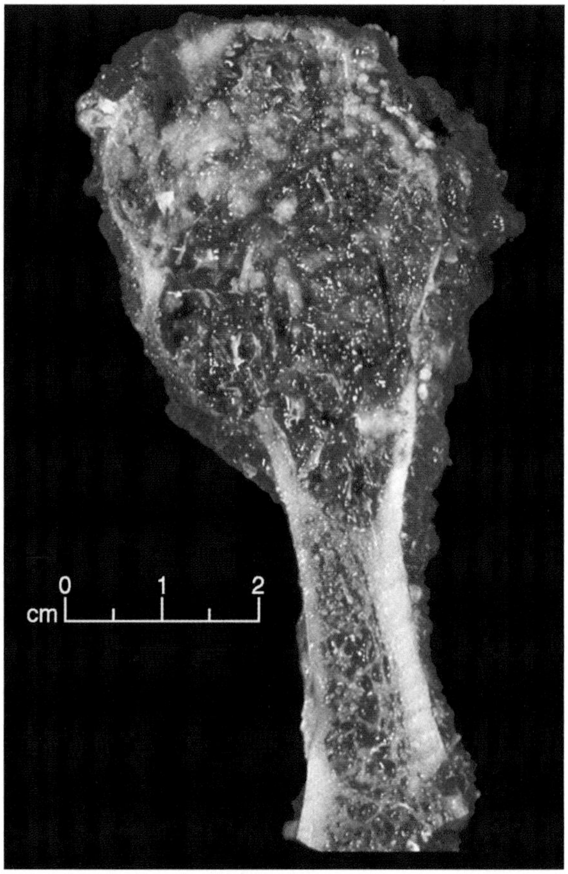

Figure 10-26

EPITHELIOID HEMANGIOENDOTHELIOMA

The lobulated, dark red neoplasm involves the ilium of a 30-year-old man. (Fig. 23-8B from Unni KK. Dahlin's bone tumors: general aspects and data on 11,087 cases, 5th ed. Philadelphia: Lippincott-Raven; 1996:320. By permission of Mayo Foundation.)

Sites. Any portion of the skeleton may be involved. As with conventional hemangioendothelioma, multicentricity is a feature of epithelioid hemangioendothelioma. Kleer et al. (30) reported that more than 50 percent were multicentric, whereas Tsuneyoshi et al. (35) found that more than two thirds were multicentric.

Radiographic Findings. The tumors occur at or near the ends of bones (fig. 10-25). The lesions are lucent, with surrounding sclerosis. The features are nonspecific, although the presence of multiple lytic lesions in one anatomic area may suggest the diagnosis.

Gross Findings. Grossly, the tumors are soft, red nodular masses (fig. 10-26).

Microscopic Findings. Under low-power magnification, the lesion appears lobulated. The center contains nodules of tumor embedded in a myxoid matrix. The periphery of the lobules may contain clusters of benign giant cells (fig. 10-27). The tumor cells are arranged in cords within the myxoid-chondroid matrix. The tumor cells have abundant pink cytoplasm and contain vacuoles that represent intracellular vessel formation (fig. 10-28). The vacuoles frequently indent the nucleus, giving the cell a signet ring appearance. The matrix may undergo calcification or even bone formation.

The tumor cells stain with CD31 (fig. 10-29). Keratin stains also tend to be positive.

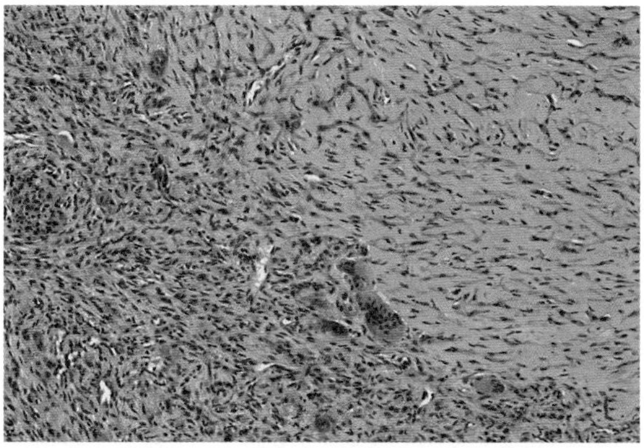

Figure 10-27

EPITHELIOID HEMANGIOENDOTHELIOMA

At low power, the tumor has a lobulated growth pattern. The cells within the lobule are arranged in cords. Multinucleated giant cells are seen at the periphery of the lobule.

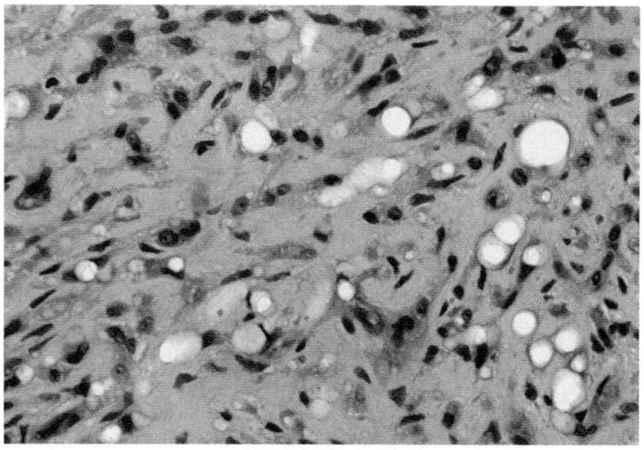

Figure 10-28

EPITHELIOID HEMANGIOENDOTHELIOMA

The tumor cells are embedded in a pale blue chondroid or myxoid matrix. Cytoplasmic vacuoles produce a signet ring appearance.

Genetics and Other Special Techniques. An identical chromosomal translocation involving chromosomes 1 and 3 [t(1;3)(p36.3;q25)] has been described in two cases of epithelioid hemangioendothelioma (one arising in the liver and the other in the soft tissue of an extremity), possibly representing a characteristic rearrangement for this histopathologic entity (31). Only one case of hemangioendothelioma of bone has been subjected to cytogenetic analysis, and this study did not demonstrate any chromosomal abnormalities in addition to the constitutional supernumerary marker chromosome observed in the peripheral blood of the patient (33). The presence of clonal karyotypic abnormalities supports a neoplastic origin for the epithelioid variant of hemangioendothelioma. Identification of the 1;3 translocation may be useful diagnostically for epithelioid hemangioendothelioma. Should additional studies confirm these data, this could lead to the identification of the gene(s) central to this neoplastic process.

Differential Diagnosis. The myxoid matrix may cause diagnostic difficulties. Chondromyxoid fibroma also tends to have a lobular growth pattern. However, the cells in chondromyxoid fibroma are stellate or spindle shaped and lack the cording seen in epithelioid hemangioendothelioma. Calcification in the matrix may suggest chondrosarcoma, especially myxoid chondrosarcoma. The typical epithelioid cell with cytoplasmic vacuoles is not seen in myxoid chondrosarcomas. Reactive new bone may suggest a bone-forming tumor, especially osteoblastoma. Osteoblastoma is characterized by prominent osteoblasts lining bony trabeculae. In epithelioid hemangioendothelioma, clusters of tumor cells are seen in the intertrabecular spaces.

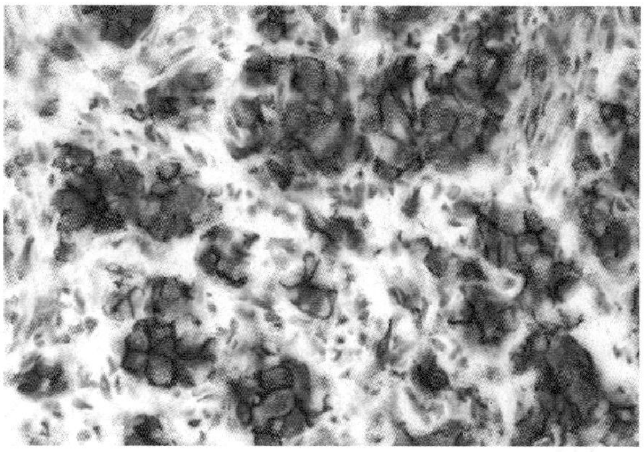

Figure 10-29

EPITHELIOID HEMANGIOENDOTHELIOMA

The epithelioid tumor cells are immunoreactive with antibodies to CD31. This immunostain and other endothelial markers such as factor VIII–related antigen and CD34 can be helpful in differentiating epithelioid hemangioendothelioma from metastatic carcinoma.

Treatment and Prognosis. When feasible, complete but conservative resection is the treatment of choice. Radiotherapy may be helpful

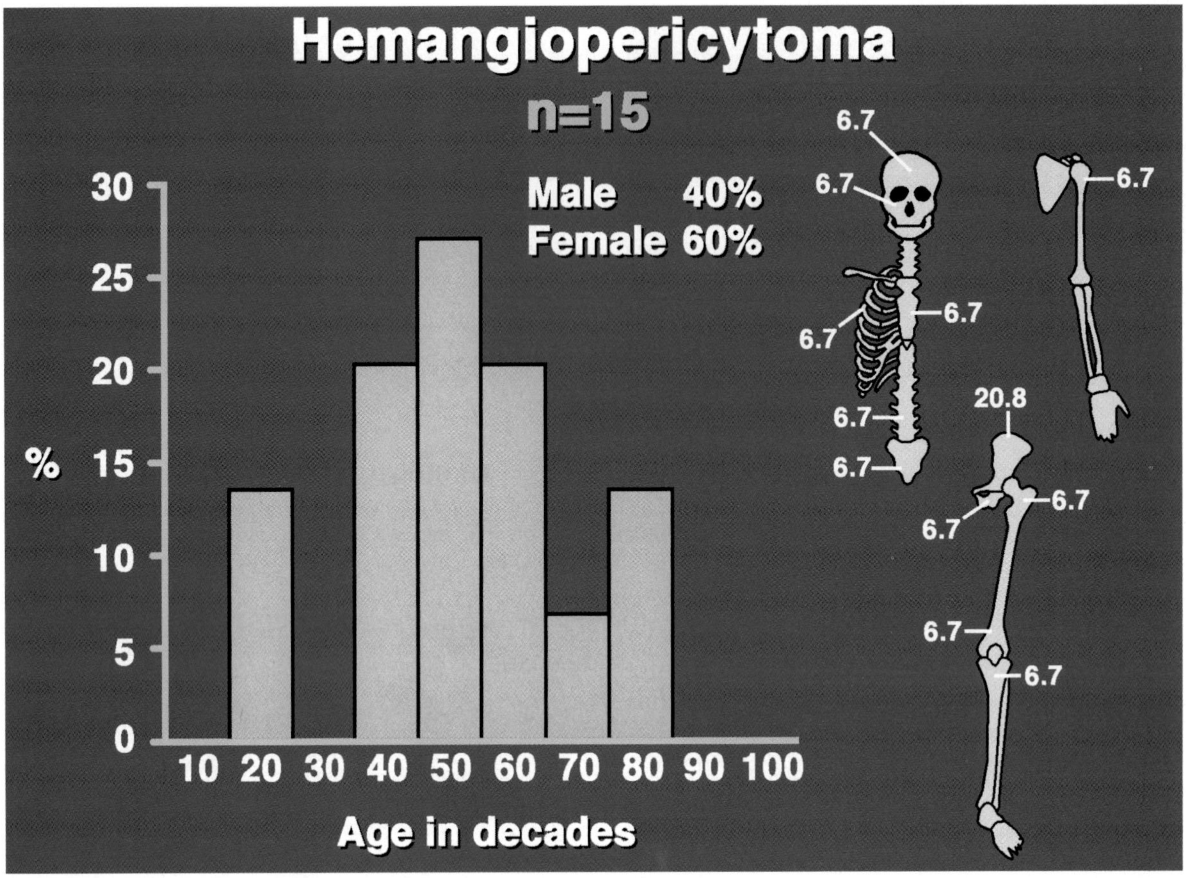

Figure 10-30

HEMANGIOPERICYTOMA

Distribution of hemangiopericytoma according to the age and sex of the patient and the site of the lesion.

for multicentric disease. The prognosis depends on whether the viscera are involved. The lungs, liver, and pleura may be involved in addition to the skeleton. These probably represent a manifestation of multicentricity rather than metastasis. In the series reported by Kleer et al. (30), 7 of the 8 patients who died of disease had visceral involvement. None of the 14 patients reported by Tsuneyoshi et al. (35) died, although a metastatic focus developed in the abdominal wall of one patient.

Hemangiopericytoma

Definition. Hemangiopericytoma is a tumor composed of oval to spindle-shaped cells arranged around vascular spaces.

General Features. Hemangiopericytoma has become a controversial subject and its very existence is being questioned. Many other tumors (especially sarcomas) can have a hemangiopericytomatous appearance, notably, synovial sarcoma, solitary fibrous tumor, endometrial stromal sarcoma, and mesenchymal chondrosarcoma. This has led to the suggestion that hemangiopericytoma is only a pattern and not a specific entity. We believe that hemangiopericytoma is an extremely uncommon but definite entity. Hemangiopericytoma is one of the rarest of all primary bone neoplasms. The Mayo Clinic files contain the records of only 15 cases (fig. 10-30).

Clinical Features. Patients present with pain. Adults are usually affected, and there is no sex predilection.

Sites. The bones of the pelvis are involved most commonly.

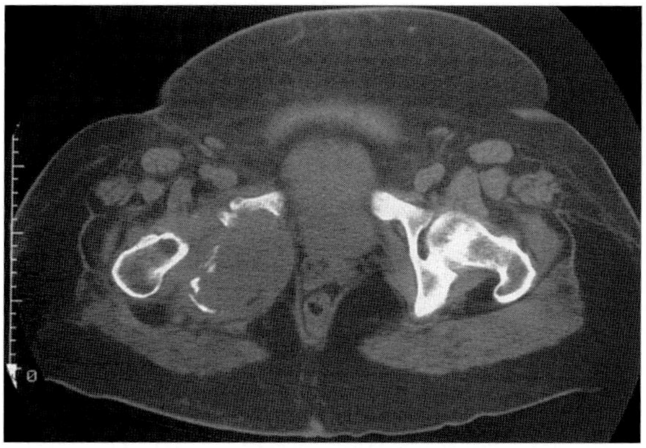

Figure 10-31

HEMANGIOPERICYTOMA

CT shows an expansive and destructive nonmineralized lesion of the right acetabulum. (Fig. 23-17B from Unni KK. Dahlin's bone tumors: general aspects and data on 11,087 cases, 5th ed. Philadelphia: Lippincott-Raven; 1996:329. By permission of Mayo Foundation.)

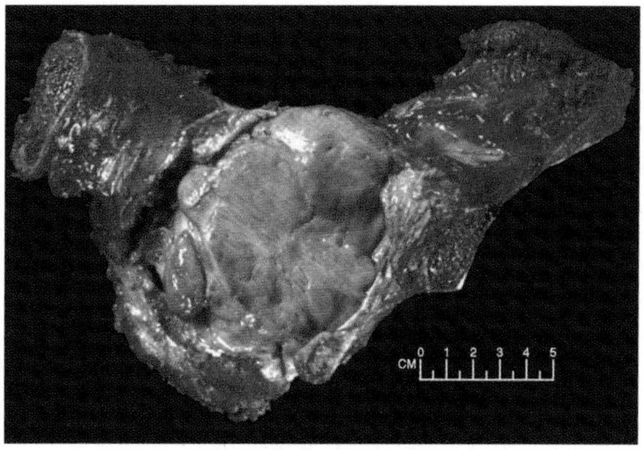

Figure 10-32

HEMANGIOPERICYTOMA

A well-demarcated, firm, rubbery, tan-gray tumor forms a destructive mass in the acetabulum of a 48-year-old woman. (Fig. 23-17C from Unni KK. Dahlin's bone tumors: general aspects and data on 11,087 cases, 5th ed. Philadelphia: Lippincott-Raven; 1996:329. By permission of Mayo Foundation.)

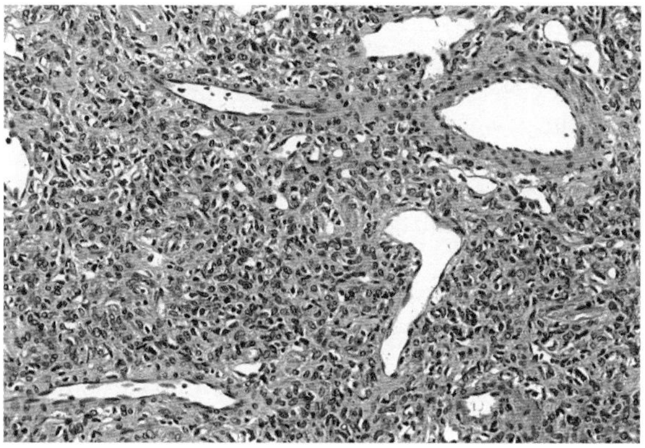

Figure 10-33

HEMANGIOPERICYTOMA

A branching stag-horn pattern of vascular spaces is apparent at low-power magnification.

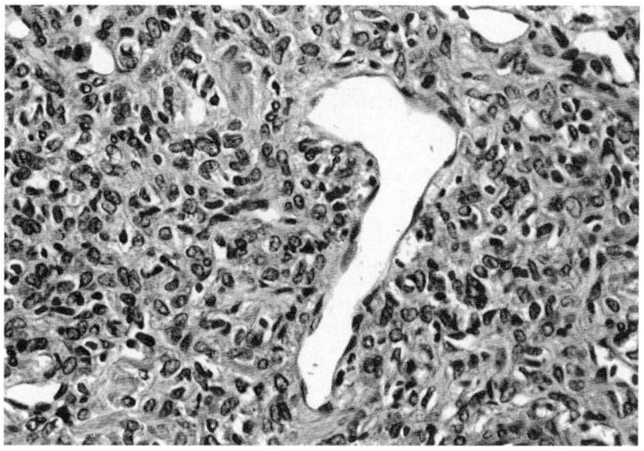

Figure 10-34

HEMANGIOPERICYTOMA

Oval to spindle-shaped cells with minimal cytologic atypia occupy the intervascular stroma.

Radiographic Findings. The lesions are usually purely lytic. Periosteal new bone formation is absent (fig. 10-31).

Gross Findings. The tumor is firm, gray to white, and rubbery (fig. 10-32). There may be considerable bleeding during surgical removal.

Microscopic Findings. Hemangiopericytoma is a vascular neoplasm; however, the vessels may be prominent or occult. When prominent, they have a sinusoidal quality and tend to branch, producing the appearance of deer antlers (fig. 10-33). The tumor cells cluster outside the vessels and tend to deform the spaces. The tumor cells are oval and have pale-staining nuclei (fig. 10-34). Nucleoli are not prominent; mitotic activity is variable. If tumor cells show pleomorphism, the diagnosis is not valid; hence, histologic grading is not practical.

Differential Diagnosis. As indicated above, many tumors have a focal hemangiopericytomatous pattern. The cytologic features and the vascular pattern should be present throughout the lesion to avoid mistaking a high-grade sarcoma for a hemangiopericytoma. Hemangiopericytoma of the meninges has a peculiar tendency to metastasize to the skeleton (38). A clinical history of meningioma should alert one to this possibility.

Treatment and Prognosis. Complete surgical removal is the treatment of choice. The prognosis is unpredictable but generally poor (39). Wold et al. (41) reported on 15 cases; follow-up information was available for 14. Eight patients died and 3 were alive with disease. Only 3 patients appeared to have survived. Some patients survive for a long time before metastases develop (40).

REFERENCES

Hemangioma

1. Dorfman HD, Steiner GC, Jaffee HL. Vascular tumors of bone. Hum Pathol 1971;2:349–76.
2. Karlin CA, Brower AC. Multiple primary hemangiomas of bone. AJR Am J Roentgenol 1977;129:162–4.
3. Kenan S, Abdelwahab IF, Klein MJ, Lewis MM. Hemangiomas of the long tubular bone. Clin Orthop 1992;280:256–60.
4. O'Connell JX, Kattapuram SV, Mankin HJ, Bhan AK, Rosenberg AE. Epithelioid hemangioma of bone. A tumor often mistaken for low-grade angiosarcoma or malignant hemangioendothelioma. Am J Surg Pathol 1993;17:610–7; comment: 1994;18:1270–1.
5. Paley D, Evans DC. Angiomatous involvement of an extremity. A spectrum of syndromes. Clin Orthop 1986;206:215–8.
6. Robbins LR, Fountain EM. Hemangioma of cervical vertebras with spinal-cord compression. N Engl J Med 1958;258:685–7.
7. Ross JS, Masaryk TJ, Modic MT, Carter JR, Mapstone T, Dengel FH. Vertebral hemangiomas: MR imaging. Radiology 1987;165:165–9.
8. Wold LE, Swee RG, Sim FH. Vascular lesions of bone. Pathol Annu 1985;20:101–37.
9. Unni KK. Dahlin's bone tumors: general aspects and data on 11,087 cases, 5th ed. Philadelphia: Lippincott-Raven; 1996:307–16.

Massive Osteolysis

10. Bullough PG. Massive osteolysis. N Y State J Med 1971;71:2267–78.
11. Fechner RE, Mills SE. Tumors of the bones and joints. Atlas of Tumor Pathology, 3rd Series, Fascicle 8. Washington, DC: Armed Forces Institute of Pathology; 1993:133–5.
12. Halliday DR, Dahlin DC, Pugh DG, Young HH. Massive osteolysis and angiomatosis. Radiology 1964;82:637–44.
13. Johnson PM, McClure JG. Observations on massive osteolysis: a review of the literature and report of a case. Radiology 1958;71:28–42.
14. Shives TC, Beabout JW, Unni KK. Massive osteolysis. Clin Orthop 1993;294:267–76.
15. Turra S, Gigante C, Scapinelli R. A 20-year follow-up study of a case of surgically treated massive osteolysis. Clin Orthop 1990;250:297–302.

Glomus Tumor

16. Pambakian H, Smith MA. Glomus tumours of the coccygeal body associated with coccydynia. A preliminary report. J Bone Joint Surg Br 1981;63:424–6.
17. Rozmaryn LM, Sadler AH, Dorfman HD. Intraosseous glomus tumor in the ulna. A case report. Clin Orthop 1987;220:126–9.

Angiosarcoma

18. Baron AL, Steinbach LS, LeBoit PE, Mills CM, Gee JH, Berger TG. Osteolytic lesions and bacillary angiomatosis in HIV infection: radiologic differentiation from AIDS-related Kaposi sarcoma. Radiology 1990;177:77–81.
19. Campanacci M, Boriani S, Giunti A. Hemangioendothelioma of bone: a study of 29 cases. Cancer 1980;46:804–14.
20. Case records of the Massachusetts General Hospital. Weekly clinicopathological exercises. Case 13-1989. A 76-year-old woman with multiple bone lesions and thrombocytopenia. N Engl J Med 1989;320:854–60.

21. De Young BR, Wick MR, Fitzgibbon JF, Sirgi KE, Swanson PE. CD31: an immunospecific marker for endothelial differentiation in human neoplasms. Appl Immunohistochem 1993;1:97–100.
22. Dorfman HD, Steiner GC, Jaffe HL. Vascular tumors of bone. Hum Pathol 1971;2:349–76.
23. LeBoit PE, Berger TG, Egbert BM, Beckstead JH, Yen TS, Stoler MH. Bacillary angiomatosis. The histopathology and differential diagnosis of a pseudoneoplastic infection in patients with human immunodeficiency virus disease. Am J Surg Pathol 1989;13:909–20.
24. O'Connell JX, Kattapuram SV, Mankin HJ, Bhan AK, Rosenberg AE. Epithelioid hemangioma of bone. A tumor often mistaken for low-grade angiosarcoma or malignant hemangioendothelioma. Am J Surg Pathol 1993;17:610–7.
25. Stout AP. Hemangio-endothelioma: a tumor of blood vessels featuring vascular endothelial cells. Ann Surg 1943;118:445–64.
26. Unni KK. Dahlin's bone tumors: general aspects and data on 11,087 cases, 5th ed. Philadelphia: Lippincott-Raven; 1996.
27. Volpe R, Mazabraud A. Hemangioendothelioma (angiosarcoma) of bone: a distinct pathologic entity with an unpredictable course? Cancer 1982;49:727–36.
28. Wold LE, Unni KK, Beabout JW, Ivins JC, Bruckman JE, Dahlin DC. Hemangioendothelial sarcoma of bone. Am J Surg Pathol 1982;6:59–70.

Epithelioid Hemangioendothelioma

29. Bhagavan BS, Dorfman HD, Murthy MS, Eggleston JC. Intravascular bronchiolo-alveolar tumor (IVBAT). A low-grade sclerosing epithelioid angiosarcoma of lung. Am J Surg Pathol 1982;6:41–52.
30. Kleer CG, Unni KK, McLeod RA. Epithelioid hemangioendothelioma of bone. Am J Surg Pathol 1996;20:1301–11.
31. Mendlick MR, Nelson M, Pickering D, et al. Translocation t(1;3)(p36.3;q25) is a nonrandom aberration in epithelioid hemangioendothelioma. Am J Surg Pathol 2001;25:684–7.
32. Mirra JM, Kameda N. Case report 366: myxoid angioblastomatosis of bone (disseminated). Skeletal Radiol 1986;15:323–6.
33. Rogatto SR, Rainho CA, Zhang ZM, et al. Hemangioendothelioma of bone in a patient with a constitutional supernumerary marker. Cancer Genet Cytogenet 1999;110:23–7.
34. Tsang WY, Chan JK. The family of epithelioid vascular tumors. Histol Histopathol 1993;8:187–212.
35. Tsuneyoshi M, Dorfman HD, Bauer TW. Epithelioid hemangioendothelioma of bone. A clinicopathologic, ultrastructural, and immunohistochemical study. Am J Surg Pathol 1986;10:754–64.
36. Unni KK. Dahlin's bone tumors: general aspects and data on 11,087 cases, 5th ed. Philadelphia: Lippincott-Raven; 1996:317–31.
37. Weiss SW, Enzinger FM. Epithelioid hemangioendothelioma: a vascular tumor often mistaken for a carcinoma. Cancer 1982;50:970–81.

Hemangiopericytoma

38. Dahlin DC. Case report 160. Skeletal Radiol 1981;6:303–5.
39. Tang JS, Gold RH, Mirra JM, Eckardt J. Hemangiopericytoma of bone. Cancer 1988;62:848–59.
40. Unni KK, Ivins JC, Beabout JW, Dahlin DC. Hemangioma, hemangiopericytoma, and hemangioendothelioma (angiosarcoma) of bone. Cancer 1971;27:1403–14.
41. Wold LE, Unni KK, Cooper KL, Sim FH, Dahlin DC. Hemangiopericytoma of bone. Am J Surg Pathol 1982;6:53–8.

11 GIANT CELL TUMOR

GIANT CELL TUMOR

Definition. Giant cell tumor is a primary neoplasm of bone that is composed of round to oval mononuclear cells and more or less uniformly distributed osteoclast-like giant cells. The tumors usually are situated at the ends of long bones in skeletally mature patients.

General Features. The histogenesis of giant cell tumors is unclear. Osteoclast-like giant cells are seen in various bone lesions, both neoplastic and non-neoplastic. Whether the giant cells are part of the neoplasm or a reaction to the mononuclear cells is debatable. In the rare examples of metastatic giant cell tumor, the distant deposits contain giant cells, suggesting that they should be considered neoplastic. The morphology of the tumor has led Dahlin (16) to suggest that the giant cells arise from the fusion of the mononuclear cells. The results of immunohistochemical studies suggest that both mononuclear and giant cells are derived from histiocytes (6,20,25,37).

Giant cell tumor has been described in association with Paget's disease (23,26,44,45,63). In a series reported by Jacobs et al. (26), 3 of 4 patients with Paget's disease and giant cell tumors were related and traced their ancestry to a town in northern Italy. Patients who have giant cell tumor with Paget's disease tend to be older and to have a propensity for tumors in the jawbones. The tumors also have the peculiarity of responding to dexamethasone therapy, which suggests that they should not be considered true neoplasms but examples of giant cell reparative granuloma.

The exact site of origin of a giant cell tumor has led to controversy. It generally is recognized that in long bones, giant cell tumors extend to the end of the bone. This supports an epiphyseal origin of the tumor. However, as pointed out by Campanacci et al. (12) and McDonald et al. (36), giant cell tumors also always involve the metaphysis. Moreover, purely metaphyseal giant cell tumors occur (12,16,17), usually in children with open epiphyseal plates. This suggests that giant cell tumors arise in the metaphysis and extend to involve the epiphysis. However, the practical consideration is that when a giant cell tumor is diagnosed, it nearly always involves the epiphyseal region.

Giant cell tumors account for about 5 percent of primary bone tumors and 20 percent of benign tumors (18). In China, however, the tumors constitute about 10 percent of all bone tumors (59). The Mayo Clinic files contain 627 cases of giant cell tumors (21.9 percent of benign tumors) (fig. 11-1).

Clinical Features. Most patients who have a giant cell tumor are in the third or fourth decade of life, with the highest incidence (39 percent) in the third decade (16). Most reports confirm a slight but definite female predominance. Dahlin (16) reported a female predominance of 56 percent, but this increased to 72 percent for patients younger than 20 years. The probable explanation for this higher percentage is that females attain skeletal maturity earlier than males.

Pain is the most common symptom. Pathologic fracture is rare. Even rarer is the incidental discovery of a giant cell tumor on radiographs. Tumors involving the sacrum and the vertebrae may cause neurologic symptoms. The majority of patients note a swelling.

Sites. Most giant cell tumors occur at the ends (epiphyses) of long bones. The distal femur is the most common site, followed by the proximal tibia. These two sites account for 46 percent of all giant cell tumors recorded in the Mayo Clinic files. The distal end of the radius is the third most common site and the sacrum is the fourth. Vertebrae, about the level of the sacrum, are involved less often. The majority of giant cell tumors of vertebrae involve the body alone or the body and posterior elements (51). Only a small proportion involve the posterior elements alone. Although the proximal femur is an uncommon site, the greater trochanter or head may be involved.

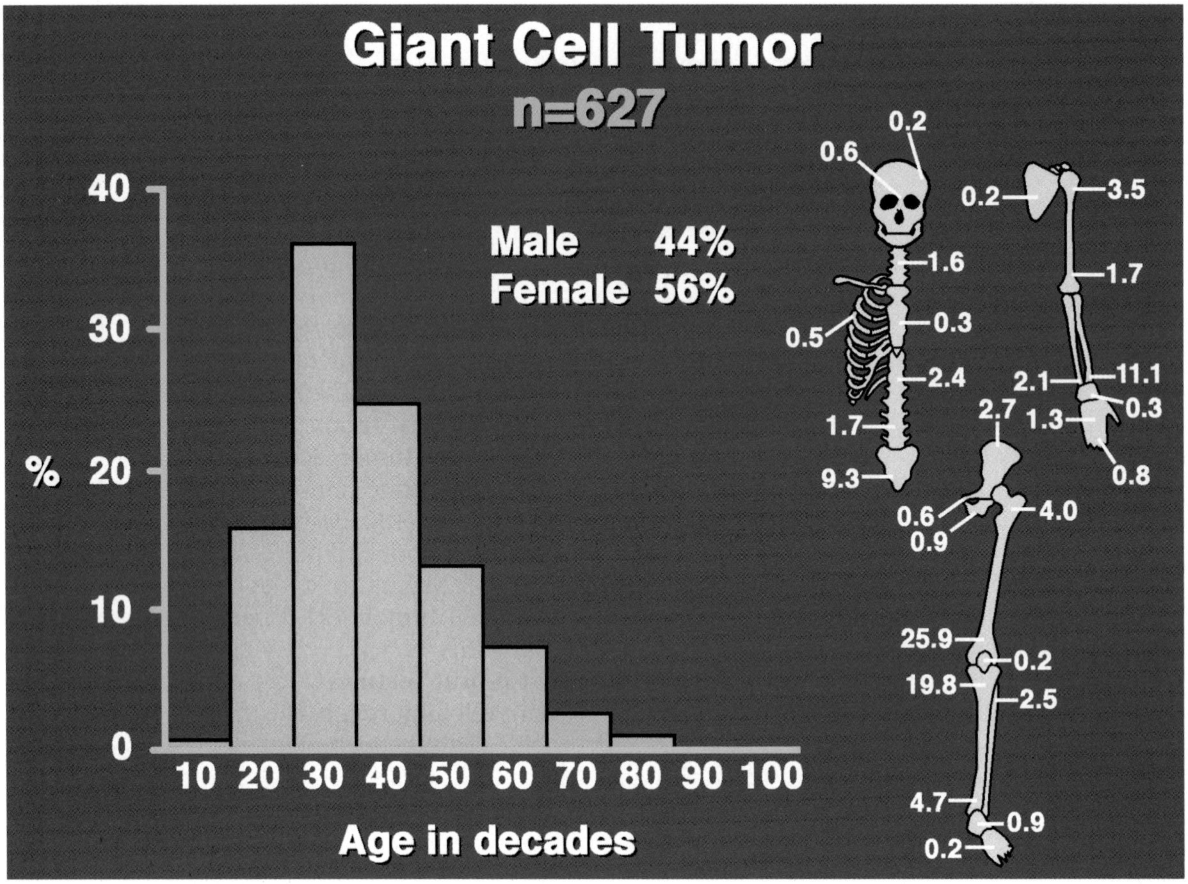

Figure 11-1

GIANT CELL TUMOR

Distribution of giant cell tumor according to the age and sex of the patient and the site of the lesion.

The flat bones are uncommon sites of involvement. In the ilium, the tumor may be periacetabular or in the wing. Involvement of the sternum, ribs, or scapula should suggest other diagnoses such as aneurysmal bone cyst or osteosarcoma. In the rare instances of giant cell tumor of the skull, the sphenoid bone is the predominant site (4).

Giant cell tumors can involve the small bones of the hands and feet. The patients tend to be younger and the process more aggressive (5,66).

Multicentric giant cell tumors are rare; in two large series, they formed about 1 percent of all giant cell tumors (15,57). Multicentric lesions tend to involve the small bones but are otherwise typical (42).

Radiographic Findings. In long bones, giant cell tumors typically occur as an eccentric, purely lytic lesion involving the end of the bone (fig. 11-2). McDonald et al. (36) found that more than 50 percent of the tumors extended to the articular cartilage and the rest had a rim of residual subchondral bone. About 5 percent invade the joint (12). Although the lesion is usually well marginated, rarely does it have a rim of sclerosis (fig. 11-3). The cortex is frequently destroyed, and the lesion expands to the soft tissues, where it is covered with a thin shell of reactive new bone. Periosteal new bone formation in the form of a Codman's triangle is rarely seen. About one fourth of giant cell tumors produce a poorly defined, aggressive-appearing lesion that cannot be differentiated from a sarcoma on radiographs (fig. 11-4).

When a giant cell tumor occurs in an unusual location, the diagnosis is less obvious. In the

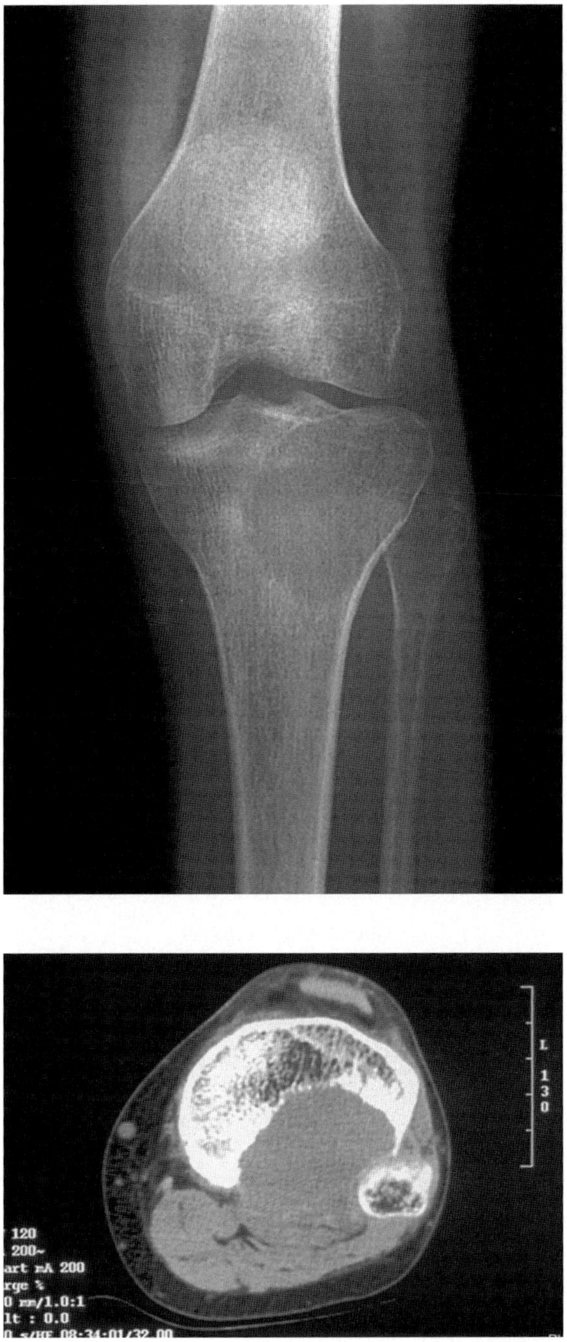

Figure 11-2

GIANT CELL TUMOR

Top: Radiograph of a giant cell tumor involving the proximal tibia of a 23-year-old man. It is a lytic tumor that extends to the end of the bone.

Bottom: Computerized tomography (CT) is helpful in identifying the extent of the tumor and size of the soft tissue mass. (Courtesy of Dr. U. Raju, Detroit, MI.)

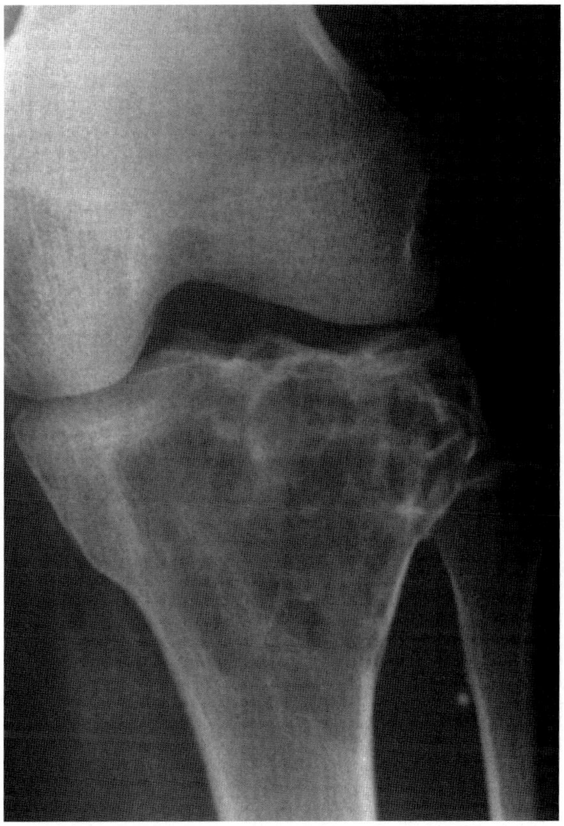

Figure 11-3

GIANT CELL TUMOR

This tumor in the proximal tibia is purely lytic, although it has a partial sclerotic rim.

vertebrae, the bodies are involved most often and the lesion may form a large destructive mass that presents as a posterior mediastinal tumor.

Classically, giant cell tumors are considered incapable of producing sclerosis, but it is well recognized that extension of the tumor into soft tissue produces an eggshell of new bone. Tumors that recur in soft tissues typically produce a rind of ossification of variable thickness that encircles the mass (fig. 11-5) (14). Not all giant cell tumors that recur in soft tissue ossify (14,33). Lung metastases tend to ossify. Some giant cell tumors in bone may show sclerosis, either at the periphery or in the center (fig. 11-6).

Computerized tomography (CT) and magnetic resonance imaging (MRI) do not show features specific for giant cell tumors (fig. 11-7). As with many other neoplasms, T_1-weighted images tend to be dark and T_2-weighted images, bright.

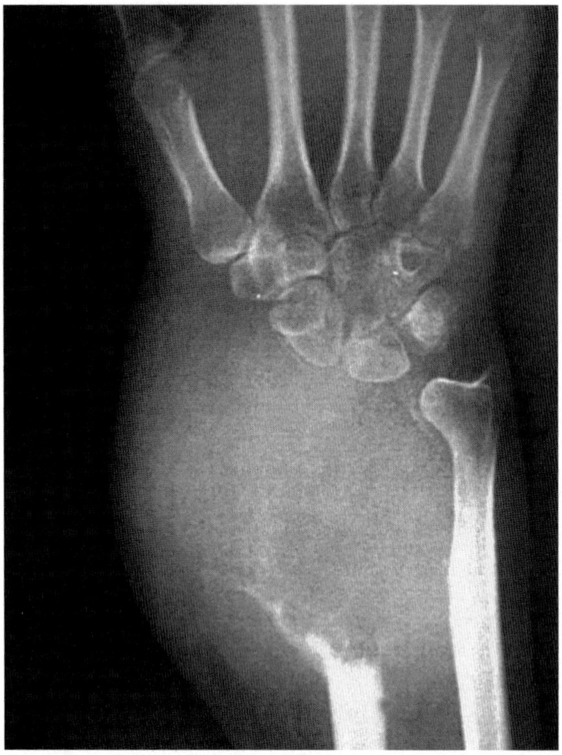

Figure 11-4

GIANT CELL TUMOR

The tumor arises in the distal radius and forms a large destructive mass. The treatment was amputation. (Courtesy of Dr. K. Allen, Jackson, MS.)

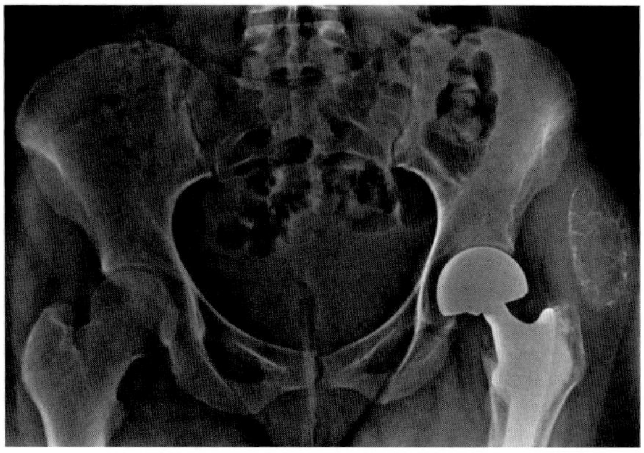

Figure 11-5

GIANT CELL TUMOR

Soft tissue recurrence in a 28-year-old woman who had surgery 18 months earlier for a giant cell tumor of the proximal femur. The soft tissue mass shows peripheral mineralization, resembling an eggshell. (Fig. 19-18 from Unni KK. Dahlin's bone tumors: general aspects and data on 11,087 cases, 5th ed. Philadelphia: Lippincott-Raven; 1996:272. By permission of Mayo Foundation.)

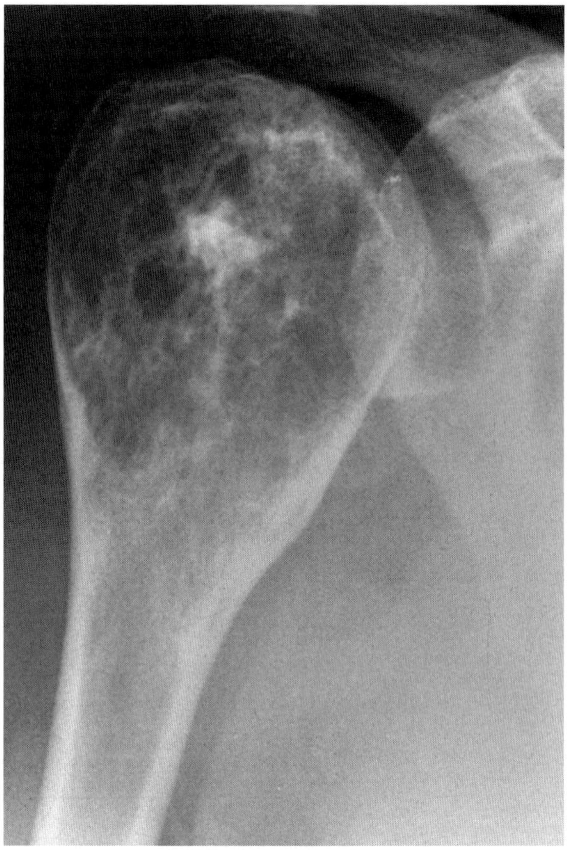

Figure 11-6

GIANT CELL TUMOR

Only rarely do giant cell tumors such as this one in the proximal humerus of a 58-year-old woman show focal radiographic evidence of mineralization. (Courtesy of Dr. F. Azizi, Fontana, CA.)

Campanacci et al. (12) proposed the following radiologic staging system for giant cell tumor: grade 1, a well-defined lesion with a thin sclerotic rim. The cortex is intact. Only 3 percent of giant cell tumors belong to this group; grade 2, a well-defined tumor but without a sclerotic rim. The cortex is thinned but intact. Seventy percent of all giant cell tumors fit this category; and grade 3, a poorly marginated, permeative, and aggressive-appearing lesion. The cortex is destroyed, and the tumor bulges into the soft tissue. Twenty-seven percent of giant cell tumors are considered to be stage 3. The authors stressed that grading does not correlate with prognosis but does offer a guide to surgical management.

Gross Findings. Specimens of giant cell tumors usually are received as fragments from

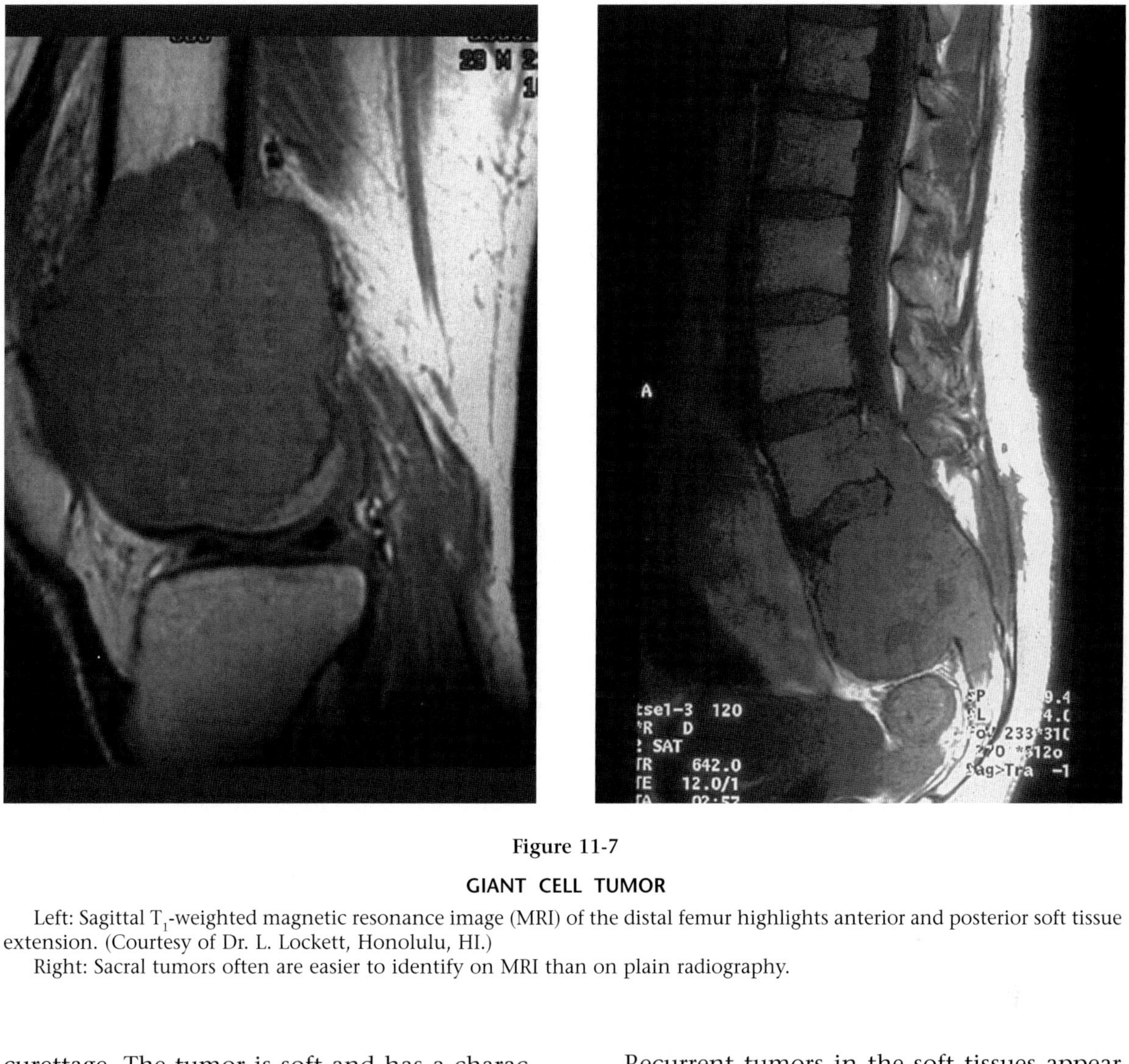

Figure 11-7

GIANT CELL TUMOR

Left: Sagittal T_1-weighted magnetic resonance image (MRI) of the distal femur highlights anterior and posterior soft tissue extension. (Courtesy of Dr. L. Lockett, Honolulu, HI.)

Right: Sacral tumors often are easier to identify on MRI than on plain radiography.

curettage. The tumor is soft and has a characteristic dark brown color (fig. 11-8). Areas of yellow discoloration are common (fig. 11-9).

In resected specimens, the tumor usually is situated eccentrically at the end of the bone. Large or small cystic areas may be seen (fig. 11-8, right). The cortex is usually thinned, and the lesion expands into the soft tissue (fig. 11-10). Although the lesion appears deceptively well circumscribed, small red pockets of tumor are frequently seen burrowing into the interstices of the cortex. Although typically dark brown, some giant cell tumors are white and fleshy, simulating a sarcoma (fig. 11-11). Tuli et al. (61) and Vistnes and Vermuelen (65) have documented the enormous sizes that neglected tumors can attain.

Recurrent tumors in the soft tissues appear as dark brown, well-circumscribed masses with a shell of reactive new bone (fig. 11-12).

Microscopic Findings. Giant cell tumors are composed of mononuclear cells and giant cells (fig. 11-13, top). The mononuclear cells have round or oval nuclei with uniformly distributed chromatin and indistinct nucleoli (fig. 11-13, bottom) (46). Mitotic figures are always present and may be abundant but never atypical (fig. 11-14). The cytoplasm is amphophilic to eosinophilic, and the borders are indistinct. The giant cells are distributed more or less uniformly and contain a variable number of nuclei, usually 40 to 60. The nuclear features are remarkably similar to those of mononuclear cells. It is often difficult to know where mononuclear cells stop

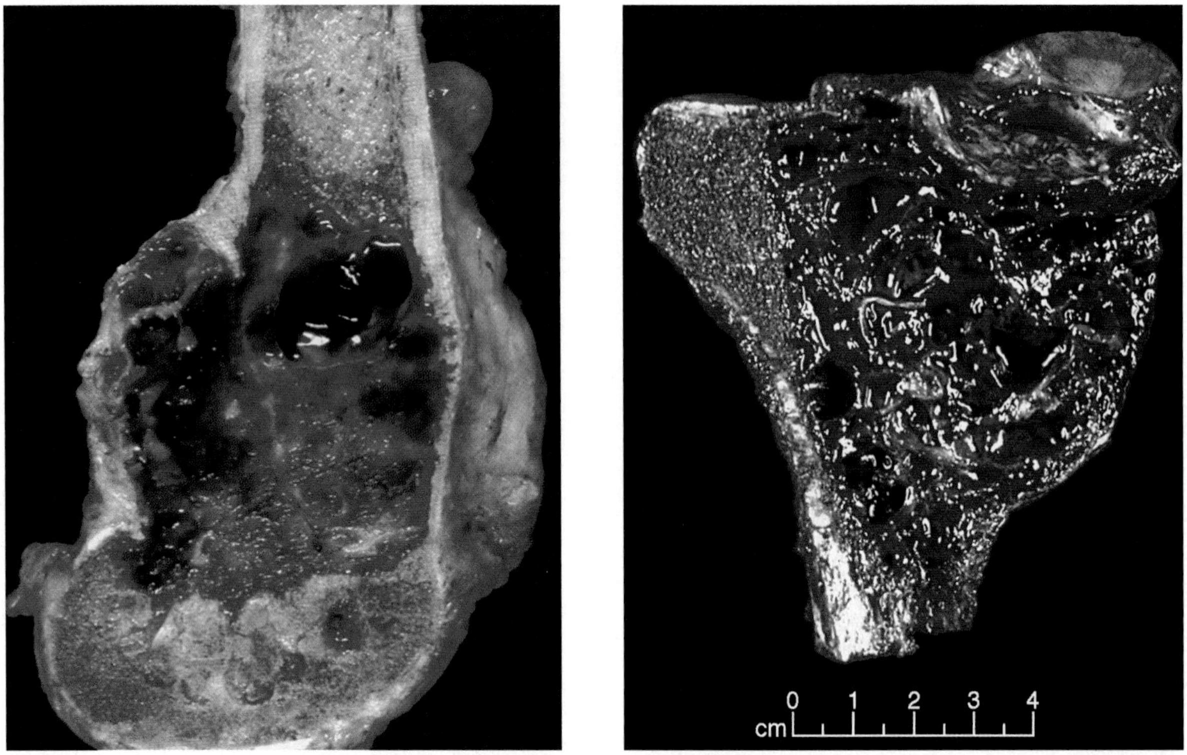

Figure 11-8

GIANT CELL TUMOR

Left: The lesion involving the entire distal femur has the typical dark brown appearance of a giant cell tumor. Focal cystic change and cortical destruction are also present.

Right: A giant cell tumor in the proximal tibia. The tumor is predominantly cystic because of a component of secondary aneurysmal bone cyst. (Fig. 19-14 from Unni KK. Dahlin's bone tumors: general aspects and data on 11,087 cases, 5th ed. Philadelphia: Lippincott-Raven; 1996:270. By permission of Mayo Foundation.)

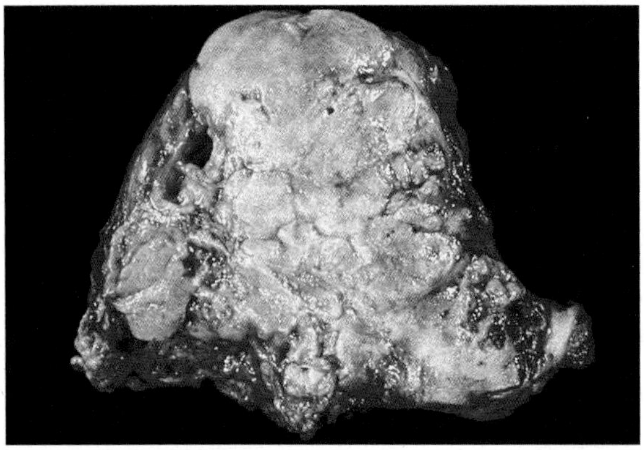

Figure 11-9

GIANT CELL TUMOR

The tumor involves the pubis and is predominately yellow-white, corresponding to degenerative changes, with numerous foam cells and fibrosis.

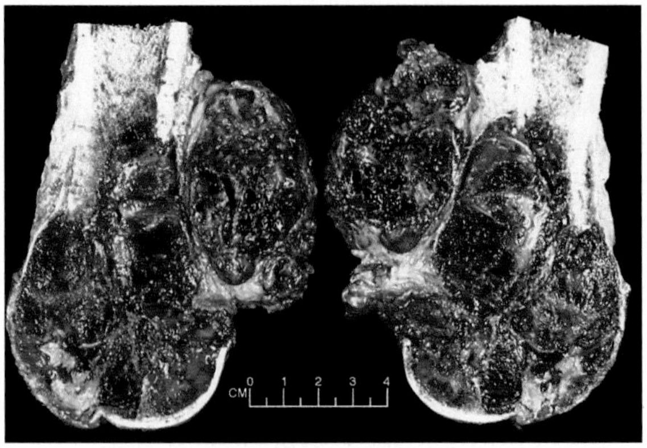

Figure 11-10

GIANT CELL TUMOR

A tan-brown tumor has destroyed the cortex and formed a large soft tissue mass. (Fig. 19-11 from Unni KK. Dahlin's bone tumors: general aspects and data on 11,087 cases, 5th ed. Philadelphia: Lippincott-Raven; 1996:269. By permission of Mayo Foundation.)

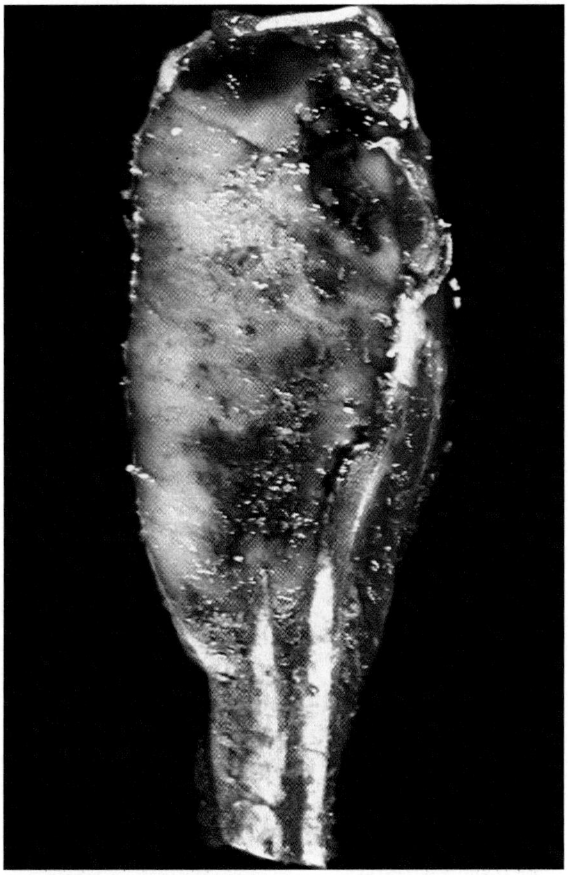

Figure 11-11

GIANT CELL TUMOR

Occasionally, giant cell tumors have a fleshy appearance and may simulate the appearance of a sarcoma.

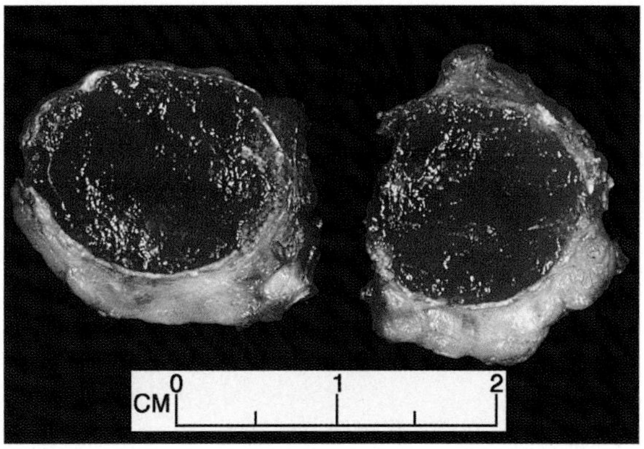

Figure 11-12

RECURRENT GIANT CELL TUMOR

The tumor involves soft tissue and forms a well-circumscribed mass with a thin, peripheral shell of ossification.

and giant cells begin. Mitotic figures are never found in giant cells. The mononuclear cells and giant cells are arranged in a compact fashion. Typically, there is no collagen formation.

The description above is that of a typical giant cell tumor; many variations are possible. Frequently, these variations are focal, associated with more typical areas.

The mononuclear cells may spindle and be arranged in a storiform pattern, suggesting a fibrohistiocytic tumor (fig. 11-15). These areas may contain only a few inconspicuous giant cells.

Clusters of foam cells are frequently present, and some giant cell tumors have a large number of these cells (fig. 11-16). The cytoplasm of neoplastic mononuclear cells may appear vacuolated, and the giant cells may have the appearance of Touton giant cells, as in some xanthomas.

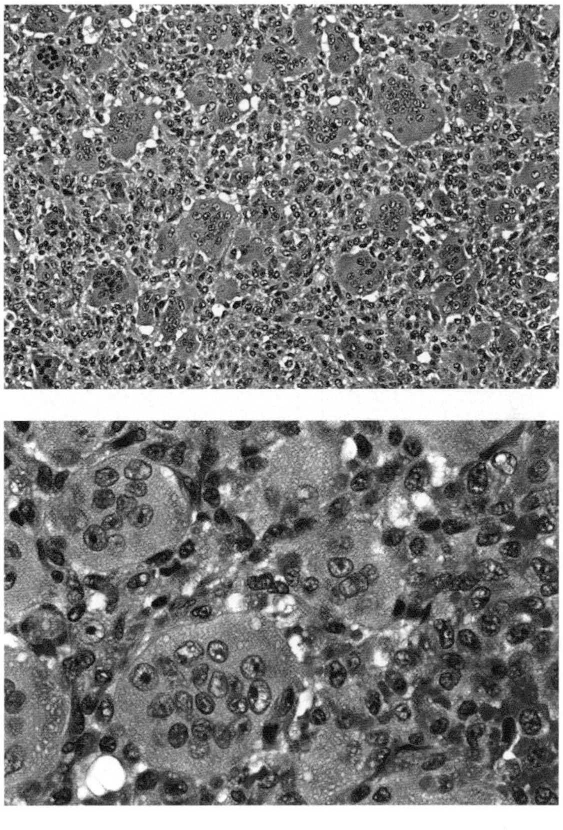

Figure 11-13

GIANT CELL TUMOR

Top: Numerous multinucleated giant cells are scattered uniformly throughout the tumor.

Bottom: The mononuclear cells between the multinucleated giant cells contain round to oval nuclei with small nucleoli. Eosinophilic cytoplasm surrounds the nuclei.

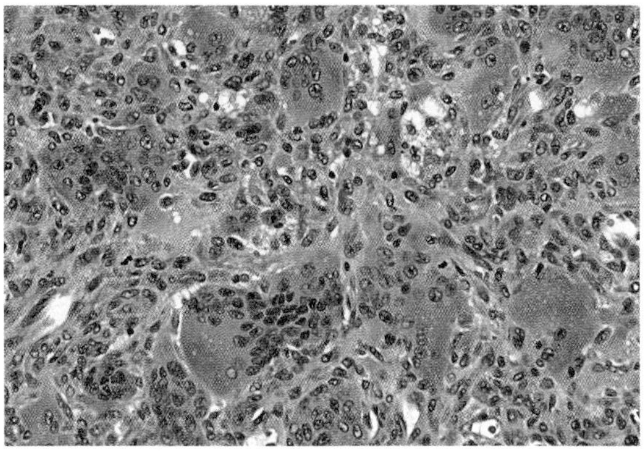

Figure 11-14

GIANT CELL TUMOR

Mitotic figures are easily identified in the tumor. However, atypical mitotic figures are not present.

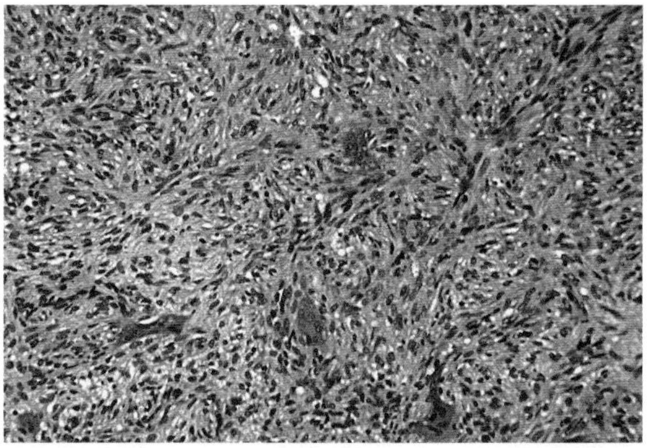

Figure 11-15

GIANT CELL TUMOR

Whorling fascicles of oval to spindle-shaped mononuclear cells create a fibrohistiocytic pattern.

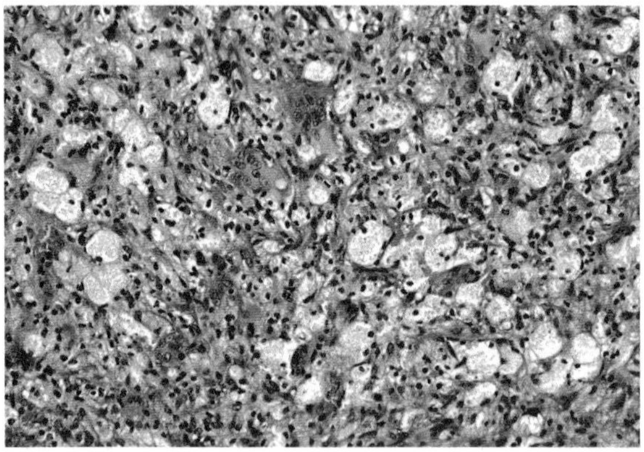

Figure 11-16

GIANT CELL TUMOR

Numerous foamy histiocytes are interspersed between the stromal cells and multinucleated giant cells.

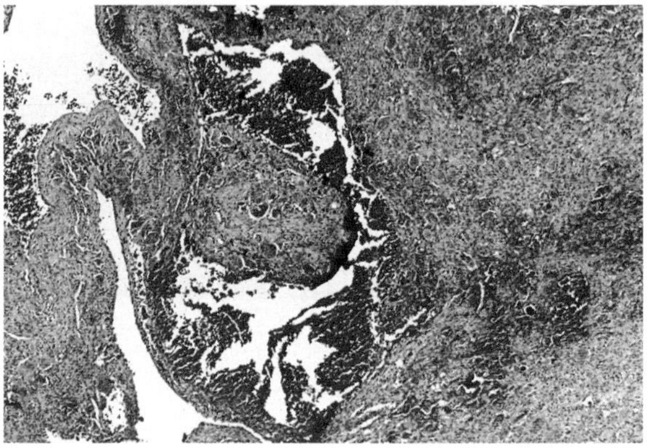

Figure 11-17

GIANT CELL TUMOR

Secondary aneurysmal bone cyst (left) merges with a typical giant cell tumor (right).

Secondary aneurysmal bone cysts are not uncommon. They may be present as microscopic cysts or the entire lesion may appear cystic, with only mural nodules of giant cell tumor (fig. 11-17).

Reactive bone formation may be focal or abundant. It usually is in the form of seams of osteoid, with prominent osteoblastic rimming (fig. 11-18). New bone formation is especially prominent in giant cell tumors of vertebrae (51).

Cartilage formation is uncommon. Microscopic nodules or hypocellular cartilage may be embedded within the tumor. Calcification in the stroma is also uncommon; when present it is usually coarse and "chunky."

The cytologic features of mononuclear cells vary. Some nuclei may be enlarged, irregular, and hyperchromatic (fig. 11-19) (32).

Areas of infarct-like necrosis are common (fig. 11-20). Ghost outlines of the mononuclear cells and giant cells persist, and there usually is no inflammatory response. Rarely, almost the entire tumor is infarcted.

Vascular invasion in the form of plugs of tumor in capillaries may be found in the soft tissues surrounding a giant cell tumor (fig. 11-21).

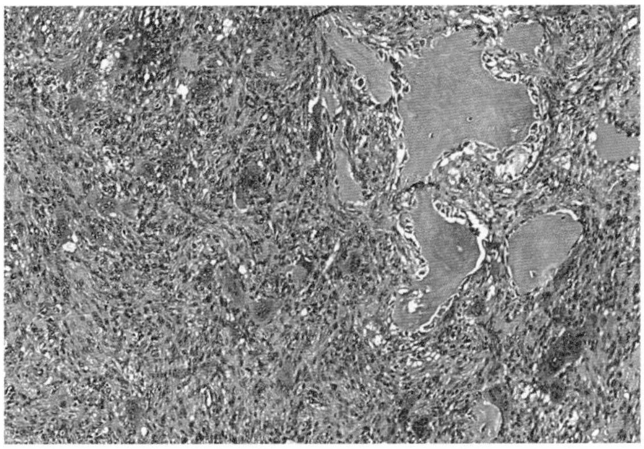

Figure 11-18

GIANT CELL TUMOR

There is focal reactive new bone formation with prominent osteoblastic rimming. The mononuclear stromal cells in giant cell tumors do not produce osteoid; thus, this reactive bone production is a secondary phenomenon.

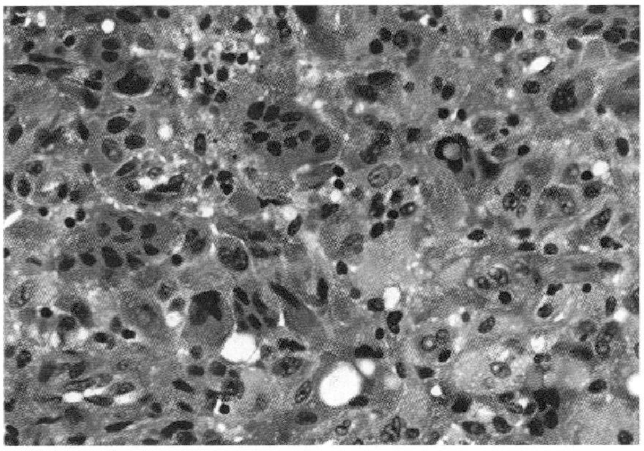

Figure 11-19

GIANT CELL TUMOR

The tumor contains several enlarged, irregularly shaped nuclei surrounded by abundant eosinophilic cytoplasm. Occasional intranuclear vacuoles are also present. These are features of degenerative atypia.

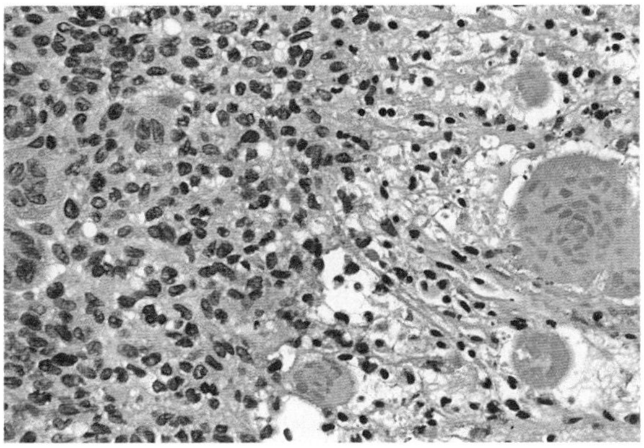

Figure 11-20

GIANT CELL TUMOR

Necrosis in the giant cell tumor results in multinucleated giant ghost cells (right) surrounded by karyolytic debris.

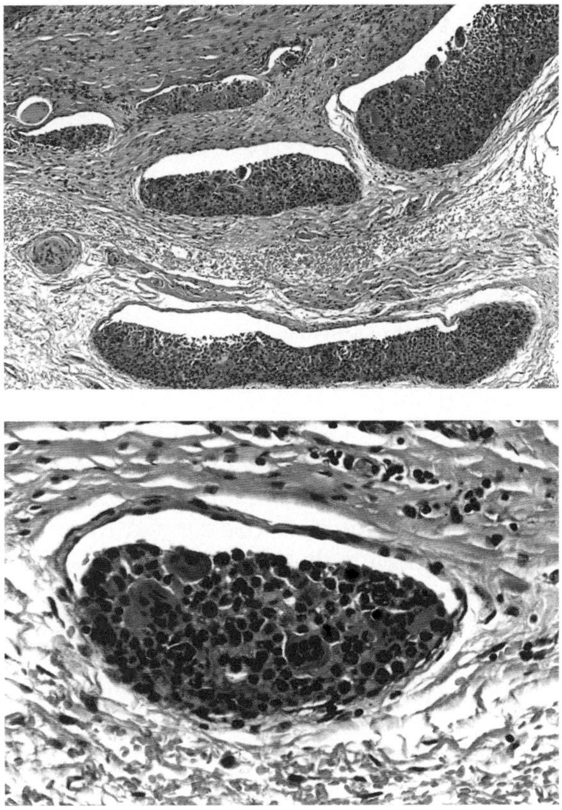

Figure 11-21

GIANT CELL TUMOR

Low- (top) and high-power (bottom) views of tumor filling the vascular channels within soft tissue at the periphery of a typical giant cell tumor.

It is not known how frequent this is or whether it correlates with pulmonary metastases.

Cytologic Findings. Giant cell tumor of bone typically yields very cellular aspirates that contain coherent cell clusters, often arranged around delicate vessels, as well as dispersed single cells. Two main cell types are recognized in variable proportions: large, multinucleated, benign-appearing osteoclasts and polygonal or short spindle cells with a single nucleus (58,64). The osteoclasts characteristically have abundant, densely staining cytoplasm that may be

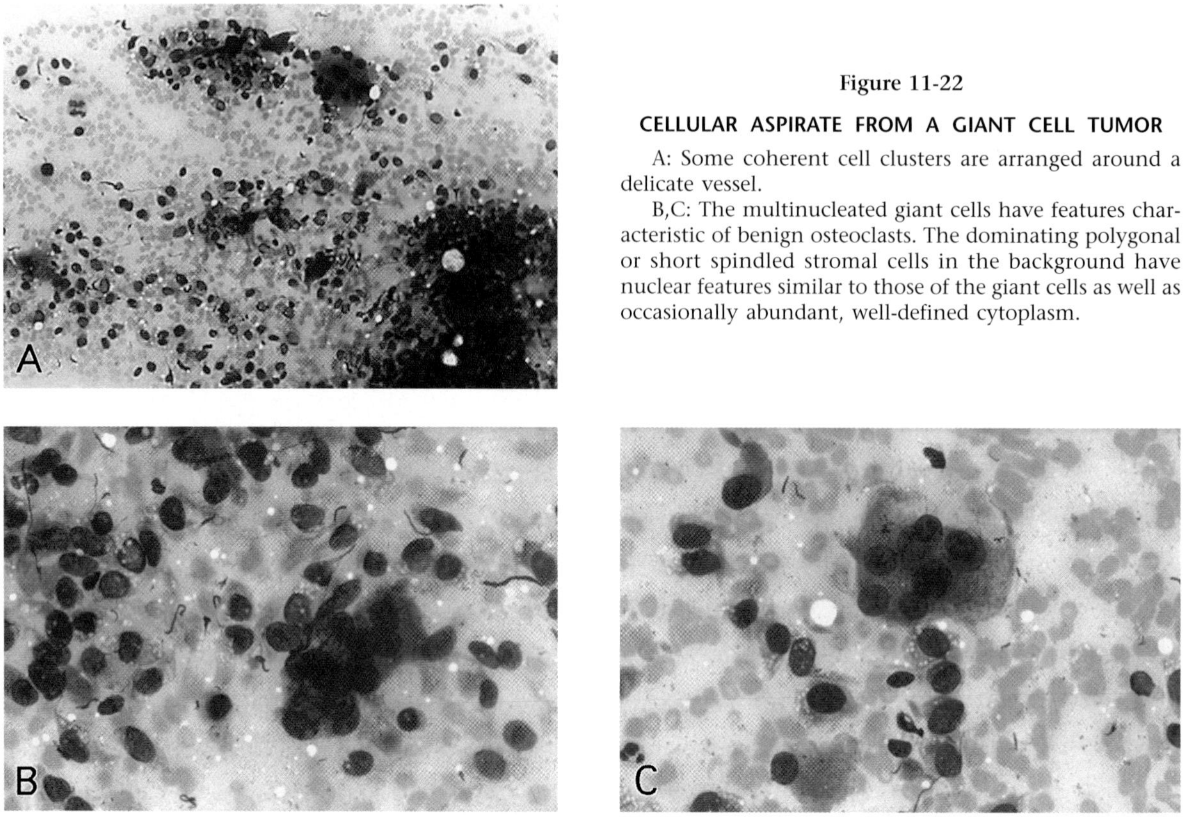

Figure 11-22

CELLULAR ASPIRATE FROM A GIANT CELL TUMOR

A: Some coherent cell clusters are arranged around a delicate vessel.

B,C: The multinucleated giant cells have features characteristic of benign osteoclasts. The dominating polygonal or short spindled stromal cells in the background have nuclear features similar to those of the giant cells as well as occasionally abundant, well-defined cytoplasm.

finely granular and rather large nuclei with coarse, dense chromatin and prominent nucleoli. The nuclei of mononuclear stromal cells are similar to those of multinucleated giant cells (fig. 11-22).

The fine-needle aspiration (FNA) diagnosis of giant cell tumor should never be based solely on the presence of numerous osteoclasts. Rather, it is the presence of the appropriate stromal cell background in the context of multinucleated giant cells and the clinical setting that should suggest the diagnosis. Giant cell tumors usually can be differentiated from several other giant cell–rich lesions such as osteoblastoma, chondroblastoma, and giant cell–rich osteosarcoma. However, its distinction from solid aneurysmal bone cyst, brown tumor of hyperparathyroidism, giant cell reparative granuloma, and giant cell reaction of bone may be impossible based on FNA findings alone.

Genetics and Other Special Techniques. Giant cell tumor of bone is characterized cytogenetically by the presence of an unusual phenomenon defined as "telomeric associations" (tas) (fig. 11-23) (7–9,53–55). Telomeric associations represent the end-to-end fusions of cytogenetically appearing "whole" or "intact" chromosomes. Normally capping the distal ends of linear chromosomes, telomeres are guanine-rich structures that contain variable quantities of a repeat TTAGGG sequence (38). Proximal to this simple repeat sequence is a complex assortment of telomere-associated repeats. Although some of these repeats appear to be unique in the genome, the majority are shared among several chromosomal termini. In situ hybridization studies have demonstrated a polymorphic distribution in the telomeric repeats in different persons (10).

The role of telomeric association in giant cell tumor and the molecular consequences of this phenomenon have not been fully elucidated. Telomeres have a protective function in the prevention of aberrant chromosomal recombination and exonucleolytic DNA degradation. Also, the maintenance of telomere integrity is fundamental in order for a cell to repeatedly undergo mitosis and for a neoplastic cell to propagate its transformed phenotype. A decrease in

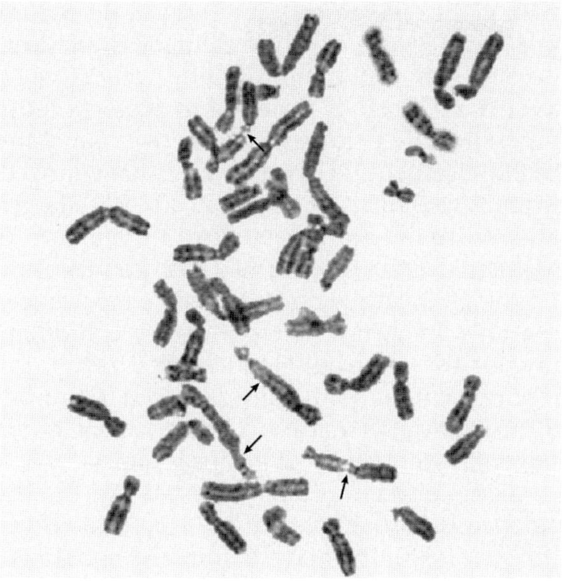

Figure 11-23

GIANT CELL TUMOR

Partial metaphase cell of a giant cell tumor demonstrates the following telomeric associations: tas(X;16)(q28;q24), tas(7;19)(q36;q13,4), and tas(13;17)(p13;q25)x2 (arrows).

telomere length (average loss of 500 bp), contributing to genetic instability, has been demonstrated in giant cell tumor when compared with leukocytes from the same patient (11). The telomeres most commonly affected include, in decreasing order of frequency, 19q, 11p, 15p, 21p, 20q, and 18p (9). Notably, other types of structural rearrangements are observed in giant cell tumor and appear predominantly to involve the short and long arms of chromosomes 11 and 19, respectively (35). These same chromosomal regions have also been described as aberrant in malignant giant cell tumor (7). Occasionally, a secondary aneurysmal bone cyst is documented in some giant cell tumors. Cytogenetic studies of these combined giant cell tumors and aneurysmal bone cyst lesions suggest that each component retains its own karyotypic baggage (aneurysmal bone cysts are characterized by rearrangements of 16q22 and 17p11-13 and giant cell tumor, by telomeric associations) (43,55).

Prognostic Markers and Other Genetic Markers. Histologic and radiographic grading and staging systems have been developed to predict the biologic behavior of giant cell tumors. However, these systems have limited prognostic value and have been abandoned by many clinicians. Various molecular markers have been examined recently to determine their value in predicting clinical behavior of giant cell tumors.

Investigation of the *c-myc* and *c-fos* proto-oncogenes in giant cell tumor has shown a strong correlation between the overexpression of c-myc mRNA and protein, and the occurrence of metastases in giant cell tumor, suggesting that the overexpression may serve as a powerful prognosticator in this tumor (21). The production of urokinase plasminogen activator (u-PA) in the tumor cells of giant cell tumor has been postulated to correlate with bone destruction and local tumor invasion, and amplification of the *u-PA* gene, its receptor (*u-PAR*), and its inhibitor (*PAI-1*) may be associated with a higher biological aggressiveness (22,67). In addition, overexpression of the hepatocyte growth factor receptor (a transmembrane tyrosine kinase encoded by the *met* proto-oncogene) may be associated with recurrent or locally aggressive giant cell tumors (19). Some investigators have suggested that an imbalance of matrix metalloproteinases and tissue inhibitors of metalloproteinases, substances that have essential roles in wound healing and neoplastic invasion and metastasis, may be of prognostic value in this neoplasm (47,48,52,62). In addition, the levels of vascular endothelial growth factor gene expression in giant cell tumors appear to correlate positively with advanced disease, and *p53* and *H-ras* mutations may correspond with malignant transformation (29,39,68). In contrast, it is unlikely that the D cyclins can be used to predict clinical behavior of giant cell tumor because overexpression of cyclins D1 and D3 is nearly universal in this neoplasm (27).

Giant cell tumors constitutively express all the signals that currently are understood to be necessary for the differentiation of osteoclasts from precursor cells (1,24,50). Osteoprotegerin ligand (OPGL), a factor essential for osteoclastogenesis, is involved in the tumor cell–induced osteoclast-like cell formation in giant cell tumor. The gene expression ratio of OPGL to its decoy receptor OPG in tumor cells contributes to the degree of osteoclastogenesis and bone resorption (1,24). Giant cell tumors also express several cytokines known to have a central role in osteoclastogenesis, namely interleukins 1, 6, 11, and 17 and tumor necrosis factor-alpha (TNF-α). Importantly, giant cell tumors of bone express high levels of macrophage colony-stimulating factor mRNA, a cytokine that is an essential cofactor of OPGL, and a survival factor for mature and developing osteoclasts (24).

Differential Diagnosis. Because nearly all bone lesions can have giant cells, the differential diagnosis of giant cell tumor involves many entities. However, only a few important ones are considered here.

Chondroblastoma. Both chondroblastoma and giant cell tumor involve the ends of long bones. In chondroblastoma, the epiphyseal plate is open, but it is closed in giant cell tumor. Typical pink cartilage and "chicken-wire" calcification are diagnostic of chondroblastoma. In chondroblastoma, the nuclei are cleaved, but they are round and regular in giant cell tumor.

Aneurysmal Bone Cyst. Aneurysmal bone cyst occurs in skeletally immature patients and is predominantly metaphyseal. The mononuclear cells are spindled and, most importantly, produce collagen. The loose granulation tissue appearance typical of aneurysmal bone cyst is not a feature of giant cell tumor in diagnostic areas.

Osteosarcoma with Giant Cells. This is discussed in chapter 5. Most osteosarcomas with giant cells occur in the metaphysis. Obvious anaplasia in the mononuclear cells rules out giant cell tumor.

Metaphyseal Fibrous Defect. Metaphyseal fibrous defects are metaphyseal (or rarely diaphyseal) and occur in children. The lesion is composed predominantly of spindle cells with a loose storiform pattern. Some metaphyseal fibrous defects contain a large number of giant cells and resemble giant cell tumor focally.

Brown Tumor of Hyperparathyroidism. It is rare to find large destructive tumors in patients with hyperparathyroidism. The tumors usually have an abundance of new bone formation and collagen. In the rare instance of a brown tumor at the end of a bone, the differential diagnosis can be difficult. Other radiographic features of hyperparathyroidism, such as subperiosteal bone resorption and biochemical abnormalities, are helpful in the diagnosis.

Treatment and Prognosis. Surgical management is the mainstay of treatment for patients with giant cell tumors. The surgical procedure selected depends on the extent of the lesion. Because giant cell tumors usually occur close to a joint, curettage is preferred to preserve joint function. The defect is filled with bone chips or bone cement. Recurrence rates have ranged from 25 to 50 percent (12,31,36,40). With larger and recurrent lesions, resection of the involved segment of bone is performed with good results. Histologic features do not predict recurrence; the only important criterion is the thoroughness of the removal. Good results have been reported with radiotherapy delivered to tumors difficult to treat surgically (13). No postradiation sarcomas were reported in this group.

Giant cell tumors rarely metastasize: the incidence is probably less than 3 percent. Until the year 2000, the Mayo Clinic files contained 19 cases of benign metastasizing giant cell tumor (of a total of 627). If they do metastasize, it usually is to the lungs, but other sites such as mediastinal lymph nodes have been affected (2,3,28,30,34,41,49,56,60). Neither histologic features nor ploidy status helps predict which tumors will metastasize (30,41). The prognosis is unpredictable, but about 25 percent of patients die with progressive disease (49). Wedge resection of the metastatic nodules is the treatment of choice. Some patients become long-term survivors even after inadequate treatment (56). Spontaneous regression of metastatic nodules has also been reported (3).

MALIGNANCY IN GIANT CELL TUMORS

Definition. Malignancy in giant cell tumor is a sarcoma arising in a giant cell tumor or at a site where a giant cell tumor has previously been documented.

General Features. The term *malignant giant cell tumor* is better established than *malignancy in giant cell tumor* but has led to confusion in the literature. Many kinds of sarcomas, especially osteosarcoma and malignant fibrous histiocytoma with a component of giant cells, have been mistaken for sarcoma arising in giant cell tumor. The term *malignant giant cell tumor* is used in this chapter for convenience. The sarcoma arising within a giant cell tumor has been termed *primary malignant giant cell tumor* and that arising at the site of a previously diagnosed giant cell tumor has been termed *secondary*

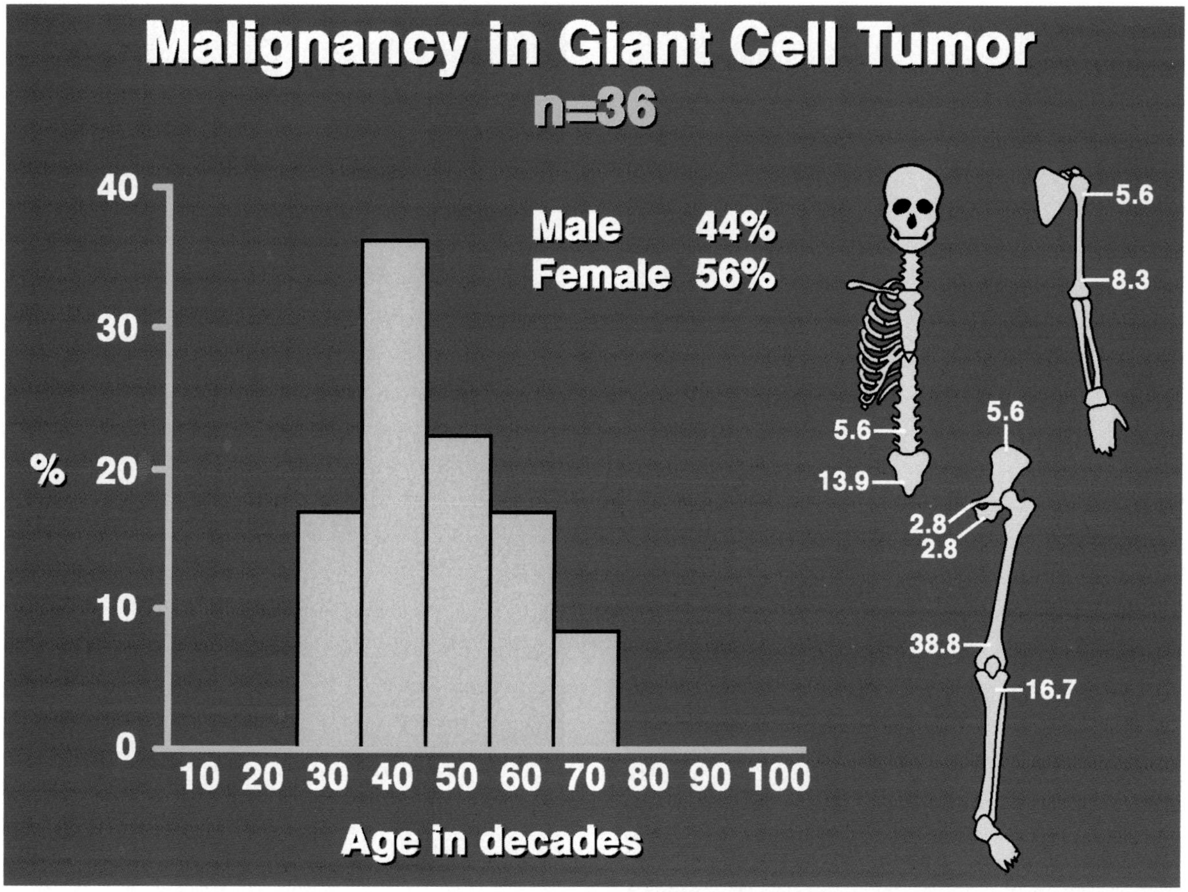

Figure 11-24

MALIGNANCY IN GIANT CELL TUMOR

Distribution of malignancy in giant cell tumor according to the age and sex of the patient and the site of the lesion.

malignant giant cell tumor (72). The term *dedifferentiated giant cell tumor* has also been used for primary malignant giant cell tumor (70).

Until the year 2000, the Mayo Clinic files contained 36 examples of malignant giant cell tumor (fig. 11-24). During the same period, the files contained 627 examples of giant cell tumor. Thirty-one cases were considered secondary and only 5 were considered primary. Of the 31 patients with secondary malignant giant cell tumor, 25 had received radiotherapy as part of the treatment of the original giant cell tumor.

Clinical Features. Patients with malignant giant cell tumor are about a decade older than those with giant cell tumor. There is a slight female predominance. The recurrence of symptoms after a long delay following treatment of a giant cell tumor should arouse suspicion of malignant change because most giant cell tumors recur within 2 years after treatment.

Sites. Malignant giant cell tumors occur at the sites of preference for giant cell tumors, that is, at the ends of long bones. Tumors in the region of the knee, including the distal femur and the proximal tibia, account for more than half of all cases. Sarcomatous change in a soft tissue recurrence has been described (69).

Radiographic Findings. Radiographs show a lesion in an epiphyseal location. A primary malignant giant cell tumor may appear remarkably similar to a giant cell tumor (fig. 11-25). Occasionally, destructive areas with mineralization are juxtaposed to a typical giant cell tumor, suggesting the possibility of a malignancy. Secondary malignant giant cell tumors have features of malignancy with destructive

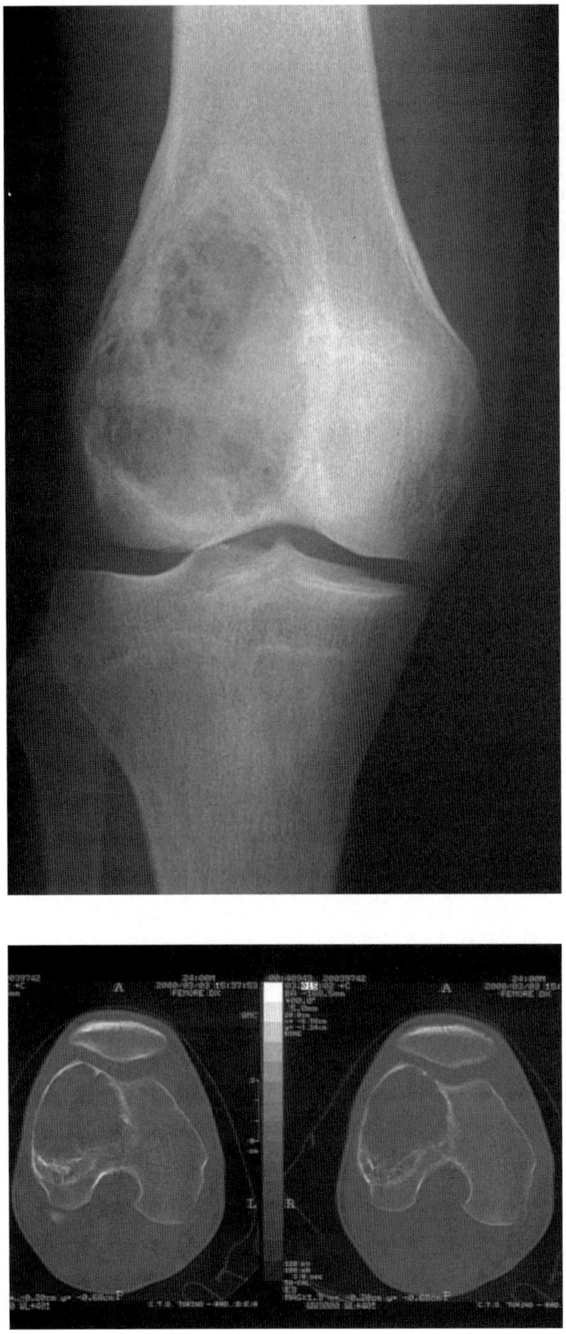

Figure 11-25

MALIGNANCY IN GIANT CELL TUMOR

Primary malignant giant cell tumor in a 24-year-old man. Anteroposterior radiograph (top) and CT (bottom) show an eccentric lytic lesion that is within the lateral femoral condyle and is confined to bone. These features suggest a benign process. Histologically, the tissue contained areas of classic giant cell tumor in addition to conventional high-grade osteosarcoma. (Courtesy of Dr. F. Bertoni, Bologna, Italy.)

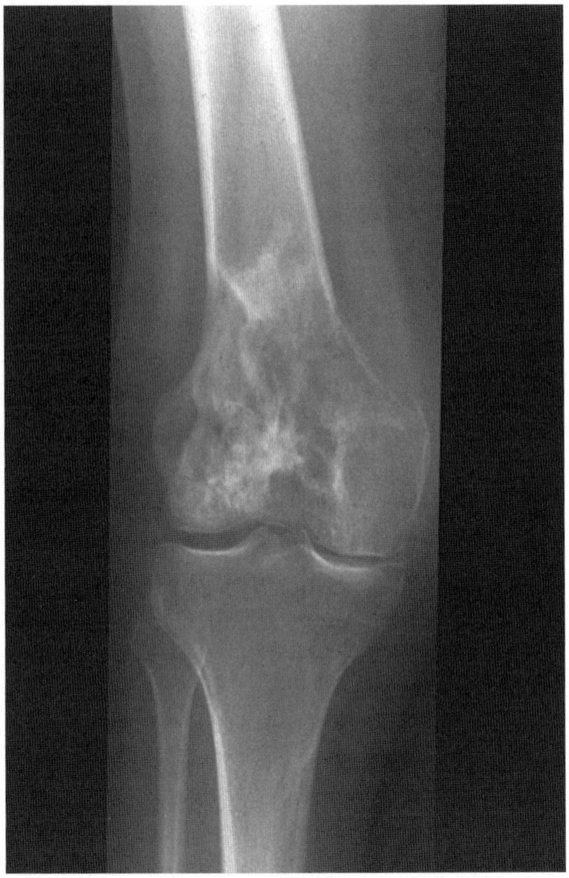

Figure 11-26

MALIGNANCY IN GIANT CELL TUMOR

Secondary malignant giant cell tumor in a 34-year-old woman. Anteroposterior radiograph shows a destructive lesion involving the distal femur. The resected tumor was a grade 4 fibrosarcoma. Fourteen years earlier, a benign giant cell tumor at this site was treated with surgery and irradiation.

changes (fig. 11-26). Calcification from previous radiation may be visible.

Gross Findings. Primary malignant giant cell tumors have the gross appearance typical of a giant cell tumor. Secondary malignant giant cell tumors have the fleshy appearance common to sarcomas (fig. 11-27).

Microscopic Findings. Primary malignant giant cell tumors have areas of typical giant cell tumor with benign-appearing mononuclear cells and more or less uniformly distributed giant cells (fig. 11-28). Juxtaposed to these areas are malignant-appearing spindle cells, with or without matrix formation. Secondary malignant giant cell tumors do not contain areas of

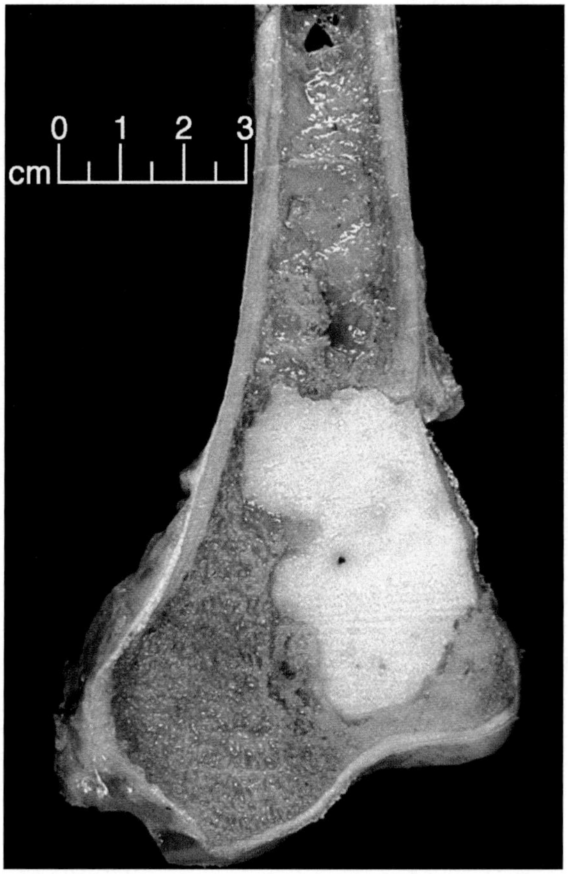

Figure 11-27

MALIGNANCY IN GIANT CELL TUMOR

Secondary malignant giant cell tumor in the distal femur of a 25-year-old woman. A giant cell tumor was removed from this location by curettage 5 years earlier. The patient did not receive radiotherapy. The recurrent gray fleshy tumor surrounding the cement was a high-grade fibroblastic osteosarcoma. (Courtesy of Dr. J. Stroh, San Pedro, CA.)

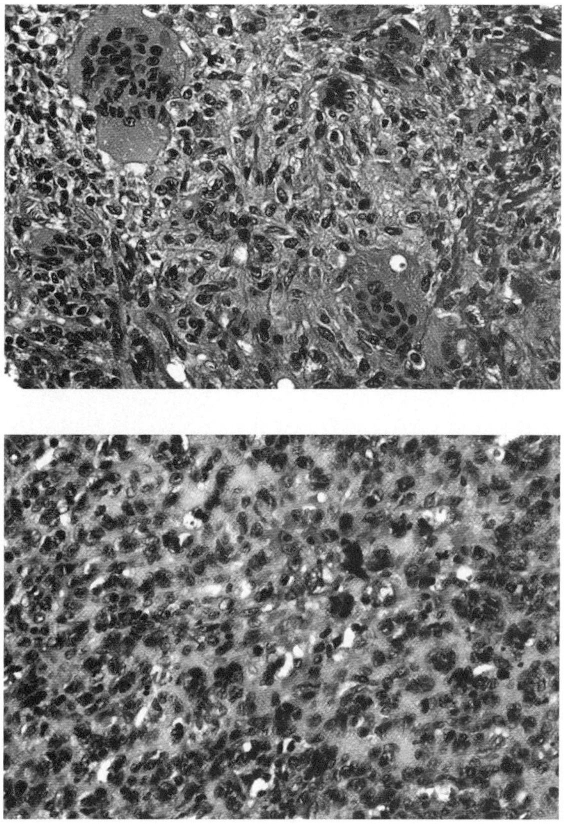

Figure 11-28

MALIGNANCY IN GIANT CELL TUMOR

Primary malignant giant cell tumor in the proximal tibia of a 44-year-old man.

Top: This area within the tumor has the histologic features of a benign giant cell tumor.

Bottom: In other parts of the same tumor, however, the mononuclear stromal cells had marked cytologic atypia indicative of sarcoma.

typical giant cell tumor. Rather, they consist of high-grade spindle cell sarcoma throughout (fig. 11-29). The correct diagnosis is possible only from the history.

Differential Diagnosis. The diagnosis of primary malignant giant cell tumor can be extremely difficult. Some giant cell tumors have pleomorphic nuclei and spindle cells toward the periphery. It is easy to mistake these tumors for malignant giant cell tumor.

Treatment and Diagnosis. Most patients whose cases have been reported have been treated surgically. The experience with neoadjuvant chemotherapy is not sufficient to make any informed remarks. An overall survival rate of 30 percent has been reported for patients with secondary malignant giant cell tumor (72). One report has suggested that patients with primary malignant giant cell tumor have an excellent prognosis (71).

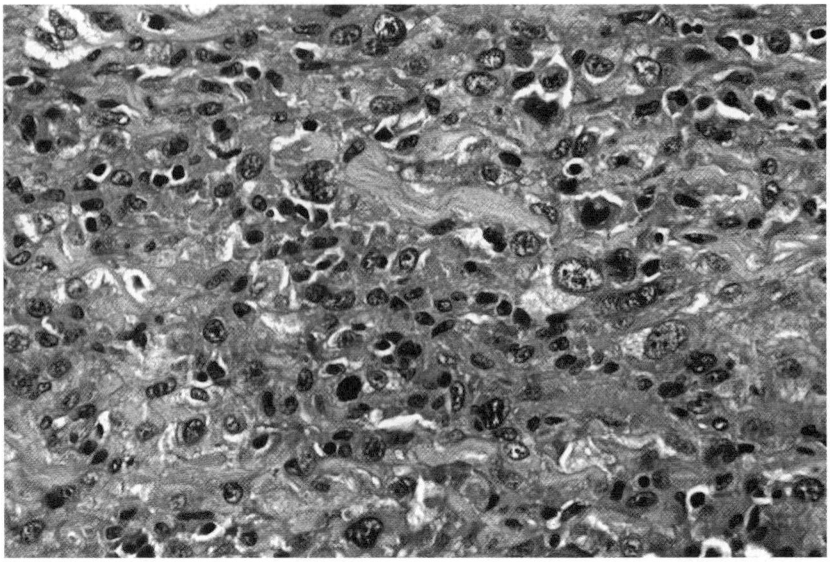

Figure 11-29

MALIGNANCY IN GIANT CELL TUMOR

Secondary malignant giant cell tumor. Pleomorphic spindle cell sarcoma occurs at the site of a benign giant cell tumor that had been treated 15 years previously with irradiation and surgery.

REFERENCES

Giant Cell Tumor

1. Atkins GJ, Haynes DR, Graves SE, et al. Expression of osteoclast differentiation signals by stromal elements of giant cell tumors. J Bone Miner Res 2000;15:640–9.
2. Bertoni F, Present D, Enneking WF. Giant-cell tumor of bone with pulmonary metastases. J Bone Joint Surg Am 1985;67:890–900.
3. Bertoni F, Present D, Sudanese A, Baldini N, Bacchini P, Campanacci M. Giant-cell tumor of bone with pulmonary metastases. Six case reports and a review of the literature. Clin Orthop 1988;237:275–85.
4. Bertoni F, Unni KK, Beabout JW, Ebersold MJ. Giant cell tumor of the skull. Cancer 1992;70:1124–32.
5. Biscaglia R, Bacchini P, Bertoni F. Giant cell tumor of the bones of the hand and foot. Cancer 2000;88:2022–32.
6. Brecher ME, Franklin WA, Simon MA. Immunohistochemical study of mononuclear phagocyte antigens in giant cell tumor of bone. Am J Pathol 1986;125:252–7.
7. Bridge JA, Mouron BJ, Neff JR, Bhatia PS. Significance of chromosomal abnormalities in a malignant giant cell tumor of bone. Cancer Genet Cytogenet 1991;57:87–92.
8. Bridge JA, Neff JR, Bhatia PS, Sanger WG, Murphey MD. Cytogenetic findings and biologic behavior of giant cell tumors of bone. Cancer 1990;65:2697–703.
9. Bridge JA, Neff JR, Mouron BJ. Giant cell tumor of bone. Chromosomal analysis of 48 specimens and review of the literature. Cancer Genet Cytogenet 1992;58:2–13.
10. Brown WR, MacKinnon PJ, Villasante A, Spurr N, Buckle VJ, Dobson MJ. Structure and polymorphism of human telomere-associated DNA. Cell 1990;63:119–32.
11. Butler MG, Sciadini M, Hedges LK, Schwartz HS. Chromosome telomere integrity of human solid neoplasms. Cancer Genet Cytogenet 1996;86:50–3.
12. Campanacci M, Baldini N, Boriani S, Sudanese A. Giant-cell tumor of bone. J Bone Joint Surg Am 1987;69:106–14.
13. Chakravarti A, Spiro IJ, Hug EB, Mankin HJ, Efird JT, Suit HD. Megavoltage radiation therapy for axial and inoperable giant-cell tumor of bone. J Bone Joint Surg Am 1999;81:1566–73.
14. Cooper KL, Beabout JW, Dahlin DC. Giant cell tumor: ossification in soft-tissue implants. Radiology 1984;153:597–602.
15. Cummins CA, Scarborough MT, Enneking WF. Multicentric giant cell tumor of bone. Clin Orthop 1996;322:245–52.
16. Dahlin DC. Caldwell Lecture. Giant cell tumor of bone: highlights of 407 cases. AJR Am J Roentgenol 1985;144:955–60.
17. Fain JS, Unni KK, Beabout JW, Rock MG. Nonepiphyseal giant cell tumor of the long bones. Clinical, radiologic, and pathologic study. Cancer 1993;71:3514–9.

18. Fechner RE, Mills SE. Tumors of the bones and joints. Atlas of Tumor Pathology, 3rd Series, Fascicle 8. Washington, DC: Armed Forces Institute of Pathology; 1993:173–81.
19. Ferracini R, Scotlandi K, Cagliero E, et al. The expression of Met/hepatocyte growth factor receptor gene in giant cell tumors of bone and other benign musculoskeletal tumors. J Cell Physiol 2000;184:191–6.
20. Fornasier VL, Protzner K, Zhang I, Mason L. The prognostic significance of histomorphometry and immunohistochemistry in giant cell tumors of bone. Hum Pathol 1996;27:754–60.
21. Gamberi G, Benassi MS, Bohling T, et al. Prognostic relevance of C-myc gene expression in giant-cell tumor of bone. J Orthop Res 1998;16:1–7.
22. Gamberi G, Benassi MS, Ragazzini P, et al. Proteases and interleukin-6 gene analysis in 92 giant cell tumors of bone. Ann Oncol 2004;15:498–503.
23. Gebhart M, Vandeweyer E, Nemec E. Paget's disease of bone complicated by giant cell tumor. Clin Orthop 1998;352:187–93.
24. Huang L, Xu J, Wood DJ, Zheng MH. Gene expression of osteoprotegerin ligand, osteoprotegerin, and receptor activator of NF-kappaB in giant cell tumor of bone: possible involvement in tumor cell-induced osteoclast-like cell formation. Am J Pathol 2000;156:761–7.
25. Huang TS, Green AD, Beattie CW, Das Gupta TK. Monocyte-macrophage lineage of giant cell tumor of bone. Establishment of a multinucleated cell line. Cancer 1993;71:1751–60.
26. Jacobs TP, Michelsen J, Polay JS, D'Adamo AC, Canfield RE. Giant cell tumor in Paget's disease of bone: familial and geographic clustering. Cancer 1979;44:742–7.
27. Kauzman A, Li SQ, Bradley G, Bell RS, Wunder JS, Kandel R. Cyclin alterations in giant cell tumor of bone. Mod Pathol 2003;16:210–8.
28. Kay RM, Eckardt JJ, Seeger LL, Mirra JM, Hak DJ. Pulmonary metastasis of benign giant cell tumor of bone. Six histologically confirmed cases, including one of spontaneous regression. Clin Orthop 1994;302:219–30.
29. Kumta SM, Huang L, Cheng YY, Chow LT, Lee KM, Zheng MH. Expression of VEGF and MMP-9 in giant cell tumor of bone and other osteolytic lesions. Life Sci 2003;73:1427–36.
30. Ladanyi M, Traganos F, Huvos AG. Benign metastasizing giant cell tumors of bone. A DNA flow cytometric study. Cancer 1989;64:1521–6.
31. Lausten GS, Jensen PK, Schiodt T, Lund B. Local recurrences in giant cell tumour of bone. Long-term follow up of 31 cases. Int Orthop 1996;20:172–6.
32. Layfield LJ, Bentley RC, Mirra JM. Pseudoanaplastic giant cell tumor of bone. Arch Pathol Lab Med 1999;123:163–6.
33. Lee FY, Montgomery M, Hazan EJ, Keel SB, Mankin HJ, Kattapuram S. Recurrent giant-cell tumor presenting as a soft-tissue mass. A report of four cases. J Bone Joint Surg Am 1999;81:703–7.
34. Lewis JJ, Healey JH, Huvos AG, Burt M. Benign giant-cell tumor of bone with metastasis to mediastinal lymph nodes. A case report of resection facilitated with use of steroids. J Bone Joint Surg Am 1996;78:106–10.
35. McComb EN, Johansson SL, Neff JR, Nelson M, Bridge JA. Chromosomal anomalies exclusive of telomeric associations in giant cell tumor of bone. Cancer Genet Cytogenet 1996;88:163–6.
36. McDonald DJ, Sim FH, McLeod RA, Dahlin DC. Giant-cell tumor of bone. J Bone Joint Surg Am 1986;68:235–42.
37. Medeiros LJ, Beckstead JH, Rosenberg AE, Warnke RA, Wood GS. Giant cells and mononuclear cells of giant cell tumor of bone resemble histiocytes. Appl Immunohistochem 1993;1:115–22.
38. Moyzis RK, Buckingham JM, Cram LS, et al. A highly conserved repetitive DNA sequence, (TTAGGG)n, present at the telomeres of human chromosomes. Proc Natl Acad Sci U S A 1988;85:6622–6.
39. Oda Y, Sakamoto A, Saito T, et al. Secondary malignant giant-cell tumour of bone: molecular abnormalities of p53 and H-ras gene correlated with malignant transformation. Histopathology 2001;39:629–37.
40. O'Donnell RJ, Springfield DS, Motwani HK, Ready JE, Gebhardt MC, Mankin HJ. Recurrence of giant-cell tumors of the long bones after curettage and packing with cement. J Bone Joint Surg Am 1994;76:1827–33.
41. Osaka S, Toriyama M, Taira K, Sano S, Saotome K. Analysis of giant cell tumor of bone with pulmonary metastases. Clin Orthop 1997;335:253–61.
42. Peimer CA, Schiller AL, Mankin HJ, Smith RJ. Multicentric giant-cell tumor of bone. J Bone Joint Surg Am 1980;62:652–6.
43. Pfeifer FM, Bridge JA, Neff JR, Mouron BJ. Cytogenetic findings in aneurysmal bone cysts. Genes Chromosomes Cancer 1991;3:416–9.
44. Potter GD, McClennan BL. Malignant giant cell tumor of the sphenoid bone and its differential diagnosis. Cancer 1970;25:167–70.
45. Potter HG, Schneider R, Ghelman B, Healey JH, Lane JM. Multiple giant cell tumors and Paget disease of bone: radiographic and clinical correlations. Radiology 1991;180:261–4.

46. Present D, Bertoni F, Hudson T, Enneking WF. The correlation between the radiologic staging studies and histopathologic findings in aggressive stage 3 giant cell tumor of bone. Cancer 1986;57:237–44.
47. Rao VH, Singh RK, Delimont DC, et al. Interleukin-1beta upregulates MMP-9 expression in stromal cells of human giant cell tumor of bone. J Interferon Cytokine Res 1999;19:1207–17.
48. Rao VH, Singh RK, Delimont DC, et al. Transcriptional regulation of MMP-9 expression in stromal cells of human giant cell tumor of bone by tumor necrosis factor-alpha. Int J Oncol 1999;14: 291–300.
49. Rock MG, Pritchard DJ, Unni KK. Metastases from histologically benign giant-cell tumor of bone. J Bone Joint Surg Am 1984;66:269–74.
50. Roux S, Amazit L, Meduri G, Guiochon-Mantel A, Milgrom E, Mariette X. RANK (receptor activator of nuclear kappa B) and RANK ligand are expressed in giant cell tumors of bone. Am J Clin Pathol 2002;117:210–6.
51. Sanjay BK, Sim FH, Unni KK, McLeod RA, Klassen RA. Giant-cell tumours of the spine. J Bone Joint Surg Br 1993;75:148–54.
52. Schoedel KE, Greco MA, Stetler-Stevenson WG, et al. Expression of metalloproteinases and tissue inhibitors of metalloproteinases in giant cell tumor of bone: an immunohistochemical study with clinical correlation. Hum Pathol 1996;27:1144–8.
53. Schwartz HS, Butler MG, Jenkins RB, Miller DA, Moses HL. Telomeric associations and consistent growth factor overexpression detected in giant cell tumor of bone. Cancer Genet Cytogenet 1991;56:263–76.
54. Schwartz HS, Jenkins RB, Dahl RJ, Dewald GW. Cytogenetic analyses on giant-cell tumors of bone. Clin Orthop 1989;240:250–60.
55. Sciot R, Dorfman H, Brys P, et al. Cytogenetic-morphologic correlations in aneurysmal bone cyst, giant cell tumor of bone and combined lesions. A report from the CHAMP study group. Mod Pathol 2000;13:1206–10.
56. Siebenrock KA, Unni KK, Rock MG. Giant-cell tumour of bone metastasising to the lungs. A long-term follow-up. J Bone Joint Surg Br 1998;80:43–7.
57. Sim FH, Dahlin DC, Beabout JW. Multicentric giant-cell tumor of bone. J Bone Joint Surg Am 1977;59:1052–60.
58. Sneige N, Ayala AG, Carrasco CH, Murray J, Raymond AK. Giant cell tumor of bone. A cytologic study of 24 cases. Diagn Cytopathol 1985;1:111–7.
59. Sung HW, Kuo DP, Shu WP, Chai YB, Liu CC, Li SM. Giant-cell tumor of bone: analysis of two hundred and eight cases in Chinese patients. J Bone Joint Surg Am 1982;64:755–61.
60. Tubbs WS, Brown LR, Beabout JW, Rock MG, Unni KK. Benign giant-cell tumor of bone with pulmonary metastases: clinical findings and radiologic appearance of metastases in 13 cases. AJR Am J Roentgenol 1992;158:331–4.
61. Tuli SM, Varma BP, Srivastava TP. Giant-cell tumour of bone. A study of natural course. Int Orthop (SICOT) 1978;2:207–14.
62. Ueda Y, Imai K, Tsuchiya H, et al. Matrix metalloproteinase 9 (gelatinase B) is expressed in multinucleated giant cells of human giant cell tumor of bone and is associated with vascular invasion. Am J Pathol 1996;148:611–22.
63. Upchurch KS, Simon LS, Schiller AL, Rosenthal DI, Campion EW, Krane SM. Giant cell reparative granuloma of Paget's disease of bone: a unique clinical entity. Ann Intern Med 1983;98:35–40.
64. Vetrani A, Fulciniti F, Boschi R, et al. Fine needle aspiration biopsy diagnosis of giant-cell tumor of bone. An experience with nine cases. Acta Cytol 1990;34:863–7.
65. Vistnes LM, Vermuelen WJ. The natural history of a giant-cell tumor. Case report. J Bone Joint Surg Am 1975;57:865–7.
66. Wold LE, Swee RG. Giant cell tumor of the small bones of the hands and feet. Semin Diagn Pathol 1984;1:173–84.
67. Zheng MH, Fan Y, Panicker A, et al. Detection of mRNAs for urokinase-type plasminogen activator, its receptor, and type 1 inhibitor in giant cell tumors of bone with in situ hybridization. Am J Pathol 1995;147:1559–66.
68. Zheng MH, Xu J, Robbins P, et al. Gene expression of vascular endothelial growth factor in giant cell tumors of bone. Hum Pathol 2000;31:804–12.

Malignancy of Giant Cell Tumors

69. Hefti FL, Gachter A, Remagen W, Nidecker A. Recurrent giant-cell tumor with metaplasia and malignant change, not associated with radiotherapy. A case report. J Bone Joint Surg Am 1992;74:930–4.
70. Meis JM, Dorfman HD, Nathanson SD, Haggar AM, Wu KK. Primary malignant giant cell tumor of bone: "dedifferentiated" giant cell tumor. Mod Pathol 1989;2:541–6.
71. Nascimento AG, Huvos AG, Marcove RC. Primary malignant giant cell tumor of bone: a study of eight cases and review of the literature. Cancer 1979;44:1393–402.
72. Rock MG, Sim FH, Unni KK, et al. Secondary malignant giant-cell tumor of bone. Clinicopathological assessment of nineteen patients. J Bone Joint Surg Am 1986;68:1073–9.

12 ADAMANTINOMA OF LONG BONES

ADAMANTINOMA

Definition. Adamantinoma is a low-grade neoplasm with epithelial differentiation and a striking predilection to involve the tibia.

General Features. The term *adamantinoma* is used because the tumor resembles the better known adamantinoma (ameloblastoma) of the jawbones. Electron microscopic and immunohistochemical studies have demonstrated an epithelial phenotype for the tumor (1,11,12,16,22). Although some histologic features have suggested an endothelial origin (15), the bimorphic pattern and the cytology of the spindle cells are strikingly similar to those of synovial sarcoma. The unusual tendency to involve the cortex of the tibia and, less frequently, the fibula is puzzling.

Baker et al. (3) and Cohen et al. (7) pointed out the association of fibrous dysplasia-like areas in adamantinoma. Some studies have demonstrated a zonal phenomenon, with a fibrous dysplasia-like area in the periphery and epithelial cells in the center of the lesion (7,12). More recently, it has been suggested that the fibro-osseous portion is similar to osteofibrous dysplasia (2,4,23). The radiographic features and the preferential involvement of the tibia also suggest some relationship between osteofibrous dysplasia and adamantinoma. On the basis of a study of the basement membrane material around the epithelial cells, Hazelbag et al. (13) suggested the transformation of fibrous tissue to epithelial cells and, as a corollary, suggested that the development of epithelial cells was a form of tumor progression in osteofibrous dysplasia. Two large studies (21,25) found keratin-positive cells in osteofibrous dysplasia but not fibrous dysplasia. However, neither study included an example of adamantinoma developing in osteofibrous dysplasia. Hazelbag et al. (12) have described two cases originally interpreted as osteofibrous dysplasia recurring as adamantinoma.

Czerniak et al. (8) studied 25 cases of adamantinoma and proposed dividing them into two groups: classic and differentiated. The classic group had all the features of osteofibrous dysplasia except for the presence of rare epithelial cells. They thought that some, if not all, examples of osteofibrous dysplasia began as adamantinoma and regressed, with the fibro-osseous process being reparative. Ishida et al. (16) supported this concept and reported that keratin-positive cells occurred singly in osteofibrous dysplasia and in clusters in osteofibrous dysplasia-like adamantinoma.

Adamantinoma is one of the rarest of bone tumors, accounting for less than 1 percent of malignant primary bone tumors reported in the Mayo Clinic files. At the beginning of 2000, these files included 40 examples of adamantinoma (fig. 12-1).

Clinical Features. Most patients are adolescents and young adults. In a review of the literature, Moon and Mori (20) reported the average age of the patients was 32.9 years (range, 4 to 74 years). There is a slight female predominance. Patients present with swelling, with or without pain. The symptoms are usually of long duration, ranging up to 50 years. More than 10 percent of patients have had symptoms for more than a decade (26) and 33 percent have had symptoms for more than 5 years (18).

Sites. The tibia is involved almost exclusively. In the cases in the Mayo Clinic files, 34 of 40 lesions involved the tibia. In two cases, the ipsilateral fibula was also involved. In the large review of Moon and Mori (20), 84.5 percent of all tumors involved the tibia. Practically all bones have been reported to be involved, including small tubular bones (20). Some tumors reported in sites other than the tibia and fibula have had unusual histologic features (16) and may not represent the same neoplasm. Similar neoplasms have been reported in pretibial soft tissues (18,19).

Radiographic Findings. The typical radiographic appearance is that of multiple, sharply circumscribed, lucent zones within the cortex of the mid-portion of the tibia (fig. 12-2). The lucencies are of different size and are surrounded

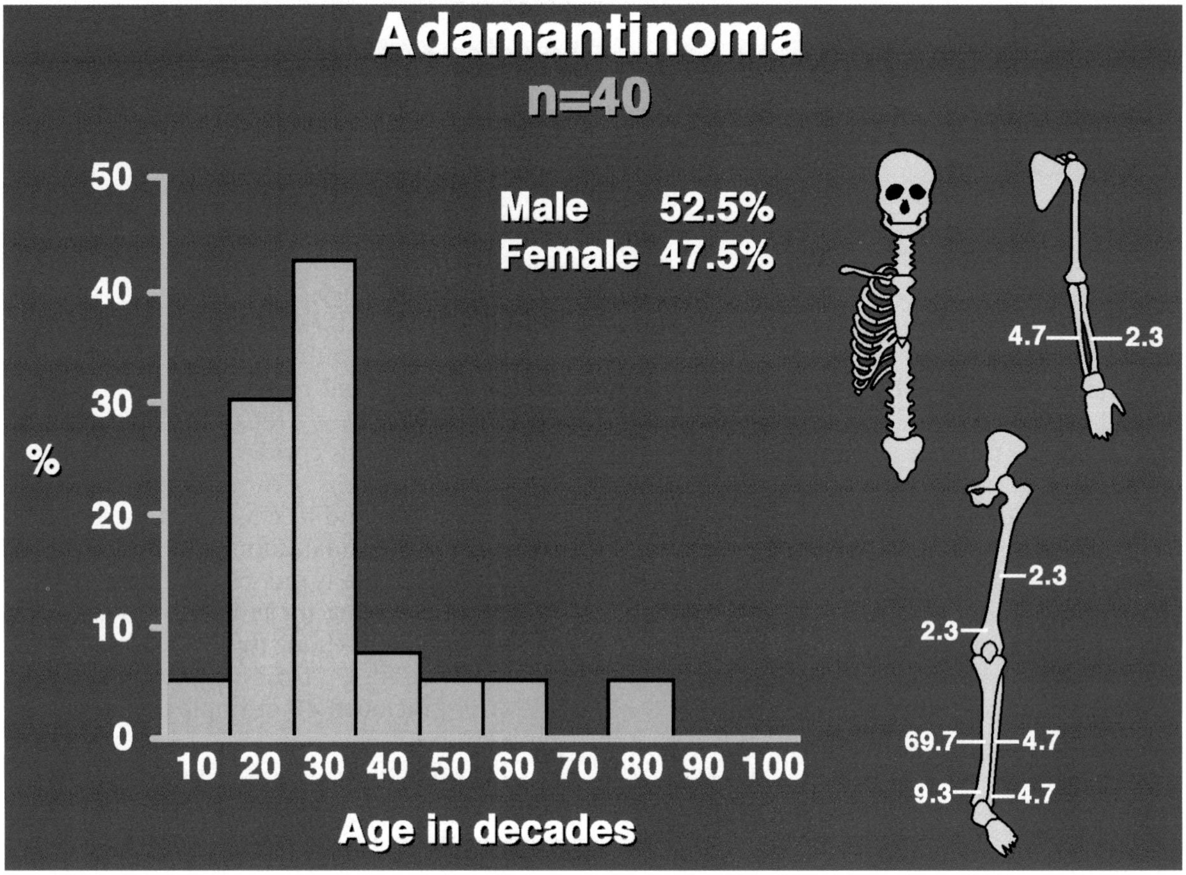

Figure 12-1

ADAMANTINOMA

Distribution of adamantinoma according to the age and sex of the patient and the site of the lesion.

by bony sclerosis. The sclerosis extends above and below the lucencies to produce a tapering appearance. One of the lucencies, typically in the middle of the process, is larger and appears more destructive (fig. 12-3). When the lesion involves the fibula, the appearance is invariably as described above. Rarely, the lucencies are within the medullary cavity, with a zone of irregular sclerosis at the periphery (fig. 12-4). Occasionally, the tumor forms a large, multiloculated, cystic lesion, creating a "soap-bubble" appearance. The cortex is usually thinned but intact. Tumors in unusual sites present as destructive lesions in the medullary cavity.

Gross Findings. Adamantinomas are soft to firm, gray-white tumors that are located in the cortex and form lobulated masses (figs. 12-5, 12-6). The tumor may extend into the medullary cavity or it may be located predominantly within the medulla (fig. 12-7). Some tumors are partly cystic.

Microscopic Findings. Adamantinomas always show epithelial differentiation. However, the histologic appearance varies greatly. Weiss and Dorfman (27) described four patterns. 1) A basaloid pattern—this consists of nests or larger masses of cells with peripheral palisading of tumor cells. This may be considered the classic pattern; it closely resembles that of ameloblastoma (fig. 12-8). The central cells are small, spindled, and have uniform nuclei without significant atypia. There may be some microcystic change similar to the stellate reticulum described in ameloblastomas. 2) A spindle cell pattern—this is similar to the basaloid pattern except for the lack of palisading cells at the periphery. The

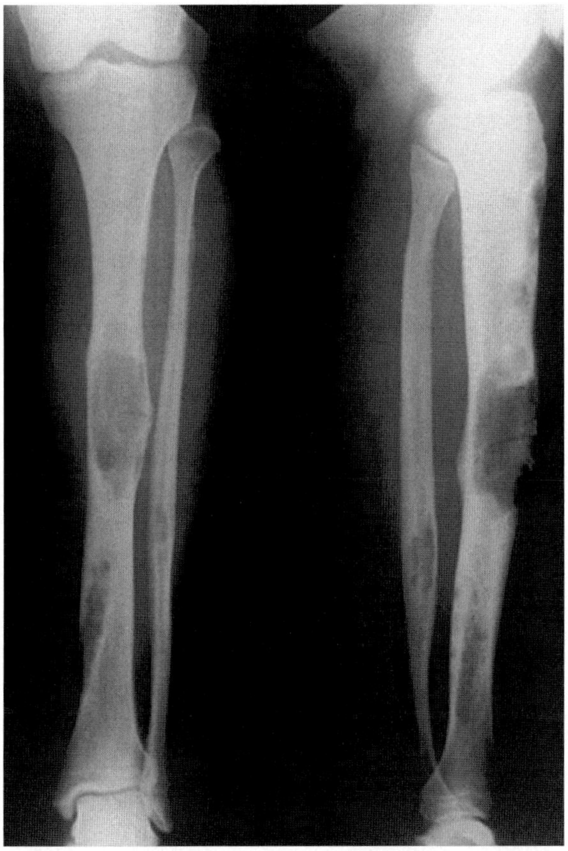

Figure 12-2

ADAMANTINOMA

Extensive lesions involving both the tibia and fibula. The cortex is involved. There are multiple lucencies with sclerosis. The lytic area in the middle is large and has a destructive appearance. (Fig. 24-2A from Unni KK. Dahlin's bone tumors: general aspects and data on 11,087 cases, 5th ed. Philadelphia: Lippincott-Raven; 1996:334. By permission of Mayo Foundation.)

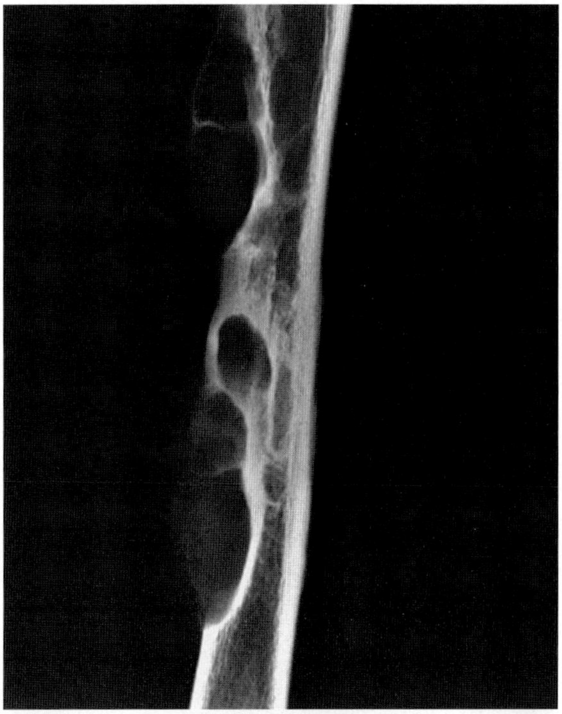

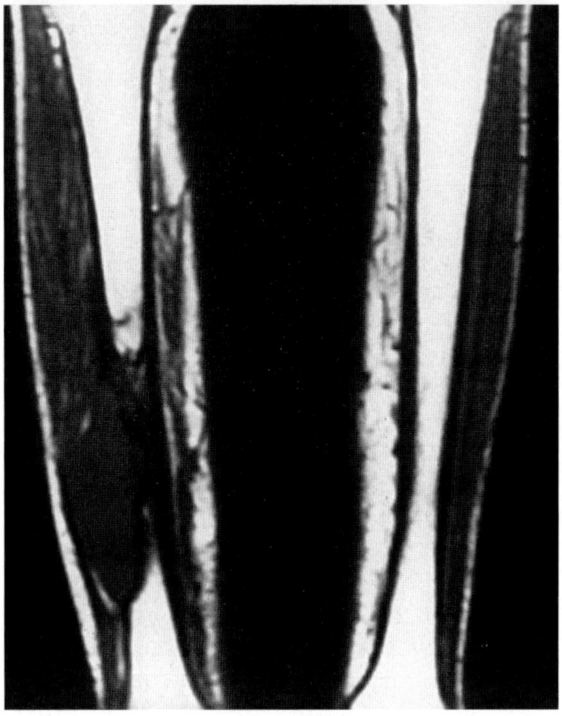

Figure 12-3

ADAMANTINOMA

Top: Large diaphyseal lesion of the tibia involves predominantly the cortex.

Bottom: Magnetic resonance image (MRI) shows a fairly large soft tissue mass.

cells may occur in islands merging into a hypocellular spindle cell stroma or the entire lesion may be spindled (fig. 12-9). This pattern is reminiscent of the pattern seen in monophasic synovial sarcoma. 3) A tubular pattern—clusters of small epithelial cells form tubular structures in a fibrous stroma. Occasionally, the epithelial cells line sinusoidal spaces, suggesting a vascular neoplasm (fig. 12-10). Such spaces tend to merge into epithelial islands. 4) A squamous pattern—this is seen within the basaloid pattern, in which individual cells show cytoplasmic keratinization or have the appearance of prickle cells. Keratin pearls are seen, but rarely (fig. 12-11).

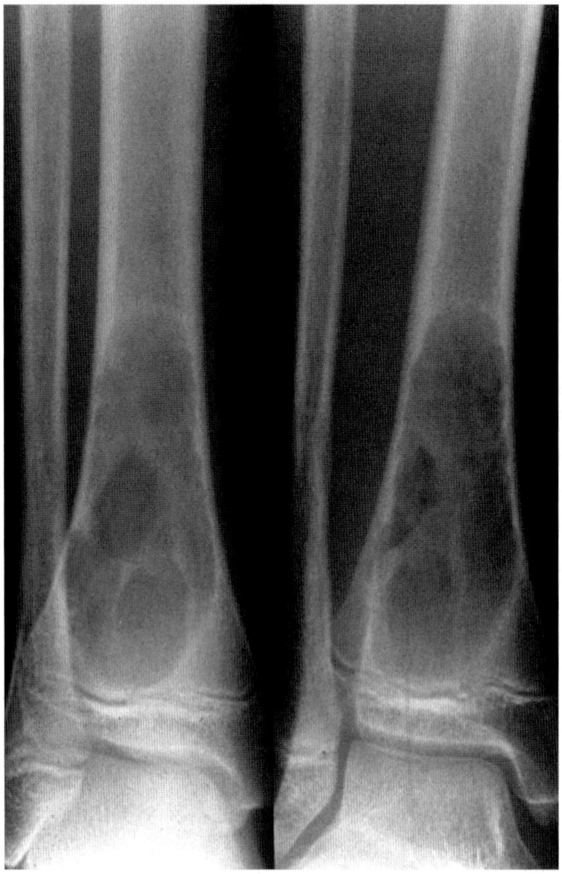

Figure 12-4

ADAMANTINOMA

This lesion, which involves the distal tibia, is almost purely lytic and involves the medulla. The appearance is not typical of adamantinoma.

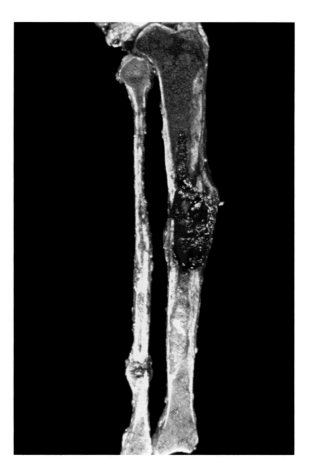

Figure 12-5

ADAMANTINOMA

Long lesion in the tibia with cortical involvement. The mid-portion shows destructive tumor in the medulla. The distal fibula is also involved.

Whatever the pattern of the epithelial cells, there is no marked cytologic atypia. As indicated above, fibrous dysplasia or osteofibrous dysplasia-like areas are frequently seen (fig. 12-12).

Immunohistochemical and electron microscopic studies have confirmed the epithelial nature of the neoplasm (fig. 12-13) (4,11,16,22,26). Hazelbag et al. (11) showed that keratins 8 and 18, usually present in synovial sarcoma and metastatic carcinoma, are absent in adamantinoma.

Genetics and Other Special Techniques. Cytogenetic and molecular cytogenetic studies of adamantinoma have demonstrated that extra copies of chromosomes 7, 8, 12, 19, and 21 are recurrent in this neoplasm (fig. 12-14) (5,14,17,24). Extra copies of one or more of these same chromosomes, except for chromosome 19, have also been seen in osteofibrous dysplasia, lending support to a relationship between osteofibrous dysplasia and adamantinoma. However, structural anomalies, including translocations, deletions, inversions, and marker chromosomes, have been detected in both differentiated and classic adamantinomas but not in osteofibrous dysplasia (fig. 12-15). The latter observation suggests that adamantinomas are slightly more complex karyotypically than osteofibrous dysplasia. Often, these structural changes are in addition to the common numerical changes (+7, +8, +12, and +21) seen in both adamantinoma and osteofibrous dysplasia. It has been hypothesized that the expansion of the abnormal clone to include structural changes might parallel a progression of

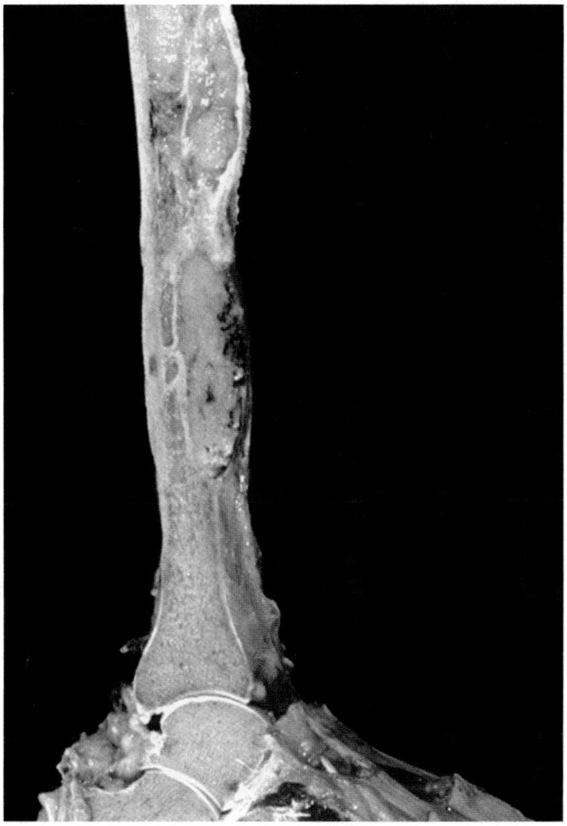

Figure 12-6

ADAMANTINOMA

Fleshy white tumor involves predominantly the cortex but also the medulla.

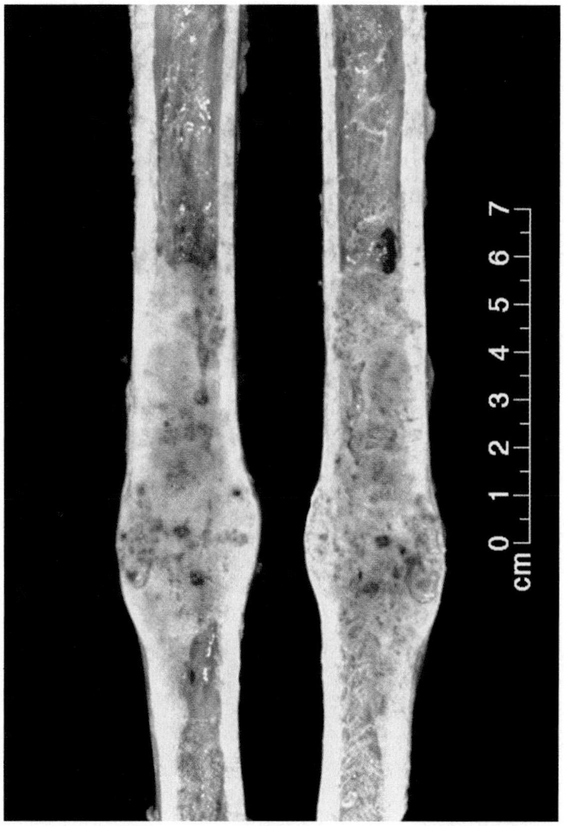

Figure 12-7

ADAMANTINOMA

This gross specimen shows involvement of the tibial diaphysis. The tumor appears fibrous and lacks the fleshy appearance of the usual sarcoma.

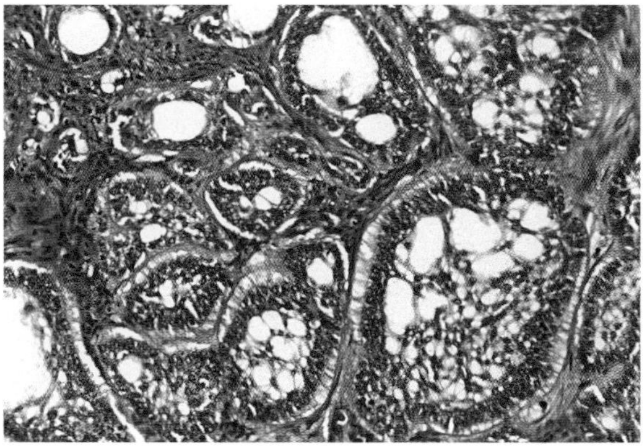

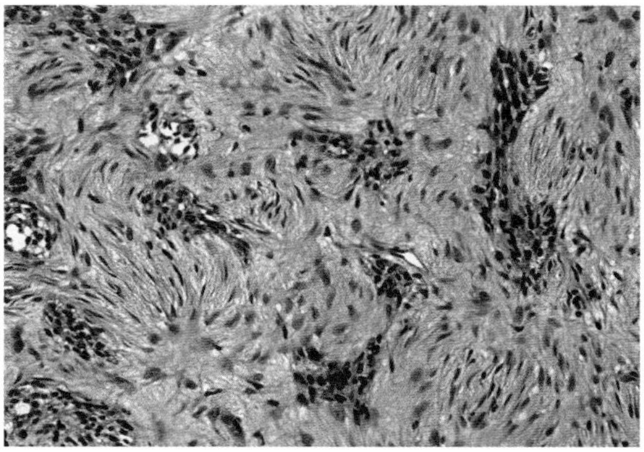

Figure 12-8

ADAMANTINOMA

Left: Basaloid pattern with peripheral palisading of cuboidal and columnar tumor cells which create cystic spaces containing central stellate-shaped cells. These features resemble those of ameloblastomas.

Right: Basaloid pattern shows clusters of cuboidal cells without marked atypia surrounded by a spindle cell stroma.

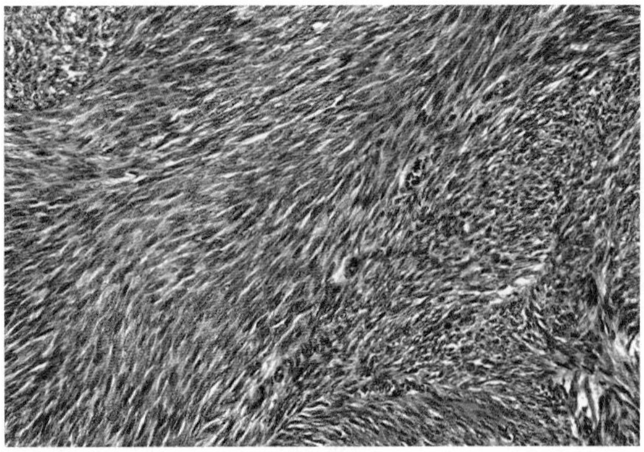

Figure 12-9

ADAMANTINOMA

Spindle cell pattern shows fascicles of spindle-shaped cells with elongated nuclei. This pattern resembles features seen in monophasic synovial sarcoma and fibrosarcoma.

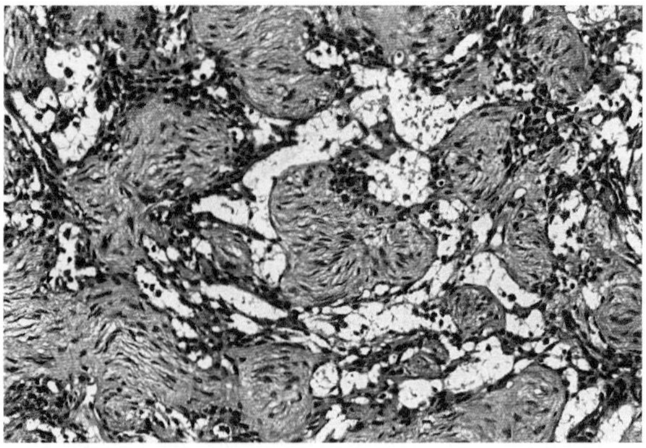

Figure 12-10

ADAMANTINOMA

Tubular pattern shows cystic spaces lined by small cuboidal epithelial cells. The appearance suggests a vascular neoplasm.

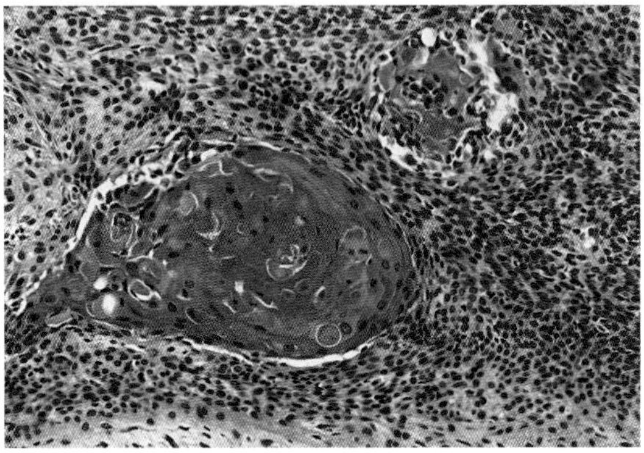

Figure 12-11

ADAMANTINOMA

Squamous differentiation with keratin pearl formation.

an osteofibrous dysplasia lesion to an adamantinoma (17).

Examination of the epithelial and mesenchymal components of adamantinoma by DNA flow and image cytometry, p53 immunohistochemistry, and polymerase chain reaction (PCR)-based loss of heterozygosity (LOH) studies has shown that aneuploidy, p53 immunoreactivity, and LOH at the p53 locus are restricted to the epithelial component (10). The authors of that study proposed that these results suggest that either adamantinoma consists of a malignant epithelial part with a reactive osteofibrous stroma

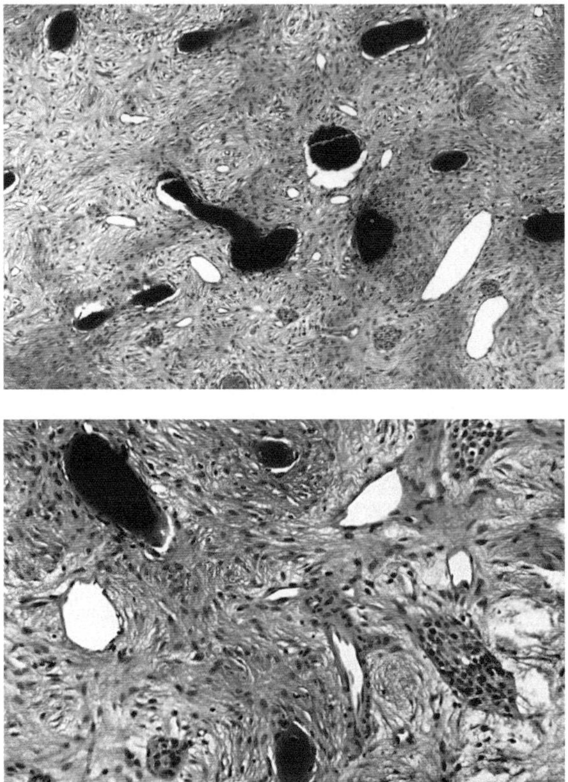

Figure 12-12

ADAMANTINOMA

Top: The pattern seen at low-power magnification has features of fibrous dysplasia.

Bottom: Higher-power view shows islands of epithelial cells.

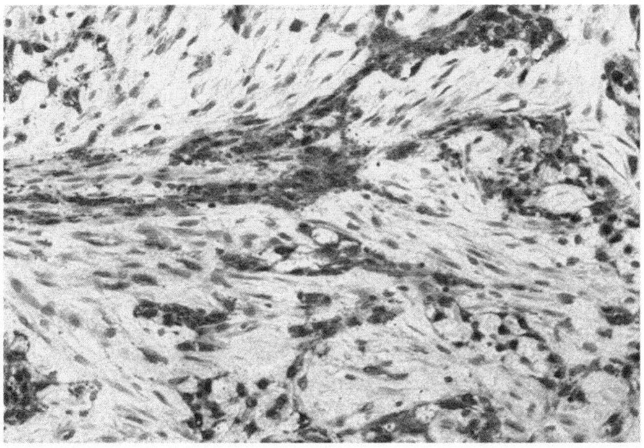

Figure 12-13

ADAMANTINOMA

Nests of keratin-positive cells in a fibrous stroma.

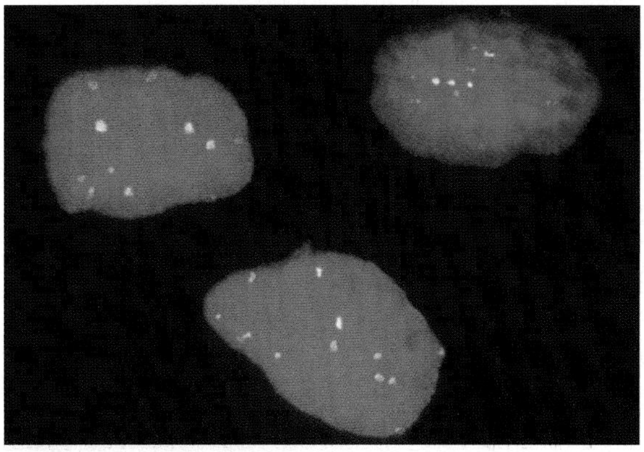

Figure 12-14

FLUORESCENCE IN SITU HYBRIDIZATION OF CLASSIC ADAMANTINOMA

The analysis was performed on a cytologic touch preparation of a classic adamantinoma arising in the tibia of a 14-year-old boy. It shows five to eight hybridization signals for chromosome 8 (red) and four hybridization signals for chromosome 12 (green). (Fig. 5C from Kanamori M, Antonescu CR, Scott M, et al. Extra copies of chromosomes 7, 8, 12, 19, and 21 are recurrent in adamantinoma. J Mol Diagn 2001;3:19.)

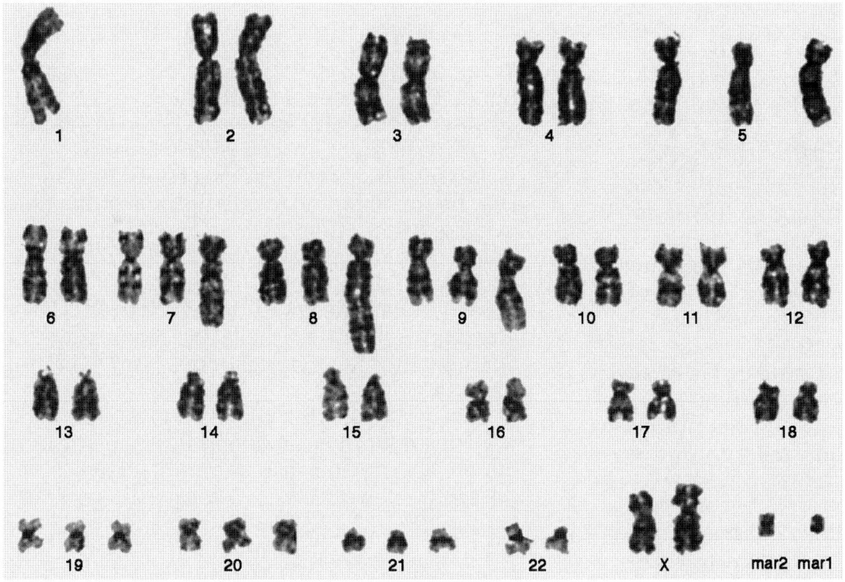

Figure 12-15

GTG-BANDED KARYOTYPE OF A CLASSIC ADAMANTINOMA

The tumor arose in the tibia of a 37-year-old woman. The karyotype was 54,XX,-1,+5, +der(7)t(?1;7)(?q21;q22), +der(8)t(1;8)(q21;q24.3),+der(9) t(1;9)(p32;q34),+19,+20,+21,+mar1, +mar2. (Fig. 3 from Kanamori M, Antonescu CR, Scott M, et al. Extra copies of chromosomes 7, 8, 12, 19, and 21 are recurrent in adamantinoma. J Mol Diagn 2001;3:19.)

or the malignant epithelial cells develop next to a proliferating benign fibrous component.

Differential Diagnosis. The main differential diagnostic consideration is metastatic carcinoma. In most cases, the location in the tibia and the relatively young age of the patients should suggest the correct diagnosis. Metastatic carcinomas usually have more cytologic atypia than seen in adamantinoma.

The adamantinoma with a purely spindle cell pattern may be mistaken for fibrosarcoma. Unlike fibrosarcomas, adamantinomas do not form collagen. Synovial sarcoma is identical to adamantinoma with a spindle cell pattern.

However, knowing that the tumor is a primary bone tumor should prevent mistaking it for synovial sarcoma.

Treatment And Prognosis. Treatment is complete surgical removal. In the past, this usually meant above-the-knee amputation because of the extensive tumor in the tibia. Advances in technique, however, have allowed resection with allograft reconstruction. Gebhardt et al. (9) reported no recurrences in nine patients who had allograft reconstruction. There is not enough experience with radiotherapy or chemotherapy to make meaningful statements.

The prognosis is unpredictable, but the course is usually indolent. Hazelbag et al. (12) reported a local recurrence rate of 32 percent and a metastatic rate of 29 percent, whereas Campanacci et al. (6) did not report any instance of distant metastasis. Of the nine patients reported by Weiss and Dorfman (27), two developed metastatic disease. Moon and Mori (20) reviewed the literature and found that 18 percent of patients reported had died, but it is not clear whether all of them died of tumor. Keeney et al. (18) reported a local recurrence rate of 31 percent at intervals ranging from 3 months to more than 19 years. Pulmonary metastases developed in 15 of these patients and lymph node metastases in 7. Metastases may be long delayed (7). Histologic features do not correlate with prognosis (18).

REFERENCES

1. Albores-Saavedra J, Diaz Gutierrez D, Altamirano Dimas M. Adamantinoma de la tibia: observaciones ultraestructurales. Rev Med Hosp Gral Mex 1968;31:241–52.
2. Alguacil-Garcia A, Alonso A, Pettigrew NM. Osteofibrous dysplasia (ossifying fibroma) of the tibia and fibula and adamantinoma. A case report. Am J Clin Pathol 1984;82:470–4.
3. Baker PL, Dockerty MB, Coventry MB. Adamantinoma (so-called) of the long bones: review of the literature and a report of three new cases. J Bone Joint Surg Am 1954;36:704–20.
4. Benassi MS, Campanacci L, Gamberi G, et al. Cytokeratin expression and distribution in adamantinoma of the long bones and osteofibrous dysplasia of tibia and fibula. An immunohistochemical study correlated to histogenesis. Histopathology 1994;25:71–6.
5. Bridge JA, Dembinski A, DeBoer J, Travis J, Neff JR. Clonal chromosomal abnormalities in osteofibrous dysplasia. Implications for histopathogenesis and its relationship with adamantinoma. Cancer 1994;73:1746–52.
6. Campanacci M, Giunti A, Bertoni F, Laus M, Gitelis S. Adamantinoma of the long bones. The experience at the Istituto Ortopedico Rizzoli. Am J Surg Pathol 1981;5:533–42.
7. Cohen DM, Dahlin DC, Pugh DG. Fibrous dysplasia associated with adamantinoma of the long bones. Cancer 1962;15:515–21.
8. Czerniak B, Rojas-Corona RR, Dorfman HD. Morphologic diversity of long bone adamantinoma. The concept of differentiated (regressing) adamantinoma and its relationship to osteofibrous dysplasia. Cancer 1989;64:2319–34.
9. Gebhardt MC, Lord FC, Rosenberg AE, Mankin HJ. The treatment of adamantinoma of the tibia by wide resection and allograft bone transplantation. J Bone Joint Surg Am 1987;69:1177–88.
10. Hazelbag HM, Fleuren GJ, Cornelisse CJ, van den Broek LJ, Taminiau AH, Hogendoorn PC. DNA aberrations in the epithelial cell component of adamantinoma of long bones. Am J Pathol 1995;147:1770–9.
11. Hazelbag HM, Fleuren GJ, vd Broek LJ, Taminiau AH, Hogendoorn PC. Adamantinoma of the long bones: keratin subclass immunoreactivity pattern with reference to its histogenesis. Am J Surg Pathol 1993;17:1225–33.
12. Hazelbag HM, Taminiau AH, Fleuren GJ, Hogendoorn PC. Adamantinoma of the long bones. A clinicopathological study of thirty-two patients with emphasis on histological subtype, precursor lesion, and biological behavior. J Bone Joint Surg Am 1994;76:1482–99.
13. Hazelbag HM, Van den Broek LJ, Fleuren GJ, Taminiau AH, Hogendoorn PC. Distribution of extracellular matrix components in adamantinoma of long bones suggests fibrous-to-epithelial transformation. Hum Pathol 1997;28:183–8.

14. Hazelbag HM, Wessels JW, Mollevangers P, van den Berg E, Molenaar WM, Hogendoorn PC. Cytogenetic analysis of adamantinoma of long bones: further indications for a common histogenesis with osteofibrous dysplasia. Cancer Genet Cytogenet 1997;97:5–11.
15. Huvos AG, Marcove RC. Adamantinoma of long bones. A clinicopathological study of fourteen cases with vascular origin suggested. J Bone Joint Surg Am 1975;57:148–54.
16. Ishida T, Iijima T, Kikuchi F, et al. A clinicopathological and immunohistochemical study of osteofibrous dysplasia, differentiated adamantinoma, and adamantinoma of long bones. Skeletal Radiol 1992;21:493–502.
17. Kanamori M, Antonescu CR, Scott M, et al. Extra copies of chromosomes 7, 8, 12, 19, and 21 are recurrent in adamantinoma. J Mol Diagn 2001;3:16–21.
18. Keeney GL, Unni KK, Beabout JW, Pritchard DJ. Adamantinoma of long bones. A clinicopathologic study of 85 cases. Cancer 1989;64:730–7.
19. Mills SE, Rosai J. Adamantinoma of the pretibial soft tissue. Clinicopathologic features, differential diagnosis, and possible relationship to intraosseous disease. Am J Clin Pathol 1985; 83:108–14.
20. Moon NF, Mori H. Adamantinoma of the appendicular skeleton—updated. Clin Orthop 1986;204:215–37.
21. Park YK, Unni KK, McLeod RA, Pritchard DJ. Osteofibrous dysplasia: clinicopathologic study of 80 cases. Hum Pathol 1993;24:1339–47.
22. Rosai J. Adamantinoma of the tibia. Electron microscopic evidence of its epithelial origin. Am J Clin Pathol 1969;51:786–92.
23. Schajowicz F, Santini-Araujo E. Adamantinoma of the tibia masked by fibrous dysplasia. Report of three cases. Clin Orthop 1989;238:294–301.
24. Sozzi G, Miozzo M, Di Palma S, et al. Involvement of the region 13q14 in a patient with adamantinoma of the long bones. Hum Genet 1990;85:513–5.
25. Sweet DE, Vinh TN, Devaney K. Cortical osteofibrous dysplasia of long bone and its relationship to adamantinoma. A clinicopathologic study of 30 cases. Am J Surg Pathol 1992;16:282–90.
26. Unni KK, Dahlin DC, Beabout JW, Ivins JC. Adamantinomas of long bones. Cancer 1974;34:1796–805.
27. Weiss SW, Dorfman HD. Adamantinoma of long bone. An analysis of nine new cases with emphasis on metastasizing lesions and fibrous dysplasia-like changes. Hum Pathol 1977;8:141–53.

13 MISCELLANEOUS TUMORS

NEURILEMMOMA OF BONE

Definition. Neurilemmoma is a benign neoplasm of Schwann cell origin located within the medullary cavity of bone.

General Features. Neurogenic tumors are rare in bone. Half of the patients with neurofibromatosis have skeletal changes that are apparent on radiographs (4). Neurofibromas, however, are distinctly uncommon within bone. The Mayo Clinic files contain only 18 cases of neurilemmoma, accounting for less than 1 percent of all benign bone tumors.

Clinical Features. Many patients with neurilemmoma are asymptomatic, and the tumor is an incidental radiographic finding. Some tumors are painful and produce swelling. Most patients are in the second or third decade of life, and there is a slight female predominance.

Sites. The mandible and sacrum are the sites most commonly involved, although other bones such as the skull and ribs have been reported to be involved (8). In the sacrum and spine, it is often difficult to determine whether the tumor truly originates from bone or arises from the nerve roots and involves bone secondarily.

Radiographic Findings. Neurilemmomas present as well-defined lucencies, occasionally with a sclerotic border (figs. 13-1, 13-2).

Gross Findings. Neurilemmomas are soft, gray-white, well-circumscribed tumors. They usually have flecks of yellow, and the lesion may be partly cystic (fig. 13-3).

Microscopic Findings. Neurilemmomas are encapsulated spindle cell tumors. The nuclei are spindle shaped and have a wavy appearance (fig. 13-4A). Palisading may be prominent. Areas of hypercellularity (Antoni A) alternate with areas of hypocellularity (Antoni B). Vessels have a thick

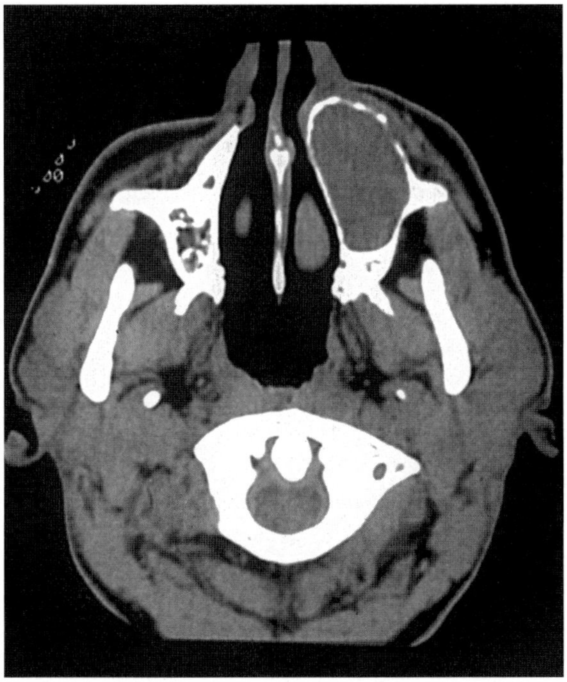

Figure 13-1

NEURILEMMOMA

An expansile mass within the maxillary bone of a 37-year-old man. (Courtesy of Dr. S. Dachs, Great Falls, MT.)

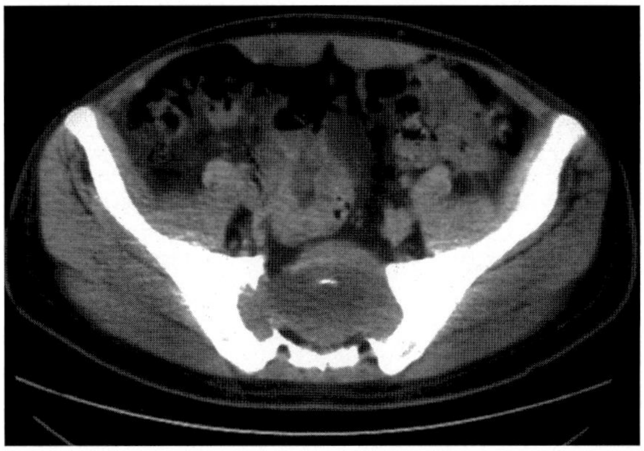

Figure 13-2

NEURILEMMOMA

Computerized tomography (CT) shows an expansile upper sacral mass involving the midline in a 40-year-old man. In the sacrum, neurilemmomas can attain a large size. The patient had experienced back pain for 2 years.

hyaline wall (fig. 13-4B). The nuclei may be enlarged and hyperchromatic focally, but cells show no mitotic activity. With immunoperoxidase stains, the cells stain strongly and uniformly with S-100 protein (fig. 13-4C).

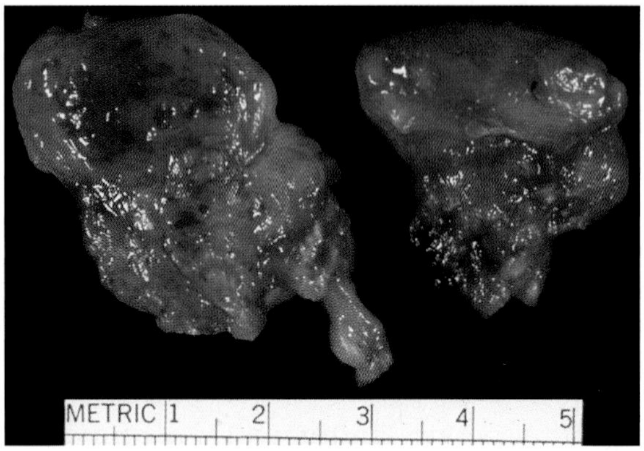

Figure 13-3

NEURILEMMOMA

This lobulated tumor involved the right distal tibia and fibula. It has a yellow-gray, glistening cut surface with areas of hemorrhagic cystic change.

Genetics and Other Special Techniques. Neurilemmomas occur sporadically or in association with neurofibromatosis 2 (NF2), an autosomal dominant disorder that predisposes to multiple neurilemmomas, meningiomas, and spinal ependymomas; bilateral vestibular neurilemmomas are the classic feature. Multiple neurilemmomas in the absence of other NF2 features are characteristic of a rare condition termed *schwannomatosis* (8).

Inactivating mutations of the *NF2* gene, accompanied by loss of the remaining wild-type allele on the long arm of chromosome 22 (which harbors the *NF2* gene), are found in approximately 60 percent of bilateral acoustic neurilemmomas of patients with NF2 and in unilateral sporadic tumors, advocating its tumor suppressor role in the pathogenesis of neurilemmoma (2,5,9,10). Most *NF2* mutations are small frameshift mutations that result in a truncated protein product, merlin. Merlin exhibits homology with the ezrin-radixin-moesin family of membrane-cytoskeleton–linking proteins (11). Merlin inhibits the action of p21-activated kinase 1 *(PAK1)* (6). *PAK1* appears to be essential for the malignant growth of NF2-deficient cells,

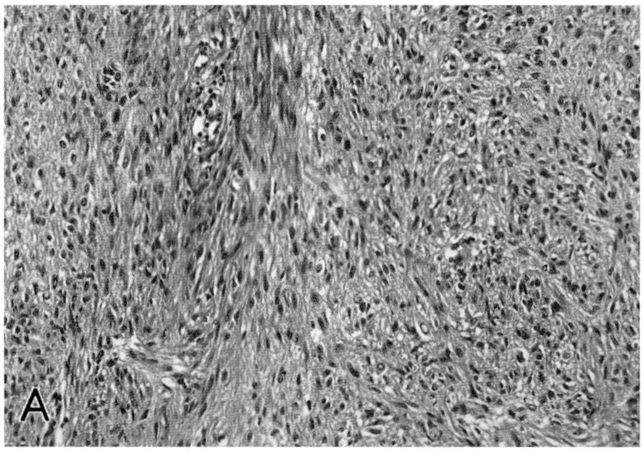

Figure 13-4

NEURILEMMOMA

A: This tumor from the mandible is composed of cells with spindle-shaped nuclei and wavy eosinophilic cytoplasm.

B: The walls of many vessels within the tumor contain thick eosinophilic hyaline material.

C: The tumor cells are immunoreactive with antibodies to S-100 protein.

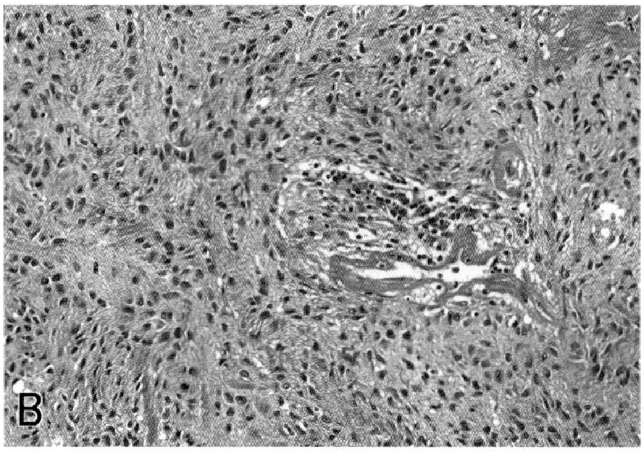

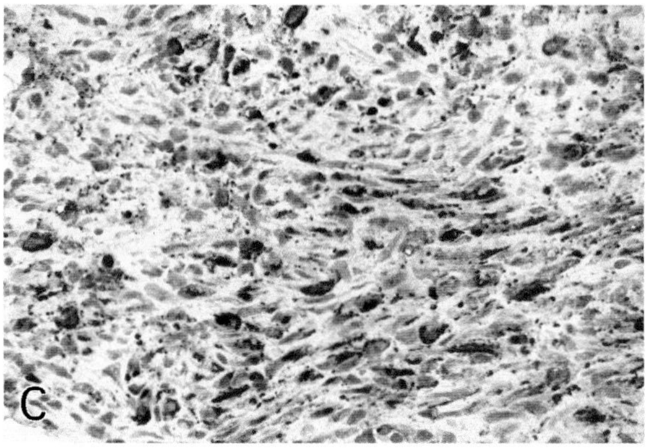

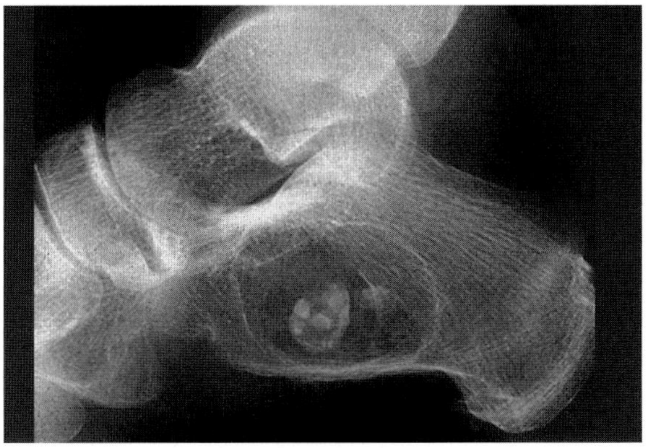

Figure 13-5

LIPOMA

This lipoma of the calcaneus is seen as a well-demarcated lucency. The target-like calcification, which represents infarct-like changes in the lesion, is typical. (Fig. 26-2 from Unni KK. Dahlin's bone tumors: general aspects and data on 11,087 cases, 5th ed. Philadelphia: Lippincott-Raven; 1996:350. By permission of Mayo Foundation.)

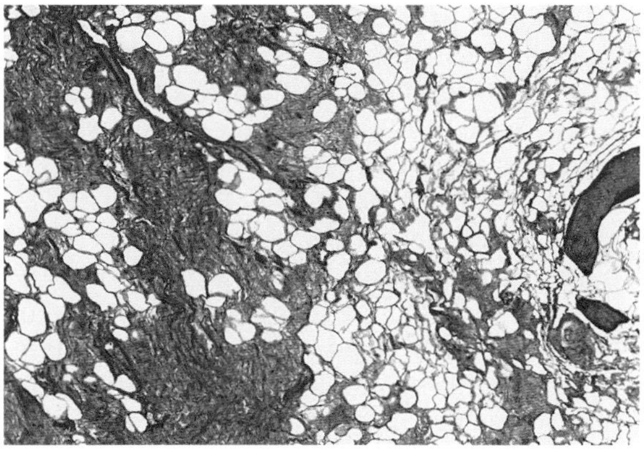

Figure 13-6

LIPOMA

Mature fat and fibrous tissue surround residual atrophic bone.

and thus, *PAK1* blocking drugs may be potentially useful for the treatment of neurilemmoma (3). No consistent secondary abnormalities have been detected in neurilemmoma (1,7).

Differential Diagnosis. Neurilemmomas may be mistaken for well-differentiated fibrosarcoma. The nonpermeative appearance of the lesion, the virtual absence of mitotic activity, and the presence of thick-walled vessels support the diagnosis of neurilemmoma. Diffuse staining with S-100 protein is also a helpful feature.

Treatment and Prognosis. Conservative surgical removal is appropriate therapy, and the prognosis is excellent.

LIPOMA OF BONE

Definition. Lipoma of bone is a medullary tumor composed of mature adipocytes.

General Features. In spite of the abundance of fat in bone, lipomas are rare. The largest series (61 cases) was reported by Milgram (16), who suggested that intraosseous lipomas may undergo involution and can be divided into three stages: in stage 1, the lesion is composed of mature adipocytes; in stage 2, there is focal fat necrosis and dystrophic calcification; in stage 3, the whole lesion has undergone fat necrosis and calcification. The Mayo Clinic files contain the cases of only eight lipomas.

Clinical Features. The lesion usually does not cause symptoms and is an incidental radiographic finding.

Sites. Any bone may be involved. In the large series reported by Milgram (16), the proximal femur was the most common site, followed by the calcaneus. In the Mayo Clinic series, many bones were affected, but in the authors' consultation files (CY Inwards, LE Wold, Mayo Clinic), the calcaneus is the preferred site.

Radiographic Findings. Lipoma appears as a well-defined area of lucency, with or without a sclerotic rim. There frequently is focal calcification in the center (fig. 13-5). Computerized tomography (CT) and magnetic resonance imaging (MRI) help confirm the fatty nature of the lesion. On CT, the central calcification has a target-like configuration.

Gross Findings. Lipomas are well demarcated and yellow. Central chalky calcification may be apparent.

Microscopic Findings. It is easy to overlook a lipoma because fat is normally a prominent part of the bone marrow. Moreover, lipomas frequently contain fragments of bony trabeculae (fig. 13-6). The lesion is usually curetted, and in these fragments, it is particularly difficult to recognize a lipoma without the advantage of the knowledge of the images. Amorphous calcification, similar to that seen in bone infarcts, is frequent (fig. 13-7).

Genetics and Other Special Techniques. Lipomas of soft tissue have been well characterized cytogenetically. Rearrangements of 12q13-15 are most common, followed by rearrangements of 6p or 13q (or both) (11,14). An identical translocation, t(11;16)(q13;p12-13), has been detected in three cases of chondroid lipoma (a rare histologic subtype exhibiting vacuolated cells embedded in a mixed stroma of mature fat, myxoid, and chondroid material and partly hyalinized fibrous tissue), suggesting that the translocation may be specific for this entity (12,14,19).

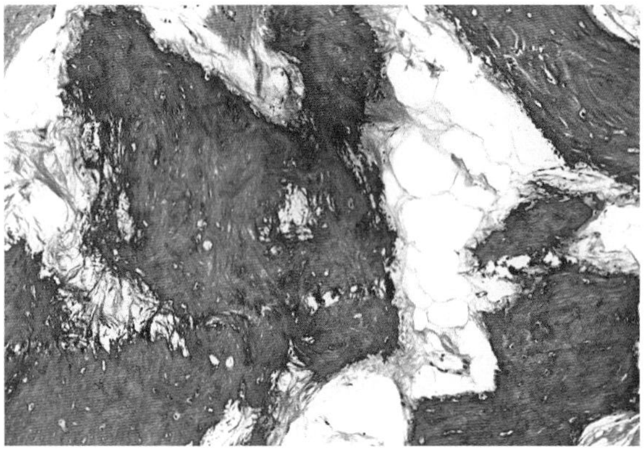

Figure 13-7

LIPOMA

Dystrophic calcification is commonly seen in intraosseous lipomas. Radiographically, such calcification usually occurs in an area of sclerosis.

Only one case of parosteal lipoma has been subjected to cytogenetic analysis (13). This case exhibited a 3;12 translocation [t(3;12)(q28;q14)] (fig. 13-8). Notably, 3q28 is the most frequently observed translocation partner of 12q14-15 in ordinary soft tissue lipomas. A member of the family of high mobility group proteins (HMG), *HMGIC* (also known as *HMGA2*), at 12q14 and a member of the LIM protein gene family, *LPP*, at 3q28 are affected by the 3;12 translocation, and as a direct result, the *HMGIC/LPP* fusion transcript is expressed. The reciprocal *LPP/HMGIC* transcript is occasionally expressed. Reverse transcriptase polymerase chain reaction (RT-PCR) and nucleotide sequence analyses of the parosteal lipoma have demonstrated *HMGIC/LPP* and *LPP/HMGIC* fusion transcripts identical to those of soft tissue lipomas characterized by the 3;12 translocation (17). These findings support a common histopathogenesis between lipomas of soft tissue and of parosteal origin.

Differential Diagnosis. Imaging findings are most helpful in arriving at the diagnosis, otherwise the lipoma may be overlooked. The calcification is similar to that seen in infarcts and fibrous dysplasia, but imaging studies resolve the problem.

Treatment and Prognosis. Lipomas do not require treatment.

Figure 13-8

PAROSTEAL LIPOMA

Partial karyotype and schematic illustrates the t(3;12)(q28;q14) observed in parosteal lipoma.

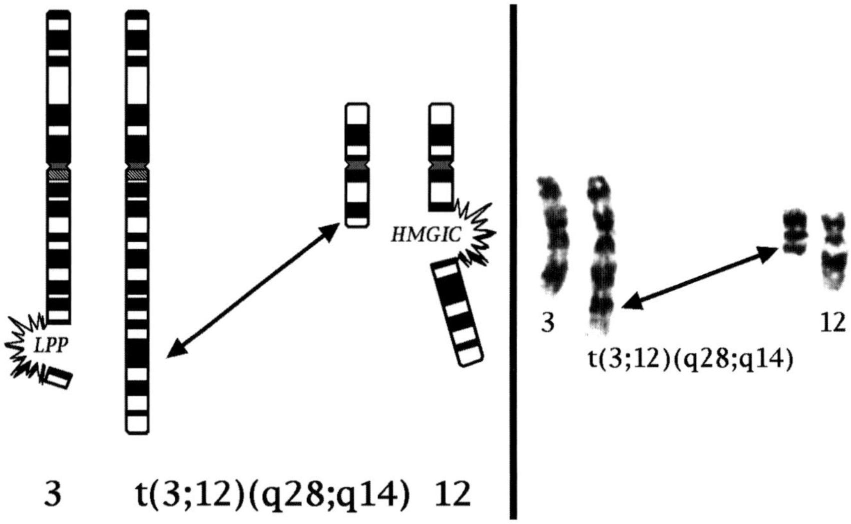

LIPOSARCOMA

Definition. Liposarcoma is a malignant tumor with differentiation toward adipocytes.

General Features. Although liposarcomas are relatively common in soft tissues, they are extraordinarily rare in bone. Metastatic liposarcomas are more common than primary liposarcomas in the skeleton. The Mayo Clinic files contain only one well-documented example of primary liposarcoma of bone. Milgram (24) has reported four cases.

Clinical Features. The clinical features are nonspecific and suggestive of malignancy.

Sites. Long bones are usually involved (24).

Gross Findings. The tumor is soft, fleshy, and may have bright yellow areas.

Microscopic Findings. Most cases reported have been pleomorphic sarcomas with focal lipoblastic differentiation. The one case in the Mayo Clinic files is a myxoid liposarcoma with round cell areas (fig. 13-9).

Genetics and Other Special Techniques. No genetic studies have been conducted on liposarcoma of bone. This is unfortunate because some of the histologic variants of soft tissue liposarcoma are associated with distinct cytogenetic and molecular genetic alterations. Well-differentiated liposarcomas of the soft tissue are characterized cytogenetically by the presence of supernumerary ring chromosomes, giant marker chromosomes, or both containing amplified sequences derived from different chromosomes, particularly chromosome 12. There is preferential amplification of 12q14-15 sequences and the following genes localized to this chromosomal region: *HDM2, HMGIC, SAS,* and *CDK4* (20,22, 26,27). The cytogenetic hallmark of myxoid and round cell liposarcoma is the chromosomal translocation t(12;16)(q13;p11) or its variant t(12;22)(q13;q12). The 12;16 translocation leads to a fusion between the *CHOP* gene on 12q13 (involved in adipocyte differentiation) with the *FUS* (or *TLS*) gene on 16p11 (encodes for a nuclear RNA binding protein), and the 12;22 translocation results in an *EWS/CHOP* hybrid gene (21,23,25). The *FUS* and *EWS* genes are homologous in both structure and function.

Differential Diagnosis. The differential diagnosis includes other pleomorphic sarcomas. It is necessary to identify lipoblasts to make the correct diagnosis.

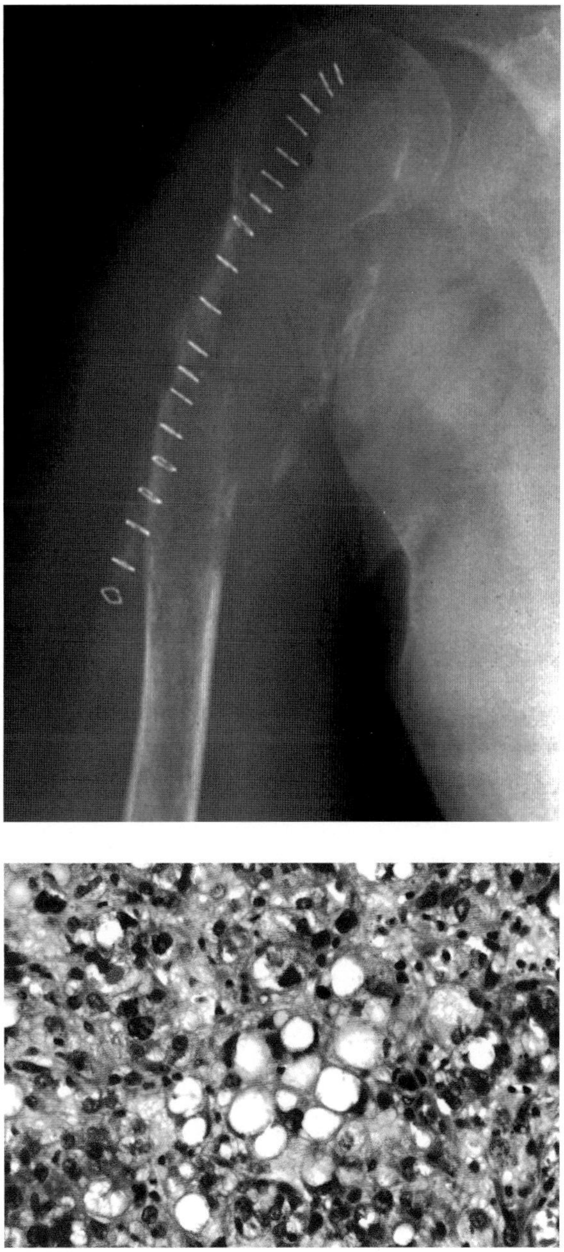

Figure 13-9

LIPOSARCOMA

Top: A lytic destructive lesion involves the proximal one third of the humerus of a 54-year-old woman.

Bottom: Microscopically, the tumor contained many vacuolated lipoblasts in addition to areas with a round cell appearance.

Treatment and Prognosis. Treatment is radical surgical removal. There is not enough experience to predict prognosis.

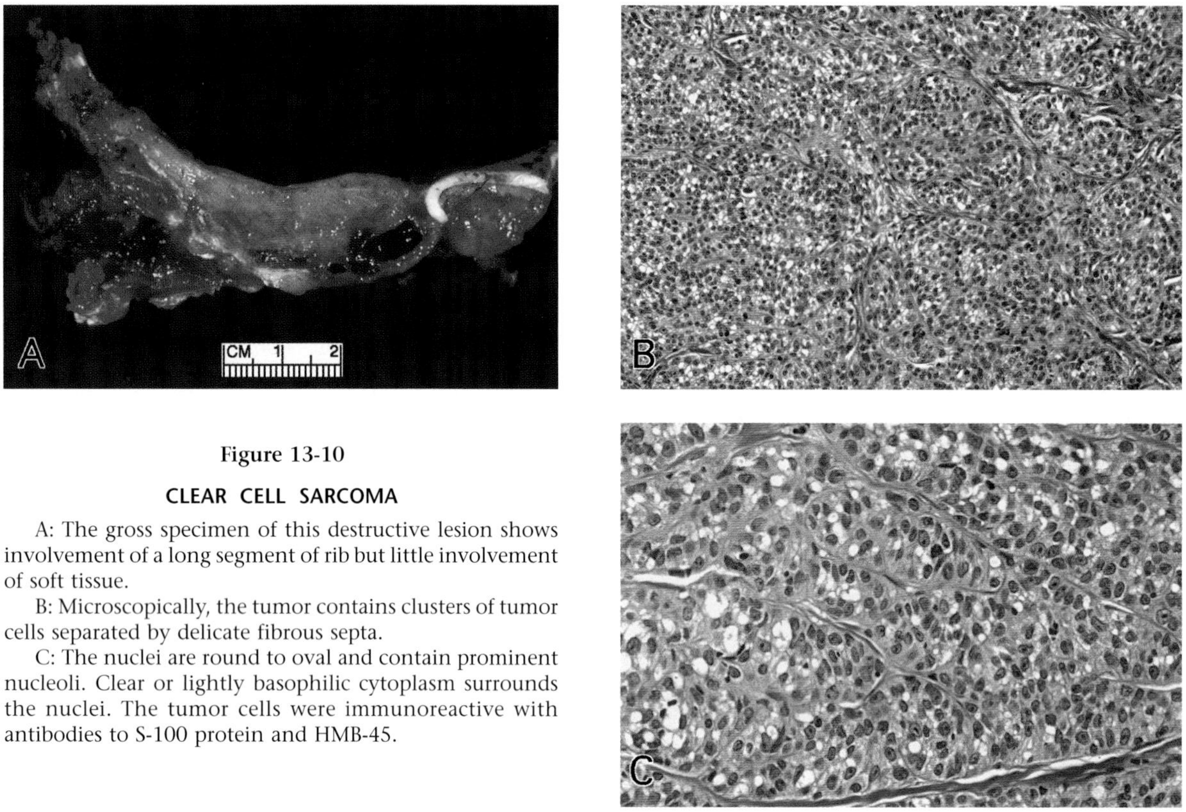

Figure 13-10

CLEAR CELL SARCOMA

A: The gross specimen of this destructive lesion shows involvement of a long segment of rib but little involvement of soft tissue.

B: Microscopically, the tumor contains clusters of tumor cells separated by delicate fibrous septa.

C: The nuclei are round to oval and contain prominent nucleoli. Clear or lightly basophilic cytoplasm surrounds the nuclei. The tumor cells were immunoreactive with antibodies to S-100 protein and HMB-45.

CLEAR CELL SARCOMA

Definition. Clear cell sarcoma is an uncommon primary tumor of tendon sheaths with melanocytic differentiation.

General Features. Clear cell sarcoma is one of the rarest of soft tissue sarcomas. The presence of melanin in the cytoplasm of tumor cells and positive staining with S-100 protein and HMB-45 suggest that the tumors are of melanocytic derivation. The term *melanoma of soft parts* is becoming increasingly popular.

Clinical Features. The clinical features are nonspecific. The case in the Mayo Clinic files is that of a patient who had a lesion of the rib and presented with pain.

Sites. The one case reported in the Mayo Clinic files involved the rib.

Radiographic Findings. The main role of radiology is to confirm that the lesion is truly a bone tumor and not a soft tissue tumor that has invaded bone secondarily. Radiographs of the rib lesion showed clearly that the epicenter of the lesion was in the bone and appeared aggressive, but otherwise the features were not specific.

Gross Findings. The tumor is fleshy and white (fig. 13-10A).

Microscopic Findings. Clear cell sarcomas are spindle cell tumors in which the tumor cells are arranged in clusters (fig. 13-10B). The nuclei are uniform and have prominent nucleoli (fig. 13-10C). The cytoplasm may contain melanin. Clusters of benign giant cells are commonly seen. On immunoperoxidase stains, both S-100 protein and HMB-45 are positive.

Genetics and Other Special Techniques. The cytogenetic translocation characteristic of clear cell sarcoma, t(12;22)(q13;q12), was first described in 1990 (28). The presence of extra copies of chromosome 8 is reportedly a common secondary event in this neoplasm (31). In clear cell sarcoma, a balanced t(12;22)(q13;q12) results in a gene fusion between the 5' portion of the *EWS* and 3' portion of the *ATF1* genes and in the production of a fusion protein in which the N-terminal 325 amino acids of EWS are fused to the C-terminal 206 amino acids of the activating transcription factor 1 (ATF1) (33). *EWS/ATF1* functions as a potent constitutive

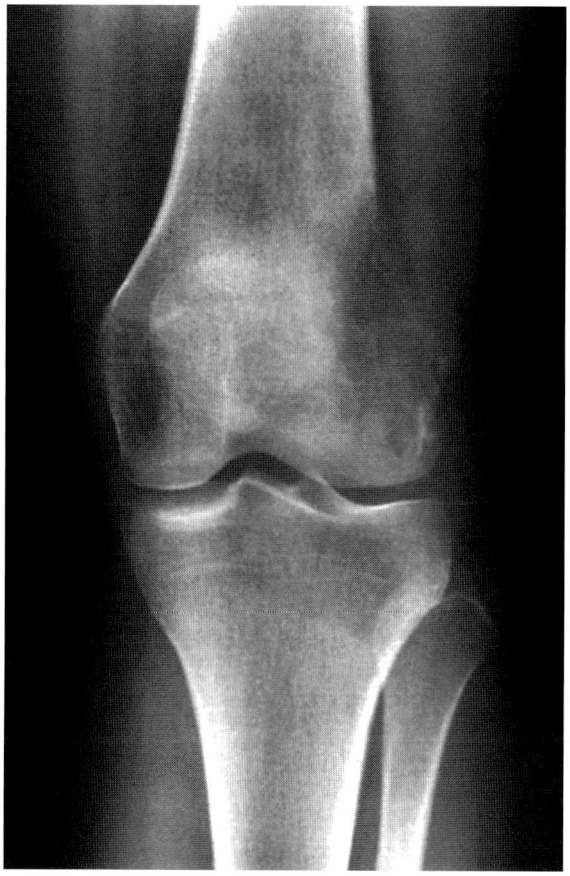

Figure 13-11

ALVEOLAR SOFT PART SARCOMA

A destructive lesion of the distal femur is seen. No other lesions have been identified, and the patient is a long-term survivor.

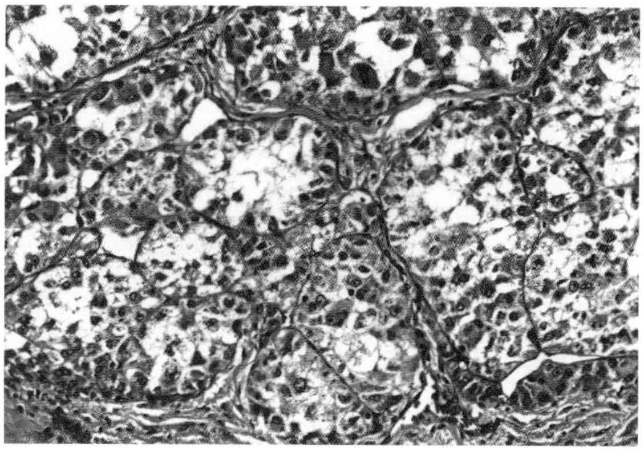

Figure 13-12

ALVEOLAR SOFT PART SARCOMA

This tumor is from the proximal tibia. Nests of tumor cells with loss of cellular cohesion create a pseudoalveolar appearance. Prominent nucleoli are present, and the cytoplasm is granular, eosinophilic, or clear. The tumor eventually metastasized to the lungs.

activator of several cyclic adenosine monophosphate (cAMP)-inducible promoters when assayed by transfection in cells that lack *EWS/ATF1* (29,30). Identification of the t(12;22)(q13;q12), its associated fusion gene, *EWS/ATF1*, or both is of value diagnostically, that is, in differentiating clear cell sarcoma from a metastasis of a cutaneous melanoma in the absence of a known primary source for the latter (31).

Differential Diagnosis. Because of its rarity, the diagnosis is not usually considered. Metastatic melanoma needs to be ruled out clinically.

Treatment and Prognosis. Treatment consists of radical surgical removal. The expected prognosis is the same as for patients with the soft tissue counterpart (32).

ALVEOLAR SOFT PART SARCOMA

Definition. Alveolar soft part sarcoma is an uncommon neoplasm, usually primary in the soft tissues, of unknown histogenesis but with a very characteristic alveolar arrangement of tumor cells.

General Features. Alveolar soft part sarcoma of soft tissue occurs in the buttock and thigh regions. The pattern of growth has suggested a paraganglioma or tumor of skeletal muscle (35).

Clinical Features. The patients are young adults, with a slight female predominance. Patients present with local pain (39).

Radiographic Findings. The radiographic appearance is that of a lucency, poorly marginated, that destroys the cortex and extends into soft tissue (fig. 13-11).

Gross Findings. The tumor is gray-white and fleshy.

Microscopic Findings. The tumor cells are arranged in an alveolar pattern, with clusters of cells separated by sinusoidal vascular spaces. The tumor cells have rounded nuclei and prominent nucleoli (fig. 13-12). The cytoplasm is granular or clear. The periodic acid–Schiff (PAS) stain shows rhomboid crystals within the cytoplasm.

Genetics and Other Special Techniques. Cytogenetic studies of alveolar soft part sarcoma have documented a recurrent derivative chromosome 17 [der(17)] due to a nonreciprocal translocation [der(17)t(X;17)(p11.2;q25)] in this sarcoma (36,37). Ladanyi et al. (38) demonstrated that this translocation fuses the *TFE3* transcription factor gene at Xp11 to a novel gene at 17q25, designated *ASPL*, implicating transcriptional deregulation in the pathogenesis of this tumor. *ASPL* is widely expressed in all adult tissues and encodes a predicted protein of unknown function containing a conserved domain possibly related to the ubiquitylation pathway. Because of the unbalanced nature of the X;17 translocation [der(17)t(X;17)(p11.2; q25)], almost all alveolar soft part sarcomas harbor genomic loss of 17q25 sequences telomeric to *ASPL*, and most show a gain of Xp sequences telomeric to *TFE3* (representing most of the short arm). Thus, this nonreciprocal structure of the *ASPL/TFE3* rearrangement suggests a special biologic feature in alveolar soft part sarcoma that combines fusion protein formation with pathogenetic losses or gains (or both) of other as yet uncharacterized genes (38). The der(17)t(X;17)(p11.2;q25) and the associated fusion gene *ASPL/TFE3* in alveolar soft part sarcoma represent translocation-based genetic markers of clinical usefulness. Aberrant nuclear immunoreactivity for TFE3 protein is also detectable in alveolar soft part sarcomas characterized by chromosome translocations involving the *TFE3* gene at Xp11.2 (34).

Differential Diagnosis. Metastatic renal cell carcinoma can be a difficult diagnostic problem. Demonstration of PAS-positive crystals helps confirm the diagnosis of alveolar soft part sarcoma.

Treatment and Prognosis. Although the behavior of alveolar soft part sarcoma of soft tissue is indolent, the long-term prognosis is poor. Metastasis involves the lungs and brain. This peculiar tendency to brain metastasis was present in the bone tumors reported by Park et al. (39); only 2 of 6 patients were alive and free of disease at the time of the report.

LEIOMYOSARCOMA

Definition. Leiomyosarcoma is a primary spindle cell malignancy of bone in which the tumor cells have the nuclear and cytoplasmic features associated with leiomyosarcomas in other locations.

General Features. Until recently, bone tumors have not frequently been diagnosed as leiomyosarcoma. The advent of electron microscopy and immunohistochemistry has helped to reclassify some of the tumors that previously would have been classified as fibrosarcoma. As pointed out by Young et al. (44), the diagnosis of leiomyosarcoma requires that metastasis, especially from the genital or gastrointestinal tract, has been ruled out. The incidence of primary leiomyosarcoma of bone is not known because only a few cases have been reported and there are no large-scale studies of all spindle cell sarcomas examined at a large institution.

Clinical Features. The symptoms are nonspecific and usually consist of pain. Pathologic fracture has been described. Patients are generally young or older adults, although the age range is wide. One patient had a history of bilateral retinoblastoma (41). Males and females are affected about equally.

Radiographic Findings. Radiographs show a purely lytic destructive defect with poorly defined margins (fig. 13-13). Although the features are nonspecific, they suggest a malignant neoplasm.

Gross Findings. The tumor has been described as firm and gray or soft and jelly-like (45).

Microscopic Findings. The hallmark of leiomyosarcoma is the presence of interlacing fascicles of spindle cells with a myogenic quality; that is, nuclei that are blunt-ended or cigar-shaped and eosinophilic cytoplasm that is tapered (fig. 13-14). Most studies have used electron microscopy to confirm smooth muscle differentiation (40,43). These studies have demonstrated intermediate filaments, dense bodies, and pinocytic vesicles in the cytoplasm. Immunoperoxidase studies have shown that the cells stain with desmin and actin (45).

Differential Diagnosis. Metastatic leiomyosarcoma has to be ruled out clinically. The spindle cells of a fibrosarcoma form a herringbone pattern and do not have eosinophilic cytoplasm.

Treatment and Prognosis. Not enough information has been reported for statements to be made about treatment and prognosis. Complete surgical ablation seems indicated. The role of chemotherapy is unclear. In the series of Myers et al. (43), 2 of 5 patients died, 1 was alive with disease, and 2 were alive (disease state unknown). In another series, prognosis was better but follow-up was short (42).

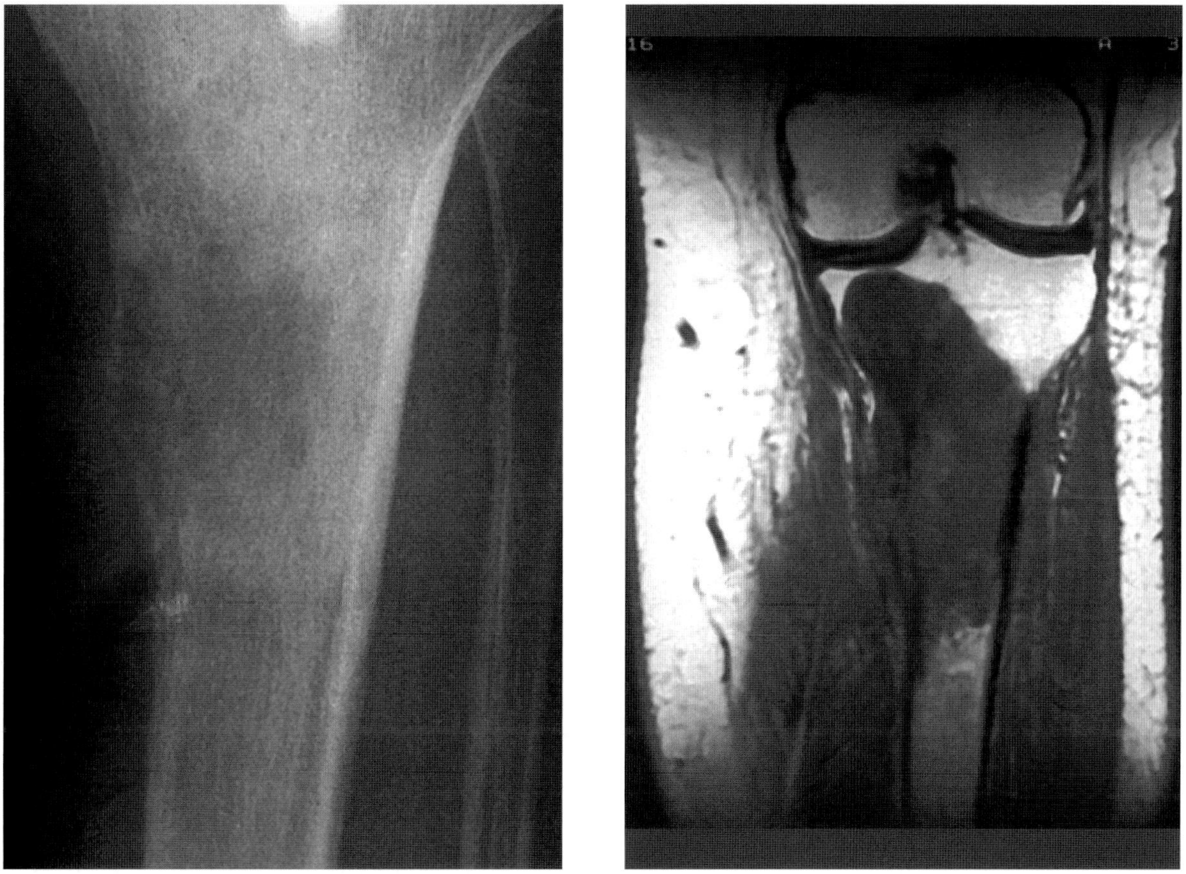

Figure 13-13

LEIOMYOSARCOMA

Left: Plain radiograph shows a lytic lesion involving the proximal tibia.
Right: Magnetic resonance image (MRI) shows extension into the subchondral region and soft tissue.

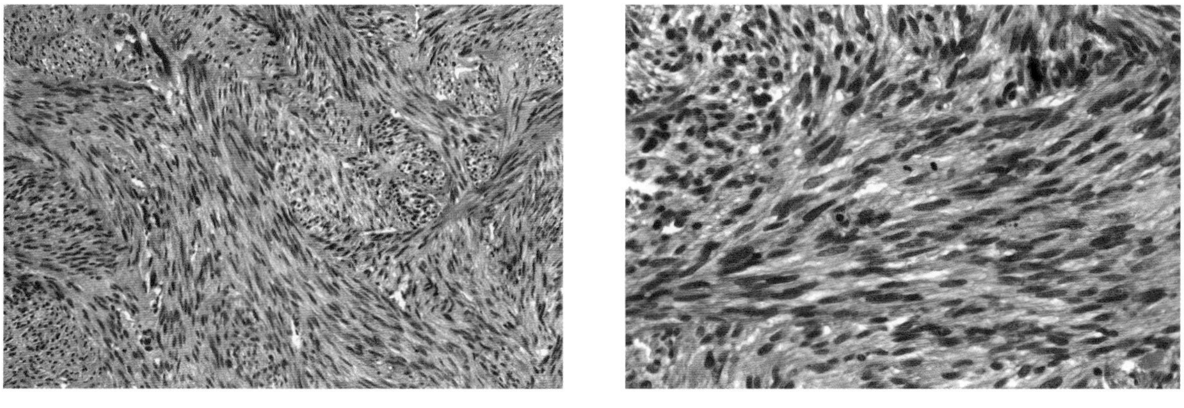

Figure 13-14

LEIOMYOSARCOMA

Left: Intersecting fascicles of spindle cells.
Right: Cytologic features include eosinophilic cytoplasm and blunt-ended nuclei. Mitotic activity is also seen.

REFERENCES

Neurilemmoma of Bone

1. Antinheimo J, Sallinen SL, Sallinen P, et al. Genetic aberrations in sporadic and neurofibromatosis 2 (NF2)-associated schwannomas studied by comparative genomic hybridization (CGH). Acta Neurochir 2000;142:1099–104.
2. Bijlsma EK, Brouwer-Mladin R, Bosch DA, Westerveld A, Hulsebos TJ. Molecular characterization of chromosome 22 deletions in schwannomas. Genes Chromosomes Cancer 1992;5:201–5.
3. Hirokawa Y, Tikoo A, Huynh J, et al. A clue to the therapy of neurofibromatosis type 2: NF2/merlin is a PAK1 inhibitor. Cancer J 2004;10:20–6.
4. Hunt JC, Pugh DG. Skeletal lesions in neurofibromatosis. Radiology 1961;76:1–20.
5. Jacoby LB, MacCollin M, Barone R, Ramesh V, Gusella JF. Frequency and distribution of NF2 mutations in schwannomas. Genes Chromosomes Cancer 1996;17:45–55.
6. Kissil JL, Wilker EW, Johnson KC, Eckman MS, Yaffe MB, Jacks T. Merlin, the product of the Nf2 tumor suppressor gene, is an inhibitor of the p21-activated kinase, Pak1. Mol Cell 2003;12:841–9.
7. Leone PE, Bello MJ, Mendiola M, et al. Allelic status of 1p, 14q, and 22q and NF2 gene mutations in sporadic schwannomas. Int J Mol Med 1998;1:889–92.
8. MacCollin M, Woodfin W, Kronn D, Short MP. Schwannomatosis: a clinical and pathologic study. Neurology 1996;46:1072–9.
9. Rey JA, Bello MJ, de Campos JM, et al. Abnormalities of chromosome 22 in human brain tumors determined by combined cytogenetic and molecular genetic approaches. Cancer Genet Cytogenet 1993;66:1–10.
10. Wolff RK, Frazer KA, Jackler RK, Lanser MJ, Pitts LH, Cox DR. Analysis of chromosome 22 deletions in neurofibromatosis type 2-related tumors. Am J Hum Genet 1992;51:478–85.
11. Xiao GH, Chernoff J, Testa JR. NF2: the wizardry of merlin. Genes Chromosomes Cancer 2003;38:389–99.

Lipoma of Bone

12. Ballaux F, Debiec-Rychter M, De Wever I, Sciot R. Chondroid lipoma is characterized by t(11;16)(q13;p12–13). Virchows Arch 2004;444:208–10.
13. Bridge JA, DeBoer J, Walker CW, Neff JR. Translocation t(3;12)(q28;q14) in parosteal lipoma. Genes Chromosomes Cancer 1995;12:70–2.
14. Gisselsson D, Domanski HA, Hoglund M, et al. Unique cytological features and chromosome aberrations in chondroid lipoma: a case report based on fine-needle aspiration cytology, histopathology, electron microscopy, chromosome banding, and molecular cytogenetics. Am J Surg Pathol 1999;23:1300–4.
15. Mandahl N, Hoglund M, Mertens F, et al. Cytogenetic aberrations in 188 benign and borderline adipose tissue tumors. Genes Chromosomes Cancer 1994;9:207–15.
16. Milgram JW. Intraosseous lipomas. A clinicopathologic study of 66 cases. Clin Orthop 1988;231:277–302.
17. Petit MM, Swarts S, Bridge JA, Van de Ven WJ. Expression of reciprocal fusion transcripts of the HMGIC and LPP genes in parosteal lipoma. Cancer Genet Cytogenet 1998;106:18–23.
18. Sreekantaiah C, Leong SP, Karakousis CP, et al. Cytogenetic profile of 109 lipomas. Cancer Res 1991;51:422–33.
19. Thomson TA, Horsman D, Bainbridge TC. Cytogenetic and cytologic features of chondroid lipoma of soft tissue. Mod Pathol 1999;12:88–91.

Liposarcoma

20. Berner JM, Meza-Zepeda LA, Kools PF, et al. HMGIC, the gene for an architectural transcription factor, is amplified and rearranged in a subset of human sarcomas. Oncogene 1997;14:2935–41.
21. Crozat A, Aman P, Mandahl N, Ron D. Fusion of CHOP to a novel RNA-binding protein in human myxoid liposarcoma. Nature 1993;363:640–4.
22. Gisselsson D, Hoglund M, Mertens F, Mitelman F, Mandahl N. Chromosomal organization of amplified chromosome 12 sequences in mesenchymal tumors detected by fluorescence in situ hybridization. Genes Chromosomes Cancer 1998;23:203–12.
23. Knight JC, Renwick PJ, Cin PD, Van den Berghe H, Fletcher CD. Translocation t(12;16)(q13;p11) in myxoid liposarcoma and round cell liposarcoma: molecular and cytogenetic analysis. Cancer Res 1995;55:24–7.
24. Milgram JW. Malignant transformation in bone lipomas. Skeletal Radiol 1990;19:347-52.
25. Panagopoulos I, Hoglund M, Mertens F, Mandahl N, Mitelman F, Aman P. Fusion of the EWS and CHOP genes in myxoid liposarcoma. Oncogene 1996;12:489–94.
26. Pedeutour F, Forus A, Coindre JM, et al. Structure of the supernumerary ring and giant rod chromosomes in adipose tissue tumors. Genes Chromosomes Cancer 1999;24:30–41.
27. Pedeutour F, Suijkerbuijk RF, Forus A, et al. Complex composition and co-amplification of SAS and MDM2 in ring and giant rod marker chromosomes in well-differentiated liposarcoma. Genes Chromosomes Cancer 1994;10:85–94.

Clear Cell Sarcoma

28. Bridge JA, Borek DA, Neff JR, Huntrakoon M. Chromosomal abnormalities in clear cell sarcoma. Implications for histogenesis. Am J Clin Pathol 1990;93:26–31.
29. Brown AD, Lopez-Terrada D, Denny C, Lee KA. Promoters containing ATF-binding sites are deregulated in cells that express the EWS/ATF1 oncogene. Oncogene 1995;10:1749–56.
30. Fujimura Y, Ohno T, Siddique H, Lee L, Rao VN, Reddy ES. The EWS-ATF-1 gene involved in malignant melanoma of soft parts with t(12;22) chromosome translocation, encodes a constitutive transcriptional activator. Oncogene 1996; 12:159–67.
31. Sandberg AA, Bridge JA. Updates on the cytogenetics and molecular genetics of bone and soft tissue tumors: clear cell sarcoma (malignant melanoma of soft parts). Cancer Genet Cytogenet 2001;130:1–7.
32. Weiss SW, Goldblum JR. Malignant tumors of the peripheral nerves. In: Weiss SW, Goldblum JR, eds. Enzinger and Weiss's soft tissue tumors, 4th ed. St. Louis: Mosby; 2001:1241–50.
33. Zucman J, Delattre O, Desmaze C, et al. EWS and ATF-1 gene fusion induced by t(12;22) translocation in malignant melanoma of soft parts. Nat Genet 1993;4:341–5.

Alveolar Soft Part Sarcoma

34. Argani P, Lal P, Hutchinson B, Lui MY, Reuter VE, Landanyi M. Aberrant nuclear immunoreactivity for TFE3 in neoplasms with TFE3 gene fusions: a sensitive and specific immunohistochemical assay. Am J Surg Pathol 2003;27:750–61.
35. Christopherson WM, Foote FW Jr, Stewart FW. Alveolar soft-part sarcomas: structurally characteristic tumors of uncertain histogenesis. Cancer 1952;5:100–11.
36. Heimann P, Devalck C, Debusscher C, Sariban E, Vamos E. Alveolar soft-part sarcoma: further evidence by FISH for the involvement of chromosome band 17q25. Genes Chromosomes Cancer 1998;23:194–7.
37. Joyama S, Ueda T, Shimizu K, et al. Chromosome rearrangement at 17q25 and xp11.2 in alveolar soft-part sarcoma. A case report and review of the literature. Cancer 1999;86:1246–50.
38. Ladanyi M, Lui MY, Antonescu CR, et al. The der(17)t(X;17)(p11;q25) of human alveolar soft part sarcoma fuses the TFE3 transcription factor gene to ASPL, a novel gene at 17q25. Oncogene 2001;20:48–57.
39. Park YK, Unni KK, Kim YW, et al. Primary alveolar soft part sarcoma of bone. Histopathology 1999;35:411–7.

Leiomyosarcoma

40. Angervall L, Berlin O, Kindblom LG, Stener B. Primary leiomyosarcoma of bone: a study of five cases. Cancer 1980;46:1270–9.
41. Guse TR, Weis LD. Leiomyosarcoma of the femur in a patient with a history of retinoblastoma. A case report. J Bone Joint Surg Am 1994;76:904–6.
42. Khoddami M, Bedard YC, Bell RS, Kandel RA. Primary leiomyosarcoma of bone: report of seven cases and review of the literature. Arch Pathol Lab Med 1996;120:671–5.
43. Myers JL, Arocho J, Bernreuter W, Dunham W, Mazur MT. Leiomyosarcoma of bone. A clinicopathologic, immunohistochemical, and ultrastructural study of five cases. Cancer 1991;67: 1051–6.
44. Young CL, Wold LE, McLeod RA, Sim FH. Primary leiomyosarcoma of bone. Orthopedics 1988;11:615–8.
45. Young MP, Freemont AJ. Primary leiomyosarcoma of bone. Histopathology 1991;19:257–62.

14 CONDITIONS THAT SIMULATE PRIMARY NEOPLASMS OF BONE

METASTATIC MALIGNANCY

Definition. A metastatic malignancy is a skeletal deposit of a malignant tumor from a distant site.

General Features. Metastatic involvement of the skeleton is more common than primary neoplasms of bone, but it is difficult to know the exact incidence of such metastases. In a series of 1,000 autopsies of patients with carcinoma, skeletal metastases were found in 27 percent (1). Some malignancies are likely to metastasize to the skeleton, others rarely do. Carcinomas of the breast, lung, prostate, thyroid, and kidney are considered "bone-seeking." In comparison, metastases from the colon or stomach, or melanoma, are unusual, at least in clinical practice. Although metastasis to the skeleton is found in 23 to 49 percent of patients with melanoma at the time of autopsy, it is rarely a clinical problem (3). Recurrent colon carcinoma frequently invades the sacrum by direct extension.

Although both metastatic carcinoma and Paget's disease occur in older adults, metastatic carcinoma is extremely unusual in pagetic bone (4,7). Schajowicz et al. (7) reported that of 987 patients with Paget's disease, only 6 had metastatic carcinoma to bone (compared with 62 sarcomas), and of these, only 2 actually involved bone affected by Paget's disease.

Simon and Karluk (8) reported that in 3 to 15 percent of patients with metastatic carcinoma, the primary site is not known. Rougraff et al. (6) were able to identify the primary site preoperatively in 85 percent of patients with the aid of the clinical history, physical examination, and imaging studies of the chest and abdomen.

Clinical Features. Most patients with metastatic carcinoma have a known primary malignancy, and the lesions may be identified on follow-up studies before they become symptomatic. Pain is the most common symptom; it is deep-seated and may be unrelenting. Pathologic fracture occasionally is the first manifestation of the disease. Systemic symptoms of cancer may or may not be present.

Radiographic Findings. Radioactive bone scanning is frequently the first imaging modality used to identify metastatic deposits. The findings are almost always positive at multiple sites (fig. 14-1). Plain radiographs may show a solitary or, more often, multiple lesions. The lesions usually start in the medullary cavity and are poorly defined; the cortex is frequently

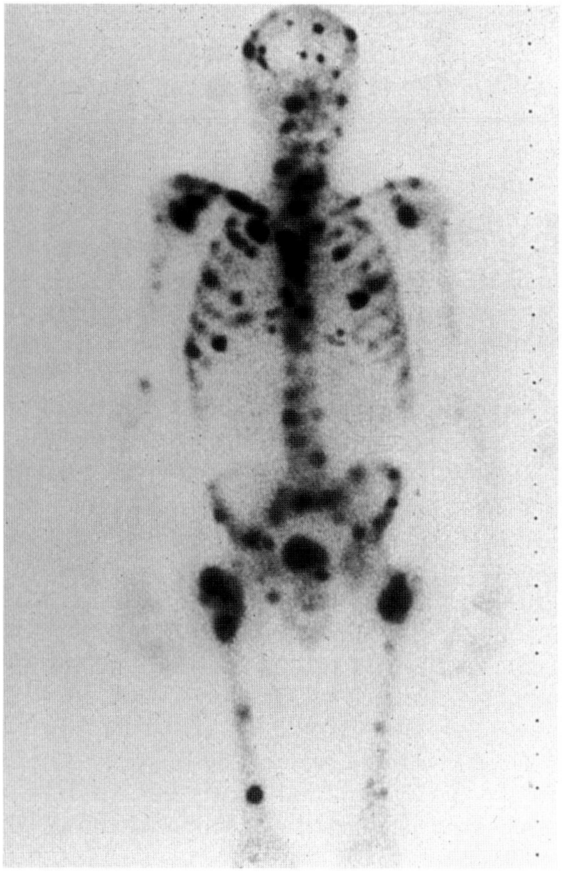

Figure 14-1

METASTATIC CARCINOMA

Radioisotope bone scan shows numerous hot spots in the skeleton of a man with metastatic prostate carcinoma.

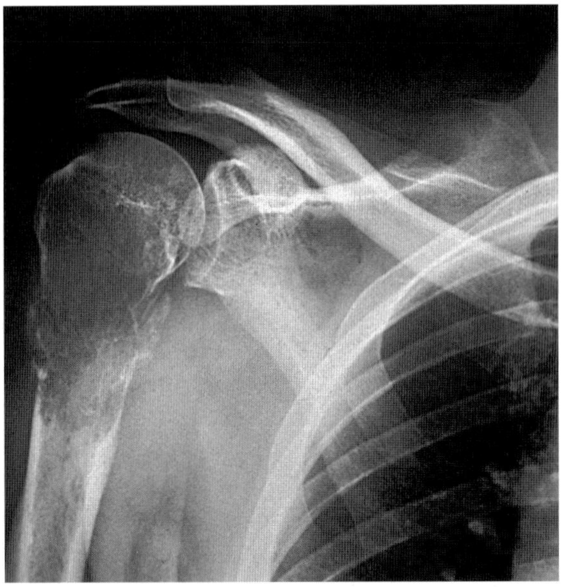

Figure 14-2

METASTATIC CARCINOMA

Metastatic renal cell carcinoma produces a lytic mass in the proximal humerus.

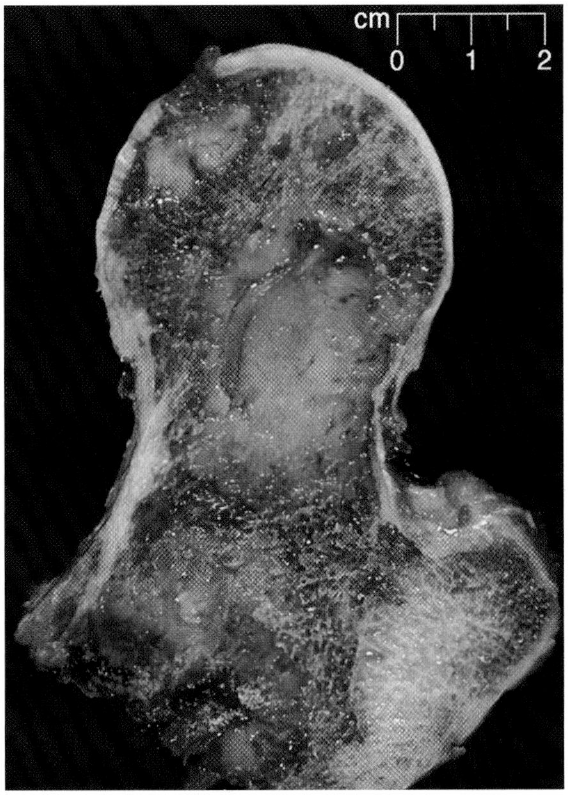

Figure 14-3

METASTATIC CARCINOMA

Proximal femur resected for extensive metastatic breast carcinoma.

destroyed, and a soft tissue mass may be present (fig. 14-2). The lesions may be purely lytic or blastic. Some tumors have a peculiar tendency to produce osteoblastic metastasis, for example, breast carcinoma and prostatic carcinoma. Metastatic hypernephromas tend to be purely lytic. Lung carcinoma may metastasize to the cortex of long bones and to the small bones of the hands and feet.

If metastatic carcinoma is purely medullary, it may be invisible on radiographs and bone scans (10). It was noted in an autopsy study of vertebrae that when metastasis involved the marrow spaces without evoking an osteoblastic response, only 7.1 percent of plain radiographs and 4 percent of bone scans were positive (10). Magnetic resonance imaging (MRI), however, showed all the lesions.

Gross Findings. No gross pathologic features are specific for metastatic carcinoma. Most metastases are soft and fleshy, with areas of necrosis (fig. 14-3). Some tumors may appear fibrotic or even bony hard. Metastatic follicular carcinoma of the thyroid may have the gross appearance of thyroid tissue, and metastatic renal cell carcinoma may have a characteristic yellow appearance.

Microscopic Findings. The microscopic appearance usually simulates the appearance of the primary neoplasm (fig. 14-4). Some metastatic carcinomas have such characteristic histologic features that the pathologist can pinpoint the primary site. Metastatic renal cell carcinoma and follicular carcinoma of the thyroid are obvious examples (fig. 14-5). Immunoperoxidase stains, for example, with prostate-specific antigen, are useful.

Some metastatic carcinomas have spindle-shaped cells and simulate a primary sarcoma; in these cases, sarcomatoid renal cell carcinoma is the usual primary tumor (fig. 14-6). Some metastatic carcinomas evoke so much osteoblastic reaction that the lesion simulates an osteosarcoma.

Cytologic Findings. Fine-needle aspiration (FNA) biopsy is a particularly useful technique for the diagnosis of metastatic bone lesions. In addition to identifying the metastatic nature of

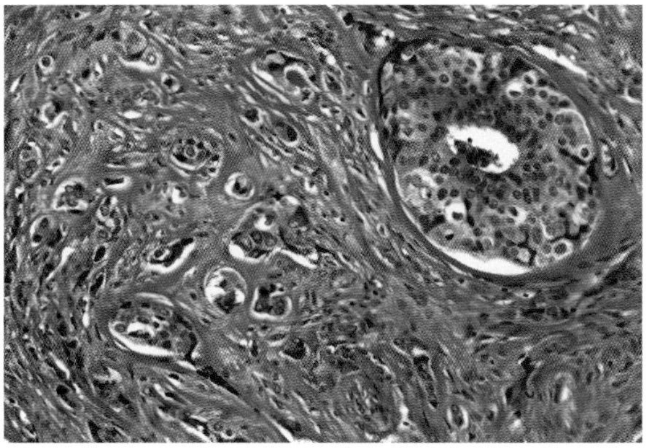

Figure 14-4

METASTATIC CARCINOMA

Metastatic breast carcinoma involves the proximal femur of a 51-year-old woman. The larger nest of tumor cells with central necrosis has features resembling ductal breast carcinoma. The tumor is associated with a fibrogenic stromal reaction.

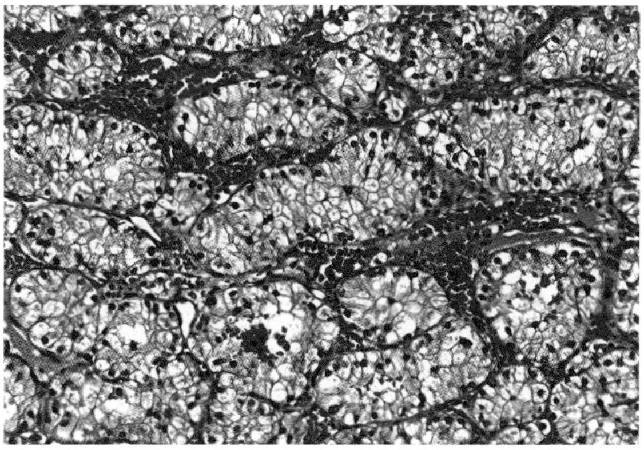

Figure 14-5

METASTATIC CARCINOMA

Metastatic renal cell carcinoma demonstrates characteristic clear cell features. The tumor is extremely vascular.

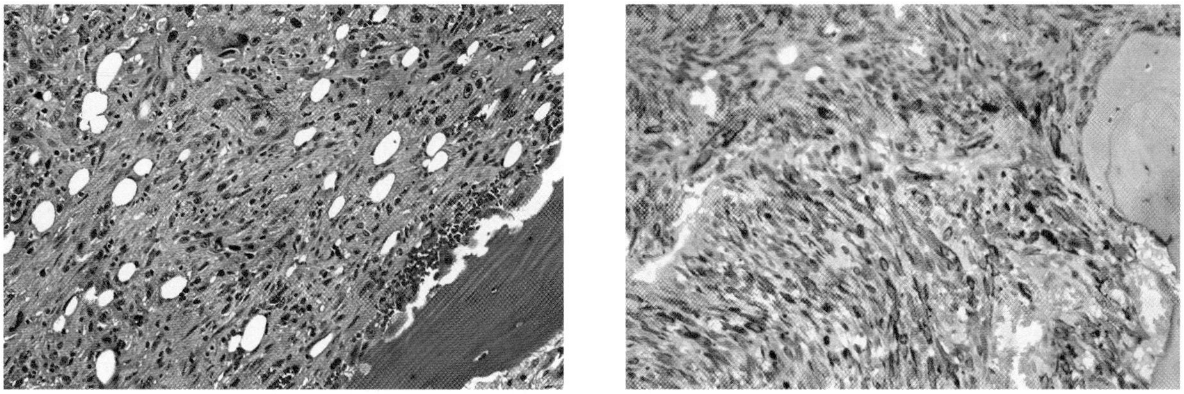

Figure 14-6

METASTATIC CARCINOMA

Left: This sarcomatoid carcinoma is composed of oval to spindle-shaped cells with prominent nucleoli. The histologic features are suggestive of a primary sarcoma involving bone.

Right: The tumor cells are immunoreactive with antibodies to keratin. This patient had a renal primary tumor with similar histologic features.

a bone lesion, FNA may also help to identify possible primary sites. Thus, the recognition of squamous, glandular, or melanocytic differentiation as well as features characteristic of small cell, signet ring, or clear cell carcinoma (the latter occurring in renal cell carcinoma) help direct further clinical and radiographic investigations (fig. 14-7) (2,5,9).

Differential Diagnosis. Most metastatic malignancies are not difficult to diagnose because the clinical features suggest the correct diagnosis. The possibility of a metastatic sarcomatoid renal cell carcinoma should be suspected in an older person with a spindle cell malignancy of bone. Sampling of the tumor usually shows the typical clear cell area; staining for epithelial markers and a thorough clinical work-up usually clarify the diagnosis. Rarely, however, one may have to report a spindle cell malignancy and suggest treatment as a fibrosarcoma if extensive work-up fails to demonstrate a primary site.

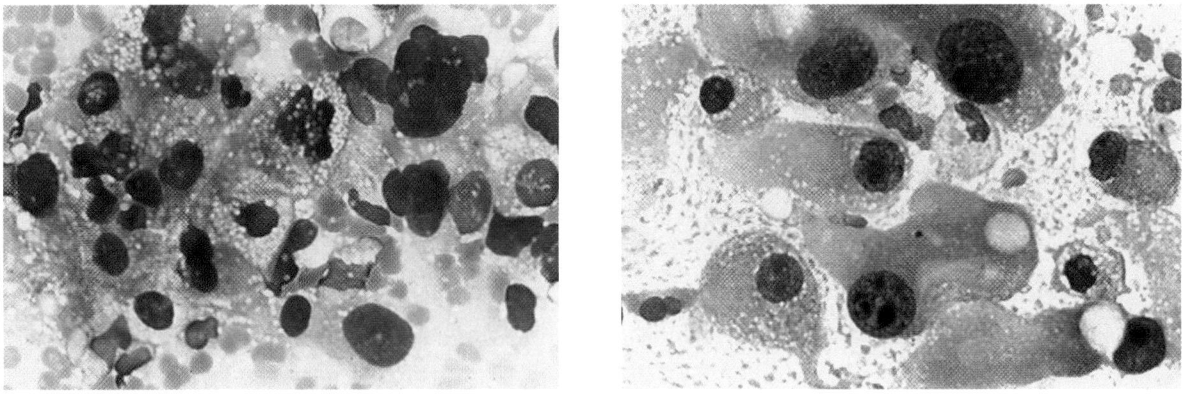

Figure 14-7

ASPIRATES FROM BONE METASTASES OF RENAL CELL CARCINOMA

Left: Atypical, pleomorphic tumor cells have epithelial features and irregular nuclei with coarse chromatin and prominent nucleoli.

Right: The large size of the tumor cells and the abundant, sometimes finely vacuolated cytoplasm superficially resemble the cytologic features of chordoma.

Some metastatic carcinomas produce large amounts of reactive bone. The reactive bone is usually trabecular (rather than the lace-like arrangement seen in high-grade osteosarcoma). Clinical features and the use of epithelial markers generally indicate the correct diagnosis.

Treatment and Prognosis. If the tumor has produced a pathologic fracture or radiographs suggest that a fracture is imminent, surgical intervention is indicated. The lesion may be curetted or the area of fracture resected. Further management depends on the primary neoplasm; hormonal manipulation is useful in cases of breast or prostatic carcinoma.

The prognosis also depends on the type of primary malignancy. Metastatic carcinoma of the breast, prostate, or thyroid may be associated with prolonged survival, but for many others (such as melanoma and lung carcinoma), skeletal metastases are terminal events.

CYSTIC LESIONS OF BONE THAT SIMULATE NEOPLASMS

Aneurysmal Bone Cyst

Definition. Aneurysmal bone cyst is a nonneoplastic, usually primary, condition of bone, which may grow at an alarming rate.

General Features. The cause of aneurysmal bone cyst is unknown, although a few have been documented to develop after a fracture (unpublished data). Because the lesions usually contain blood, it has been suggested they result from arteriovenous malformations (13,14).

It is not unusual to find aneurysmal bone cyst-like areas in other tumors and tumor-like conditions (18). These precursor lesions are almost always benign, and the aneurysmal bone cyst is a minor component of the process. However, the lesion may be predominantly cystic, and the primary lesion may be present as a mural nodule. Martinez and Sissons (19) reported that 28 percent of 123 aneurysmal bone cysts were secondary. Only primary aneurysmal bone cysts are discussed in this chapter. In the Mayo Clinic files, aneurysmal bone cysts are half as common as giant cell tumors. Until the beginning of 2000, the Mayo Clinic files contained 341 cases of aneurysmal bone cyst (fig. 14-8).

Clinical Features. Pain and swelling are the cardinal symptoms. Lesions of the spine may produce symptoms of spinal cord compression. There is a slight female predominance. Although aneurysmal bone cysts occur in any age group, most are seen in the first and second decades of life; of the cases in the Mayo Clinic files, 53 percent occurred during the second decade of life.

Sites. The region around the knee, including the distal femur and proximal tibia, is the most common site of aneurysmal bone cysts. The spine is frequently involved, most commonly the cervical spine. In the long bones, aneurysmal bone

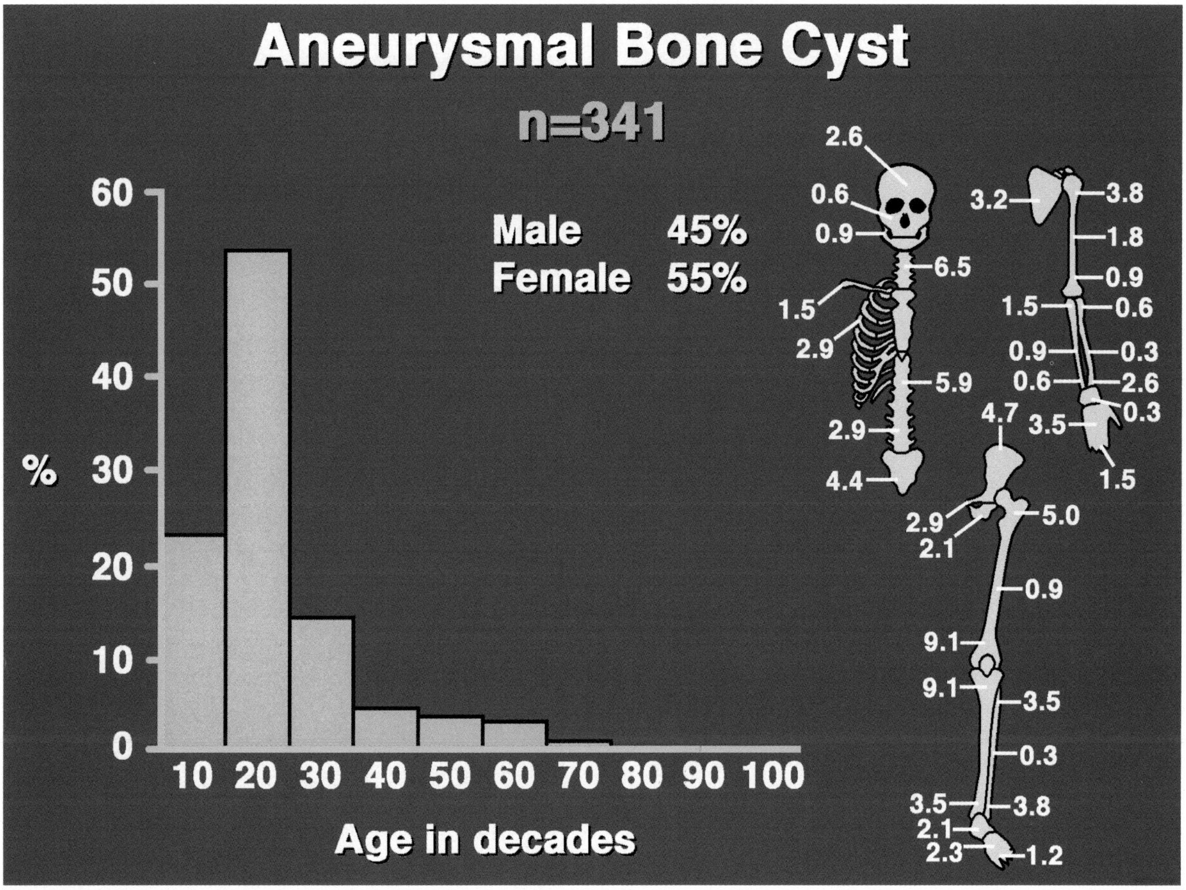

Figure 14-8

ANEURYSMAL BONE CYST

Distribution of aneurysmal bone cyst by the age and sex of the patient and the site of the lesion.

cysts tend to involve the metaphysis, whereas in the spine, they involve predominantly the posterior elements.

Radiographic Findings. The typical radiographic appearance of an aneurysmal bone cyst is an area of lucency situated eccentrically in the medullary cavity in the metaphysis of a long bone (fig. 14-9). However, the lesion may be central, cortical, or even on the surface of bone. The margins may be well or poorly defined. The lesion tends to grow rapidly; the cortex may be destroyed, and the lesion may bulge out into the soft tissue. Usually, a rim of calcification forms a shell around the soft tissue extension (fig. 14-10). The lesion is usually purely lytic, but traces of mineral may be present. Computerized tomography (CT) is helpful; it highlights the peripheral bony shell and demonstrates fluid-fluid levels in the lesion (16). Although this fluid-fluid level is highly characteristic of aneurysmal bone cysts, it is not specific. MRI demonstrates the internal septations that produce a honeycomb appearance and fluid-fluid levels (fig. 14-11).

Gross Findings. The lesions are usually curetted, and red-brown fragments are received in the laboratory (fig. 14-12). Frequently, the gross tumor is considerably smaller than expected from the dimensions seen on radiographs. If the lesion is resected, cystic spaces containing blood and separated by fibrous septa of varying thickness are found (fig. 14-13). Rarely, the entire lesion is solid, red, and granular.

Microscopic Findings. Under low-power magnification, an aneurysmal bone cyst has the appearance of multiple spaces separated by septa

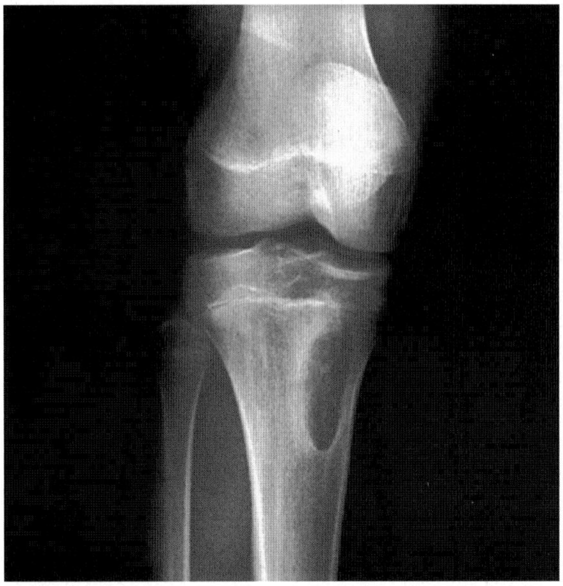

Figure 14-9

ANEURYSMAL BONE CYST

Aneurysmal bone cyst involves the proximal tibial metaphysis in a 14-year-old boy. The lesion is eccentric and purely lytic. (Courtesy of Dr. F. Shipkey, Jackson, MS.)

(fig. 14-14). The spaces contain blood or are empty. The septa lack an endothelial lining and consist of spindle cells, giant cells, capillaries, and varying amounts of matrix (fig. 14-15). The spindle cells have plump nuclei but are without hyperchromasia; mitotic figures are usually abundant. The cells are loosely arranged in a haphazard fashion. The appearance is "loose" because of capillary proliferation or edema. The giant cells are usually scattered randomly throughout the lesion, but they may form large sheets.

Osteoid and bony matrix may be prominent. Frequently, there is a thin layer of osteoid (fiber osteoid) in the septa just below the lining cells (fig. 14-16). Osteoid seams undergo calcification and mature to bony trabeculae in the more solid areas. This maturation is similar to that of heterotopic ossification.

Calcification is frequently present (fig. 14-17). The calcification is amorphous and may have a chondroid aura (25). Rarely, calcification is prominent and may form trabeculae around the septa.

A small proportion of aneurysmal bone cysts are completely solid (12,23). The histologic features are usually dominated by a loosely arranged spindle cell proliferation and prominent

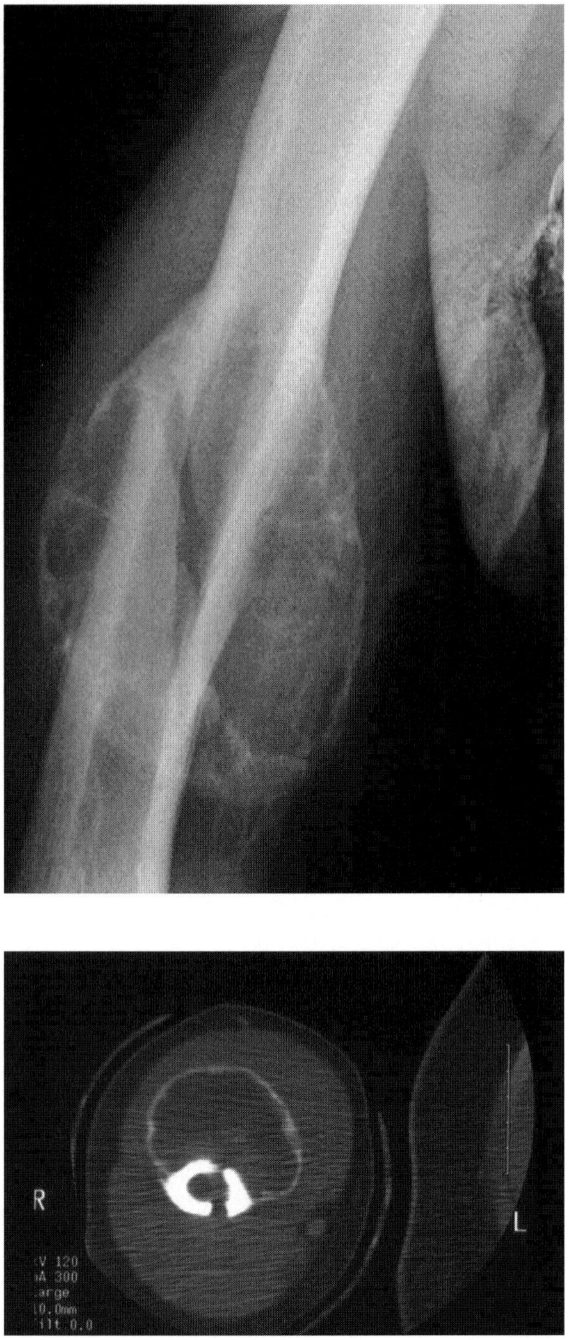

Figure 14-10

ANEURYSMAL BONE CYST

Top: Aneurysmal bone cyst, arising in the mid-humerus of a 17-year-old boy, is associated with a pathologic fracture. The lesion is outlined by a shell of ossification.

Bottom: Corresponding computerized tomography (CT) highlights the peripheral bony shell of the soft tissue component.

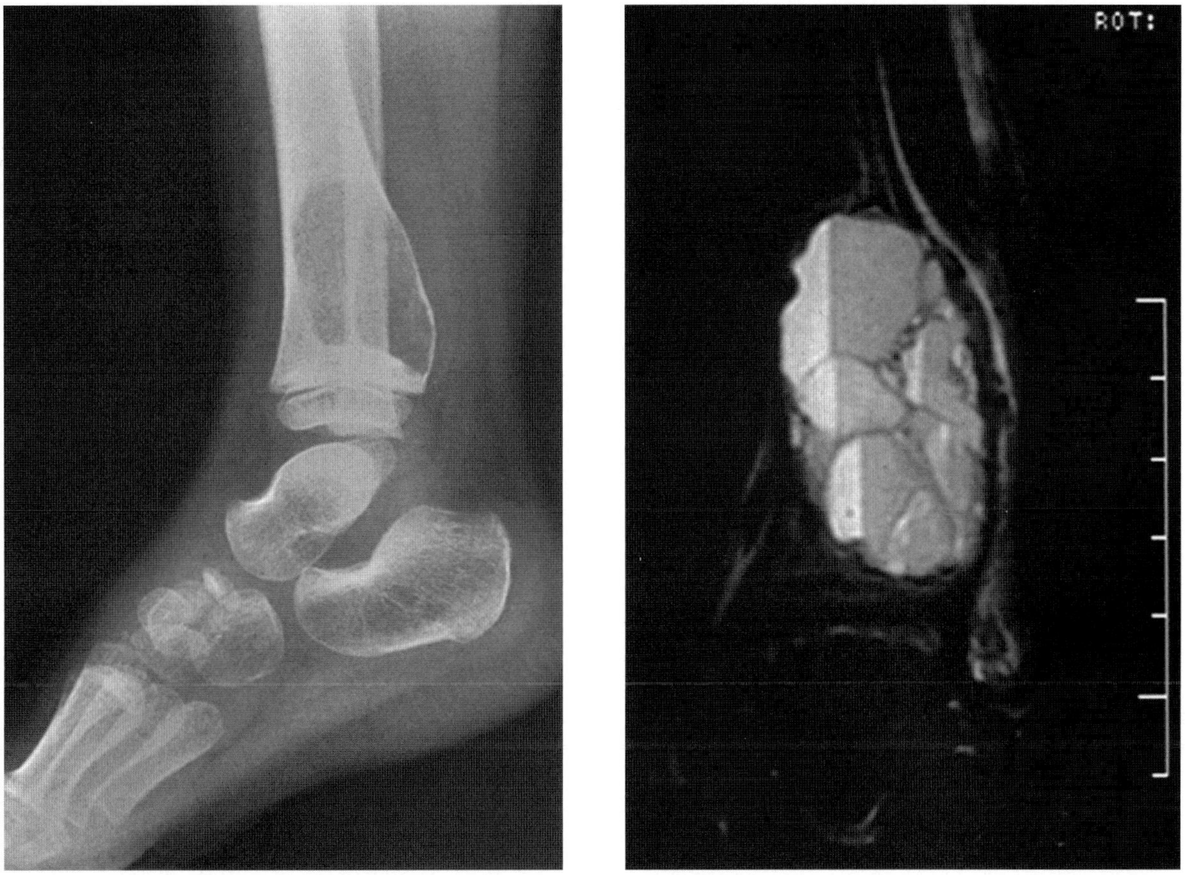

Figure 14-11

ANEURYSMAL BONE CYST

Plain radiograph (left) and corresponding magnetic resonance image (MRI) (right) of a typical aneurysmal bone cyst in a 4-year-old boy. MRI highlights septation and fluid-fluid levels. (Courtesy of Dr. S. Gurly, Phoenix, AZ.)

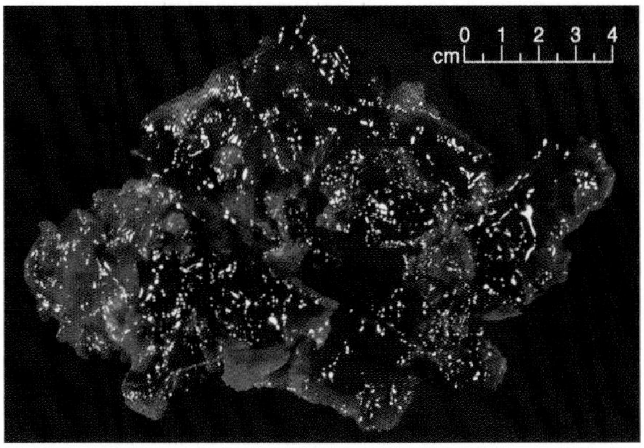

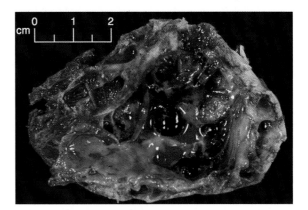

Figure 14-12

ANEURYSMAL BONE CYST

Gross specimen of lesion in figure 14-10. The curetted fragments show blood-filled spaces separated by septa.

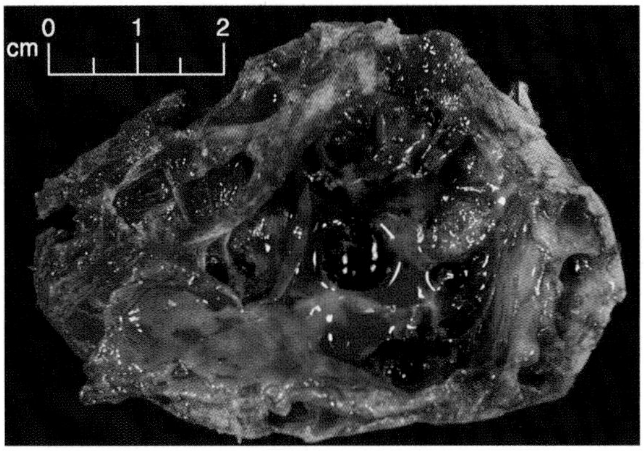

Figure 14-13

ANEURYSMAL BONE CYST

Hemicylindrical resection of the distal tibia for recurrent aneurysmal bone cyst. The cortex is thinned, and there are many delicate septa.

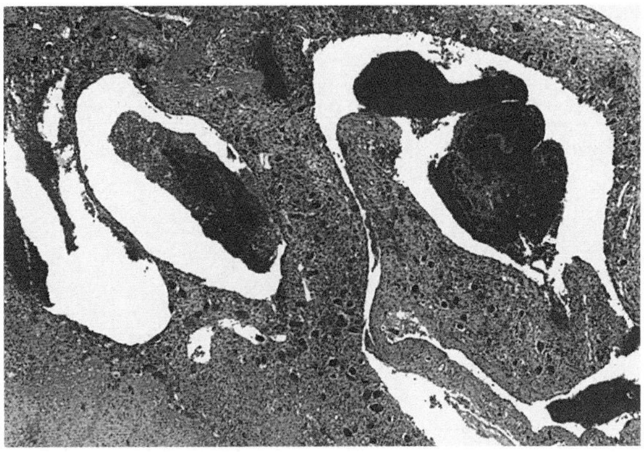

Figure 14-14

ANEURYSMAL BONE CYST

Irregularly shaped cystic spaces are surrounded by fibrous septa.

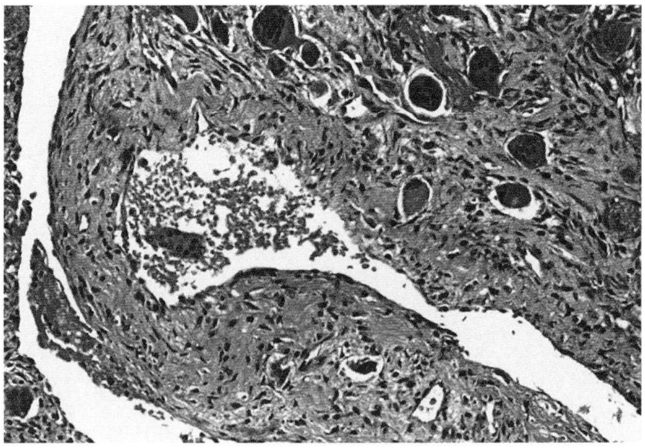

Figure 14-15

ANEURYSMAL BONE CYST

The septa contain spindle-shaped cells without cytologic atypia, multinucleated giant cells, and capillaries.

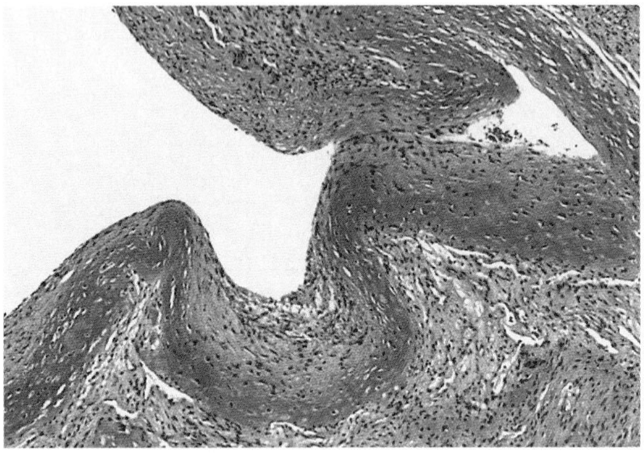

Figure 14-16

ANEURYSMAL BONE CYST

It is common to see pink parallel seams of osteoid in the septa.

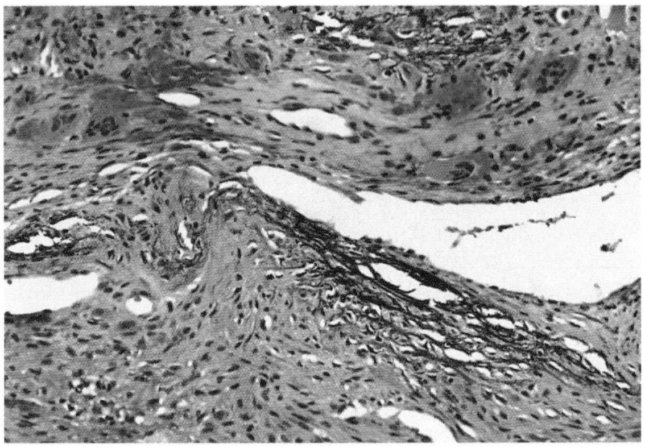

Figure 14-17

ANEURYSMAL BONE CYST

Lace-like or powdery calcification is seen within the septa.

osteoid and bone formation (fig. 14-18). The bony trabeculae tend to anastomose and to have a prominent osteoblastic rim. Deposits of blotchy purple calcification, as seen in the more conventional type of aneurysmal bone cyst, may also be present.

Genetics and Other Special Techniques. Clonal karyotypic abnormalities of chromosomal bands 16q22 and 17p13 are recurrent in aneurysmal bone cysts (including the solid variant and extraosseous forms) (fig. 14-19) (15,21, 24,26). Frequently, a reciprocal 16;17 translocation [t(16;17)(q22;p13)] is seen. In a subset of aneurysmal bone cysts, however, rearrangement of 17p13 with a chromosome partner other than 16q22 occurs and, conversely, 16q22 abnormalities exclusive of 17p13 abnormalities have also been detected (11,15,21). The chromosomal translocation t(16;17)(q22;p13) creates a chimeric gene in which the osteoblast cadherin 11 gene (*CDH11*) promoter region on 16q22 is juxtaposed to the entire ubiquitin-specific protease *USP6* (*Tre2*) coding sequence on 17p13 (20). *CDH11* is highly expressed in bone, indicating that *USP6* tumorigenic activity can result from transcription upregulation. The nonrandom alterations in aneurysmal bone cyst may serve as useful diagnostic markers of the lesion, particularly in the

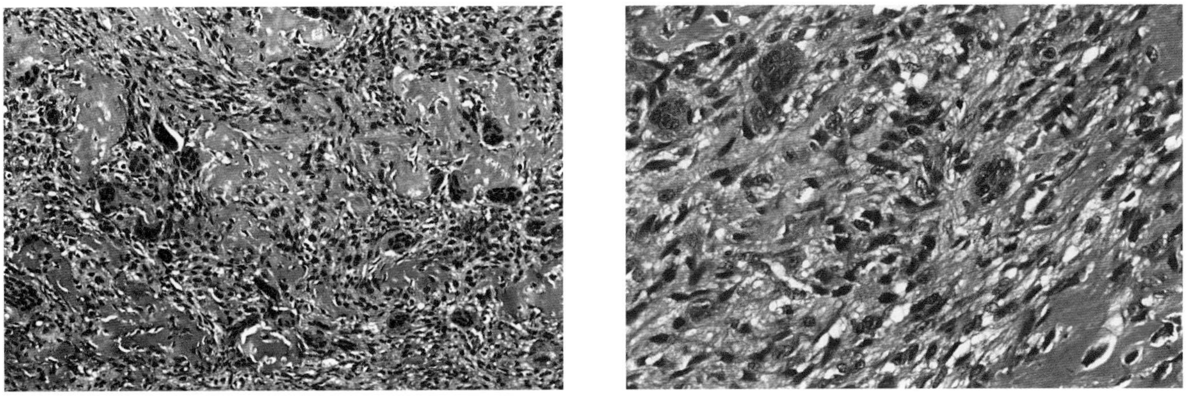

Figure 14-18

ANEURYSMAL BONE CYST

Left: A solid component of an aneurysmal bone cyst shows reactive bone production, multinucleated giant cells, and a cellular spindle cell stroma.

Right: The solid areas are mitotically active and have features similar to those of a giant cell tumor.

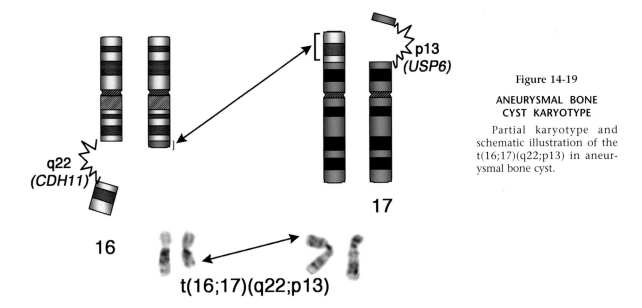

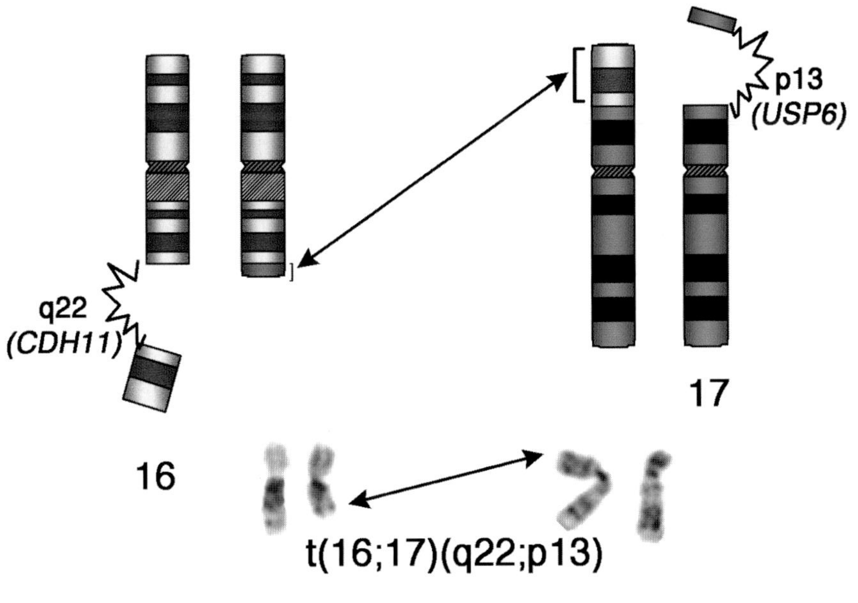

Figure 14-19

ANEURYSMAL BONE CYST KARYOTYPE

Partial karyotype and schematic illustration of the t(16;17)(q22;p13) in aneurysmal bone cyst.

differential diagnosis of telangiectatic osteosarcoma (the latter tends to exhibit numerous, complex karyotypic anomalies).

Alterations of a group of cell cycle regulator genes (*TP53, p16, RB, HDM2,* c-*myc,* and *ras*) were found to be rare in aneurysmal bone cysts and other benign osteoblastic tumors, in contrast to malignant osteoblastic tumors (22).

Differential Diagnosis. An aneurysmal bone cyst may be confused with many conditions, especially giant cell tumor, telangiectatic osteosarcoma, and low-grade osteosarcoma. The clinical presentation and radiographic features of a giant cell tumor are very different from those of an aneurysmal bone cyst. Giant cell tumors occur in skeletally mature patients and involve the ends of bones, whereas aneurysmal bone cysts occur in skeletally immature patients and are metaphyseal. Histologically, giant cell tumors are arranged compactly, whereas the tissue of aneurysmal bone cysts has a loose arrangement. The proliferating mononuclear cells in giant cell tumors are round to oval, whereas those in aneurysmal bone cysts are spindle shaped.

The clinical, radiographic, and gross features of telangiectatic osteosarcoma can be indistinguishable from those of aneurysmal bone cyst. However, the cells in the septa in telangiectatic osteosarcoma are highly pleomorphic, whereas those in aneurysmal bone cyst show no atypia.

The solid variant of aneurysmal bone cyst may be mistaken for a low-grade osteosarcoma. Paradoxically, aneurysmal bone cysts are more cellular and more active mitotically than low-grade osteosarcomas. The dense collagen between tumor cells in low-grade osteosarcomas is absent from aneurysmal bone cysts. The bony trabeculae in aneurysmal bone cysts are lined with osteoblasts, which is not a feature of low-grade osteosarcomas.

Treatment and Prognosis. Surgical excision, usually with curettage, is the treatment of choice. Recurrence is rare, and even incomplete removal may result in a cure. Malignant transformation, as reported by Kyriakos and Hardy (17), has not been reported in the cases in the Mayo Clinic files. However, the files contain three examples of postradiation sarcoma that developed after treatment of aneurysmal bone cysts.

Simple Cyst

Definition. Simple cyst, or *unicameral bone cyst*, is an intramedullary, almost invariably unilocular, cyst that contains clear yellow fluid.

General Features. The cause of simple cyst is not known. Chigira et al. (28) demonstrated that internal pressure is higher in the cyst than in normal bone marrow and suggested that venous outflow obstruction caused the cyst. Pathologists seldom receive biopsy specimens of simple cysts because they are no longer treated surgically.

Clinical Features. Simple cysts may produce pain, but a pathologic fracture usually draws attention to the lesion. Most patients are in the first two decades of life. A simple cyst may be an incidental radiographic finding in adults, especially in the calcaneus and ilium.

Sites. In children, the proximal humerus and proximal femur are the most common sites of simple cysts (27). In adults, the calcaneus and ilium are the common sites.

Radiographic Findings. Typically, a simple cyst is located centrally in the medullary cavity and abuts the epiphyseal plate (fig. 14-20). The lesion is no wider than the epiphyseal plate. The cortex is thinned but intact unless there is a pathologic fracture. The lesion appears trabeculated because of the bony ridges in the cortex. Occasionally, a fragment of bone appears to be floating within the cyst, the "fallen fragment" sign (31). In older children, the cyst may appear to be diaphyseal because of skeletal growth.

Gross Findings. Although the cyst may be empty, more often it contains clear yellow fluid. A thin membrane usually covers the bone.

Microscopic Findings. If the lesion is curetted, a few giant cells and fibroblasts are found in the membrane. Frequently, there is calcification, which has been likened to cementum (fig. 14-21). Septa that contain giant cells and spindle cells, as in aneurysmal bone cysts, may be found *(secondary aneurysmal bone cyst)* (fig. 14-22). A giant cell reaction to crystalline material may occur if the patient was treated previously with injections of corticosteroid.

Treatment and Prognosis. Scaglietti et al. (30) showed that most simple cysts can be treated successfully with aspiration of the fluid and injection of methylprednisolone acetate. Rarely, a recurrent tumor needs curettage and bone grafting. There are rare examples of sarcomas arising in simple cysts (29).

Intraosseous Ganglion

Definition. Intraosseous ganglion is a cyst that contains glairy mucinous fluid and is located next to the articular cartilage within the medullary cavity.

General Features. The gross and microscopic features resemble those of the more common ganglia of soft tissues. The features also are similar to those of cysts associated with degenerative joint disease. A ganglion of soft tissues may involve bone secondarily.

Clinical Features. Patients generally are asymptomatic and the lesions are incidental radiographic findings.

Sites. Schajowicz et al. (32) found that the hip region is the site involved most commonly by intraosseous ganglion. The distal tibia and fibula, the proximal tibia, and the carpal bones also are involved commonly.

Radiographic Findings. Radiographs show a well-defined lucency that abuts the articular cartilage and is surrounded frequently by a sclerotic rim (fig. 14-23).

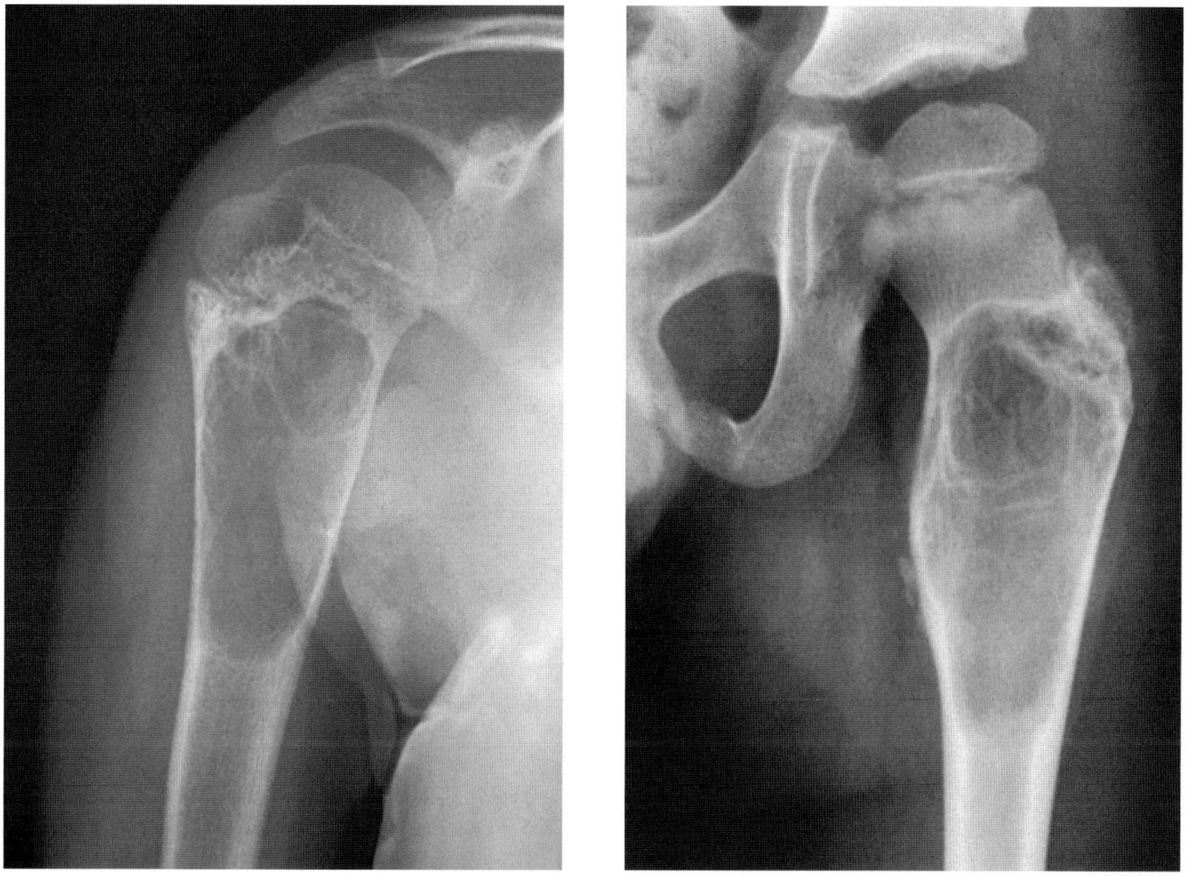

Figure 14-20

SIMPLE CYST

The simple cyst involves the most frequent sites: proximal humerus (left) and proximal femur (right). The lesion is central, extends to the epiphyseal plate, and does not widen the bone. (Left, courtesy of Dr. J. Bjornsson, Reykjavik, Iceland; right, courtesy of Dr. J. Lo, Chicago, IL.)

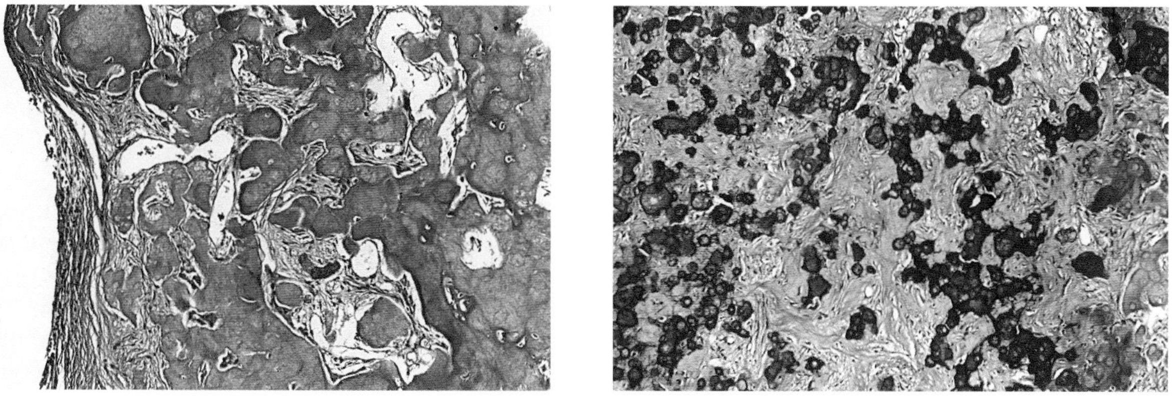

Figure 14-21

SIMPLE CYST

Left: Abundant irregular masses of degenerating fibrin are within the cyst wall.
Right: The fibrin deposits resemble cementum when they become calcified.

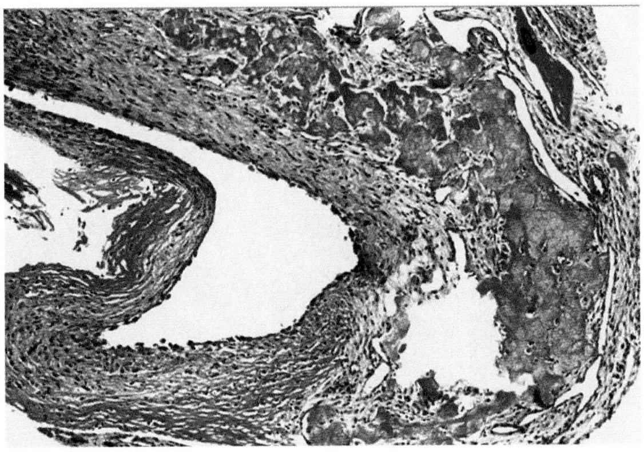

Figure 14-22

SIMPLE CYST

Occasionally, fibrous septa resemble those seen in aneurysmal bone cysts.

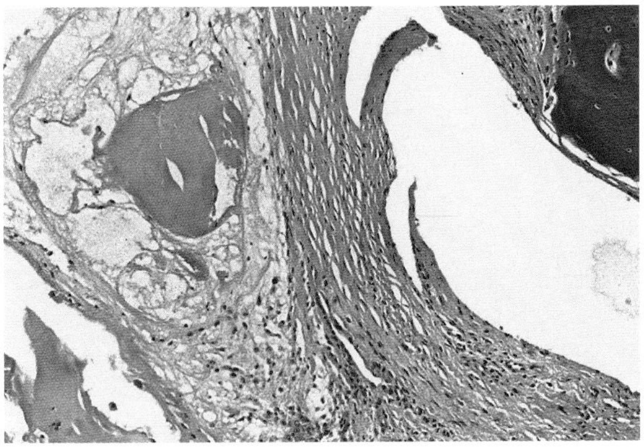

Figure 14-24

INTRAOSSEOUS GANGLION

Fibrous-walled cystic space contains mucinous material.

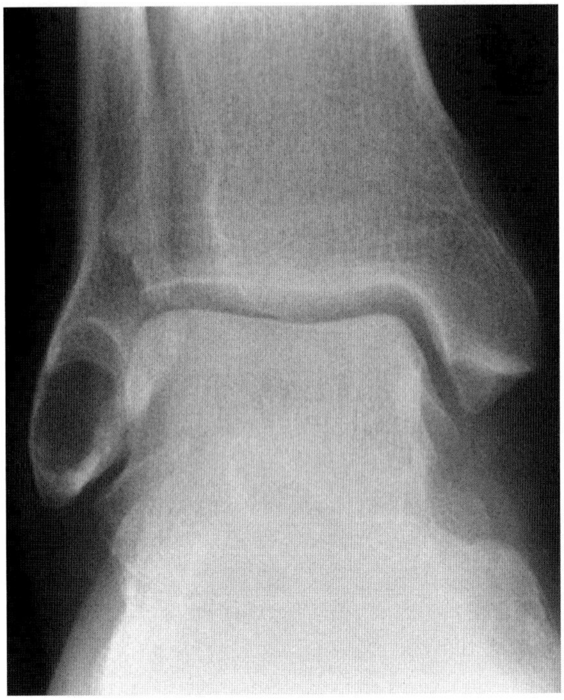

Figure 14-23

INTRAOSSEOUS GANGLION

Intraosseous ganglion presents as a well-circumscribed lucency in the distal fibula. (Fig. 27-69 from Unni KK. Dahlin's bone tumors: general aspects and data on 11,087 cases, 5th ed. Philadelphia: Lippincott-Raven; 1996:392. By permission of Mayo Foundation.)

Gross Findings. Curetted specimens show thin fibrous septa and thick mucinous material.

Microscopic Findings. The dominant microscopic feature is the acellular mucinous material (fig. 14-24). The lining may consist of a loosely arranged spindle cell proliferation in a myxoid background.

Differential Diagnosis. An intraosseous ganglion may be mistaken for other lesions containing myxoid material, for example, chondrosarcoma and chondromyxoid fibroma. Chondrosarcoma may have foci of acellular myxoid matrix, but sampling always shows typical cellular areas. Chondromyxoid fibroma has a lobulated growth pattern and rarely has a liquefied myxoid matrix. Cysts of degenerative joint disease are very similar to intraosseous ganglia; radiographic evidence of degenerative joint disease in the former is the only distinguishing feature.

Treatment and Prognosis. Surgical excision with curettage is usually curative.

Epidermoid Cyst

Definition. An epidermoid cyst is a cyst lined with squamous epithelium and filled with keratin.

General Features. Squamous-lined cysts (dentigerous cysts and keratocysts) are relatively common in the jawbones, but they are not included in this discussion. Otherwise, in the skeleton, epidermoid cysts are found only in the skull and distal phalanges (33). In the skull, they probably are developmental defects, and in the fingers, they probably represent traumatic implantation of squamous epithelium.

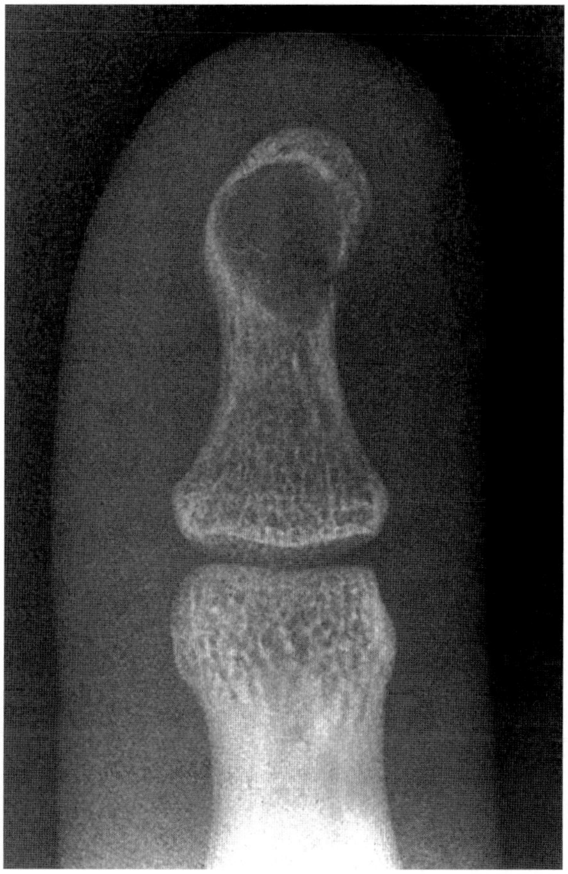

Figure 14-25

EPIDERMOID CYST

A typical location of an epidermoid cyst is in the distal phalanx of a finger. The well-demarcated lucent defect has sclerotic borders.

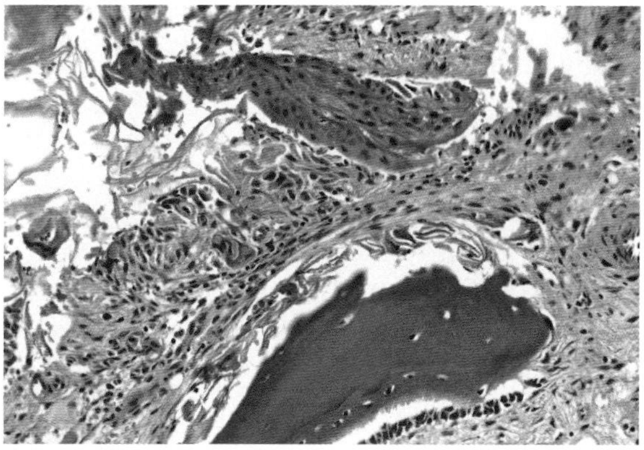

Figure 14-26

EPIDERMOID CYST

Fragments of the squamous-lined cyst wall and keratinous debris are adjacent to the surrounding bone.

Clinical Features. In the skull, epidermoid cysts may be expansile and compress the brain. In the phalanges, they are usually incidental radiographic findings.

Sites. As mentioned above, epidermoid cysts occur in the skull and distal phalanges of the hands.

Radiographic Findings. Epidermoid cysts appear as sharply demarcated lucencies with a rim of reactive sclerosis (fig. 14-25).

Gross Findings. Curetted material has the white pasty appearance of keratin.

Microscopic Findings. The cyst lining consists of mature squamous epithelium. Part of the lining may be destroyed and associated with a foreign-body giant cell reaction. The cavity contains keratinous debris (fig. 14-26).

Treatment and Prognosis. Curettage is the treatment of choice. If part of the lining is left, the cyst may recur.

Subungual Keratoacanthoma

Definition. Subungual keratoacanthoma is a proliferating squamous epithelial lesion of the nail bed with a pronounced tendency to invade the underlying bone.

Clinical Features. Patients complain of a painful, rapidly progressive swelling of the nail bed (35). On physical examination, the distal portion of the finger is swollen, indurated, and erythematous.

Sites. The distal phalanx of a toe or finger is involved.

Radiographic Findings. Subungual keratoacanthoma appears as a sharply circumscribed lytic defect (fig. 14-27) (34).

Gross Findings. The tumor contains large amounts of keratinous debris.

Microscopic Findings. The microscopic appearance is similar to that of the more common keratoacanthoma of skin. A cup-shaped depression contains keratin; large squamous cells with glassy cytoplasm proliferate at the edges (fig. 14-28).

Differential Diagnosis. Rarely, a well-differentiated squamous cell carcinoma arises in the nail bed and invades the underlying bone (36). Radiographs of a well-differentiated squamous cell sarcoma show a permeative process, whereas

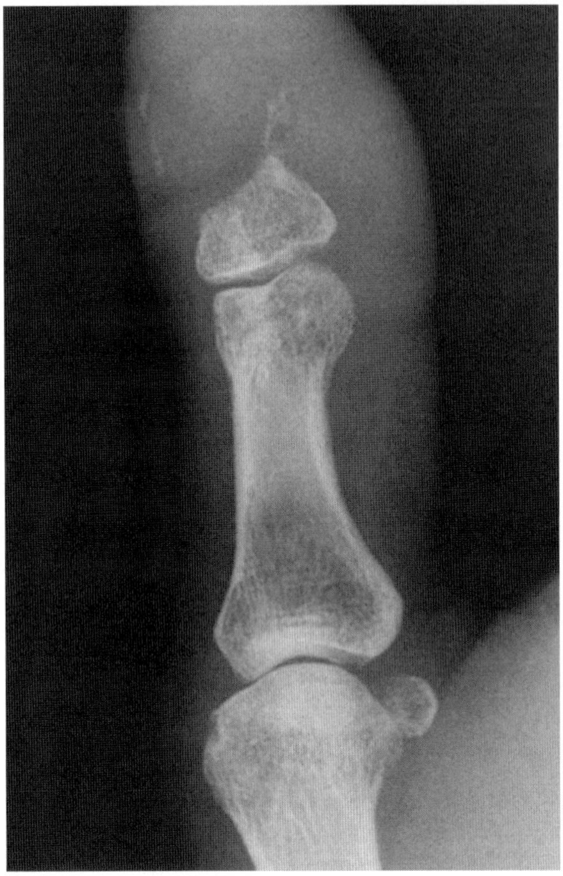

Figure 14-27

SUBUNGUAL KERATOACANTHOMA

Subungual keratoacanthoma produces a destructive lesion in the distal phalanx. Even though the appearance may be alarming, the bony outlines are maintained. (Fig. 27-76 from Unni KK. Dahlin's bone tumors: general aspects and data on 11,087 cases, 5th ed. Philadelphia: Lippincott-Raven; 1996:394. By permission of Mayo Foundation.)

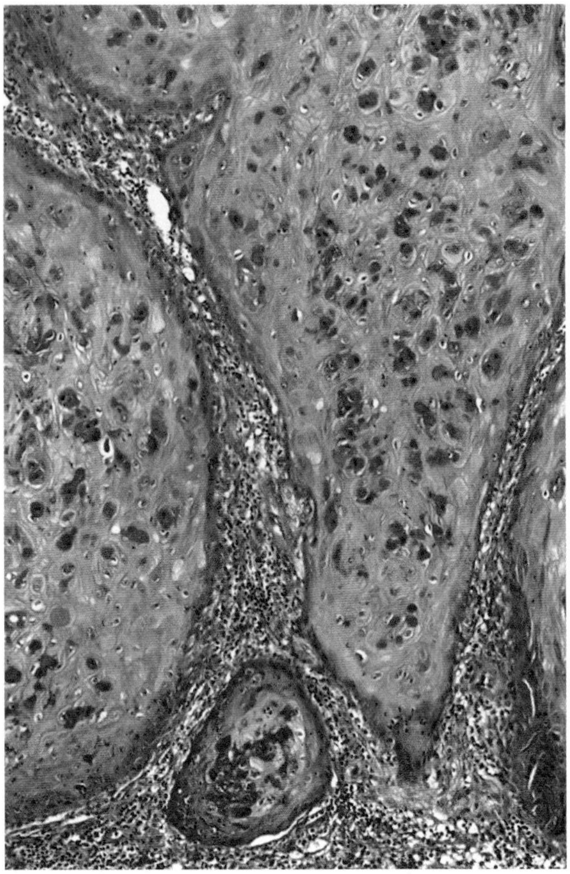

Figure 14-28

SUBUNGUAL KERATOACANTHOMA

Proliferating squamous epithelial cells with intracytoplasmic keratin.

a subungual keratoacanthoma is sharply demarcated. Microscopically, well-differentiated squamous cells permeate bony trabeculae; permeation is not found in subungual keratoacanthoma.

Treatment and Prognosis. The process is self-limited and may even regress spontaneously. If treatment is initiated, it should be conservative surgical removal.

FIBROUS LESIONS OF BONE THAT SIMULATE NEOPLASMS

Several non-neoplastic conditions of bone that are composed of predominantly spindle cells may be classified as "fibrous."

Metaphyseal Fibrous Defect

Definition. Metaphyseal fibrous defect is a spindle cell proliferation that involves the cortex or cortex and medullary cavity in the metaphysis of long bones of children; it has a tendency to resolve spontaneously.

General Features. The term *fibrous cortical defect* refers to the process confined to the cortex. If the medullary cavity is also involved, the term *nonossifying* or *nonosteogenic fibroma* has been used. The presence of foam cells and the arrangement of spindle cells in a storiform pattern have led to the term *fibroxanthoma*. That the lesion is relatively common in children and tends to resolve spontaneously suggests it is non-neoplastic and almost certainly a defect in ossification,

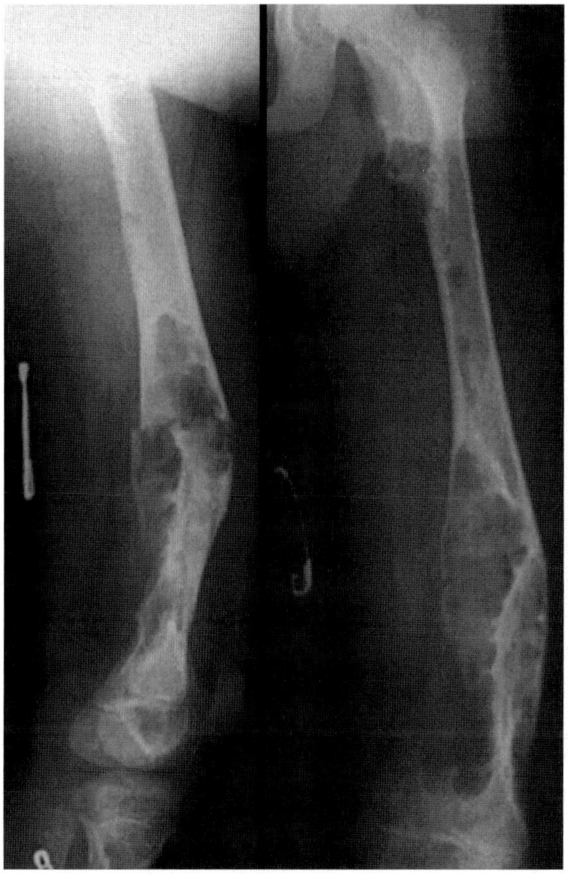

Figure 14-29

METAPHYSEAL FIBROUS DEFECT

Extensive lesions of polyostotic metaphyseal fibrous defect involve the distal femur. There is an associated pathologic fracture.

hence the term *metaphyseal fibrous defect*, which also has the advantage of pinpointing the site.

It is not unusual for a patient to have two or three lesions (38). Rarely, a patient presents with multiple lesions with bone deformities, café au lait spots, and other congenital anomalies (fig. 14-29) (39,41).

Metaphyseal fibrous defects are relatively common; it has been suggested that, based on a skeletal survey, 35 percent of children between 4 and 8 years old have a metaphyseal fibrous defect. However, patients are rarely symptomatic and, hence, the lesion is under-represented in a surgical series. Until the year 2000, the Mayo Clinic files contained the records of 137 cases of metaphyseal fibrous defect (fig. 14-30).

Clinical Features. The lesions are usually incidental radiographic findings. Rarely, localized pain is reported. Occasionally, pathologic fracture brings the lesion to attention. There is a slight male predominance. Metaphyseal fibrous defect is almost exclusively a disease of the first two decades of life. In the Mayo Clinic files, the oldest patient was 37 years.

Sites. The metaphysis of long bones around the knee is the most common site. Rarely, an identical lesion is found in a flat bone.

Radiographic Findings. In long bones, a metaphyseal fibrous defect starts in the metaphysis and is aligned along the long axis of the bone. The lesion is usually eccentric, although occasionally the entire width of the bone is involved (fig. 14-31). The lesion appears lobulated, with a sclerotic margin, creating a scalloped appearance. It may bulge into the cortex, thinning it. If the lesion is confined to the cortex, it is smaller, lucent, and sharply circumscribed. In the rare event that a metaphyseal fibrous defect is found in an adult, the process may occur in the shaft because the epiphyseal plate has grown away from the lesion. The lesion frequently appears mineralized, an attempt at healing.

Gross Findings. Rarely is a lesion removed intact; however, one may be present in a bone removed for some other process. The lesion is granular and red, with areas of brown and yellow discoloration (fig. 14-32). It is well demarcated and lobulated.

Microscopic Findings. A metaphyseal fibrous defect is composed of plump spindle cells arranged in a loose storiform pattern (fig. 14-33). Usually, benign multinucleated giant cells are scattered throughout the lesion. Rarely, the giant cells form large sheets. The spindle cells lack cytologic atypia, but mitotic activity is frequent (fig. 14-34). Foam cells are always present, either singly or in clusters, and histiocytes contain iron pigment (fig. 14-35). Although the name *nonossifying fibroma* suggests that there is no matrix formation, this is not always the case. Foci of reactive new bone may be present. In adults, much of the lesion may consist of bony trabeculae that fill in the defect. Necrosis is present only if a fracture has occurred. Geographic areas of necrosis with an infarct-like quality may be present.

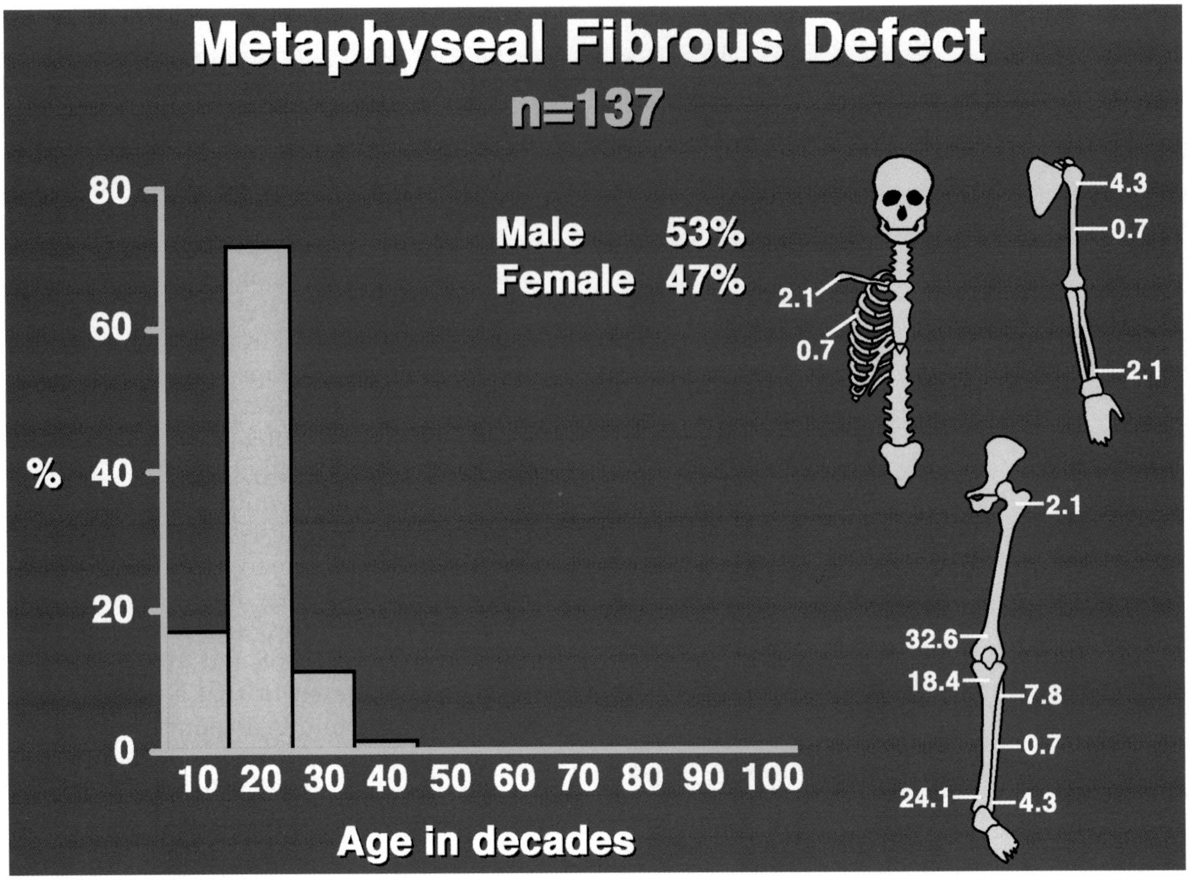

Figure 14-30

METAPHYSEAL FIBROUS DEFECT

Distribution of metaphyseal fibrous defect by the age and sex of the patient and the site of the lesion.

Genetics and Other Special Techniques. Two cases of metaphyseal fibrous defect have reportedly exhibited clonal karyotypic abnormalities: 46,XX,del(4)(p14) (43) and 46,XX, t(1;4)(p31;q34) (42).

Differential Diagnosis. The differential diagnosis involves giant cell tumor and a fibrohistiocytic neoplasm. The characteristic location in the metaphysis and the radiographic appearance of sclerotic margins are helpful features. The spindle cells with a storiform pattern so typical of metaphyseal fibrous defects are not seen in the diagnostic areas of giant cell tumors. Some authors consider a metaphyseal fibrous defect to be of fibrohistiocytic origin. The term *benign fibrous histiocytoma* is applied only if the lesion occurs in an adult and in an unusual location.

Treatment and Prognosis. No treatment is necessary unless fracture is imminent (37). In that case, simple curettage with bone grafting is adequate treatment. If a sarcoma is adjacent to a metaphyseal fibrous defect, it probably is a coincidence and not a cause-and-effect process (40).

Periosteal Desmoid (Avulsive Cortical Irregularity)

Definition. Periosteal desmoid is an irregularity of cortex found incidentally in the distal femur.

General Features. The term *periosteal desmoid* (43) was suggested because of the hypocellular spindle cell proliferation. However, the term is unfortunate because "desmoid" may suggest a true neoplasm. The term *avulsive cortical irregularity* is more appropriate. The process is considered to be the result of muscle stress from the insertion of the adductor magnus. The lesion is relatively common, but its exact incidence is not known.

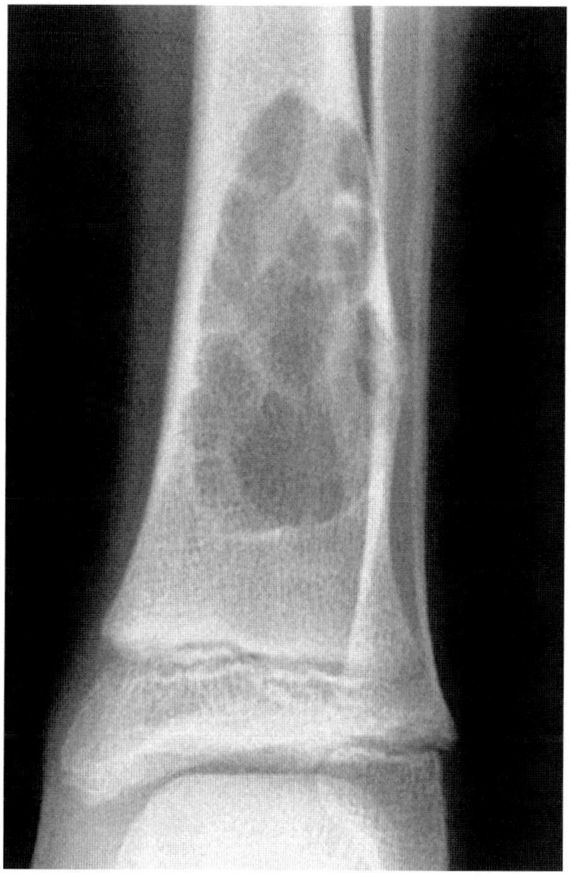

Figure 14-31

METAPHYSEAL FIBROUS DEFECT

Plain radiograph shows a well-demarcated lucency with lobulated borders.

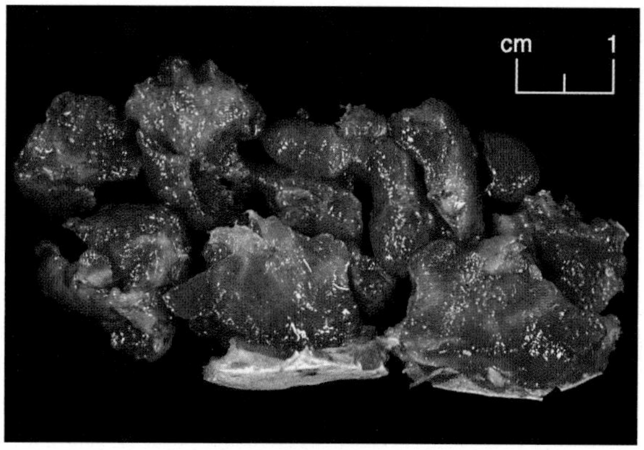

Figure 14-32

METAPHYSEAL FIBROUS DEFECT

A red-brown tumor has areas of golden yellow discoloration.

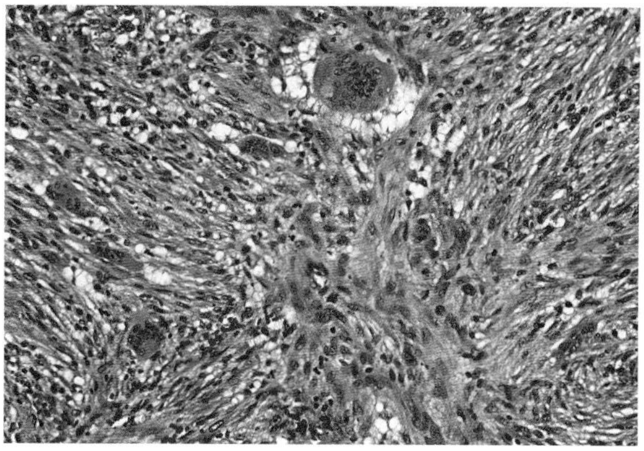

Figure 14-33

METAPHYSEAL FIBROUS DEFECT

Multinucleated giant cells are scattered throughout a spindle cell stroma, forming a storiform pattern.

Clinical Features. Most lesions are incidental findings, although some patients complain of pain. The process is found most commonly in adolescent boys (44).

Sites. The posteromedial aspect of the distal femur is the only site of involvement.

Radiographic Findings. Radiographs show a radiolucency arranged longitudinally along the posteromedial cortex of the distal femur (fig. 14-36).

Gross Findings. Grossly, the bone shows a thin strip of fibrous tissue.

Microscopic Findings. Biopsy specimens show a hypocellular spindle cell proliferation that replaces part of the cortex. The spindle cells do not have cytologic atypia.

Genetics and Other Special Techniques. Molecular cytogenetic analysis of a periosteal desmoid tumor showed extra copies of chromosomes 8 and 20, findings similar to those observed in desmoid tumor of soft tissue (45).

Differential Diagnosis. Periosteal desmoid may be mistaken for a low-grade spindle cell neoplasm. Correlation with the radiographic appearance is critical to avoid this mistake.

Treatment and Prognosis. No treatment is necessary. The process is self-healing.

Fibrous Dysplasia

Definition. Fibrous dysplasia is a defect in ossification that leads to fibrous proliferation and spicules of disorganized bone in the medullary

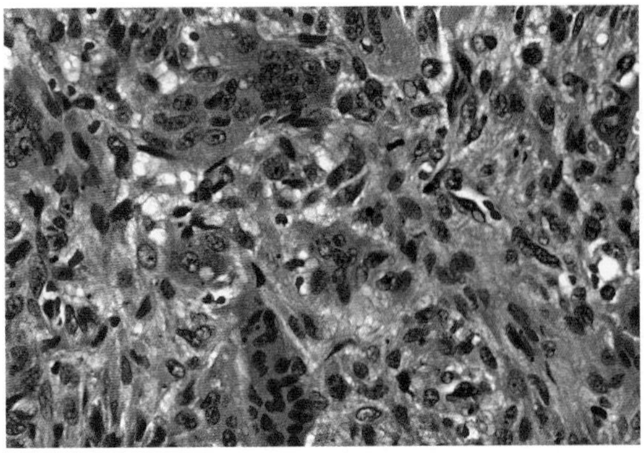

Figure 14-34

METAPHYSEAL FIBROUS DEFECT

Mitotic figures are commonly seen.

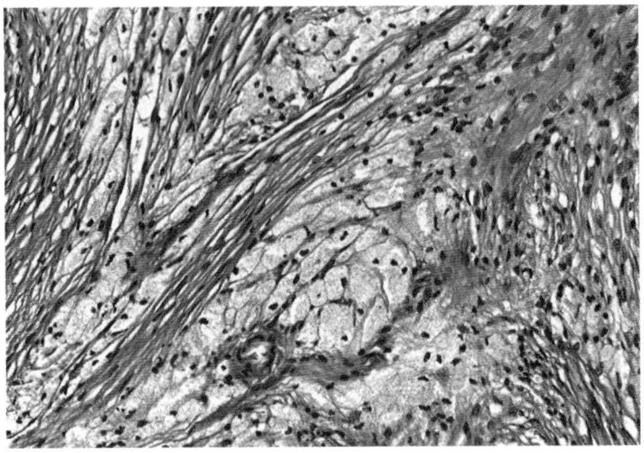

Figure 14-35

METAPHYSEAL FIBROUS DEFECT

Clusters of foam cells occur within a fibrogenic stroma.

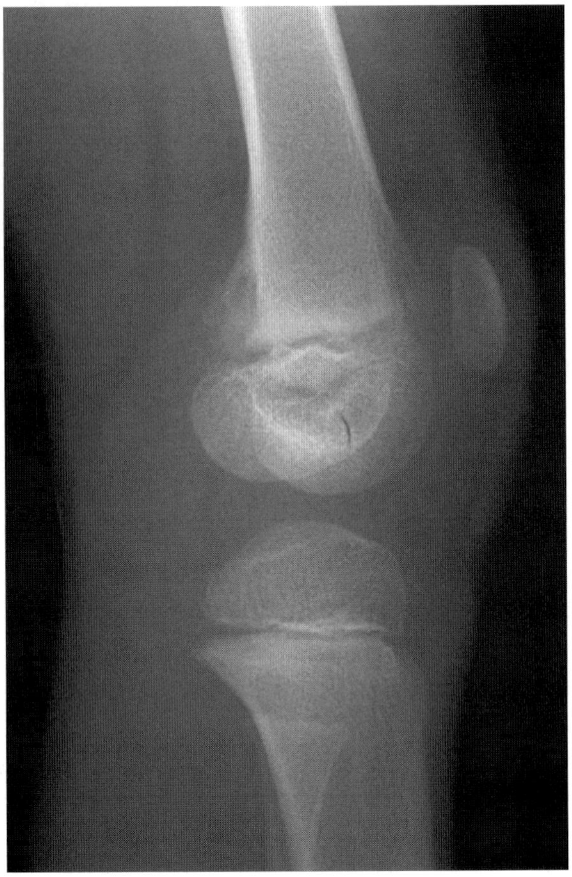

Figure 14-36

PERIOSTEAL DESMOID

The lesion presents as an area of lucency in the distal posterior cortex of the femur. (Courtesy of Dr. F. Pikul, Belleville, IL.)

cavity. It may involve a single skeletal site (monostotic) or multiple sites (polyostotic).

General Features. The cause of fibrous dysplasia is unknown. Although the term "metaplastic bone" is used for the bony trabeculae in the lesional tissue, a recent study has demonstrated that the stromal cells are not fibroblasts but preosteogenic cells (61).

The incidence of fibrous dysplasia is not known because many patients are asymptomatic. Until 1971, more than 1,500 cases had been reported (57). The Mayo Clinic files contain the records of 631 cases (fig. 14-37).

Clinical Features. The clinical features depend on the site of involvement and whether the disease is monostotic or polyostotic. In long bones, the lesions usually are incidental radiographic findings. Lesions in the region of the femoral neck may produce pathologic fracture. Patients with involvement of the jawbones have swelling or deformities. Patients with skull lesions may be asymptomatic or have swelling.

In a report from Mayo Clinic, almost half of the lesions were polyostotic (65). However, this was a surgical series, and undoubtedly polyostotic disease, which is more likely to cause symptoms, was over-represented. Nager et al. (57) reported that about 30 percent of lesions are polyostotic. Only 3 percent of patients have polyostotic disease with endocrine disturbances. Polyostotic fibrous dysplasia with endocrine disturbances, especially precocious puberty in girls, constitutes *Albright's syndrome*.

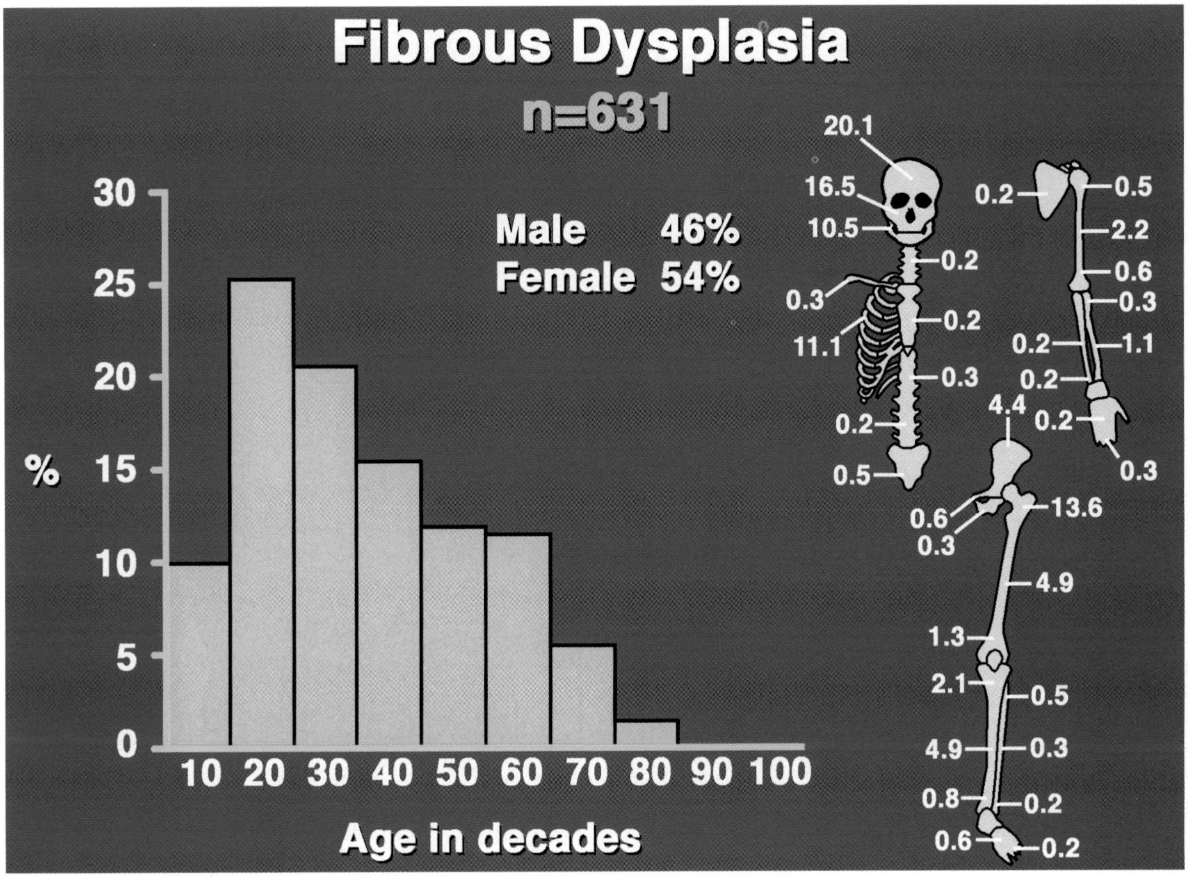

Figure 14-37

FIBROUS DYSPLASIA

Distribution of fibrous dysplasia by the age and sex of the patient and the site of the lesion.

Skin pigmentation is the most frequent extraskeletal manifestation and is rarely seen in the monostotic form. However, it occurs in about 50 percent of patients who have polyostotic disease and is almost always present in those with Albright's syndrome. Other associated disorders are hyperthyroidism, Cushing's syndrome, and hyperparathyroidism. McArthur et al. (55) described four patients who had fibrous dysplasia and hypophosphatemic osteomalacia. Kaplan et al. (54) described a patient with Albright's syndrome who experienced the rapid growth of two lesions during pregnancy. In this patient, osteogenic cells contained estrogen and progesterone receptors.

Patients usually present with disease in the first two decades of life. Patients who have polyostotic disease are younger and those with rib lesions are older (fig. 14-38). There is a slight female predominance.

Sites. The long bones are involved most commonly, with the femoral neck region being the most common site. The jawbones, skull, and ribs are involved in decreasing order.

Radiographic Findings. Fibrous dysplasia appears as a well-defined zone of rarefaction (fig. 14-39). Often, the lucency is surrounded by a thick bony rind. In the ribs, the lesions tend to be expansile; occasionally, the process becomes massive (fig. 14-40). In the jawbones, the lesions are not well defined. Often, a hazy mineralization within the lesion produces a "ground-glass" appearance. Some lesions, especially ones in the head and neck, are radiopaque. Rarely, an aggressive lytic component is present; this usually represents a superimposed aneurysmal bone cyst

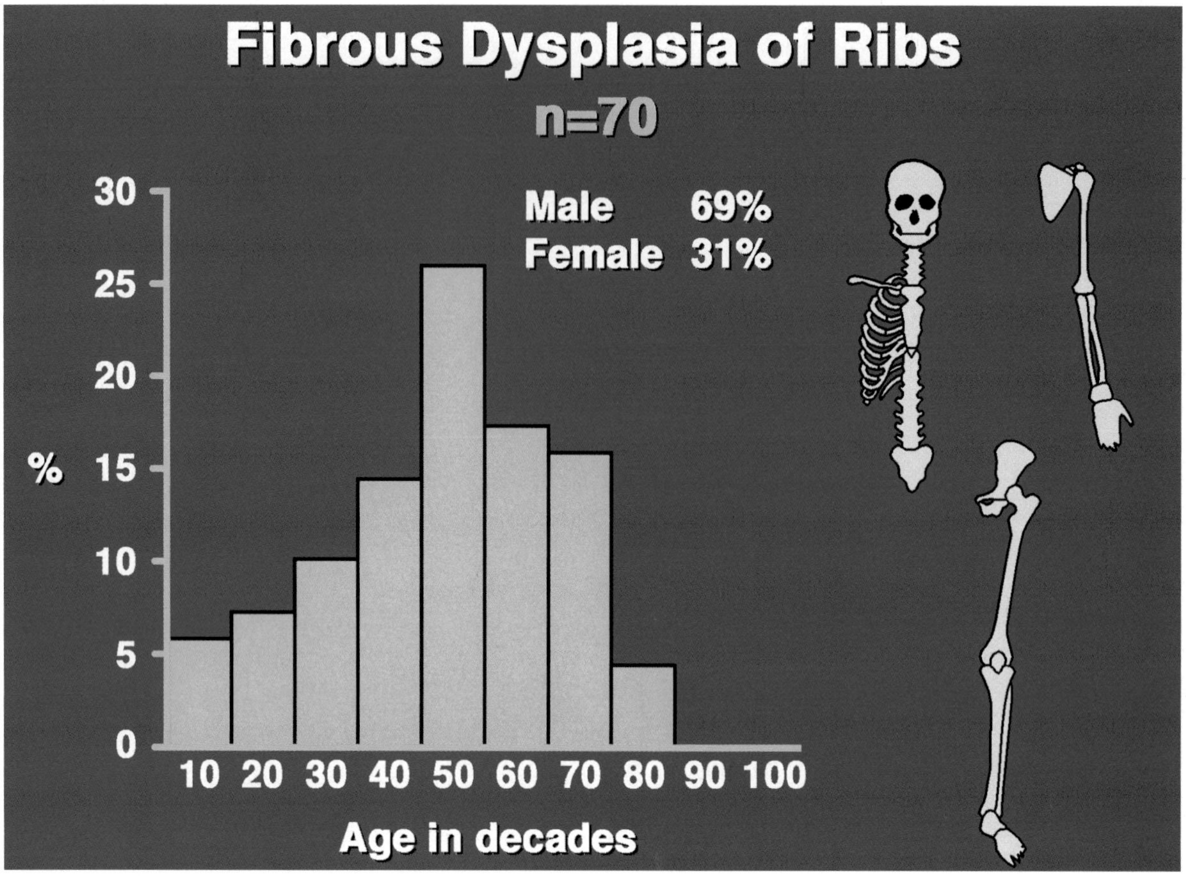

Figure 14-38

FIBROUS DYSPLASIA

Distribution of fibrous dysplasia of the ribs by the age and sex of the patient.

(fig. 14-41). Punctate calcification suggests cartilaginous areas. On MRI, the lesions show low signal intensity on T_1-weighted images and high signal intensity on T_2-weighted images (53).

Gross Findings. If the lesion is resected intact, as with rib lesions, the bone appears expanded and the cortex thinned (fig. 14-42). The bone marrow is replaced with dense, white fibrous tissue that feels gritty on sectioning due to the presence of bony spicules. Yellow areas, if present, suggest collections of foam cells. The lesion may be partly cystic.

Microscopic Findings. In fibrous dysplasia, the bone marrow is replaced with a mixture of stromal cells and bony spicules (fig. 14-43). Under low-power magnification, the lesion appears sharply demarcated from the surrounding bone marrow. The stroma is hypocellular and composed of plump spindle cells that lack the tapered nuclei typically associated with such cells (fig. 14-44). There is no cytologic atypia, and mitotic activity is rare. Bony spicules are distributed more or less evenly throughout the lesion, although there may be large areas of spindle cells without matrix. In these areas, the cells may have a storiform pattern. The bony spicules are shaped irregularly (C shaped or comma shaped) and typically show no osteoblastic rimming. However, the presence of osteoblastic activity does not rule out the diagnosis of fibrous dysplasia. The bony trabeculae typically are the woven type, although lamellar bone may occur, especially in the jawbones (fig. 14-45).

The bony spicules may be spherical and psammomatous, especially in the jawbones and base of the skull (fig. 14-46). Some authors have

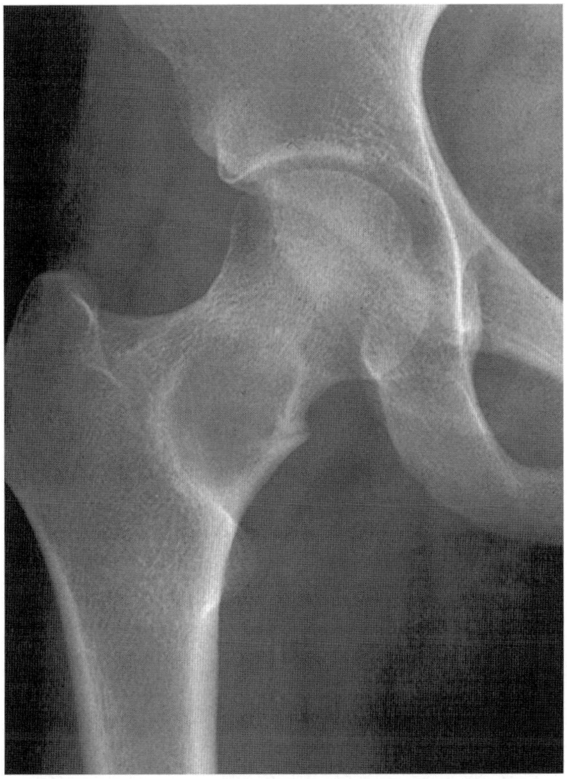

Figure 14-39

FIBROUS DYSPLASIA

Plain radiograph shows a lucent, well-marginated lesion of the femoral neck with a thick sclerotic rim and a healing pathologic fracture through the medial neck. (Courtesy of Dr. R. Gaffney, Albuquerque, NM.)

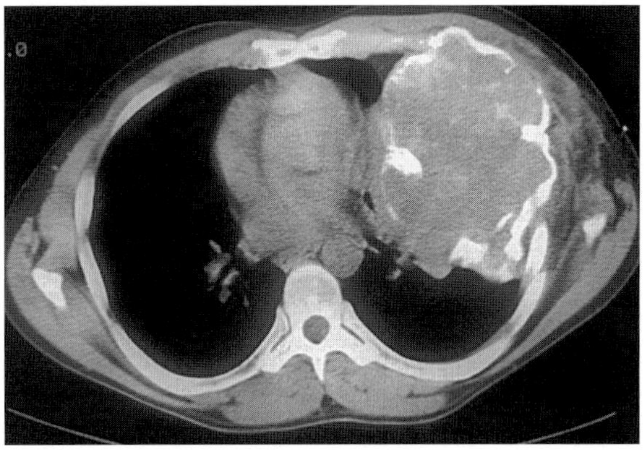

Figure 14-40

FIBROUS DYSPLASIA

Massive fibrous dysplasia of a rib. CT shows an expansile mass compressing the lung. The lesion has sclerotic borders.

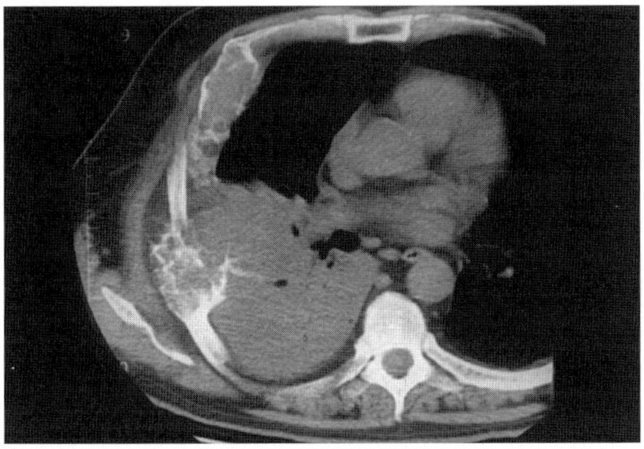

Figure 14-41

FIBROUS DYSPLASIA

Fibrous dysplasia with secondary aneurysmal bone cyst. CT shows involvement of a long segment of rib. The expansile mass was due partly to a secondary aneurysmal bone cyst. (Courtesy of Dr. R. Drake, Sylvania, OH.)

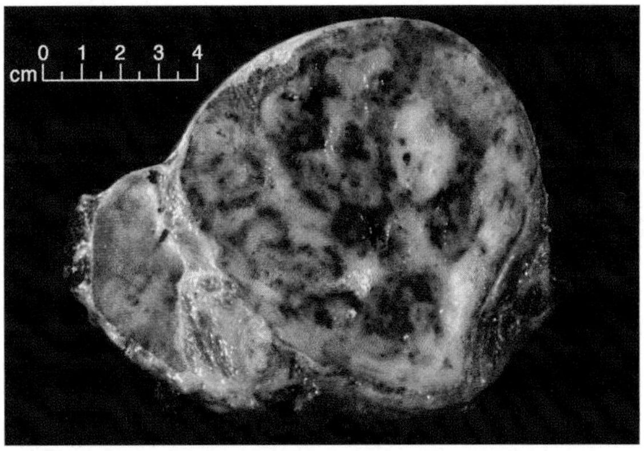

Figure 14-42

FIBROUS DYSPLASIA

The specimen corresponds to the lesion shown in figure 14-40. The tumor has a heterogeneous appearance, and is red-brown to tan-gray throughout.

suggested that these lesions may be aggressive locally (67).

Clusters of foam cells are frequently present (fig. 14-47), and benign giant cells may be present. Sometimes the stroma undergoes myxoid change (fig. 14-48). These areas may be nondiagnostic.

Large islands of cartilage may dominate the histologic features. The islands usually form round nodules and rarely, round plate-like structures resembling epiphyseal plates (fig. 14-49). Areas of secondary aneurysmal bone cyst may be present.

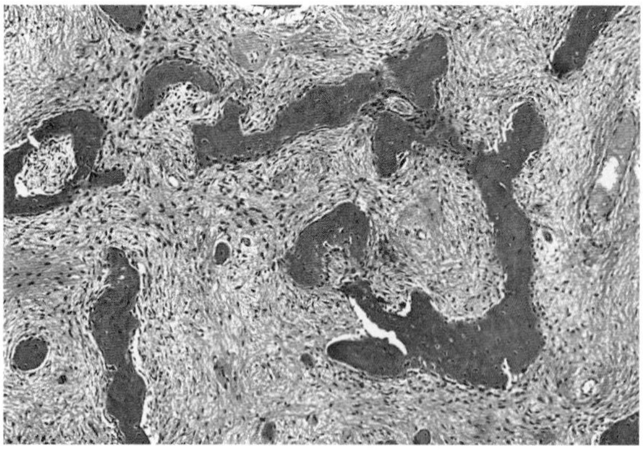

Figure 14-43

FIBROUS DYSPLASIA

Branching and anastomosing trabeculae of woven bone in a fibrous stroma.

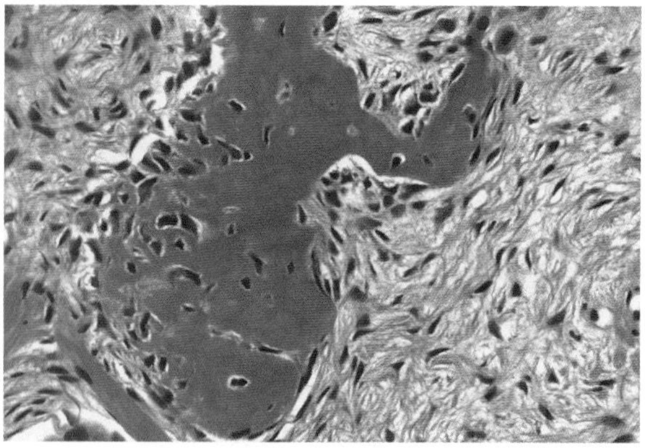

Figure 14-44

FIBROUS DYSPLASIA

The cells surrounding the bone contain oval tapered nuclei surrounded by a small amount of eosinophilic cytoplasm. There is no evidence of cytologic atypia.

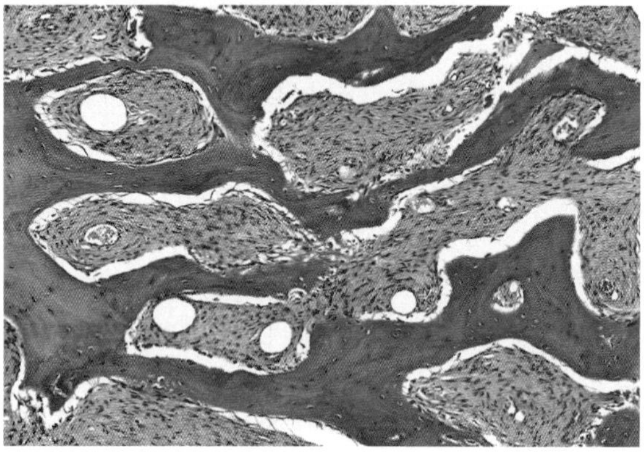

Figure 14-45

FIBROUS DYSPLASIA

The pattern of bone production in this tumor from the mandible resembles trabecular bone. Low-grade osteosarcoma is in the differential diagnosis.

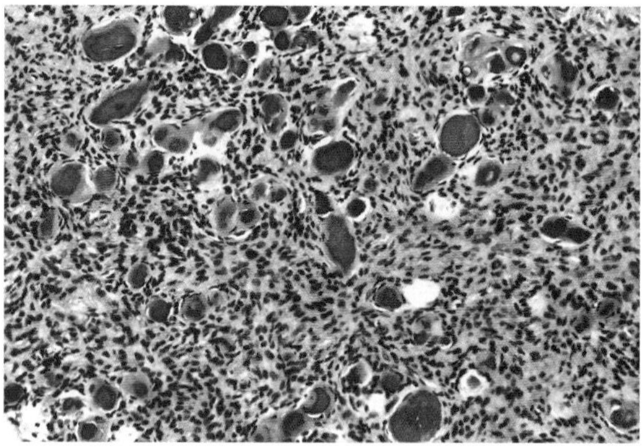

Figure 14-46

FIBROUS DYSPLASIA

Spherules of woven bone with a psammomatous appearance are seen more commonly in extragnathic sites.

Genetics and Other Special Techniques. Activating mutations of the alpha chain of the heterotrimeric signal transducer G_s disrupt the inherent guanosine triphosphatase activity of the alpha chain, stimulate adenylyl cyclase, and can result in independent cell proliferation. Such mutations of the *GNAS1* gene have been identified in fibrous dysplasia (monostotic and polyostotic forms) and in the multiple endocrinopathies of Albright's syndrome (47,48,66). In contrast, there is no evidence of $G_s\alpha$ mutations in osteofibrous dysplasia (47,63). These data suggest that fibrous dysplasia and osteofibrous dysplasia are distinct pathogenetically and that the presence or absence of a $G_s\alpha$ mutation may be used to distinguish these histologically similar lesions. The significance of a $G_s\alpha$ mutation in one of five fibrous dysplasia-like low-grade central osteosarcomas examined is not clear (60). Cytogenetic studies of fibrous dysplasia are few; however, extra copies of chromosome 2, rearrangements of 12p13, or both appear to be recurrent (49,50,59). The presence of clonal karyotypic abnormalities and the

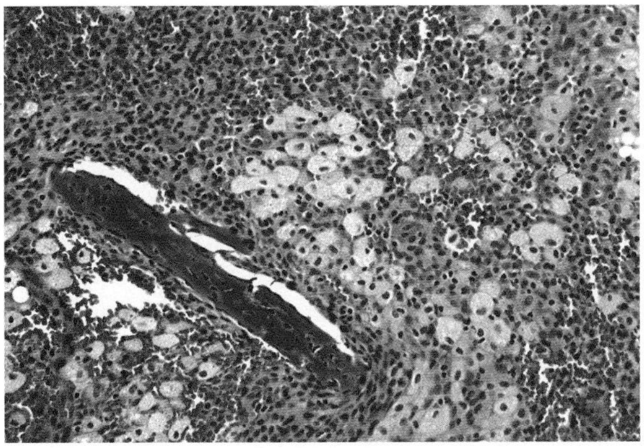

Figure 14-47

FIBROUS DYSPLASIA

Clusters of foam cells are commonly seen in fibrous dysplasia.

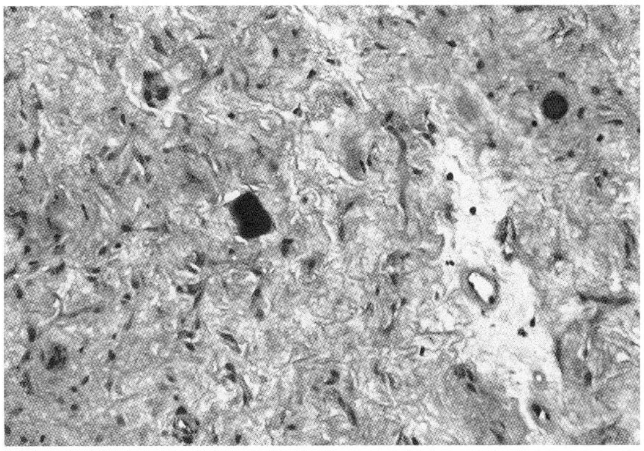

Figure 14-48

FIBROUS DYSPLASIA

Occasionally, the stroma undergoes myxoid change, either focally or diffusely.

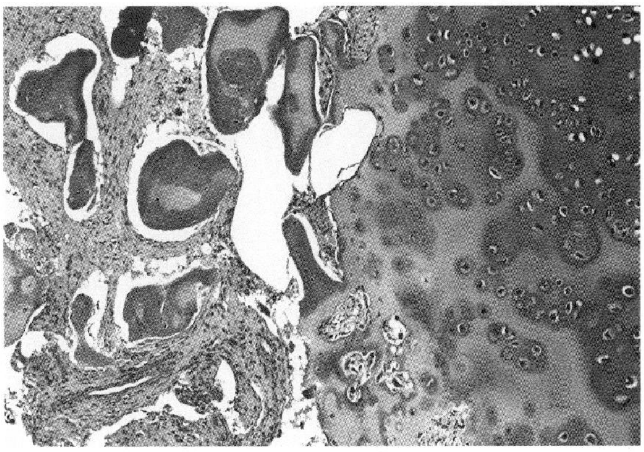

Figure 14-49

FIBROUS DYSPLASIA

Fibrocartilaginous dysplasia is rare. Irregularly shaped islands of benign cartilage are scattered throughout the tumor, which otherwise has features typical of fibrous dysplasia. When an abundant cartilage component is present, it may mask the underlying fibrous dysplasia.

identification of monoclonality for the human androgen receptor gene (*HUMARA*) by methylation-specific polymerase chain reaction analysis in fibrous dysplasia suggest that this lesion is neoplastic in nature (49,50,56,59).

Differential Diagnosis. Low-grade osteosarcoma is the most important diagnostic consideration. In low-grade osteosarcoma, the bony spicules are trabecular and the stromal cells are spindle shaped. The bone produced is usually in the form of trabeculae, as seen in parosteal osteosarcoma. The spindle cells have more elongated nuclei than those in typical fibrous dysplasia. However, most importantly, low-grade osteosarcoma permeates bone marrow fat, preexisting bony trabeculae, or soft tissue. Fibrous dysplasia with cartilage may be mistaken for chondrosarcoma. Recognition of typical areas of fibrous dysplasia prevents this mistake. Clusters of foam cells may lead to the mistaken diagnosis of metastatic hypernephroma, especially in limited samples. Foam cells have abundant bubbly cytoplasm and small nuclei with inconspicuous nucleoli, unlike the appearance of hypernephroma cells.

Treatment and Prognosis. Patients with solitary lesions have an excellent prognosis and may not require treatment. Patients with polyostotic disease occasionally have difficulty because of multiple fractures or respiratory insufficiency from involvement of the chest wall.

Sarcomas are a rare complication of fibrous dysplasia. In some series, sarcomas developed only after irradiation (64), but others have documented sarcomatous change without previous irradiation (52,62). Sarcoma may arise in the monostotic or polyostotic form. Although chondrosarcoma (51) and dedifferentiated chondrosarcoma (58) have been reported, most secondary malignancies are fibrosarcomas. The prognosis is similar to that of sarcomas arising de novo.

Osteofibrous Dysplasia

Definition. Osteofibrous dysplasia is a benign fibro-osseous process that involves the

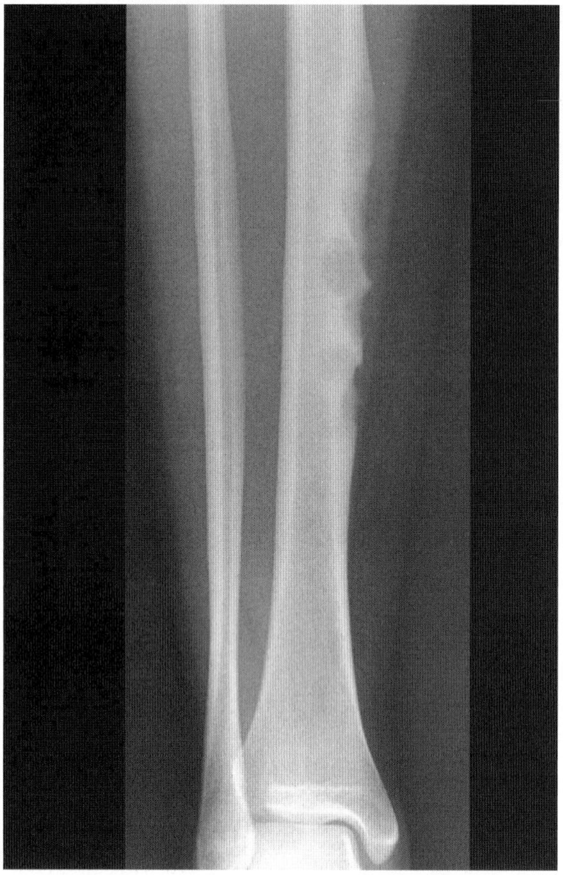

Figure 14-50

OSTEOFIBROUS DYSPLASIA

Plain radiograph shows a cortical-based lesion involving the mid-portion of the tibia. Multiple lucencies are surrounded by sclerotic bone.

cortex. It is limited to the tibia, less commonly the fibula, and, occasionally, to both.

General Features. Osteofibrous dysplasia was described by Kempson (75) as ossifying fibroma. Campanacci (71) introduced the term *osteofibrous dysplasia*. The controversy about the relationship between osteofibrous dysplasia and adamantinoma is discussed in chapter 12. Osteofibrous dysplasia is rare: until the year 2000, the Mayo Clinic files contained the records of only 10 cases, compared with 631 cases of fibrous dysplasia.

Clinical Features. Osteofibrous dysplasia is diagnosed in the first decade of life, usually before the age of 5. Patients present with anterior bowing of the tibia or pathologic fracture.

Sites. The tibia and fibula are involved exclusively.

Radiographic Findings. Radiographs show involvement of the cortex in the diaphysis. The lesions are long, lucent, and surrounded by sclerosis (fig. 14-50). Multiple lucencies with intermixed sclerosis are seen. Usually, the anterior tibia is bowed. When the fibula is involved, the appearance is similar.

Gross Findings. The process is well-demarcated and involves the outer aspect of the cortex. The lesion is white, firm, and fibrous.

Microscopic Findings. Microscopically, osteofibrous dysplasia consists of a hypocellular spindle cell stroma and bony spicules, which are lined by prominent osteoblasts (fig. 14-51). Campanacci and Laus (72) described zonation,

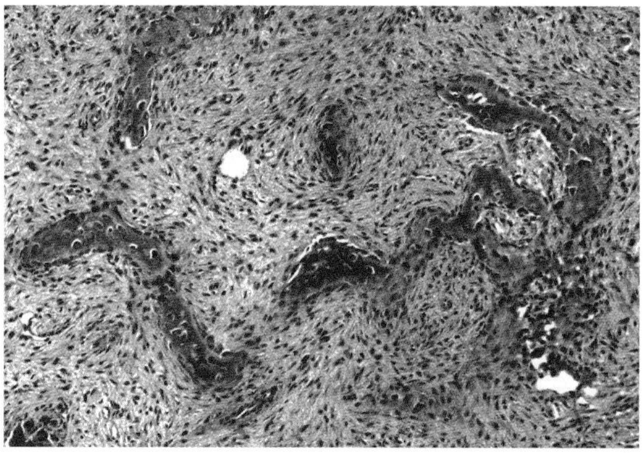

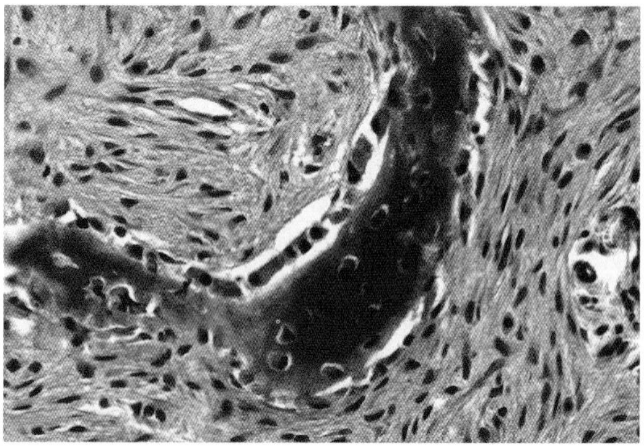

Figure 14-51

OSTEOFIBROUS DYSPLASIA

Left: Irregularly shaped bony trabeculae within a spindle cell stroma.
Right: Prominent osteoblastic rimming of bony spicules.

with more mature bony trabeculae toward the periphery. These small, cellular, lamellar-appearing spicules merge into cortical bone. Immunoperoxidase stains show single keratin-positive cells in the majority of cases (78).

Genetics and Other Special Techniques. Certain clinicopathologic features of osteofibrous dysplasia—its radiographic appearance, proclivity for the tibia, and association with fibro-osseous tissues—are similar to those of adamantinoma, supporting a relationship between these two entities. The expression of certain protooncogene products, bone matrix proteins, and the karyotypic findings of osteofibrous dysplasia and adamantinoma are also similar, extending the osteofibrous dysplasia and adamantinoma relationship (69,70,73,74,76). Extra copies of chromosome 7, 8, 12, or 21 (or some combination of these) are nonrandom aberrations in both lesions. Adamantinoma differs from osteofibrous dysplasia, however, by occasionally exhibiting extra copies of chromosome 19 as well as various structural chromosomal anomalies in addition to the common numerical changes (+7, +8, +12, and +21). Thus, karyotypically, adamantinomas are slightly more complex than osteofibrous dysplasia. It has been hypothesized that the expansion of the abnormal clone to include structural chromosomal abnormalities in adamantinoma may parallel the progression of an osteofibrous dysplastic lesion to an adamantinoma (74).

Treatment and Prognosis. Several studies have suggested a conservative approach to management (68,71,77). The lesions tend to regress with maturation of the skeleton.

Congenital Fibromatosis (Myofibromatosis)

Definition. Congenital fibromatosis, or infantile myofibromatosis, is a nodular proliferation of cells with myogenic features (myofibroblasts). Frequently, it is associated with a hemangiopericytomatous vascular proliferation.

General Features. Congenital fibromatosis is a rare condition that usually involves the soft tissues. It may be solitary, presenting as a subcutaneous nodule in infancy, or multicentric, with involvement of soft tissues and the skeleton. Visceral involvement is rare.

Clinical Features. Patients with skeletal involvement are infants or children. They usually are asymptomatic.

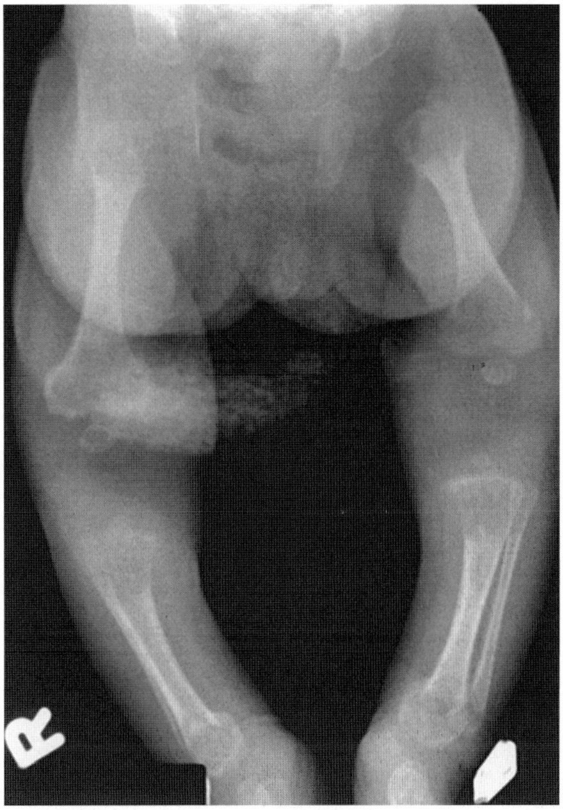

Figure 14-52

CONGENITAL FIBROMATOSIS

The plain radiograph shows bilateral symmetric lucencies involving the metaphyses of long bones.

Sites. The multicentric form involves the metaphyseal regions of the long bones. The solitary form nearly always involves the skull or jawbones (79,80).

Radiographic Findings. The lesions are lucent and well demarcated. In the multicentric form, bilateral symmetrical lesions are found in the metaphysis of long bones (fig. 14-52). In the solitary form, lucencies are surrounded by a sclerotic rim (fig. 14-53).

Gross Findings. The lesions are spherical, soft to firm, and may have central areas of calcification.

Microscopic Findings. Under low-power magnification, congenital fibromatosis has a distinctly nodular appearance (fig. 14-54). The lesion is hypocellular and consists of plump spindle cells with pink myogenic cytoplasm (fig. 14-55). Vascular proliferation is prominent,

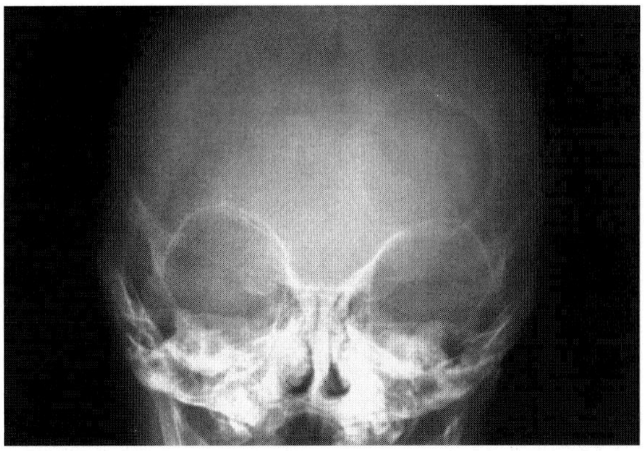

Figure 14-53

CONGENITAL FIBROMATOSIS

The lesion presents as a well-demarcated lucency in the frontal bone of a 7-year-old girl.

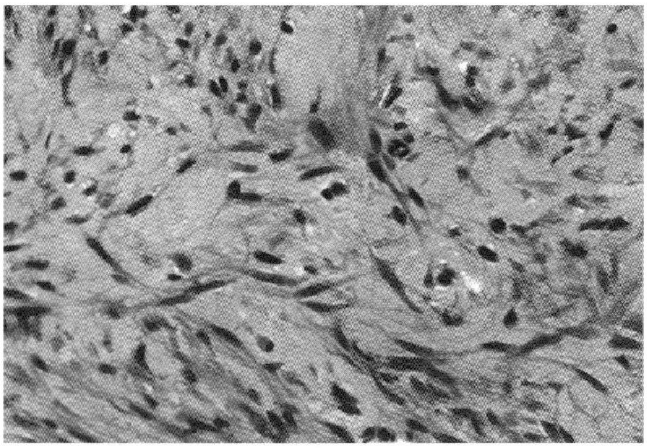

Figure 14-55

CONGENITAL FIBROMATOSIS

The myofibroblasts contain elongated tapered nuclei with pale pink cytoplasm.

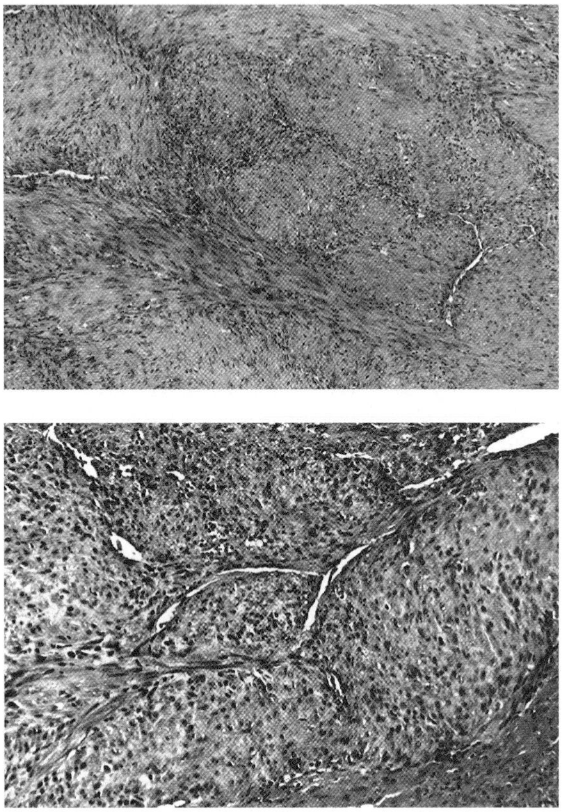

Figure 14-54

CONGENITAL FIBROMATOSIS

Top: Characteristic low-power nodular appearance. Fascicles of spindle cells sweep between the nodules.

Bottom: Occasionally, the stroma within the nodules is pale blue, imparting a pseudochondroid appearance.

with cleft-like or angulated vascular spaces. Occasionally, the vessels have a staghorn appearance; small spindle cells arranged around the vessels produce a hemangiopericytomatous pattern (fig. 14-56).

Differential Diagnosis. The vascular proliferation may suggest the diagnosis of hemangiopericytoma. The correct diagnosis is made by recognizing the characteristic nodules of myofibroblasts. Congenital fibromatosis may also be mistaken for a spindle cell sarcoma. The nodular arrangement and lack of cytologic atypia are helpful features.

Treatment and Prognosis. If the lesions are recognized clinically, no treatment is necessary. Both solitary and multiple lesions tend to resolve spontaneously. Patients with visceral involvement have a poor prognosis.

Fibrocartilaginous Mesenchymoma

Definition. Fibrocartilaginous mesenchymoma is a rare intraosseous lesion that is characterized by a proliferation of spindle cells, bony trabeculae, and cartilaginous plates, which simulate epiphyseal plates.

General Features. The cases that were the basis of the original description of Dahlin et al. (82) were separated from cases of fibrochondrodysplasia because of the unusual histologic features. Only a handful of cases have been reported (81).

Clinical Features. The lesion tends to affect young patients. There is a slight male predominance.

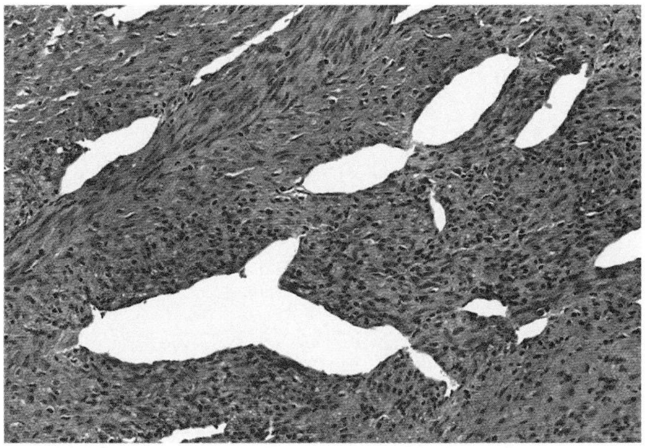

Figure 14-56

CONGENITAL FIBROMATOSIS

Distended and branching vascular spaces produce a hemangiopericytomata-like appearance.

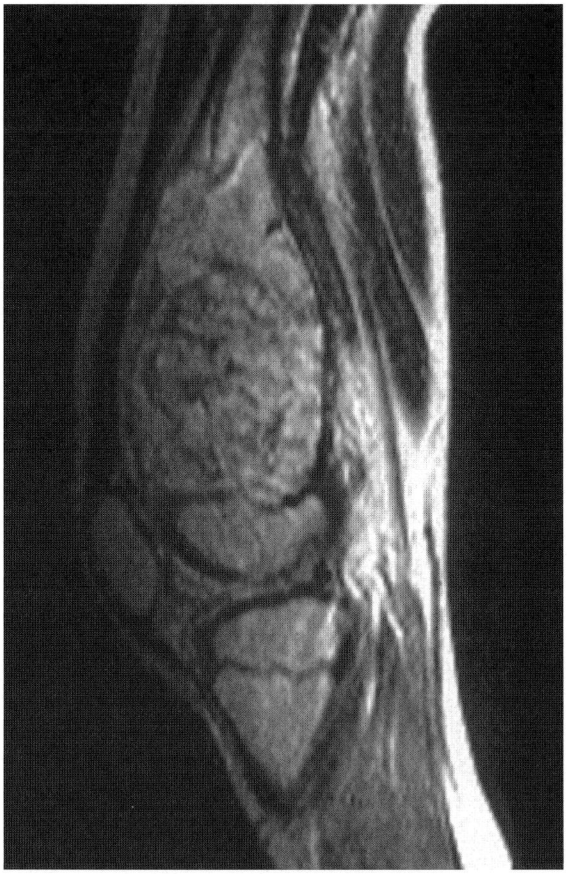

Figure 14-57

FIBROCARTILAGINOUS MESENCHYMOMA

MRI shows an expansile lesion involving the metaphysis of the femur. (Courtesy of Dr. S. Rwacan, Ankara, Turkey.)

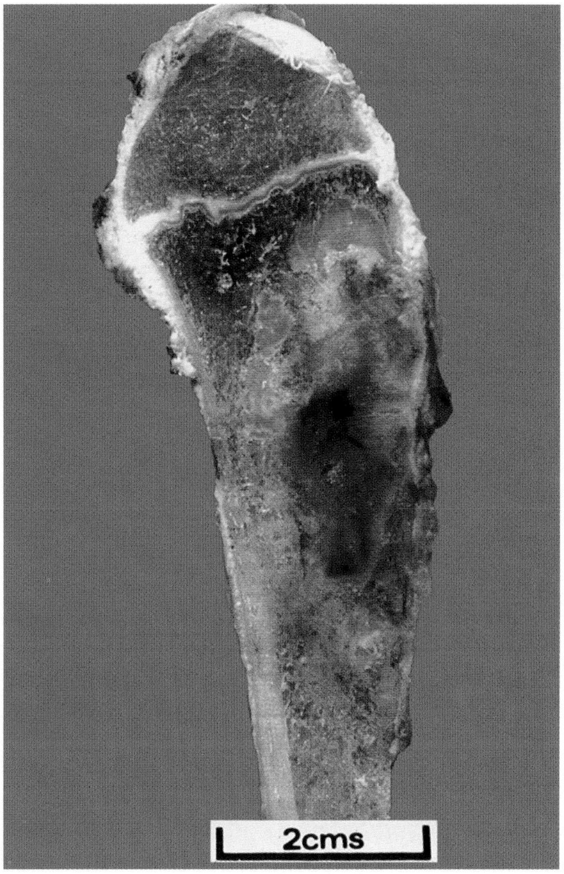

Figure 14-58

FIBROCARTILAGINOUS MESENCHYMOMA

The gross specimen shows nodules of cartilage, with calcific lines simulating epiphyseal plates. (Fig. 27-47 from Unni KK. Dahlin's bone tumors: general aspects and data on 11,087 cases, 5th ed. Philadelphia: Lippincott-Raven; 1996:379. By permission of Mayo Foundation.)

Patients present with pain or swelling, or the lesion may be an incidental radiographic finding.

Sites. Any portion of the skeleton may be involved, but the proximal fibula is the most common site.

Radiographic Findings. The lesions involve the metaphyseal portion and abut the epiphyseal plate (fig. 14-57). The bone is slightly expanded, and the lesion is predominantly lucent. Mineralization suggesting a cartilaginous component is usually present.

Gross Findings. The lesion is white and fibrous. Blue streaks, which represent plates of cartilage, may be seen (fig. 14-58).

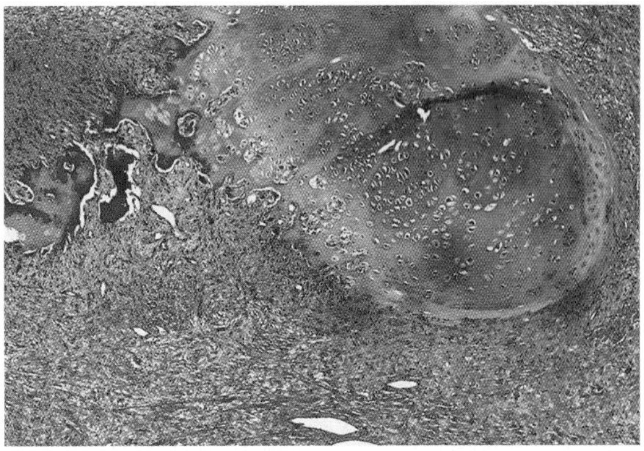

Figure 14-59

FIBROCARTILAGINOUS MESENCHYMOMA

A nodule of cartilage with enchondral bone formation is surrounded by a moderately cellular spindle cell stroma.

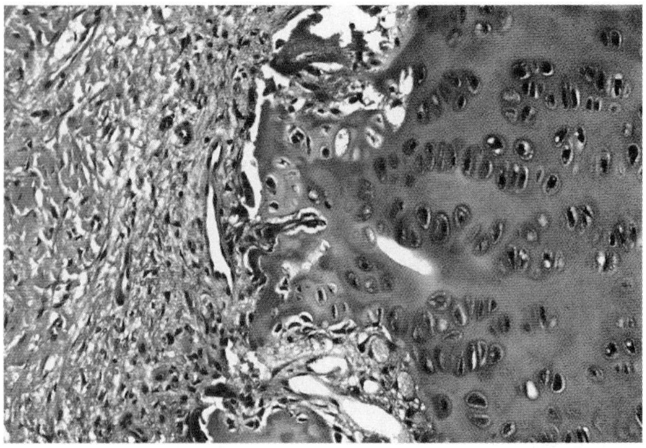

Figure 14-60

FIBROCARTILAGINOUS MESENCHYMOMA

The chondrocytes form a columnar arrangement in an area of enchondral ossification, simulating epiphyseal plate cartilage.

Microscopic Findings. Fibrocartilaginous mesenchymoma shows a mixture of bone, cartilage, and spindle cell stroma (fig. 14-59). The cartilage occurs in the form of plates, with enchondral bone formation (fig. 14-60). The bone produces trabeculae, and the intratrabecular spaces are filled with spindle cells, which show no atypia.

Differential Diagnosis. Fibrous dysplasia with cartilage also has the various elements seen in fibrocartilaginous mesenchymoma. However, in fibrous dysplasia, the cartilage is mostly in nodules and the bone produced is woven and not trabecular; also, the stromal cells are plump and not elongated.

Treatment and Prognosis. Conservative surgery is indicated. Although there have been local recurrences, no instance of malignant behavior has been reported.

BONE-FORMING LESIONS THAT SIMULATE NEOPLASMS

Several non-neoplastic conditions produce bone or osteoid.

Heterotopic Ossification

Definition. Heterotopic ossification is a reactive, self-limited condition in which fibroblasts proliferate in the soft tissues, producing bone and, occasionally, cartilage.

General Features. *Myositis ossificans* is a synonym; however, the process does not always occur in muscle and it is not associated with inflammation. A previous history of trauma may or may not be elicited. *Myositis ossificans progressiva* is a condition in which heterotopic ossification occurs in many muscle groups, is dominantly inherited, is life-threatening, and is associated with skeletal anomalies, especially of the toes and fingers (89). It is not related to the much more common solitary lesion. *Ischial apophyseolysis* (86) is a form of heterotopic ossification induced by the avulsion of the apophysis of the ischial tuberosity caused by strenuous exercise.

Clinical Features. Patients complain of a rapidly enlarging swelling, usually of a few weeks' duration. There may or may not be pain. The process affects any age group but especially young adults. There is no sex predilection. The physical examination demonstrates a well-circumscribed mass that may be crepitant.

Sites. Any part of the body may be involved, but the anterior thigh is the most common site. The soft tissues of the hands and feet are also commonly involved, and this is where the radiographic and histologic features may be distinct.

Radiographic Findings. Plain radiographs do not show any changes for the first 3 weeks or they show an ill-defined mass. In later, more typical stages, mineralization is present at the periphery and has a ring-like configuration; the center is lucent (fig. 14-61). CT highlights the peripheral ossification and central lucency (fig. 14-62). MRI shows inhomogeneous signals on both T_1- and T_2-weighted images (87). Edema

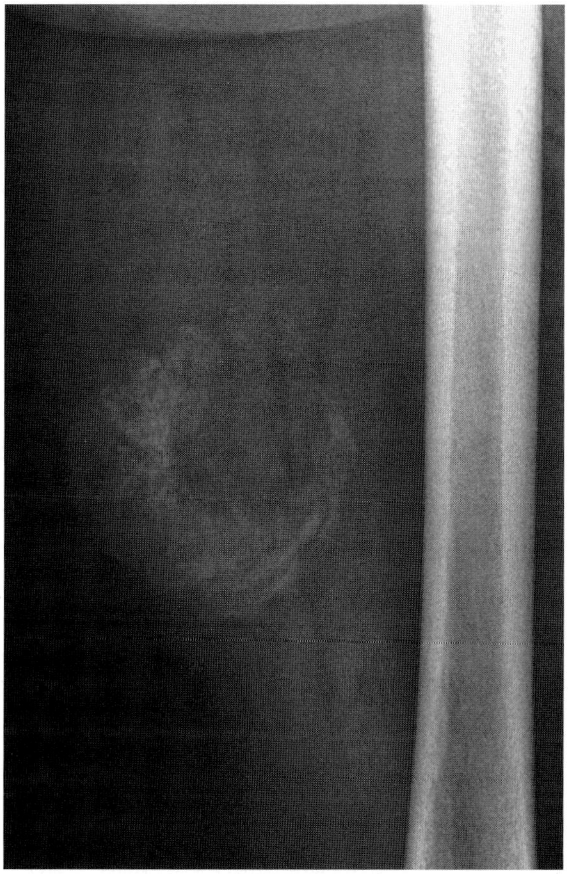

Figure 14-61

HETEROTOPIC OSSIFICATION

A well-marginated soft tissue mass has a central lucency and peripheral sclerosis.

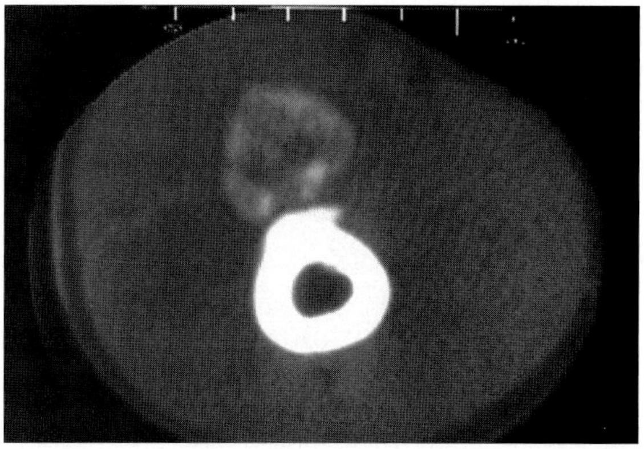

Figure 14-62

HETEROTOPIC OSSIFICATION

CT highlights a shell of ossification.

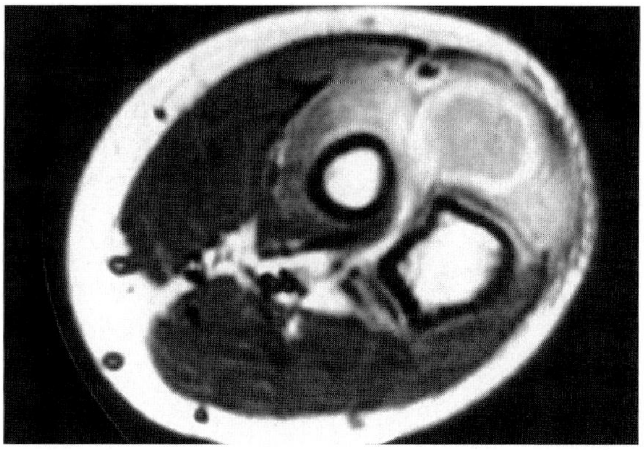

Figure 14-63

HETEROTOPIC OSSIFICATION

MRI demonstrates a well-demarcated lesion in the elbow. Signal changes around the lesion due to edema may suggest a permeative neoplasm.

surrounding the lesion may suggest that the lesion is not well demarcated; this may be alarming (fig. 14-63). The underlying cortex is not involved, and a lucent zone occurs between the lesion and bone. As the lesion matures, it becomes more mineralized and smaller and involutes. In the later stages, it may be attached to the underlying bone.

Gross Findings. The lesion is remarkably well circumscribed and, hence, easily separated from the surrounding tissues. The central zone shows edematous skeletal muscle, similar to the appearance of proliferative myositis, and the periphery shows calcification, suggesting an eggshell (fig. 14-64). There may be cystic spaces in the center or, rarely, the lesion is multicystic, with the septa simulating the appearance of an aneurysmal bone cyst (88).

Microscopic Findings. Ackerman (84) introduced the concept of zonation in the diagnosis of heterotopic ossification. He pointed out that the central portion of the lesion is composed of proliferating fibroblasts that appear less mature than those in the periphery, and the periphery is composed of more mature bone and cartilage (fig. 14-65). The spindle cells in the center are loosely arranged and do not have atypia but are mitotically active (fig. 14-66). Osteoid seams lined with prominent osteoblasts appear toward the periphery and mature into mineralized trabeculae, which contribute to the bony shell. Islands of cartilage may be present,

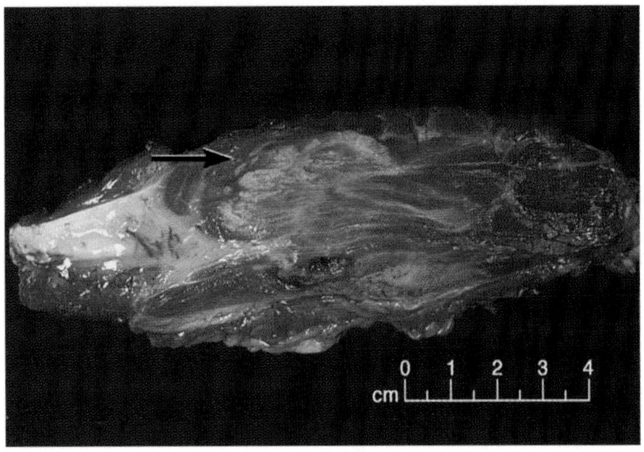

Figure 14-64

HETEROTOPIC OSSIFICATION

Edematous muscle with peripheral calcification.

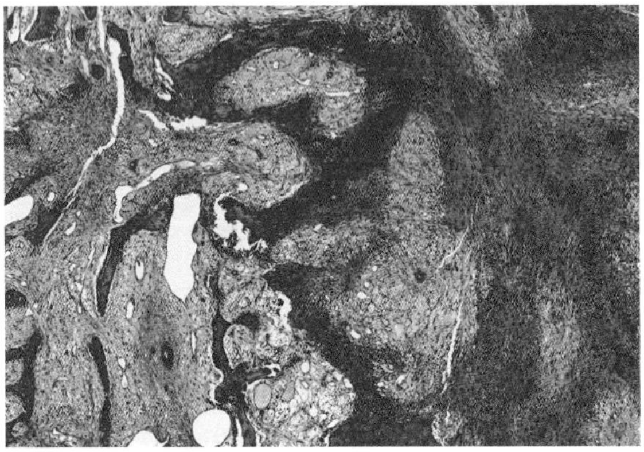

Figure 14-65

HETEROTOPIC OSSIFICATION

Zonation is evident, with immature bone and proliferating fibroblasts (right) merging into reactive new bone formation with osteoblastic rimming (left).

especially at the periphery, and have a cap-like architecture, with bony trabeculae arising from it, simulating osteochondroma. Aneurysmal bone cyst–like changes may be seen and occasionally are the dominant feature.

Differential Diagnosis. Parosteal osteosarcoma and soft tissue osteosarcoma are usually considered in the differential diagnosis of heterotopic ossification. Parosteal osteosarcoma is attached to bone, whereas heterotopic ossification is not. Parosteal osteosarcoma has a uniform architecture throughout and lacks the zonation typical of heterotopic ossification. The radiographic appearance of heterotopic ossification

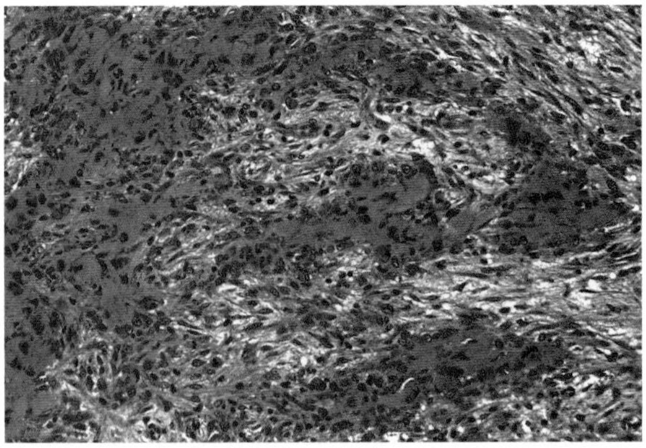

Figure 14-66

HETEROTOPIC OSSIFICATION

Cellular spindle cell stroma with mitotic activity, but no cytologic atypia. Early osteoid production is present.

can be similar to that of soft tissue osteosarcoma. However, osteosarcoma cells show pronounced anaplasia and the tumor lacks the orderliness of heterotopic ossification.

Treatment and Prognosis. If recognized clinically and radiographically, no treatment is necessary. Conservative excision is adequate therapy. Recurrences are rare, and most lesions involute spontaneously. Only two examples of sarcoma arising in heterotopic ossification have been well documented (83,85). One patient had dermatomyositis and the other had heterotopic ossification secondary to an electrical burn. Occasionally, a soft tissue osteosarcoma, in which a portion of the lesion appears more mature on radiographs and on histologic examination, may be found. However, these are difficult to document as true examples of sarcoma arising in heterotopic ossification.

Subungual Exostosis

Definition. Subungual exostosis is a proliferative process consisting of bone and cartilage, and involving the nail bed.

General Features. The term *subungual exostosis* is related to the gross and microscopic features that simulate the appearance of an osteochondroma. The lesion is rare: for the years 1910 to 1975, the Mayo Clinic files contain the records of only 44 cases (90).

Clinical Features. Subungual exostosis usually occurs in the second or third decade of life, and

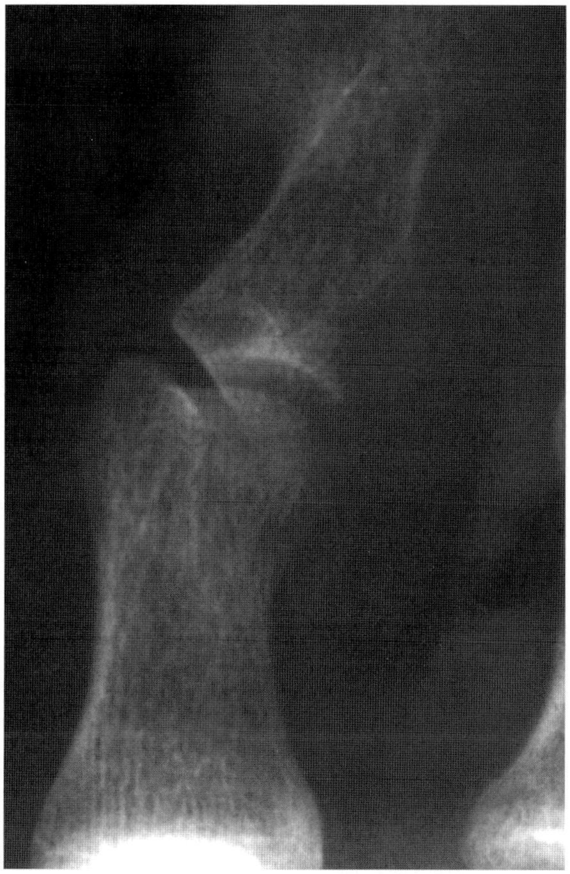

Figure 14-67

SUBUNGUAL EXOSTOSIS

A well-marginated, uniformly mineralized mass is attached to the surface of the distal phalanx. (Courtesy of Dr. R. Yio, Sacramento, CA.)

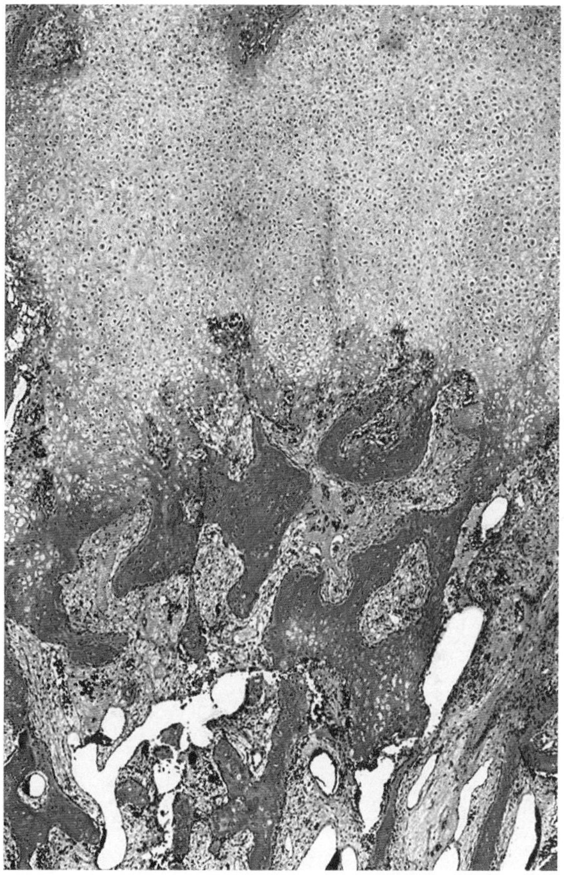

Figure 14-68

SUBUNGUAL EXOSTOSIS

Abundant cartilage matures into trabecular-appearing bone.

there is a pronounced male predominance. Patients usually present with a mass lesion that elevates the nail and sometimes causes ulceration.

Sites. The distal phalanx of the great toe is involved in more than three fourths of cases. Other toes and fingers are rarely affected.

Radiographic Findings. Radiographs show a mineralizing mass attached to the surface of the distal phalanx (fig. 14-67). The cortex and medulla of the phalanx are not continuous with the lesion.

Gross Findings. The lesion is well circumscribed and consists of a cartilage cap and bony stalk.

Microscopic Findings. Under low-power magnification, the cartilage is abundant and arranged in a plate-like fashion. Trabecular bone arises from the cartilage (fig. 14-68). Under higher-power magnification, the cartilage cap shows spindle cell proliferation on the surface. This matures into cartilage, which in turn matures into bone. The cartilage is cellular and the nuclei are enlarged (fig. 14-69). The intertrabecular spaces contain loosely arranged spindle cells.

Differential Diagnosis. The proliferating spindle cells and cartilage may lead to a mistaken diagnosis of osteosarcoma or chondrosarcoma. The orderly arrangement and maturation are important clues for recognizing the reactive nature of the lesion. Subungual melanomas can produce bone and cartilage and mimic subungual exostosis (91,92). The presence of junctional activity and the compact arrangement of the cells support a diagnosis of melanoma. In melanoma, the spindle cells are

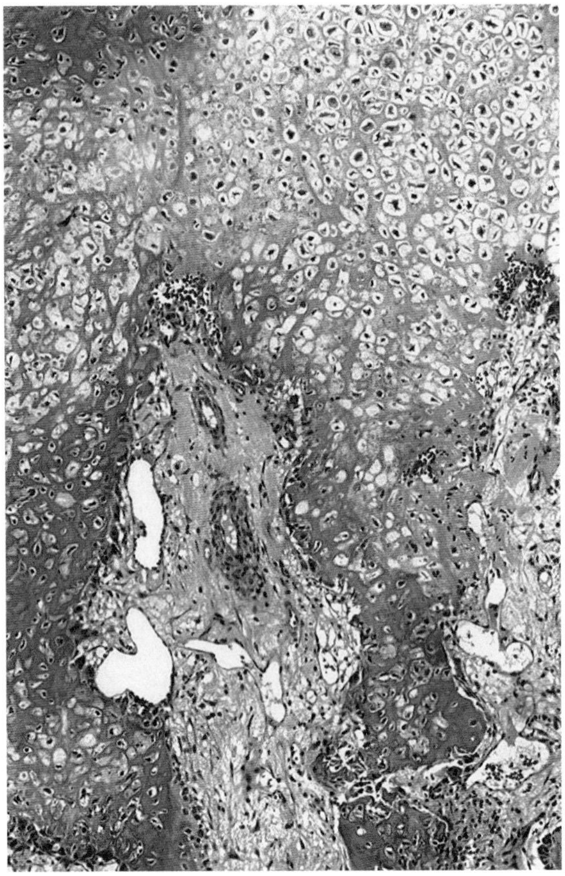

Figure 14-69

SUBUNGUAL EXOSTOSIS

The cartilage is maturing into new bone formation with prominent osteoblastic rimming. The cartilage is cellular, with some nuclear enlargement. Out of context, these features would be worrisome for malignancy.

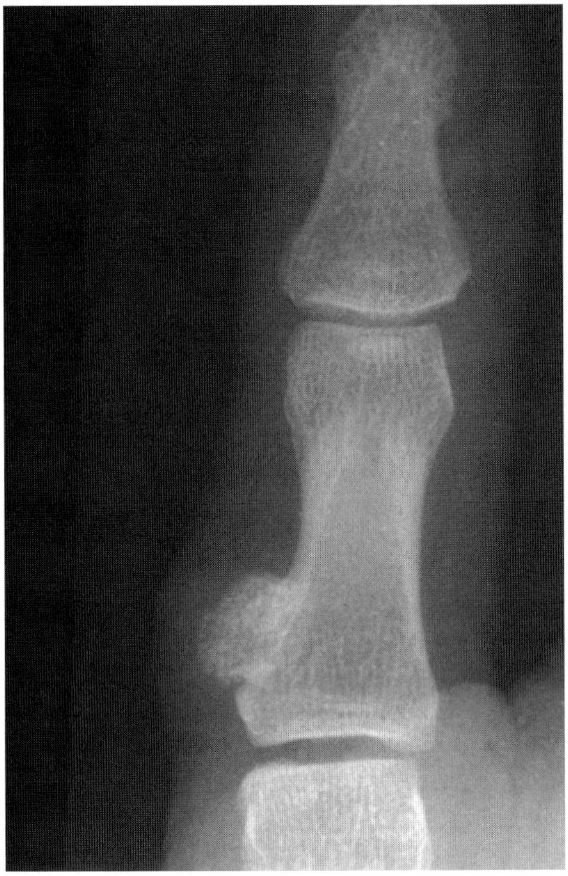

Figure 14-70

BIZARRE PAROSTEAL OSTEOCHONDROMATOUS PROLIFERATION

A uniformly mineralized mass is attached to the surface of bone.

positive for S-100 protein, whereas in subungual exostosis, only the cartilage cells are positive.

Treatment and Prognosis. Simple excision is sufficient. Recurrences are rare and are controlled by re-excision.

Bizarre Parosteal Osteochondromatous Proliferation

Definition. Bizarre parosteal osteochondromatous proliferation is a reactive process composed of bone and cartilage attached to the surface of bone.

General Features. Bizarre parosteal osteochondromatous proliferation was first described by Nora et al. (96) as a reactive proliferation involving the small bones of the hands and feet. Later studies have shown that other bones can be involved (94). The word "bizarre" was used to describe the cartilage, which can be quite proliferative.

Clinical Features. Patients are usually young adults, and males and females are affected equally. Patients complain of a swelling, with or without pain. The growth is usually rapid.

Radiographic Findings. Plain radiographs show a heavily and uniformly mineralized, well-circumscribed mass plastered onto the underlying bone (fig. 14-70). Unlike osteochondroma, there is no continuity between the cortex and medulla of the involved bone and the tumor.

Gross Findings. The lesion resembles an osteochondroma, with a cartilage cap and a stalk

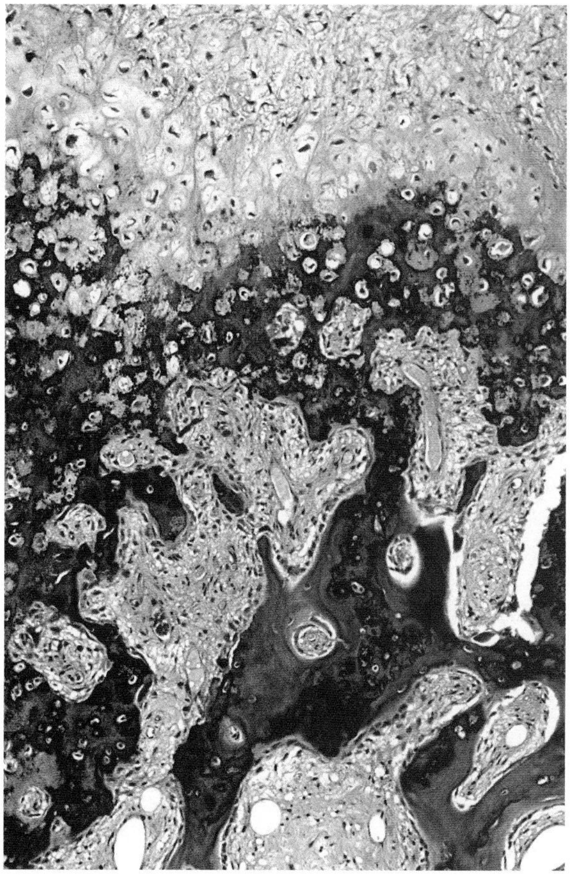

Figure 14-71

BIZARRE PAROSTEAL OSTEOCHONDROMATOUS PROLIFERATION

Cap-like cartilage (top) is maturing into trabecular bone.

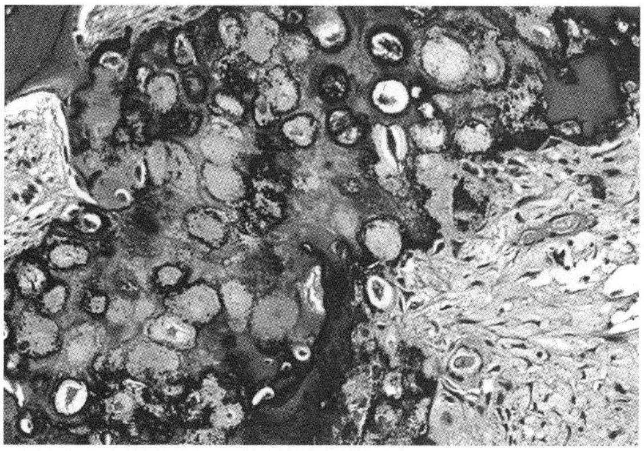

Figure 14-72

BIZARRE PAROSTEAL OSTEOCHONDROMATOUS PROLIFERATION

The matrix is dark blue to purple in areas where it is becoming mineralized.

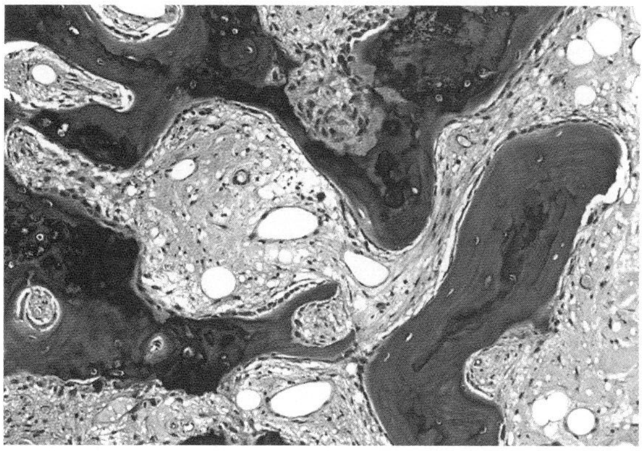

Figure 14-73

BIZARRE PAROSTEAL OSTEOCHONDROMATOUS PROLIFERATION

A spindle cell proliferation with scattered blood vessels surrounds the new bone that is being formed.

composed of bony trabeculae. Cartilage may be abundant and appear lobulated.

Microscopic Findings. Under low-power magnification, bizarre parosteal osteochondromatous proliferation resembles an osteochondroma. The cartilage plate is hypercellular and the chondrocytes appear enlarged. At the bottom of the plate is enchondral ossification (fig. 14-71). The calcification at this junction is purple or blue and has been referred to as "blue bone" (fig. 14-72). This calcification is essential for the diagnosis. The bony trabeculae have prominent osteoblastic rimming, and the intertrabecular spaces contain capillaries and loosely arranged spindle cells (fig. 14-73).

Florid, reactive periostitis describes a condition in which myositis ossificans occurs on the surface of the small bones of the hands and feet (97).

Genetics and Other Special Techniques. A t(1;17)(q32;q21) or variant translocations involving 1q32 are recurrent and unique in bizarre parosteal osteochondromatous proliferation (95). The underlying genes potentially involved with these rearrangements have not yet been identified.

Differential Diagnosis. Osteochondromas seldom occur on the small bones. Radiographs show cortical and medullary continuity. Moreover, osteochondromas do not have the blue bone typical of bizarre parosteal osteochondromatous proliferation.

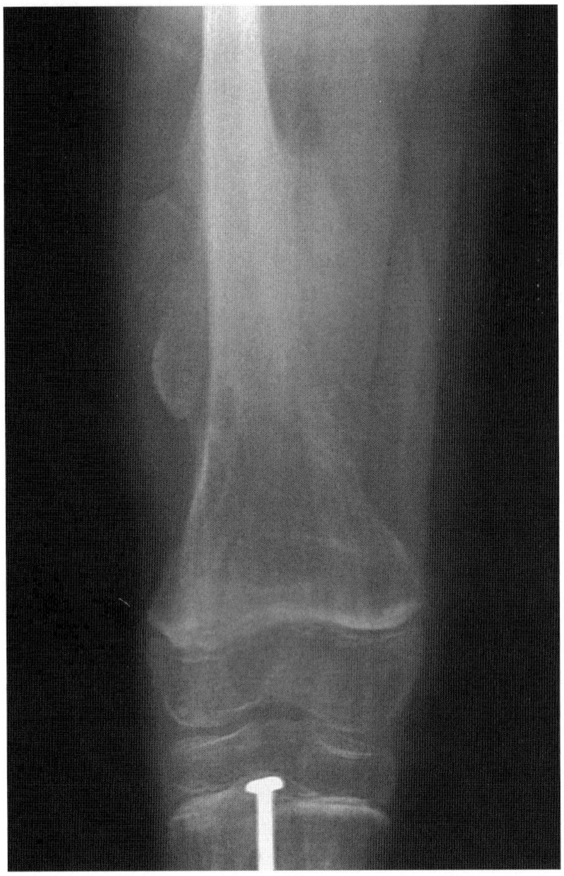

Figure 14-74

HYPERTROPHIC CALLUS

A heavily mineralized mass on the surface of bone in a patient with osteogenesis imperfecta. (Courtesy of Dr. A. Segura, Milwaukee, WI.)

Treatment and Prognosis. Simple excision is sufficient treatment. Recurrences are common but are managed adequately with re-excision (94). We are not aware of any reports of bizarre parosteal osteochondromatous proliferation involuting. There is one well-documented example of fibrosarcoma arising in association with bizarre parosteal osteochondromatous proliferation (93).

Fracture Callus

Definition. Fracture callus is a reparative process involved in bridging the gap caused by a fracture.

General Features. Fractures may be traumatic or pathologic. In patients with osteoporosis, insignificant trauma may cause fracture.

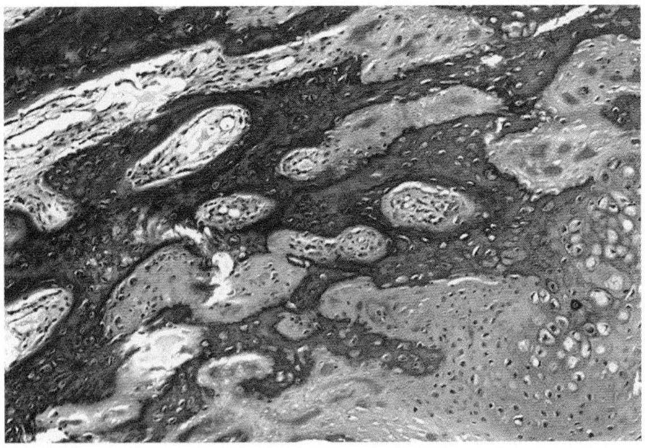

Figure 14-75

FRACTURE CALLUS

Hyperplastic cartilage and immature woven bone are arranged in an orderly pattern.

Clinical Features. Fracture associated with osteoporosis occurs predominantly in postmenopausal women. Pathologic fractures occur mostly with metastatic carcinoma and myeloma; hence, older adults are affected. Patients with osteogenesis imperfecta develop a hypertrophic callus.

Sites. Any portion of the skeleton may be involved, but the femoral neck is the site of predilection, especially in patients with osteoporosis.

Radiographic Findings. The bone involved may show features of a pathologic process, such as osteoporosis, osteogenesis imperfecta, Paget's disease, or metastatic carcinoma (fig. 14-74). In some conditions, such as Paget's disease, the fracture is horizontal, but in most other conditions, the fracture lines are irregular. The periosteum is often thickened, and mineralization occurs in the soft tissues adjacent to the fracture. In such conditions as osteogenesis imperfecta and paraplegia, the mineralized mass may be substantial.

Gross Findings. In hypertrophic callus, nodules of cartilage and bone form pronounced masses.

Microscopic Findings. The cardinal findings are loosely arranged spindle cells and new bone formation. Seams of osteoid with prominent osteoblastic rimming mature into trabecular-appearing bone (fig. 14-75). Nodules of hyperplastic cartilage may be present. Although the cartilage may be hypercellular, there is an orderly maturation into bone. Mitotic activity in the stromal cells is brisk, but there is no cytologic atypia.

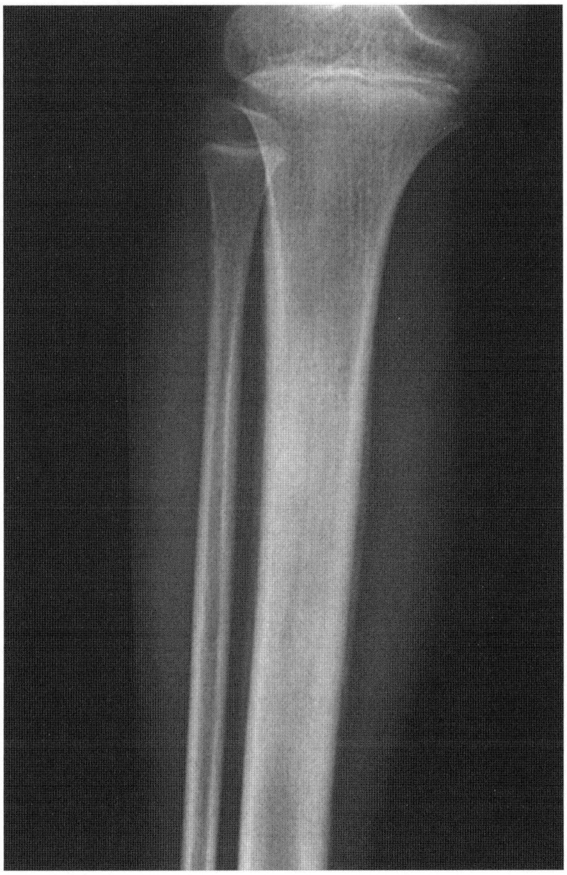

Figure 14-76

STRESS FRACTURE

Diffuse sclerosis in the proximal tibial shaft. The appearance may be mistaken for a bone-forming neoplasm. (Courtesy of Dr. W. Roseneau, San Francisco, CA.)

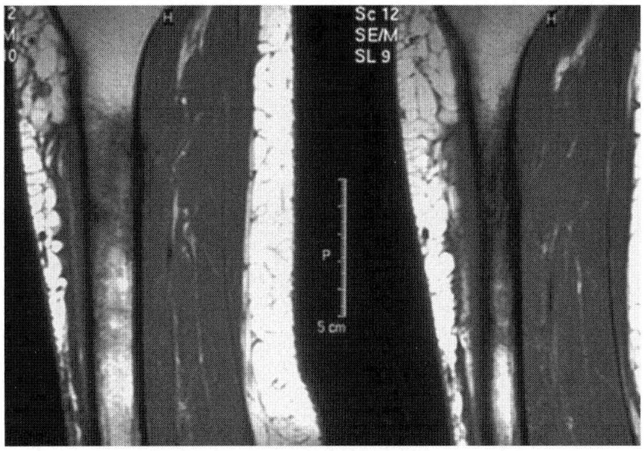

Figure 14-77

STRESS FRACTURE

MRI demonstrates abnormal bone marrow signals. This may suggest a permeative process. (Courtesy of Dr. J. Jansen, Lexington, KY.)

Differential Diagnosis. Hypertrophic callus may be mistaken for chondrosarcoma or osteosarcoma. In osteosarcoma, there is no orderliness to the proliferating tissues. Orderly maturation is the most important feature of callus.

Treatment and Prognosis. Treatment should be directed at the underlying condition.

Stress (Insufficiency) Fracture

Definition. Stress fracture occurs when the elastic resistance of bone is insufficient or inadequate to withstand the stresses of normal activity (98).

General Features. Stress fractures are usually associated with repetitive activities, such as marching and jogging. Insufficiency fractures are usually associated with osteoporosis.

Clinical Features. Patients complain of persistent pain.

Sites. The tibial shaft and metatarsals are the common sites of stress fractures. The sacral ala and the pubic rami are associated with insufficiency fractures.

Radiographic Findings. A fracture line usually is not obvious on plain radiographs. There may be diffuse periosteal new bone formation suggestive of a permeative process, such as a small cell malignancy (fig. 14-76). Plain radiographs are frequently negative, but bone scans are hot and MRI shows abnormal bone marrow signals (fig. 14-77). In insufficiency fractures of the pelvis, there is linear sclerosis of the sacral ala and increased uptake on bone scans (fig. 14-78) (98). In the pubis, areas of lysis may simulate metastatic carcinoma. CT frequently demonstrates fractures not obvious on radiographs (fig. 14-79).

Gross Findings. Biopsy specimens show fragments of cortical bone.

Microscopic Findings. Biopsy specimens from the medullary cavity show active new bone formation. Woven bone with light purple calcification is present in the bone marrow spaces and may appear permeative (fig. 14-80).

Differential Diagnosis. The permeative features of the matrix may suggest osteosarcoma, but there is no cellular proliferation to support a diagnosis of malignancy.

Treatment and Prognosis. Treatment is supportive.

Bone Island

Definition. A bone island is a nodule of cortical-appearing bone within the medullary cavity.

General Features. The cause of bone islands is unknown. Rarely, a patient has multiple lesions, in which case the term *osteopoikilosis* is used.

Clinical Features. Patients are asymptomatic.

Sites. Any portion of the skeleton may be involved.

Radiographic Findings. Bone islands appear as well-rounded, densely sclerotic masses within the medullary cavity. They are usually 1 to 2 cm in their greatest dimension, but they may be considerably larger. The edges are irregular and narrow spicules extend into surrounding bone, providing a feathery appearance (fig. 14-81).

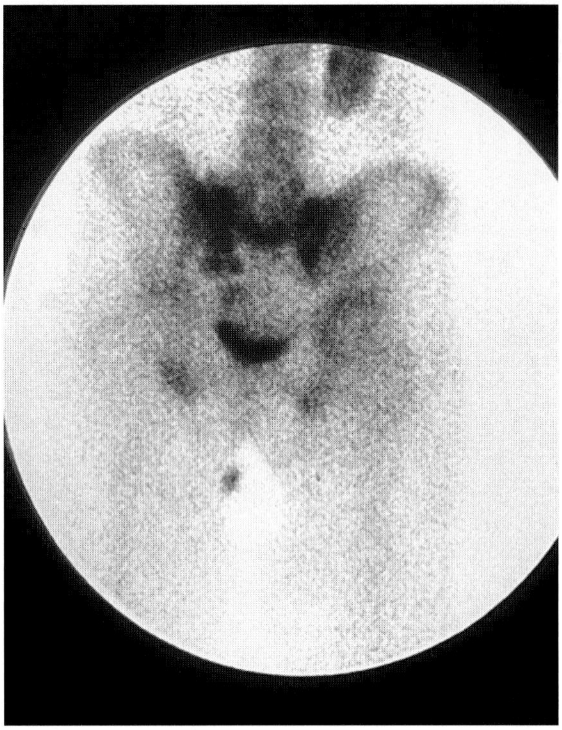

Figure 14-78

INSUFFICIENCY FRACTURE

Radioisotope bone scan shows uptake in both ala of the sacrum.

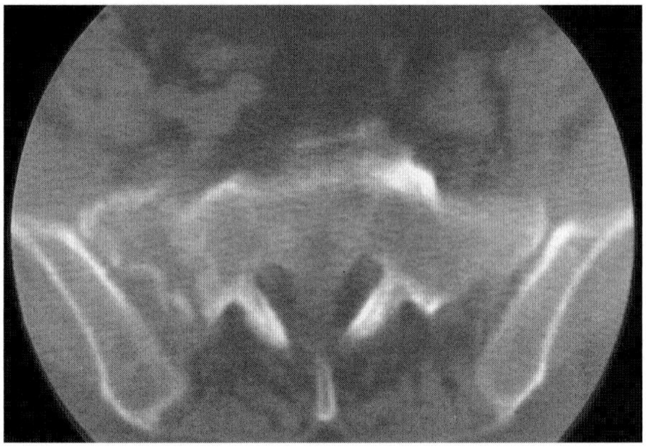

Figure 14-79

INSUFFICIENCY FRACTURE

CT clearly demonstrates a fracture in the sacrum.

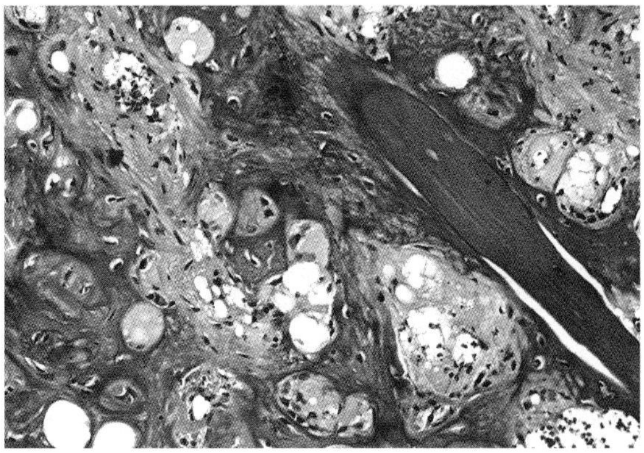

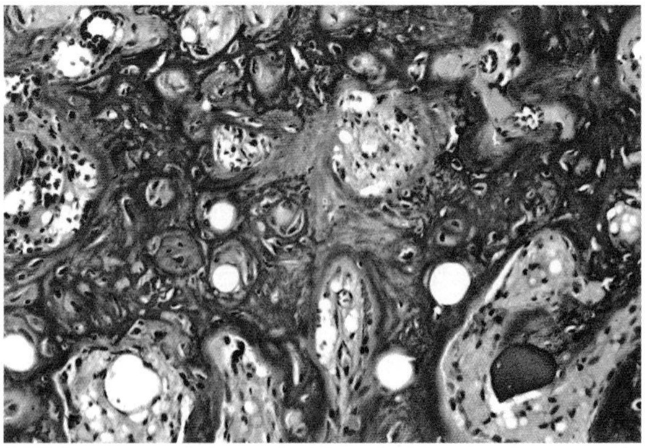

Figure 14-80

STRESS FRACTURE

Left: Reactive new bone fills the bone marrow spaces, creating a pattern that may be mistaken for a permeative osseous neoplasm.

Right: As the immature bone becomes mineralized, it takes on a blue-purple color.

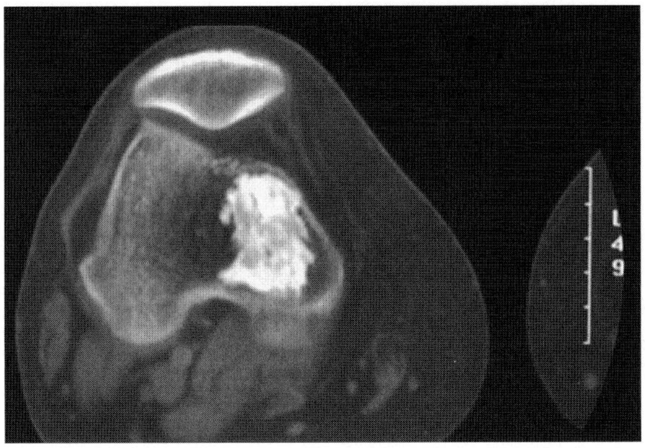

Figure 14-81

BONE ISLAND

CT demonstrates a heavily mineralized mass confined to the bone marrow. The outline is irregular.

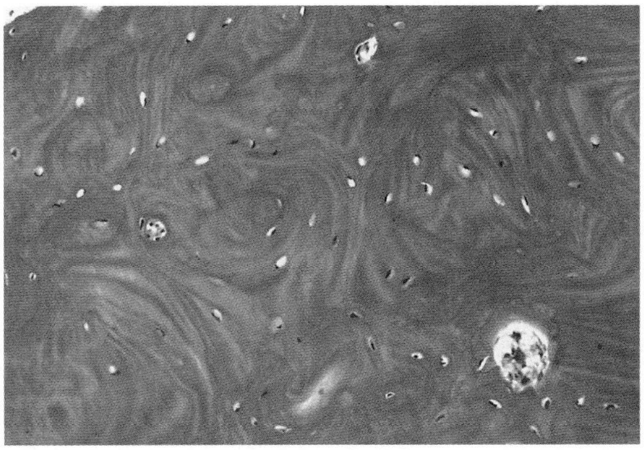

Figure 14-82

BONE ISLAND

Compact bone with haversian canals.

Gross Findings. If removed intact, bone islands appear as rounded masses of densely sclerotic bone situated within the medullary cavity.

Microscopic Findings. Cortical-appearing bone with haversian canals occurs in the medullary cavity (fig. 14-82). There is no associated spindle cell proliferation.

Differential Diagnosis. Radiographically, a bone island may be mistaken for a focus of blastic metastasis. However, microscopically, the lack of any cellular proliferation differentiates a bone island from any other process.

Treatment and Prognosis. No treatment is necessary.

MISCELLANEOUS CONDITIONS THAT SIMULATE NEOPLASM

Giant Cell Reparative Granuloma

Definition. Giant cell reparative granuloma is a reactive process consisting of giant cells, fibroblasts, and new bone formation. It is limited to the jawbones and small bones of the hands and feet.

General Features. The term *giant cell reparative granuloma* was coined by Jaffe (102) to describe a reactive process of the jawbones that he considered to be a reaction to hemorrhage. In 1962, Ackerman and Spjut (99) described two lesions in the phalanges that had similar histologic features; they used the term *giant cell reaction*. Several publications have confirmed the presence of these reactive lesions in the small bones of the hands and feet (101,103–105) and the term *giant cell reparative granuloma* is well accepted.

Clinical Features. The age distribution of patients with giant cell reparative granuloma is broad, with the mean in the third decade. Males and females are affected equally. Patients present with pain, swelling, or both.

Sites. The small bones of the hands and feet are involved exclusively. One large series reported a preference for the bones of the feet (104), but another reported a preference for the bones of the hands (105).

Radiographic Findings. Giant cell reparative granuloma is predominantly lucent. The bone is commonly expanded, the cortex may be thinned, and the process may extend into the soft tissue (fig. 14-83). The lesion usually occurs in the middle but may extend to the ends of the bone.

Gross Findings. Gross specimens consist of curetted fragments, and the tissue is friable and red.

Microscopic Findings. Giant cell reparative granuloma consists of giant cells that usually are arranged in clusters (fig. 14-84). The mononuclear cells are spindle shaped, loosely arranged, and produce collagen. Spicules of bone and osteoid, with prominent osteoblastic rimming, are present (fig. 14-85).

Genetics and Other Special Techniques. Only a single case of giant cell reparative granuloma has been reported to have been subjected to cytogenetic analysis (100). A clonal rearrangement involving the X chromosome [t(X;4)

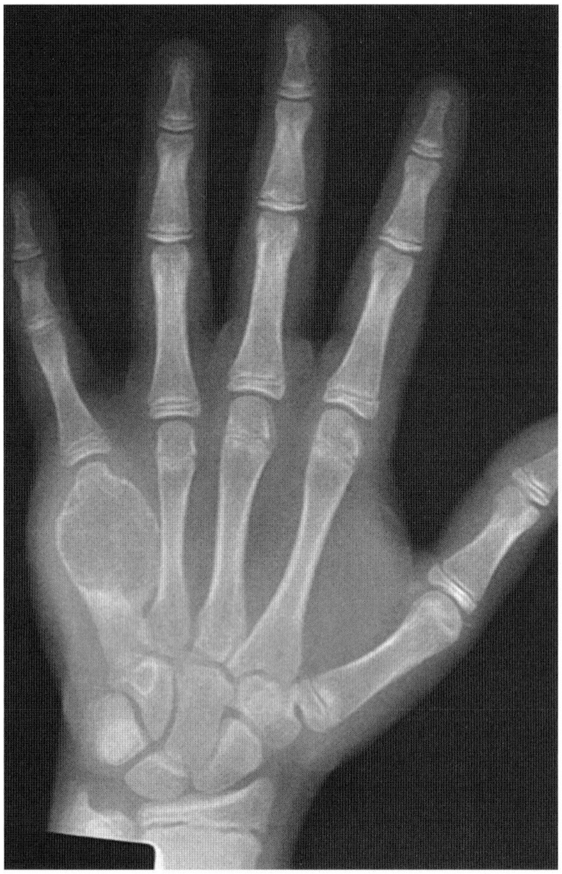

Figure 14-83

GIANT CELL REPARATIVE GRANULOMA

An expansile lucency in a metacarpal bone does not extend to the end of the bone. (Courtesy of Dr. V. Herr, Rapid City, SD.)

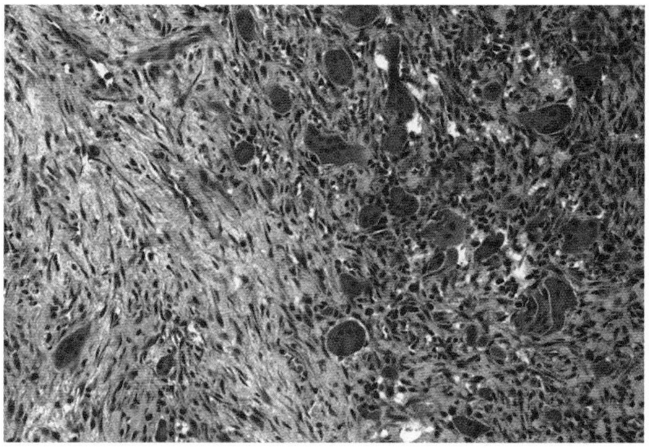

Figure 14-84

GIANT CELL REPARATIVE GRANULOMA

Numerous giant cells occur within a dense fibrous stroma that contains scattered hemosiderin-laden macrophages.

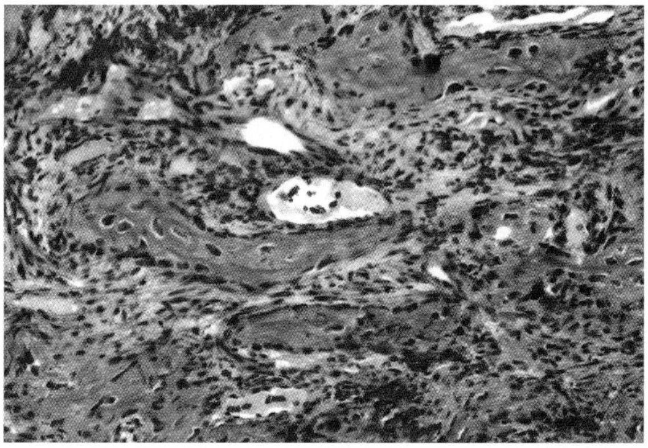

Figure 14-85

GIANT CELL REPARATIVE GRANULOMA

Reactive new bone formation is commonly seen in giant cell reparative granulomas.

(q22;q31.3)] was detected. Additional cases of giant cell reparative granuloma must be examined cytogenetically to determine the specificity and significance of these findings.

Differential Diagnosis. Differentiating a giant cell reparative granuloma from a giant cell tumor can be difficult. Their radiographic features overlap. In giant cell tumors, the giant cells are distributed more uniformly than they are in giant cell reparative granuloma, but this feature may not be useful in biopsy material. The most important features that differentiate the two are spindle cells, collagen production, and bone formation in giant cell reparative granuloma.

Treatment and Prognosis. Curettage is the treatment of choice. Recurrences are common and are managed effectively with recurettage.

Langerhans' Cell Histiocytosis (Eosinophilic Granuloma)

Definition. Langerhans' cell histiocytosis is a proliferation of Langerhans cells, usually associated with eosinophils.

General Features. In 1953, Lichtenstein (107) proposed that eosinophilic granuloma of bone, Hand-Schüller-Christian disease, and Letterer-Siwe disease are related conditions caused by the proliferation of histiocytes. He considered Letterer-Siwe disease to be an acute disseminated form with skeletal, skin, and visceral involvement; Hand-Schüller-Christian disease a

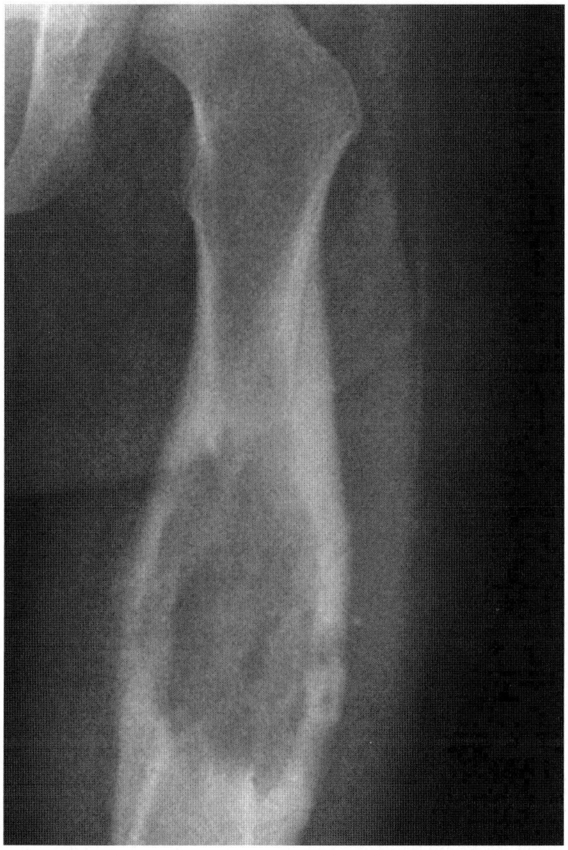

Figure 14-86

LANGERHANS' CELL HISTIOCYTOSIS

A plain radiograph shows a large lytic defect in the diaphysis of the femur. There is thick, organized, periosteal new bone formation. (Courtesy of Dr. C. Jarnes, St. Paul, MN.)

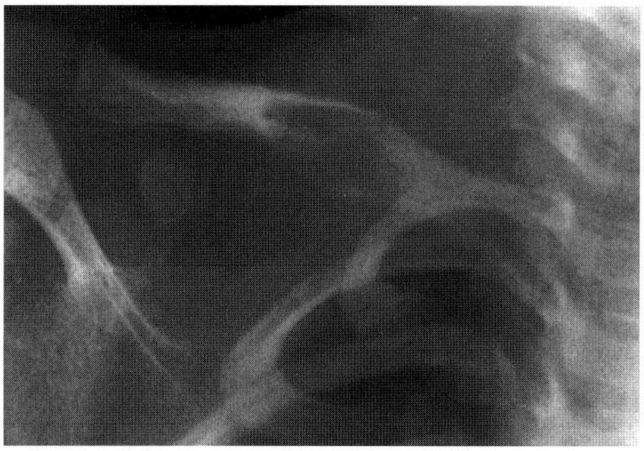

Figure 14-87

LANGERHANS' CELL HISTIOCYTOSIS

An expansile mass in the clavicle, with poor margination, suggests an aggressive process. (Courtesy of Dr. A. Filice, Redding, CA.)

chronic disseminated form with the triad of skeletal involvement, exophthalmos, and diabetes insipidus; and eosinophilic granuloma a form limited to the skeleton, usually as a single focus of involvement. This unitarian hypothesis has been questioned (108).

The cause of Langerhans' cell histiocytosis is unknown, but some studies have demonstrated monoclonality of the histiocytes, suggesting a neoplasm (110,112).

Clinical Features. Most patients with skeletal involvement are younger than 5 years of age; adults, however, account for about one third of all patients. Pain is the usual symptom, and patients with skull involvement complain of headache. Involvement of the jawbones may be associated with loose teeth or even the loss of teeth.

Sites. The skull is the site involved most commonly in both children and adults (106). The jawbones, ribs, vertebrae, and femur are also affected relatively commonly.

Radiographic Findings. Langerhans' cell histiocytosis presents as a sharply demarcated lucency, often associated with a benign-appearing thick periosteal reaction (figs. 14-86–14-88). In the skull, a "hole-in-hole" appearance results from the unequal destruction of the two tables. In the vertebrae, the body is affected, causing compression and vertebra plana.

Gross Findings. Grossly, the lesion is soft, red, and granular. Rarely, there is a greenish tint (fig. 14-89).

Microscopic Findings. The diagnostic cell (Langerhans' cell) is characterized by an oval nucleus with a longitudinal groove, producing the appearance of a coffee bean (fig. 14-90). The cytoplasm is clear or eosinophilic. Mitotic figures may be abundant. Inflammatory cells such as lymphocytes, plasma cells, and eosinophils are invariably present. Eosinophils may be abundant and produce eosinophilic abscesses. Benign giant cells are nearly always present. Foci of necrosis are common (fig. 14-91). A characteristic feature is the loose arrangement of the tissue: the histiocytes tend to form loose aggregates and not sheets (fig. 14-92).

Electron microscopic examination shows cytoplasmic inclusions called *Birbeck granules*. With

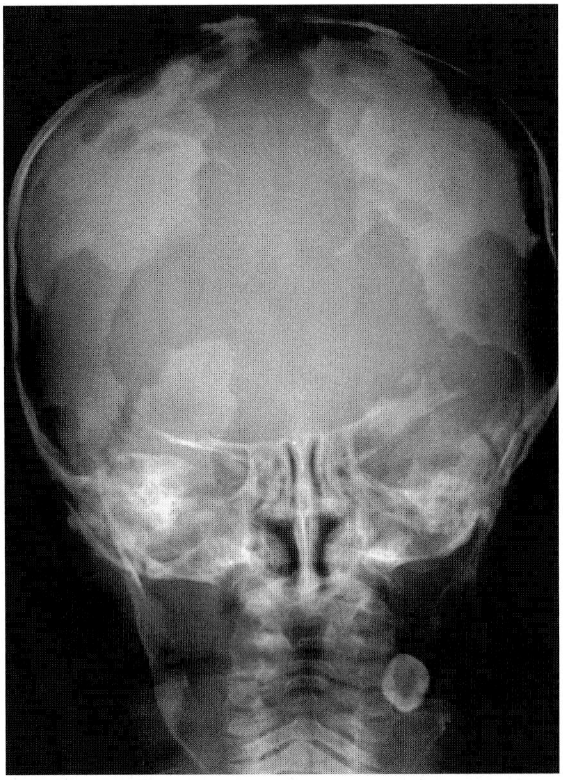

Figure 14-88

LANGERHANS' CELL HISTIOCYTOSIS

The skull of a 3-year-old boy with disseminated disease has multiple areas of lysis. (Fig. 27-102 from Unni KK. Dahlin's bone tumors: general aspects and data on 11,087 cases, 5th ed. Philadelphia: Lippincott-Raven; 1996:409. By permission of Mayo Foundation.)

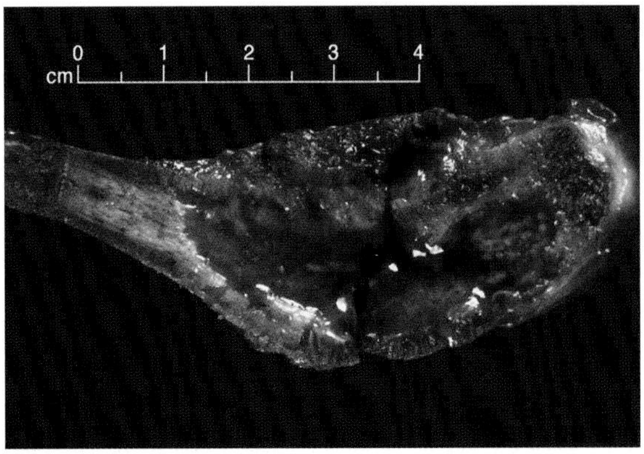

Figure 14-89

LANGERHANS' CELL HISTIOCYTOSIS

A lesion in the clavicle is soft and red, and destroys the cortex.

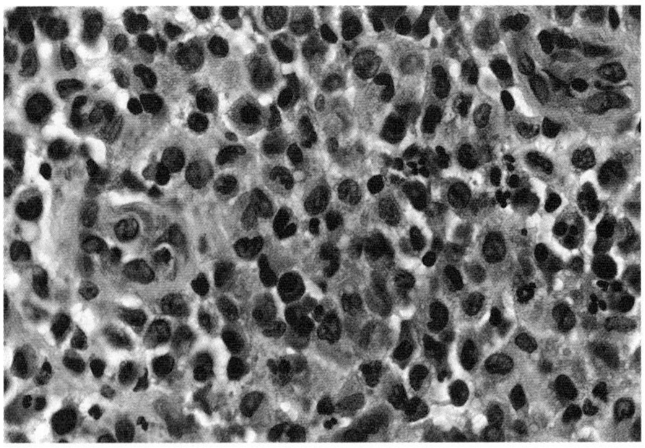

Figure 14-90

LANGERHANS' CELL HISTIOCYTOSIS

The Langerhans cells contain oval nuclei that have central grooves and often appear folded. Abundant eosinophilic cytoplasm surrounds the nuclei. Mitotic figures may be found. Eosinophils, lymphocytes, and plasma cells are scattered throughout the field.

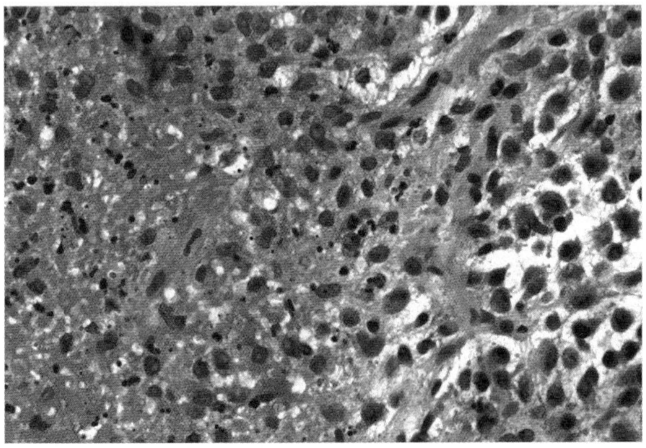

Figure 14-91

LANGERHANS' CELL HISTIOCYTOSIS

An area of necrosis in Langerhans' cell histiocytosis.

immunoperoxidase stains, the histiocytes are positive for S-100 protein and CD1a (fig. 14-93).

Cytologic Findings. In conjunction with the clinical setting and radiographic findings, the FNA features of localized Langerhans' cell histiocytosis (eosinophilic granuloma of bone) are sufficiently distinctive to allow a definite diagnosis (fig. 14-94). The hallmarks of this lesion are fairly large histiocytes with nuclei that are grooved or folded, evenly stained nuclei, and a variable admixture of eosinophils (109,111). In addition,

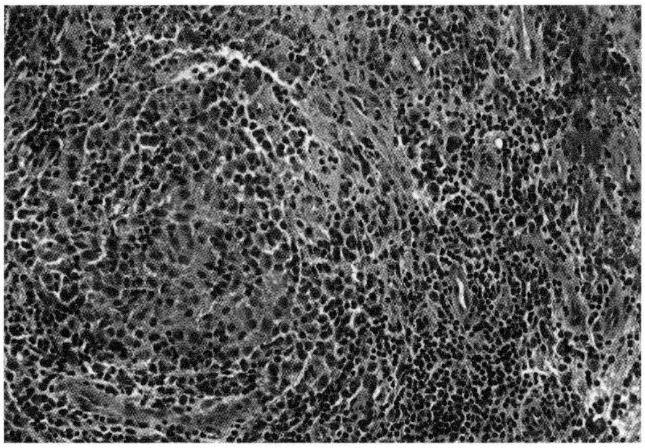

Figure 14-92

LANGERHANS' CELL HISTIOCYTOSIS

A nodular aggregate of Langerhans cells is interspersed with eosinophils. Chronic inflammatory cells and pigmented macrophages are found at the periphery of the nodule.

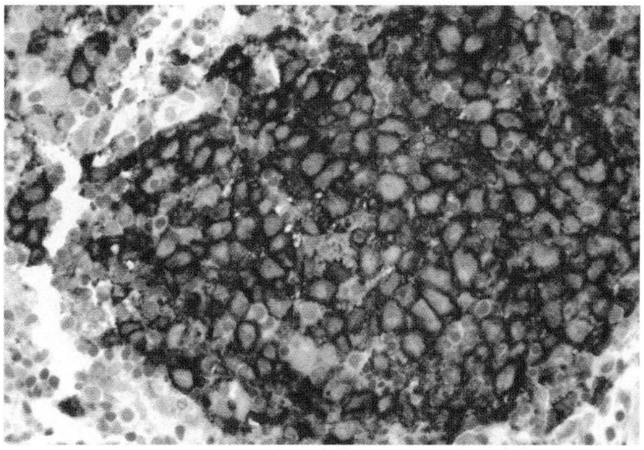

Figure 14-93

LANGERHANS' CELL HISTIOCYTOSIS

Langerhans cells are immunoreactive with CD1a.

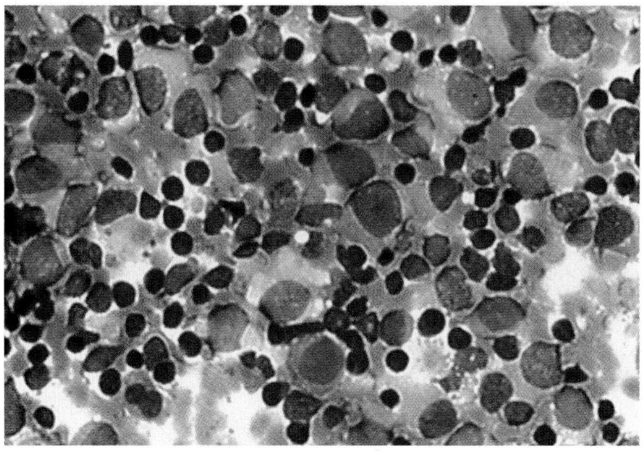

Figure 14-94

LANGERHANS' CELL HISTIOCYTOSIS ASPIRATE

Characteristic histiocytes are seen in a background of eosinophils, neutrophils, and lymphocytes.

there frequently are accompanying foamy macrophages, multinucleated giant cells, neutrophils, lymphocytes, and plasma cells. Occasionally, these cells may be so prominent that they obscure the diagnostic Langerhans cells, often leading to a misdiagnosis of osteomyelitis. However, electron microscopy can be performed on FNA material to identify Birbeck granules. Immunohistochemical demonstration of S-100 protein and CD1a in the diagnostic histiocytes may be difficult to interpret in FNA specimens.

Genetics and Other Special Techniques. X chromosome inactivation studies show that Langerhans' cell histiocytosis is clonal (110).

Differential Diagnosis. The mixture of cells is similar to the infiltrate seen in osteomyelitis. However, Langerhans' cell histiocytosis lacks the proliferation of capillaries and the appearance of granulation tissue typical of osteomyelitis. In difficult cases, immunoperoxidase stains for S-100 protein and CD1a are useful. Rarely, a lymphomatous process enters the differential diagnosis. In lymphoma, however, the histiocytic-appearing cells lack the clustering, loose arrangement typical of Langerhans' cell histiocytosis.

Treatment and Prognosis. The prognosis depends on the extent of involvement. Patients with involvement of a single skeletal site do well, and those with systemic involvement, especially hepatosplenomegaly, do not. Patients with involvement of multiple skeletal sites (more than three) are more likely to have systemic disease (106). Solitary lesions can be treated with curettage, injections of methylprednisolone, or small dose of radiation. Systemic chemotherapy may be helpful in patients with disseminated disease.

Erdheim-Chester Disease

Definition. Erdheim-Chester disease is characterized by the accumulation of foamy histiocytes in several organs, especially in long bones.

General Features. The disease was first described by Chester in 1930 (114); at that time, it was considered to be lipid granulomatosis. Its association with Langerhans' cell histiocytosis is

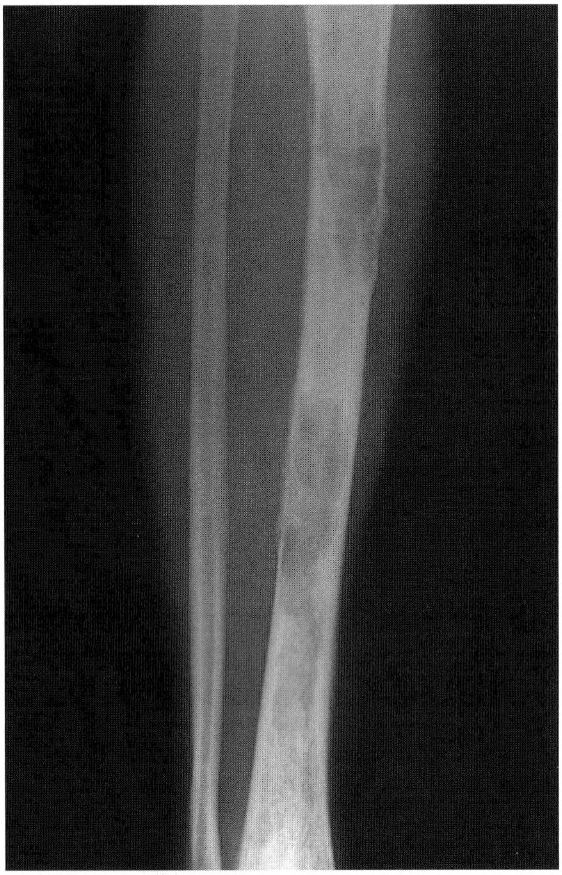

Figure 14-95

ERDHEIM-CHESTER DISEASE

A plain radiograph shows multiple areas of involvement of the tibia. Note the mixed lytic and sclerotic appearance.

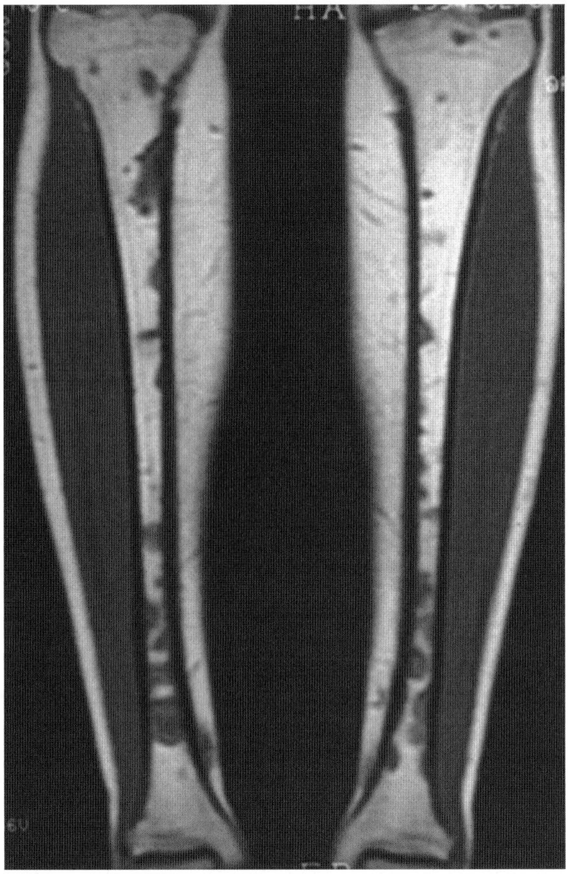

Figure 14-96

ERDHEIM-CHESTER DISEASE

MRI shows bilateral, symmetric lesions in the tibia of a 26-year-old man.

enigmatic. Erdheim-Chester disease may involve the pituitary gland (leading to diabetes insipidus), lung, and skeleton, similar to the triad in Langerhans' cell histiocytosis. However, long bones are involved in Erdheim-Chester disease, whereas the skull, jawbones, ribs, and vertebrae are primarily involved in Langerhans' cell histiocytosis. The pattern of lung involvement is also different (116). Kambouchner et al. (116) described a patient who had both Erdheim-Chester disease and Langerhans' cell histiocytosis; the authors were able to demonstrate CD1a-positive cells in the latter but not in the lesions of Erdheim-Chester disease.

Clinical Features. Patients with skeletal lesions may be asymptomatic or have pain. Extraskeletal manifestations include diabetes insipidus, retroperitoneal fibrosis, or symptoms associated with pulmonary disease. Most patients are adults, and there is a distinct male predominance.

Sites. The metaphysis and diaphysis of the long bones are involved; the lesions are usually bilateral and symmetric.

Radiographic Findings. The most common radiographic finding is medullary sclerosis of the involved bone. A mixture of medullary sclerosis and lucency (often with a honeycomb pattern) is typically seen in the long bones (figs. 14-95, 14-96). On bone scans, the uptake of isotope in the metadiaphyseal region of long bones with bilateral symmetric lesions is striking (fig. 14-97).

Microscopic Findings. The medullary bone appears thickened, and the bone marrow is replaced with fibrous tissue and foamy histiocytes (fig. 14-98). Lymphocytes and giant cells may be present.

Genetics and Other Special Techniques. Data are conflicting regarding the clonality of Erdheim-Chester disease (113,115).

Differential Diagnosis. The histologic features are typical but not diagnostic. The differential diagnosis includes many conditions with foam cells, such as fibrous dysplasia and Rosai-Dorfman disease. The radiographic appearance, however, is unmistakable.

Treatment and Prognosis. The prognosis is generally good. Some patients with extraskeletal involvement die of progressive disease.

Mast Cell Disease

Definition. Mast cell disease is a proliferation of mast cells with involvement of multiple organ systems, including the skeleton.

General Features. Involvement of the skin by urticaria pigmentosa is the most common manifestation of mast cell disease and may begin in infancy or childhood. *Systemic mastocytosis* is the term used when other organ systems are involved; this may or may not be associated with involvement of the skin.

Clinical Features. The manifestations of systemic mast cell disease may be protean. Systemic symptoms include fatigue, flushing, and syncope attacks; patients with involvement of the gastrointestinal tract may present with diarrhea. In a study of 58 patients with systemic mast cell disease, Travis et al. (118) found that

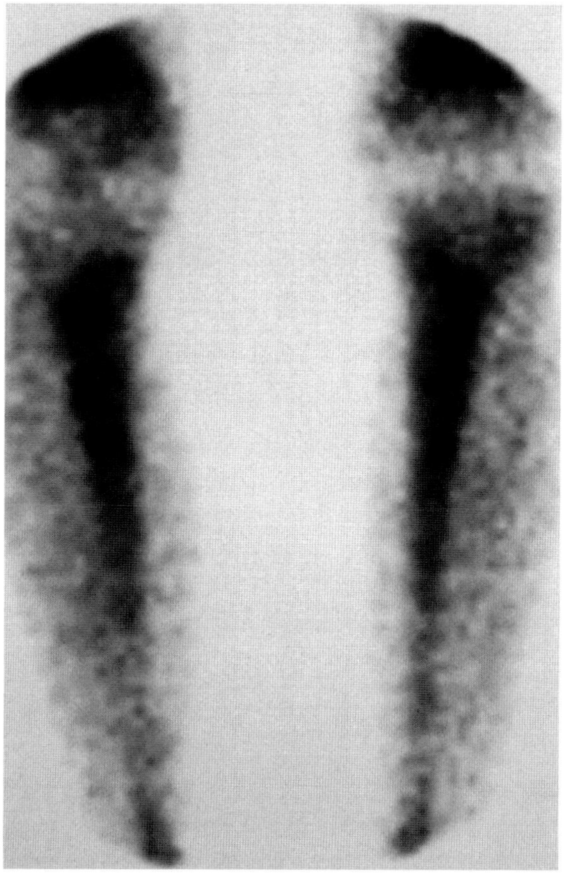

Figure 14-97

ERDHEIM-CHESTER DISEASE

A bone scan shows diffuse uptake in both tibias of a 52-year-old man who also had retroperitoneal and pulmonary disease.

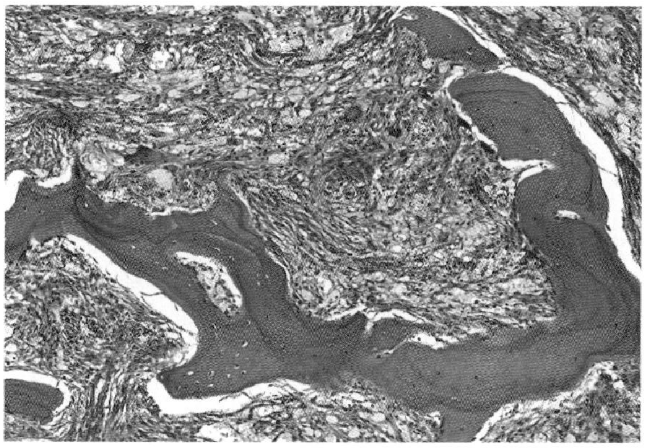

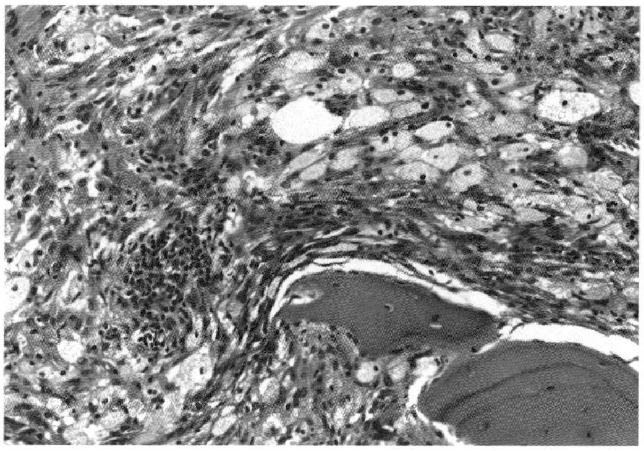

Figure 14-98

ERDHEIM-CHESTER DISEASE

Left: The bone is sclerotic.

Right: The marrow spaces contain a mixture of foamy histiocytes, lymphocytes, Touton giant cells, and loose fibrosis.

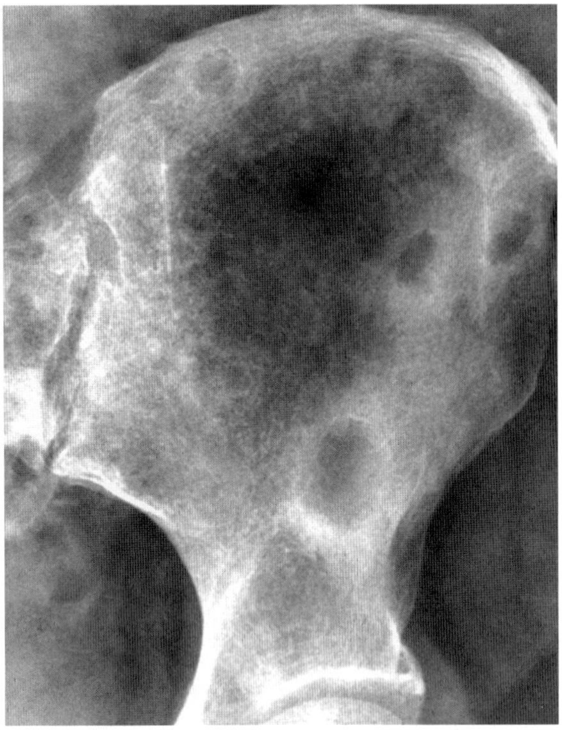

Figure 14-99

MAST CELL DISEASE

A plain radiograph shows multiple lytic areas surrounded by sclerosis.

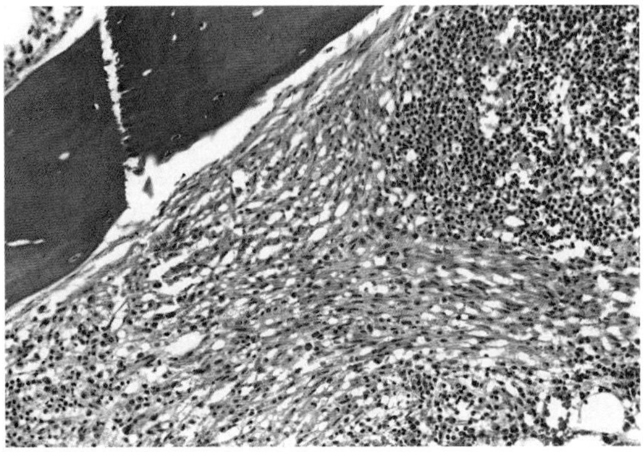

Figure 14-100

MAST CELL DISEASE

A paratrabecular aggregate of mast cells is bordered by a cluster of lymphocytes and bone marrow elements.

28 percent presented with symptoms of skeletal involvement, such as pain and fractures.

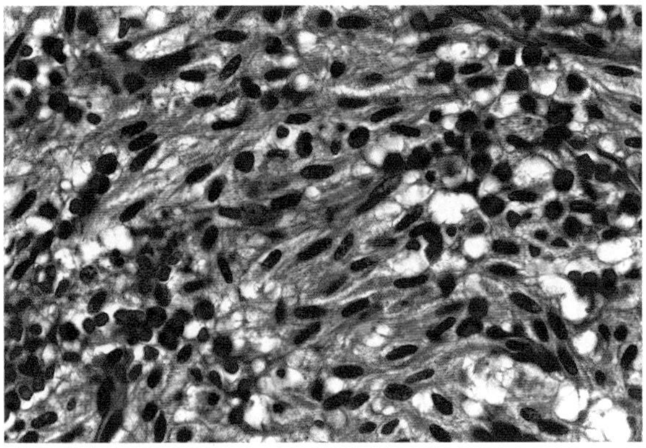

Figure 14-101

MAST CELL DISEASE

The mast cells have a bland spindle cell morphology. Eosinophils are also present.

However, radiographs showed skeletal disease in 59 percent of patients.

Radiographic Findings. Radiographs show multiple areas of medullary sclerosis, sometimes associated with lysis (fig. 14-99).

Microscopic Findings. Mast cells typically form small aggregates (microgranulomas) in the bone marrow, typically in a paratrabecular location (fig. 14-100). However, the nodules may be in the bone marrow fat or around vessels. The bony trabeculae appear thickened. The cells are small and uniform and have well-defined cytoplasmic borders (fig. 14-101). The nuclei are oval and do not have prominent nucleoli. The cytoplasm is clear or faintly granular. Eosinophils are usually present in these nodules. Metachromatic stains, such as toluidine blue, highlight the granules. Immunohistochemical demonstration of tryptase is a sensitive and specific marker for mast cells (fig. 14-102).

Genetics and Other Special Techniques. Systemic mastocytosis is a clonal neoplasm associated with gain of function mutations involving the tyrosine kinase domain of *c-kit* (117).

Differential Diagnosis. Mast cell disease is usually mistaken for metastatic carcinoma. The nodular arrangement of the mast cells and the lack of atypia should suggest the correct diagnosis.

Treatment and Prognosis. The prognosis is unpredictable. Patients who die with disease have usually developed other malignancies such as leukemia.

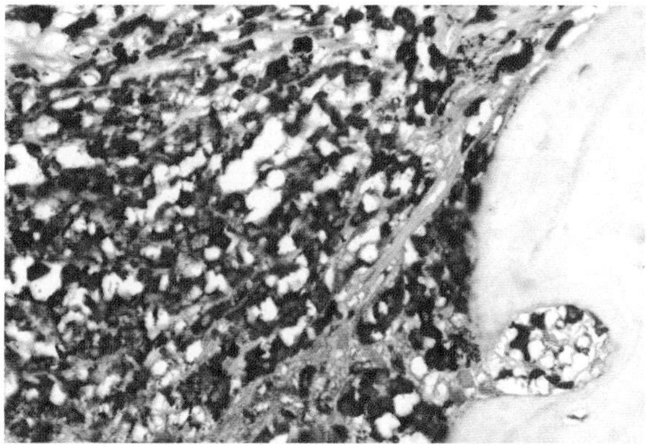

Figure 14-102

MAST CELL DISEASE

The mast cells are immunoreactive with antibodies to tryptase.

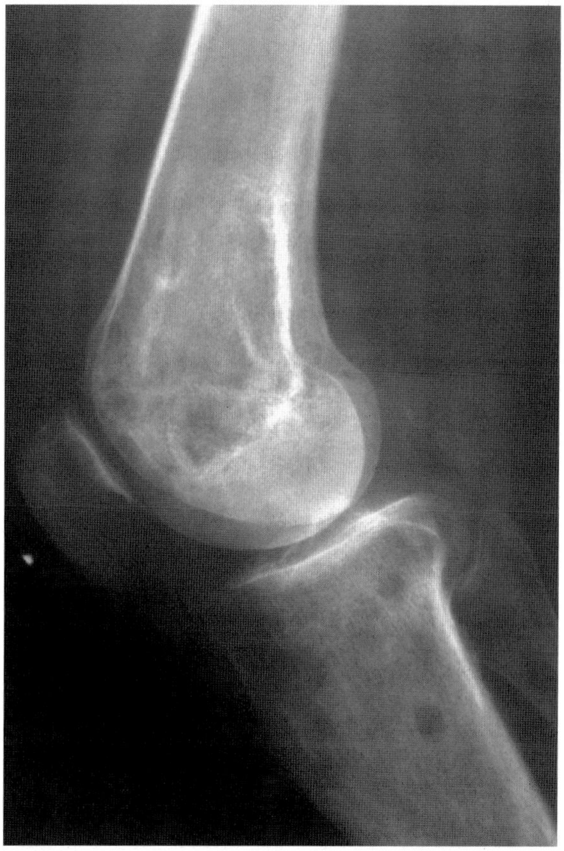

Figure 14-103

SINUS HISTIOCYTOSIS WITH MASSIVE LYMPHADENOPATHY

The lesion is a well-marginated area of lysis in the distal femur. The appearance is nonspecific.

Sinus Histiocytosis with Massive Lymphadenopathy (Rosai-Dorfman Disease)

Definition. Sinus histiocytosis with massive lymphadenopathy, of unknown cause, was first described to involve lymph nodes, but later was shown to involve multiple organ sites. It is characterized by a proliferation of histiocytes, lymphocytes, and plasma cells.

General Features. As described initially, the disease involved the cervical lymph nodes of young children (124). It is characterized by fever, increased erythrocyte sedimentation rate, and leukocytosis. The prognosis is excellent, and the enlarged lymph nodes regress spontaneously. Practically all organ systems have been reported to be involved by the disease (119).

Clinical Features. In most patients with skeletal involvement, the diagnosis is established on the basis of lymph node disease (125). In one report, fewer than 5 percent of patients with the lymph node disease developed skeletal disease (125). The skeletal lesions may be incidental radiographic findings or may be painful (120). A few patients have been reported to have bone involvement as the sole manifestation of the disease (120–122). Extraskeletal disease may develop in some of these patients (121).

Sites. Any skeletal site may be involved.

Radiographic Findings. The lesions are well-demarcated lucent defects with sclerotic margins (fig. 14-103).

Gross Findings. The bone is expanded and the marrow is replaced by a soft yellow-white mass (120).

Microscopic Findings. The microscopic features of sinus histiocytosis with massive lymphadenopathy in bone are similar to those of lymph nodes. The bone marrow is infiltrated by histiocytes, lymphocytes, and plasma cells (fig. 14-104). Because the histiocytes tend to aggregate, clear and dark areas may be identified with low-power magnification. The histiocytes have vesicular nuclei, with or without a prominent nucleolus, and abundant clear cytoplasm. The diagnostic feature is emperipolesis, that is, the presence of lymphocytes and plasma cells in the cytoplasm of the histiocytes (fig. 14-105). Fibrosis usually occurs in the background and can be prominent.

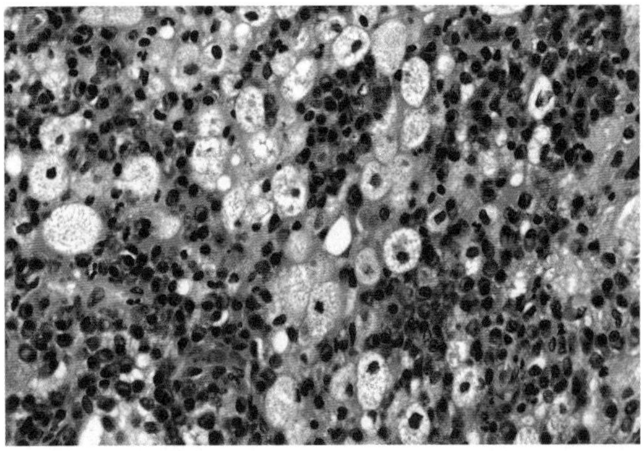

Figure 14-104

SINUS HISTIOCYTOSIS WITH MASSIVE LYMPHADENOPATHY

A lesion in the proximal tibia of a 26-year-old woman is composed predominantly of foamy histiocytes, plasma cells, and a few scattered lymphocytes.

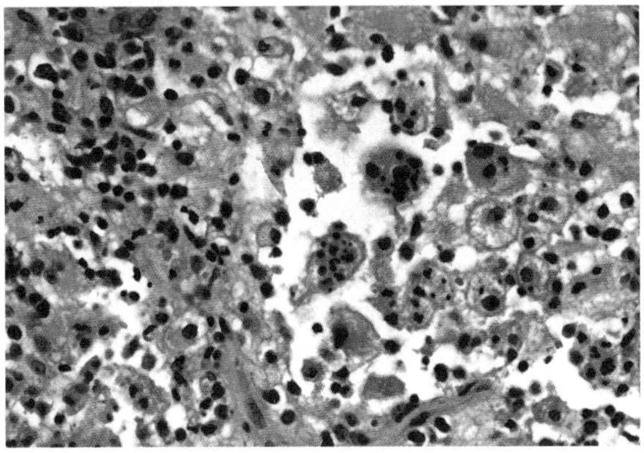

Figure 14-105

SINUS HISTIOCYTOSIS WITH MASSIVE LYMPHADENOPATHY

Emperipolesis is a diagnostic feature of sinus histiocytosis with massive lymphadenopathy.

Rarely, the bony spicules appear thickened. The histiocytes stain for S-100 protein (fig. 14-106).

Genetics and Other Special Techniques. X chromosome inactivation studies show that sinus histiocytosis with massive lymphadenopathy is polyclonal (123).

Differential Diagnosis. Histiocytes can be found in a wide variety of bone lesions. Emperipolesis, however, is not found in the histiocytes of any condition other than sinus histiocytosis with massive lymphadenopathy.

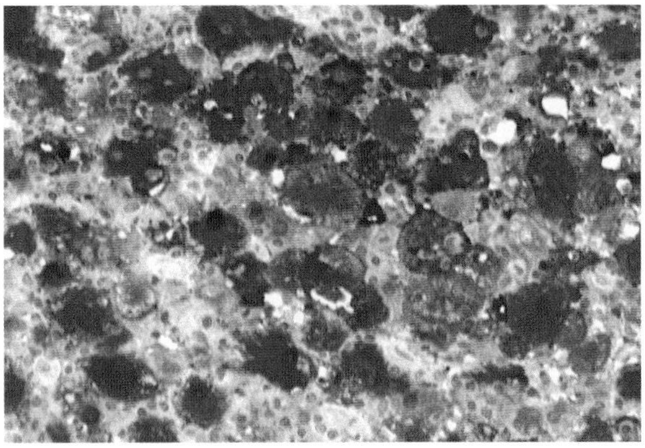

Figure 14-106

SINUS HISTIOCYTOSIS WITH MASSIVE LYMPHADENOPATHY

The histiocytes react with antibodies to S-100 protein.

Treatment and Prognosis. No treatment is known for the disease; however, the prognosis is excellent and the lesions may resolve spontaneously. Some patients with systemic disease develop amyloidosis (125).

Osteomyelitis

Definition. Osteomyelitis is an inflammatory response of bone to an infectious agent.

General Features. Osteomyelitis is relatively common and will continue to be so, especially in immunosuppressed patients. Unusual organisms may be responsible for the infection in these patients. Classically, osteomyelitis is divided into acute, subacute, and chronic forms, but there is considerable overlap in the features (134). Osteomyelitis is hematogenous in 19 percent of patients (occurring in the metaphyses of long bones in children), secondary to a contiguous focus in 47 percent (including postoperative), and associated with peripheral vascular disease in 34 percent (134).

Clinical Features. Patients present with pain and systemic symptoms such as chills and fever. Laboratory testing demonstrates anemia, leukocytosis, and an increased erythrocyte sedimentation rate. *Hematogenous osteomyelitis* affects long bones in children and the spine in adults. It is unusual for hematogenous osteomyelitis to be multifocal. *Chronic recurrent osteomyelitis* can involve multiple bones (128, 131,133). Patients with sickle cell anemia are susceptible to *Salmonella osteomyelitis* (126).

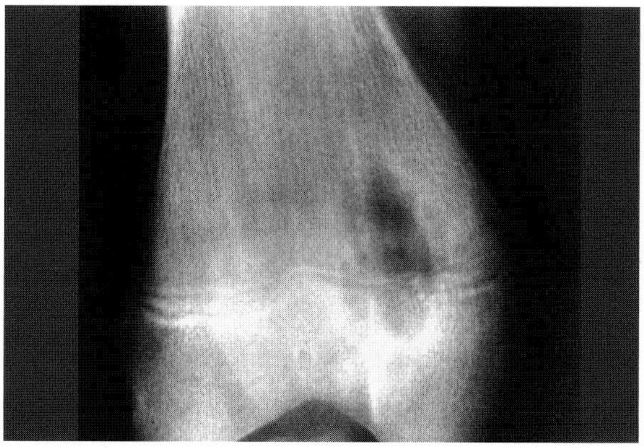

Figure 14-107

OSTEOMYELITIS

A destructive lesion involves the metaphysis and crosses the epiphyseal plate. (Courtesy of Dr. D. Forth, Walnut Creek, CA.)

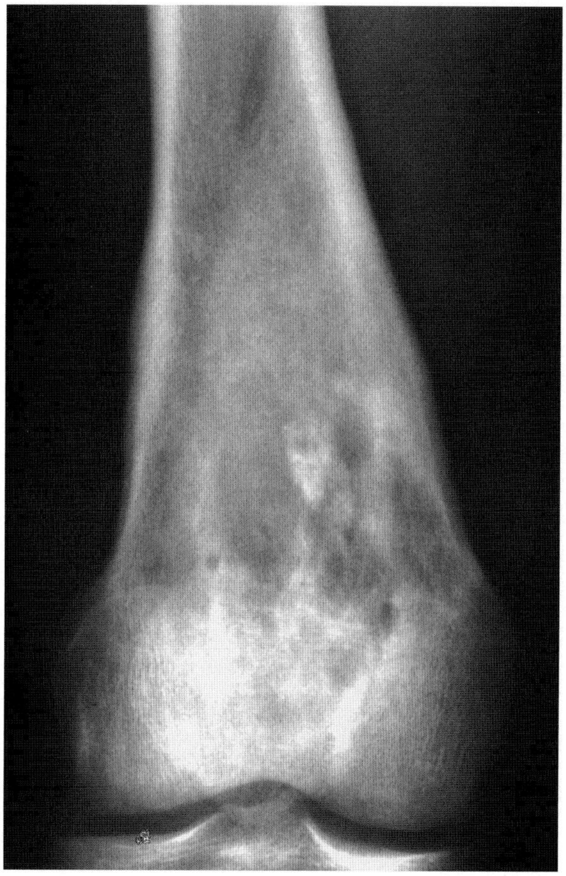

Figure 14-108

OSTEOMYELITIS

There is irregular lysis associated with sclerosis in the distal femur. The appearance is that of a long-standing process.

Sites. Any portion of the skeleton can be involved. In the spine, the disease typically involves the disk space and the bodies of the vertebrae above and below the space.

Radiographic Findings. The radiographic features can be alarming and suggest a neoplasm such as Ewing's sarcoma or malignant lymphoma (129). The earliest manifestation is irregular rarefaction, which may be associated with periosteal new bone formation (fig. 14-107). In later stages, geographic areas of destruction, with thick periosteal new bone formation, may be present (fig. 14-108). The borders may be irregular and appear aggressive. The process may produce a lucency within the cortex that is associated with reactive sclerosis, suggesting osteoid osteoma (Brodie's abscess).

Gross Findings. Grossly, the cortex may be thickened or absent focally. The bone marrow may contain obvious pus (fig. 14-109). The center of the lesion frequently contains fragments of necrotic bone (sequestrum).

Microscopic Findings. In the early stages, the bone marrow cavity is replaced with granulation tissue, accompanied by vascular proliferation and an outpouring of polymorphonuclear leukocytes (fig. 14-110). The bony trabeculae may have empty lacunae, confirming necrosis. A few poorly formed granulomas are usually present. In the later stages, the inflammatory infiltrate is composed mostly of plasma cells. Specific infections such as tuberculosis show granulomas with caseation. Special stains are needed to demonstrate the organism. In chronic sclerosing osteomyelitis, the bone marrow is replaced with a loose fibrous tissue and the bony trabeculae appear thickened.

Differential Diagnosis. The heavy plasma cell infiltrate of chronic osteomyelitis may suggest a diagnosis of myeloma. However, there is never a pure collection of plasma cells in osteomyelitis and the granulation tissue is distinctive. In difficult cases, immunoperoxidase stains for kappa and lambda light chains can determine the clonality of the plasma cells.

Chronic sclerosing osteomyelitis can be mistaken for fibrous dysplasia and low-grade osteosarcoma. In osteomyelitis, the fibrosis of the bone

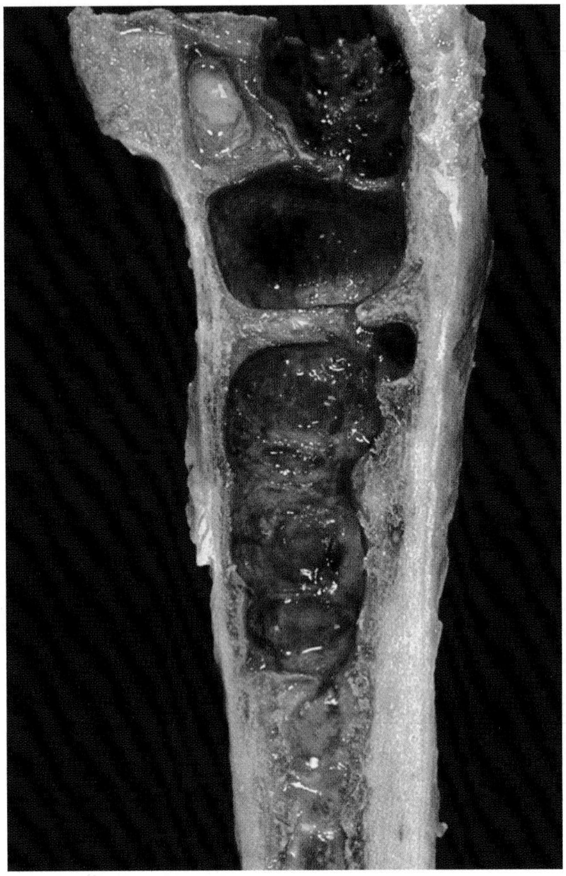

Figure 14-109

OSTEOMYELITIS

There is extensive destruction of the proximal tibia. Purulent material was found at arthroplasty.

marrow has little proliferation of spindle cells and is composed instead of loose fibrous tissue.

Treatment and Prognosis. Antibiotic treatment has improved the prognosis dramatically. In chronic osteomyelitis, the sequestrum may have to be debrided surgically; if left intact, it acts as a nidus for persistent infection. A few patients with chronic osteomyelitis and a draining sinus tract develop squamous cell carcinoma. When this occurs, patients complain of pain and an increase in a foul-smelling discharge. The carcinoma is usually grade 1 (verrucous); rarely is it high grade. The presence of squamous cells, even bland-appearing ones, in the bone marrow is diagnostic of carcinoma (130, 132). Other malignancies, such as spindle cell sarcoma, have also been reported (127). Treatment of the carcinoma consists of complete surgical removal, which may require amputation.

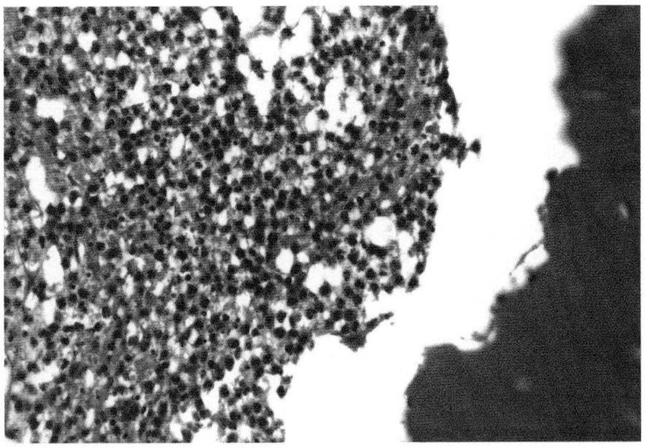

Figure 14-110

OSTEOMYELITIS

Collections of acute inflammatory cells and granulation tissue are intimately associated with trabecular bone.

Paget's Disease

Definition. Paget's disease is a disorder in which progressive deformity of the skeleton is associated with thickening of the involved bone.

General Features. The first description was made by Sir James Paget, in 1876, of a patient who had progressive deformity of the skull and long bones (Paget used the term "osteitis deformans") and who eventually developed sarcoma of the humerus. The cause of the disease is unknown; however, the detection of viral particles in the giant cells has led to the suggestion that the process is a slow-virus disease (140). The incidence of disease has a pronounced geographic variation: common in England but extremely rare in Africa and Asia (136).

Clinical Features. Paget's disease affects older persons, and there is a male predominance. Of the men in England older than 85 years, 20 percent have radiographic evidence of the disease (136). Patients present with pain and progressive deformity. Rarely, it is an incidental finding (137). Fractures occur in about 12 percent of the patients. Almost invariably, alkaline phosphatase levels are increased.

Sites. Any portion of the skeleton may be involved, but the innominate bone is the most common site, followed by the sacrum, lumbar spine, skull, femur, and tibia. The ribs and the

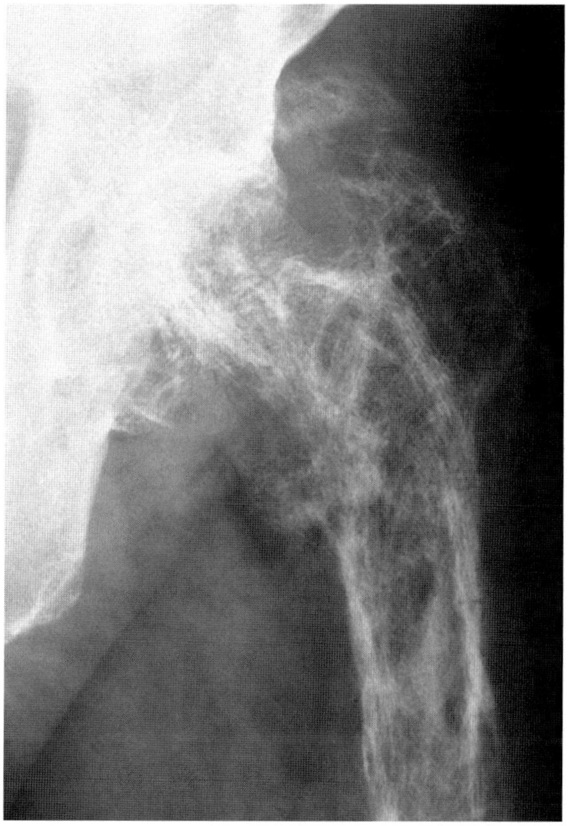

Figure 14-111

PAGET'S DISEASE

The bony trabeculae of the proximal femur are thickened and coarse. The process extends to the end of the bone.

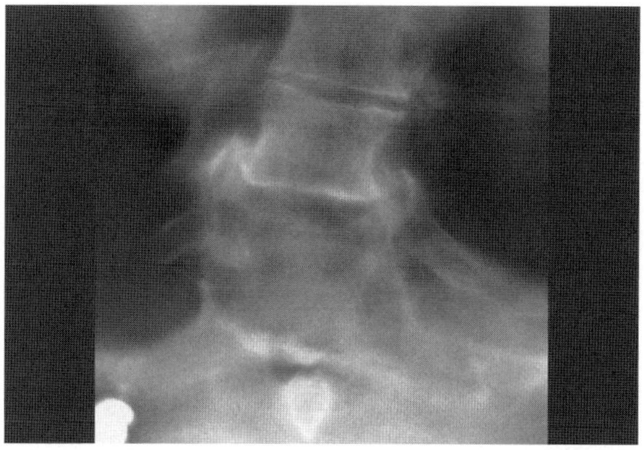

Figure 14-112

PAGET'S DISEASE

Paget's disease of the vertebral body. The entire body is enlarged. (Courtesy of Dr. R. Ramanathan, Champaign, IL.)

small bones of the hands and feet are rarely affected (139).

Radiographic Findings. Paget's disease has typical radiographic features, namely, a sharply demarcated lucency associated with thickened cortex and medullary bone (fig. 14-111). In the skull, the term *osteoporosis circumscripta* is applied to the well-defined defect. Subperiosteal bone is laid down, increasing the width of the bone (fig. 14-112). In the vertebrae, the body is involved; the lucency in the center with thick cortical outlines creates the appearance of a picture frame. Occasionally, the entire vertebral body is sclerotic (ivory vertebra). Rarely, the disease has a purely lytic pattern and the vertebral body disappears, simulating a neoplasm. In the long bones, the process almost always extends to the end of the bone and the lytic area has a tapering zone of transition; this produces a V shape that is referred to as a "flame" sign or a "blade of grass" sign (fig. 14-113) (138). Multiple fissure fractures involve the cortex. MRI confirms the thickened bone and may be useful in detecting complications (145). Pseudomalignant changes can be present because of extension of the process to the soft tissues or lytic areas (135). Radionuclide bone scans are more sensitive than radiographs for detecting the disease (fig. 14-114).

Gross Findings. The cortical bone and medullary trabeculae are coarse and thickened (fig. 14-115).

Microscopic Findings. The bony trabeculae are thickened and irregular (fig. 14-116). Multiple blue cement lines occur within the bone (fig. 14-117). Osteoblasts and osteoclasts are prominent. The bone marrow is replaced with loose connective tissue.

Genetics and Other Special Techniques. Paget's disease of bone is genetically heterogeneous. In some cases, phenotypes linked to 18q22.1 are caused by mutations in the *TNFRSF11A* gene, and phenotypes linked to 5q35 are caused by mutations in the *SQSTM1* gene (141–144).

Differential Diagnosis. The histologic appearance of Paget's disease is typical but not diagnostic. Pagetoid bone can be found in neoplasms such as osteoblastoma and osteosarcoma. Before making the diagnosis of Paget's disease, it is important to confirm that the radiographic features are consistent with the diagnosis.

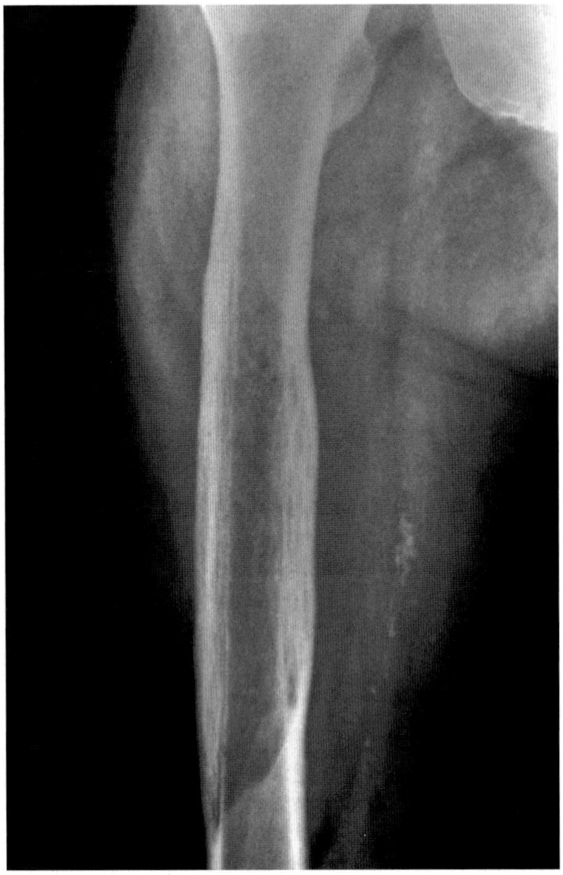

Figure 14-113

PAGET'S DISEASE

A lytic area within the femur terminates in a sharp border ("blade of grass" sign).

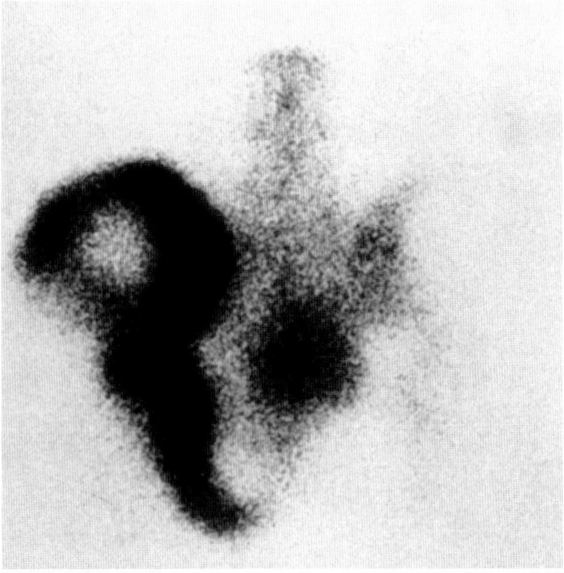

Figure 14-114

PAGET'S DISEASE

Positive bone scan of the ilium.

Treatment and Prognosis. Calcitonin and bisphosphonates have shown promise in arresting the progress of the disease (146). Development into sarcoma can be expected in fewer than 1 percent of patients (137).

Hyperparathyroidism

Definition. Hyperparathyroidism is associated with skeletal changes due to hyperfunctioning of the parathyroid glands because of neoplasm or hyperplasia.

General Features. Bony changes may result from primary or secondary hyperparathyroidism. Currently, it is unusual for hyperparathyroidism to be unrecognized and present as a bone tumor.

Clinical Features. The clinical presentation of hyperparathyroidism is extremely variable. Hypercalcemia and increased serum levels of parathyroid hormone are the best indicators of disease.

Sites. Any portion of the skeleton may show localized defects, but generally there is diffuse demineralization.

Radiographic Findings. The brown tumor of hyperparathyroidism presents as an area of lucency (fig. 14-118). A skeletal survey shows other changes typical of hyperparathyroidism, especially subperiosteal resorption of bone in the phalanges.

Gross Findings. Brown tumors are soft and red, and they produce expansile masses of bone.

Microscopic Findings. Brown tumors have a proliferation of giant cells, with a background of spindle cells and fibrosis (fig. 14-119). The giant cells usually are arranged in clusters. The bony trabeculae show increased osteoblastic and osteoclastic activity.

Differential Diagnosis. Hyperparathyroidism should be suspected if a lesion that suggests the diagnosis of giant cell tumor occurs in an unusual site, such as a rib or the metaphysis of a long bone. Serum biochemical changes and skeletal survey usually resolve the issue. Histologically, hyperparathyroidism has more fibrogenesis than a giant cell tumor.

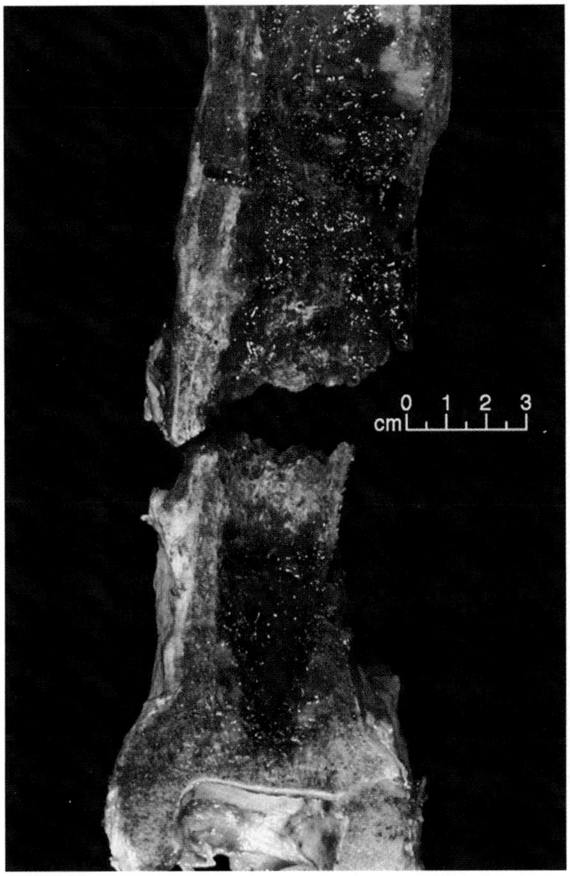

Figure 14-115

PAGET'S DISEASE

A nonhealing fracture led to amputation. The cortex is thick, and the fracture is transverse.

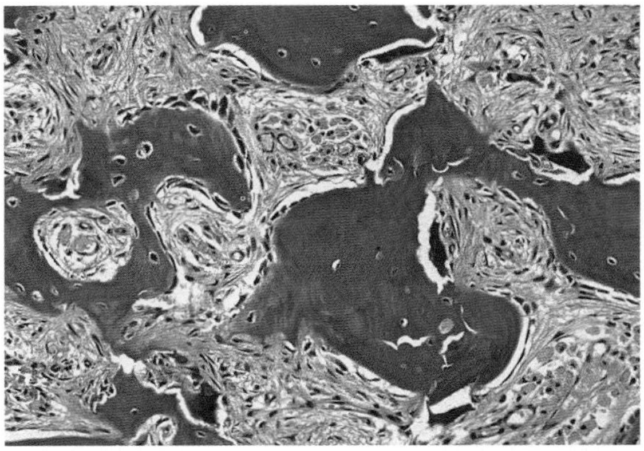

Figure 14-116

PAGET'S DISEASE

Irregularly thickened bony trabeculae with prominent osteoblastic and osteoclastic activity. The marrow space contains loose fibrovascular connective tissue.

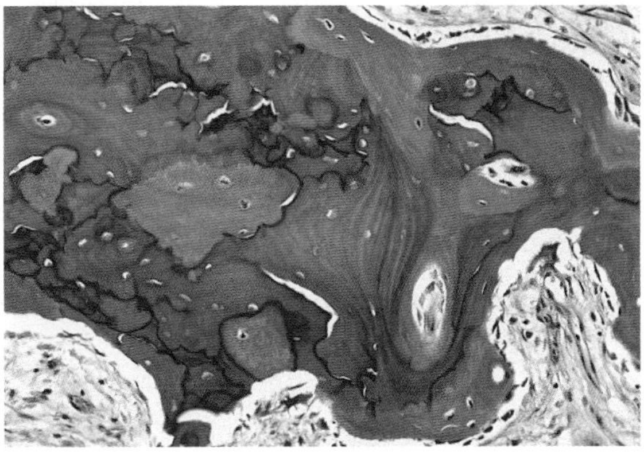

Figure 14-117

PAGET'S DISEASE

Thickened bony trabeculae with a mosaic pattern.

Treatment and Prognosis. Treatment should be directed toward surgical removal of the hyperfunctioning parathyroid gland.

Infarct of Bone

Definition. Infarct of bone is an area of necrosis in bone associated with localized ischemia.

General Features. Clinically, avascular necrosis of the femoral head is the most common type of bone infarct. The process usually is idiopathic, but it may be associated with corticosteroid use, alcohol abuse, pancreatitis, or even sickle cell anemia or decompression sickness.

Clinical Features. Patients with avascular necrosis present with pain in the hip; infarcts in other portions of the bone do not cause symptoms.

Sites. Avascular necrosis commonly involves the femoral head, but other sites such as a humeral head may be affected. Bone infarcts usually affect the metaphyseal region of long bones.

Radiographic Findings. In femoral head necrosis, an area of lucency in the subarticular region is associated with hazy sclerosis. The articular cartilage may be collapsed. In infarcts, radiographic findings are negative initially. Later, an area of lucency surrounded by calcification is apparent (figs. 14-120, 14-121).

Gross Findings. The femoral head shows collapse of articular cartilage and, underneath, a yellow semilunar-shaped area. In infarcts, the bone

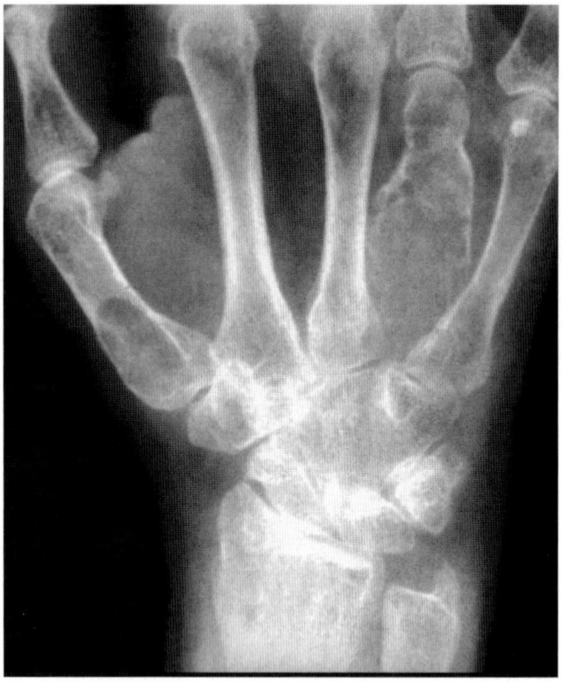

Figure 14-118

HYPERPARATHYROIDISM

Metacarpal bones contain multiple lytic areas. (Courtesy of Dr. M. Dalaker, Trondheim, Norway.)

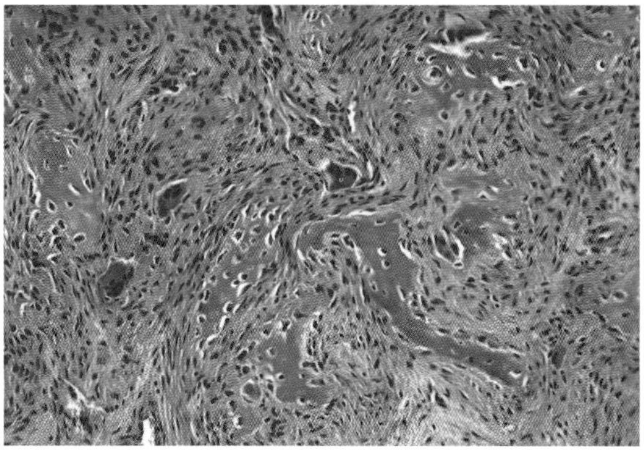

Figure 14-119

HYPERPARATHYROIDISM

Trabeculae of bone with osteoblastic rimming are surrounded by a fibrous stroma with scattered multinucleated giant cells.

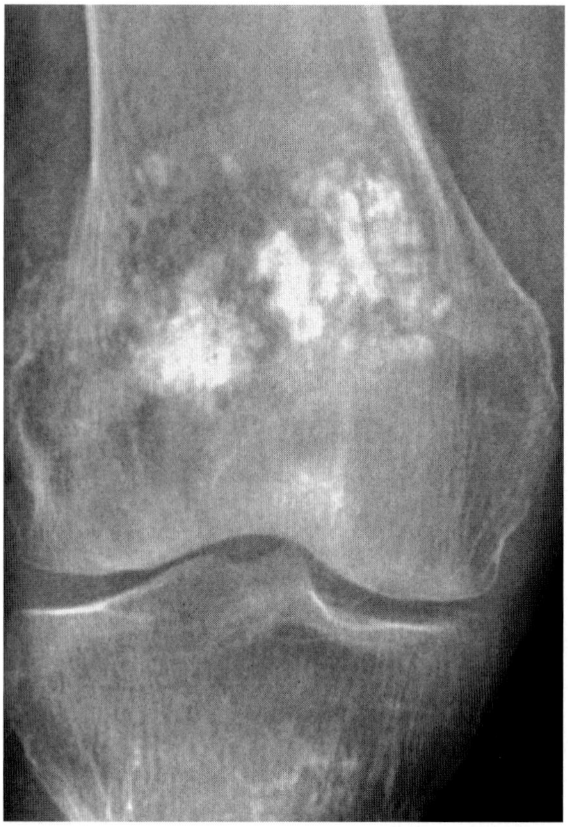

Figure 14-120

BONE INFARCT

Areas of lysis and mineralization are associated with fracture.

marrow space appears fibrotic and the surrounding area has irregular, undulating calcification.

Microscopic Findings. The bony spicules have empty osteocytic lacunae, indicating necrosis. However, this appearance may be artifactual and caused by overdecalcification. The bone marrow shows the changes of fat necrosis and calcification; these features are necessary to definitely identify infarction (fig. 14-122).

Differential Diagnosis. Calcification similar to that in bone infarcts may be seen in lipomas, fibrous dysplasia, and enchondromas. The correct diagnosis requires correlation with radiographic findings.

Treatment and Prognosis. Femoral head necrosis is treated by total hip arthroplasty. Other infarcts do not require treatment. The chance of a sarcoma arising in an infarct is small but definite (147).

Transient Osteoporosis

Definition. Transient osteoporosis is an uncommon condition in which patients complain of hip pain and radiographs show marked demineralization of the proximal femur.

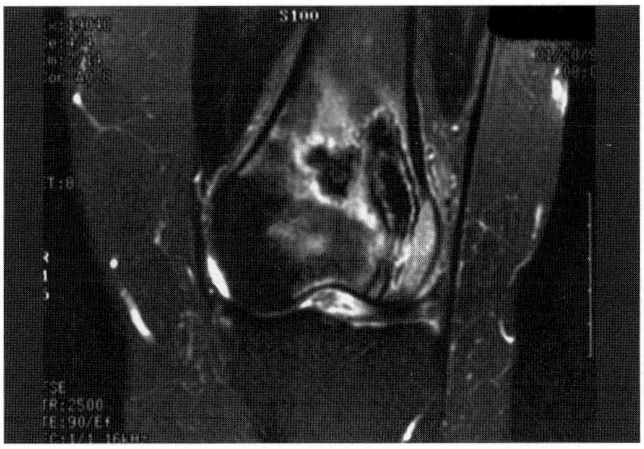

Figure 14-121

BONE INFARCT

MRI shows irregular serpiginous borders around an infarct of the distal femur. (Courtesy of Dr. D. Shuster, Royal Oak, MI.)

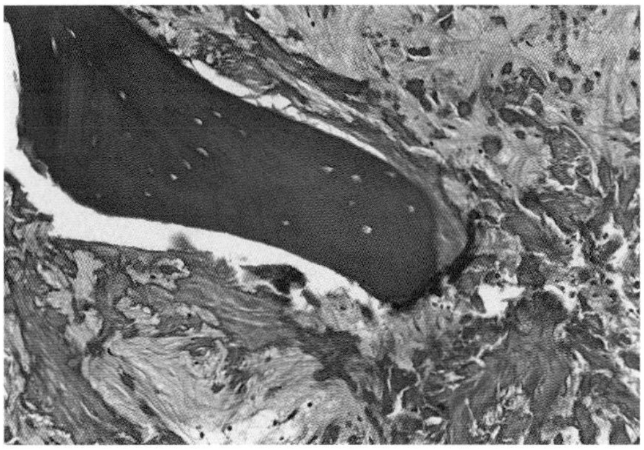

Figure 14-122

BONE INFARCT

Necrotic bone is associated with degenerative changes in the marrow space, including fat necrosis with calcification and focal fibrosis.

General Features. The condition was first described by Ravault et al. in 1947 (quoted in Bramlett et al. [148]) as transient osteoporosis characterized by the presence of severe, often incapacitating pain. Although the hip is the region affected most severely, the disease has been reported in other joints.

Clinical Features. Patients present with severe pain limited to the affected area.

Radiographic Findings. Radiographs show severe demineralization of the femoral head. Radioactive bone scans show intense uptake of isotope. These features may suggest a destructive neoplasm.

Microscopic Findings. Biopsy of the bone does not show diagnostic changes (149).

Treatment and Prognosis. The prognosis is excellent, and patients recover fully. Treatment should be symptomatic and supportive.

Traumatic Osteolysis

Definition. Traumatic osteolysis is the loss of a portion of the lateral ends of the clavicles associated with physical activity.

General and Clinical Features. Patients complain of pain in the shoulder. They may recall an injury associated with hyperextension of the joint.

Radiographic Findings. Radiographs show loss of the lateral portion of the clavicle. The process may be unilateral or bilateral.

Microscopic Findings. The biopsy does not show diagnostic changes. If the condition is recognized on radiographs, a biopsy should not be performed.

Treatment and Prognosis. The prognosis is excellent. Treatment consists of cessation of the activity that led to the development of the condition.

Chest Wall Hamartoma

Definition. Chest wall hamartoma is a congenital malformation of the chest wall that occurs in infants and produces a mass that simulates a neoplasm.

General Features. Several names have been applied to this condition, including *chest wall hamartoma of infancy* (152), *mesenchymal hamartoma of chest wall* (153), and *vascular and cartilaginous hamartoma of ribs* (151).

Clinical Features. The lesion always occurs in infancy and on the chest wall. The chest wall mass may cause mechanical problems during childbirth (152). The child is born with an obvious mass of the chest wall that may be alarming.

Radiographic Findings. Radiographs show an extrapleural mass that nearly always is mineralized. One or more ribs in the center of the lesion are destroyed, and ones at the periphery are deformed (fig. 14-123).

Gross Findings. The gross specimen shows a well-circumscribed mass, which on section has multiple cystic areas (fig. 14-124). The more solid areas contain nodules of cartilage.

Microscopic Findings. The cystic spaces have the appearance of an aneurysmal bone cyst (fig. 14-125). Cartilage nodules and plates are

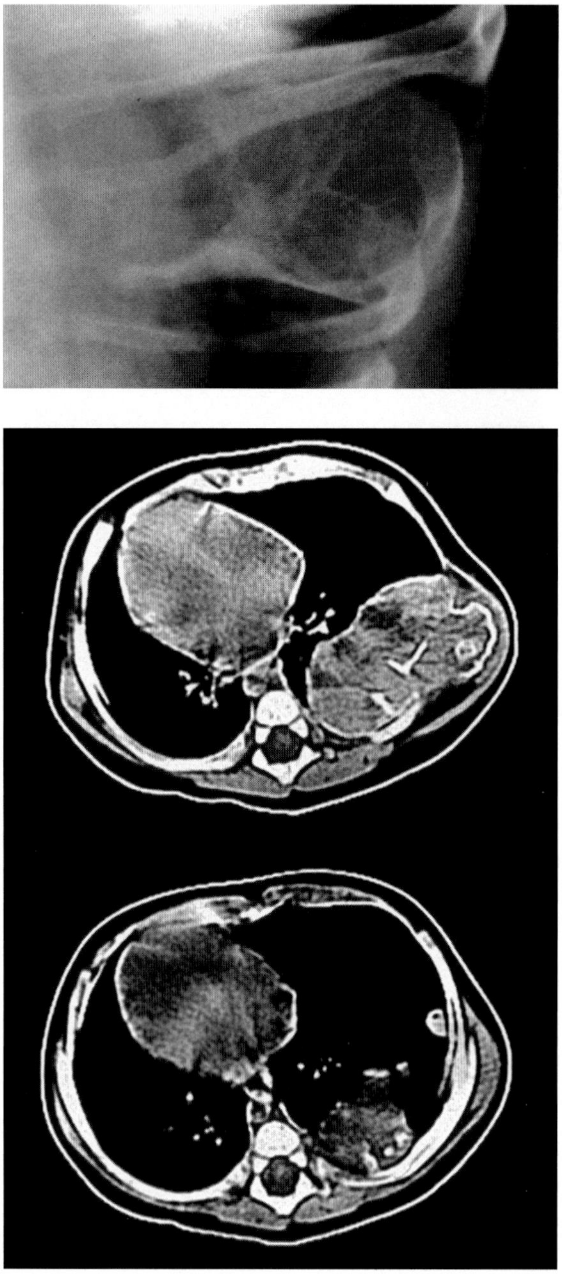

Figure 14-123

CHEST WALL HAMARTOMA

Top: A plain radiograph shows an expansile mass deforming the chest wall of a 4-month-old infant.

Bottom: CT shows that although the lesion is large and expansile, it is well demarcated. (Courtesy of Dr. E. Campinas, São Paulo, Brazil.)

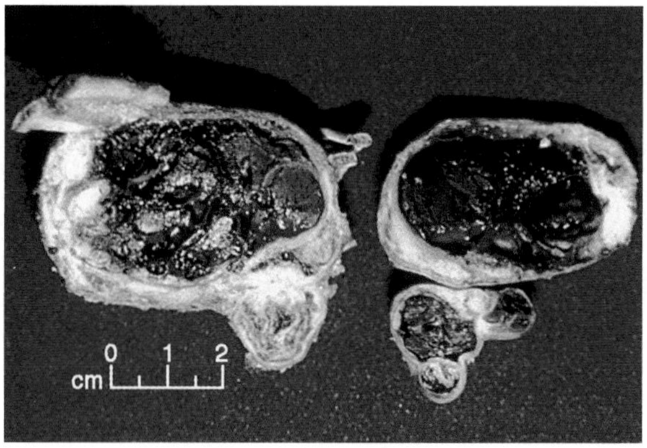

Figure 14-124

CHEST WALL HAMARTOMA

Gross specimen of the lesion shown in figure 14-123. Much of the lesion has the appearance of an aneurysmal bone cyst. Nodules of cartilage are visible.

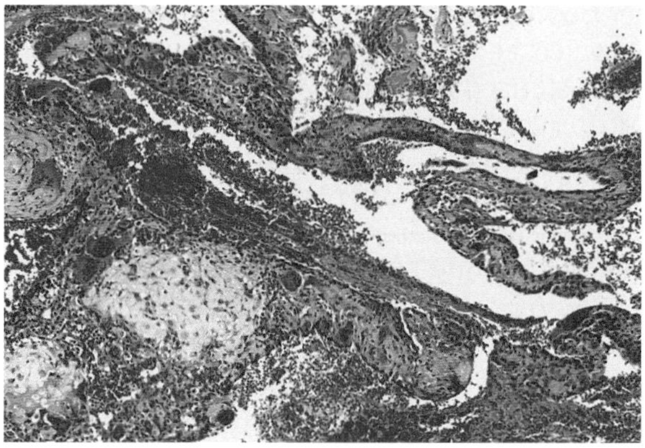

Figure 14-125

CHEST WALL HAMARTOMA

Cystic spaces have features similar to those seen in aneurysmal bone cysts.

present and may appear hypercellular. Typically, the cartilage plates undergo enchondral ossification, simulating the appearance of epiphyseal plates (fig. 14-126). The more solid areas contain loosely arranged, plump spindle cells and reactive bone with prominent osteoblastic activity (fig. 14-127).

Differential Diagnosis. If the age of the patient and the location of the lesion are known, the diagnosis is obvious. Epiphyseal plate-like cartilage is also a helpful feature.

Treatment and Prognosis. No treatment is necessary; the lesion regresses spontaneously. If surgical removal is attempted, it is important to be conservative (150).

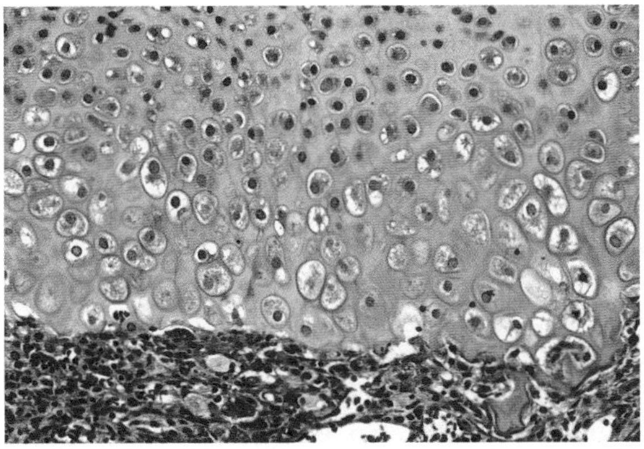

Figure 14-126

CHEST WALL HAMARTOMA

Cellular plates of cartilage show enchondral ossification.

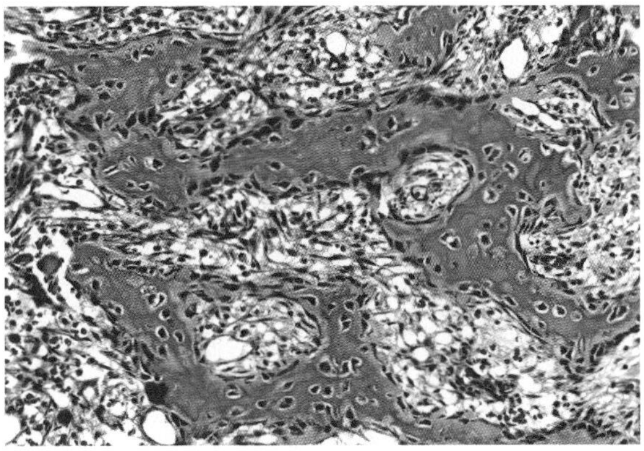

Figure 14-127

CHEST WALL HAMARTOMA

Immature bone is surrounded by plump fibroblasts.

Neuropathic Joint

Definition. Neuropathic joint is a term applied to the changes in an insensate joint caused by repetitive trauma (154).

General Features. The basic mechanism is demineralization of the joint due to any cause. The term "Charcot joint" was used initially because of the relationship to syphilis. The term *neuropathic joint* is preferred now because other causes predominate, especially diabetic neuropathy (155). Syringomyelia may also give rise to neuropathic joints.

Clinical Features. Patients present with swelling. Other changes, such as ulcers, may be present in a foot of a patient with diabetes (diabetic foot).

Radiographic Findings. Radiographs show swelling of the joint and calcific debris within the joint. In later stages, part of the bone that forms the joint, for example the femoral head or humeral head, disappears (fig. 14-128). The appearance is suggestive of a neoplasm.

Microscopic Findings. Histologically, the features are disappointing compared with the dramatic radiographic appearance. Debris from the articular cartilage and bone is scattered in the synovium, similar to severe degenerative joint disease. Often there is proliferating cartilage and bone, similar to the appearance of a callus (fig. 14-129).

Differential Diagnosis. Radiographs may be misinterpreted as a neoplasm or even as Gorham's disease. Histologically, only severe degenerative joint disease should be considered; neuropathic joint is a severe degenerative joint disease.

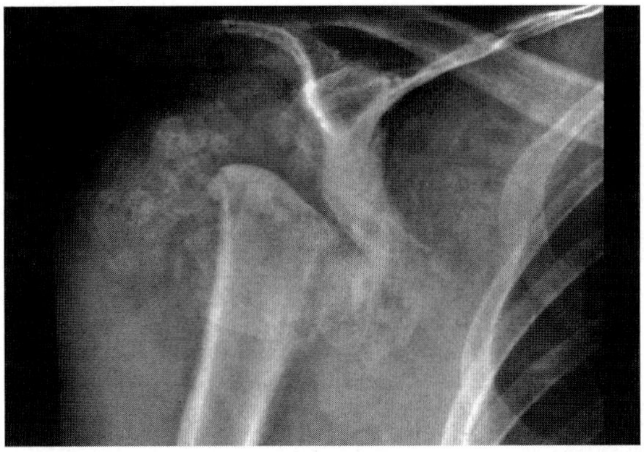

Figure 14-128

NEUROPATHIC JOINT

Neuropathic joint in a patient with syringomyelia. The head of the humerus has been destroyed, and the joint is filled with calcified debris. (Fig. 27-130 from Unni KK. Dahlin's bone tumors: general aspects and data on 11,087 cases, 5th ed. Philadelphia: Lippincott-Raven; 1996:426. By permission of Mayo Foundation.)

Calcifying Pseudoneoplasm

Definition. Calcifying pseudoneoplasm is a poorly understood calcifying process with poorly formed granulomas. It usually occurs along the neural axis.

General Features. The cause is unknown. The lesion is commonly found along the posterior aspect of the neural axis in proximity to

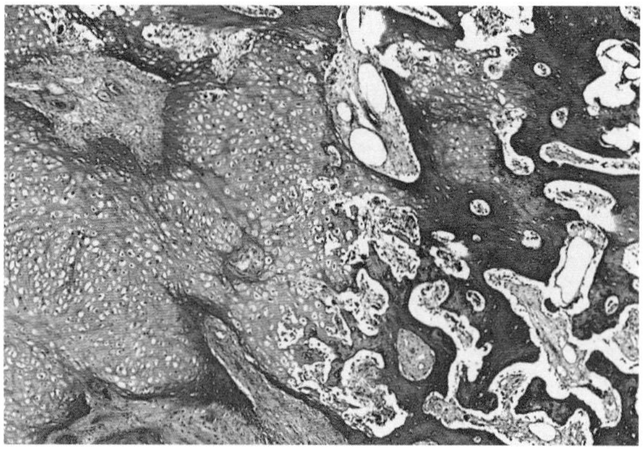

Figure 14-129

NEUROPATHIC JOINT

Synovial tissue contains debris from articular cartilage and bone.

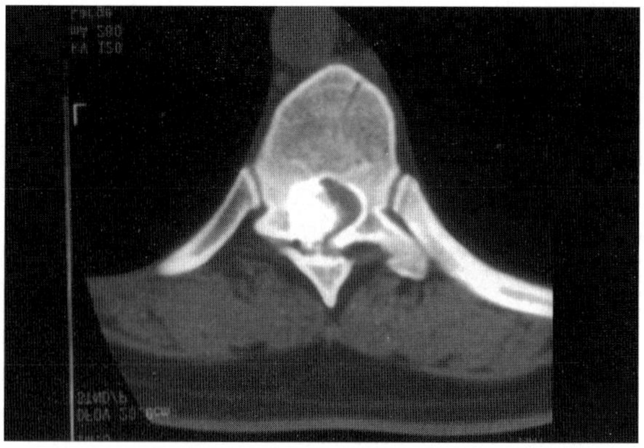

Figure 14-130

CALCIFYING PSEUDONEOPLASM

CT shows a calcified lesion impinging on the spinal canal. (Courtesy of Dr. B. Chamides, Torrance, CA.)

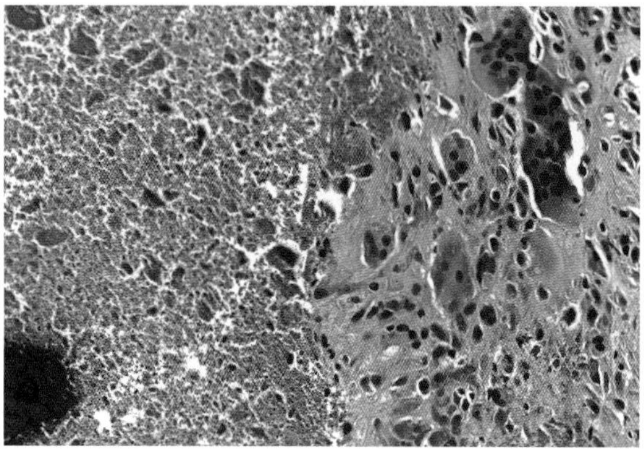

Figure 14-131

CALCIFYING PSEUDONEOPLASM

Nodular area with a granulomatous appearance. The nodules are lined by histiocytes, with scattered multinucleated giant cells.

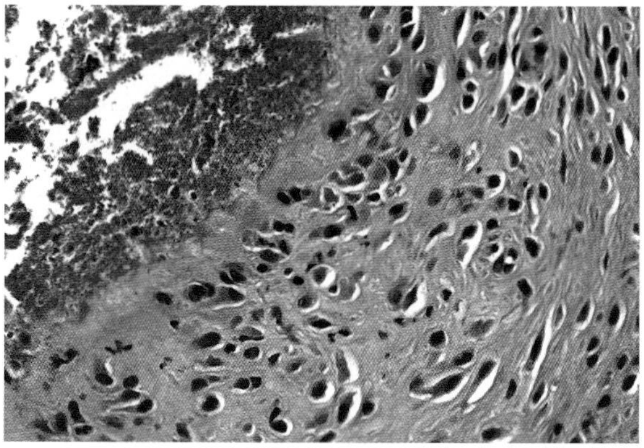

Figure 14-132

CALCIFYING PSEUDONEOPLASM

The central area of the nodules contains partially calcified acellular debris.

a disk space or facet joint, suggesting that the lesion is a reactive process due to an extruded disk or a ganglion. Because of the palisading histiocytes, the lesion may be mistaken for an infectious granuloma.

Clinical Features. Patients generally are asymptomatic and the process is discovered at the time of surgery for another disease. However, the lesion can be tumefactive and compress the spinal cord. Rarely, other sites are involved, such as the orbit, brain, or long bones (156).

Radiographic Findings. Plain radiography or CT shows a calcified extradural mass (fig. 14-130).

Gross Findings. The gross specimen consists of fibrous tissue without distinctive characteristics.

Microscopic Findings. The cardinal findings are the formation of palisading histiocytes and rare giant cells forming vague granulomas (fig. 14-131). However, instead of caseation, calcification occurs in the center (fig. 14-132). Special stains for microorganisms are always negative.

Treatment and Prognosis. Conservative surgical removal is indicated if the patient is symptomatic. We are not aware of any examples of recurrence.

REFERENCES

Metastatic Malignancy

1. Abrams HL, Spiro R, Goldstein N. Metastases in carcinoma: analysis of 1000 autopsied cases. Cancer 1950;3:74–85.
2. Bommer KK, Ramzy I, Mody D. Fine-needle aspiration biopsy in the diagnosis and management of bone lesions: a study of 450 cases. Cancer 1997;81:148–56.
3. DeBoer DK, Schwartz HS, Thelman S, Reynolds VH. Heterogeneous survival rates for isolated skeletal metastases from melanoma. Clin Orthop 1996;323:277–83.
4. Fenton P, Resnick D. Metastases to bone affected by Paget's disease. A report of three cases. Int Orthop 1991;15:397–9.
5. Phadke DM, Lucas DR, Madan S. Fine-needle aspiration biopsy of vertebral and intervertebral disc lesions: specimen adequacy, diagnostic utility, and pitfalls. Arch Pathol Lab Med 2001;125:1463–8.
6. Rougraff BT, Kneisl JS, Simon MA. Skeletal metastases of unknown origin. A prospective study of a diagnostic strategy. J Bone Joint Surg Am 1993;75:1276–81.
7. Schajowicz F, Velan O, Santini Araujo E, et al. Metastases of carcinoma in the pagetic bone. A report of two cases. Clin Orthop 1988;228:290–6.
8. Simon MA, Karluk MB. Skeletal metastases of unknown origin. Diagnostic strategy for orthopedic surgeons. Clin Orthop 1982;166:96–103.
9. Willen H. Fine needle aspiration in the diagnosis of bone tumors. Acta Orthop Scand Suppl 1997;273:47–53.
10. Yamaguchi T, Tamai K, Yamato M, Honma K, Ueda Y, Saotome K. Intertrabecular pattern of tumors metastatic to bone. Cancer 1996;78:1388–94.

Aneurysmal Bone Cyst

11. Althof PA, Ohmori K, Zhou M, et al. Cytogenetic and molecular cytogenetic findings in 43 aneurysmal bone cysts: aberrations of 17p mapped to 17p13.2 by fluorescence in situ hybridization. Mod Pathol 2004;17:518–25.
12. Bertoni F, Bacchini P, Capanna R, et al. Solid variant of aneurysmal bone cyst. Cancer 1993;71:729–34.
13. Biesecker JL, Marcove RC, Huvos AG, Mike V. Aneurysmal bone cysts. A clinicopathologic study of 66 cases. Cancer 1970;26:615–25.
14. Clough JR, Price CH. Aneurysmal bone cyst: pathogenesis and long term results of treatment. Clin Orthop 1973;97:52–63.
15. Dal Cin P, Kozakewich HP, Goumnerova L, Mankin HJ, Rosenberg AE, Fletcher JA. Variant translocations involving 16q22 and 17p13 in solid variant and extraosseous forms of aneurysmal bone cyst. Genes Chromosomes Cancer 2000;28:233–4.
16. Hudson TM. Fluid levels in aneurysmal bone cysts: a CT feature. AJR Am J Roentgenol 1984;142:1001–4.
17. Kyriakos M, Hardy D. Malignant transformation of aneurysmal bone cyst, with an analysis of the literature. Cancer 1991;68:1770–80.
18. Levy WM, Miller AS, Bonakdarpour A, Aegerter E. Aneurysmal bone cyst secondary to other osseous lesions. Report of 57 cases. Am J Clin Pathol 1975;63:1–8.
19. Martinez V, Sissons HA. Aneurysmal bone cyst. A review of 123 cases including primary lesions and those secondary to other bone pathology. Cancer 1988;61:2291–304.
20. Oliveira AM, Hsi BL, Weremowicz S, et al. USP6 (Tre2) fusion oncogenes in aneurysmal bone cysts. Cancer Res 2004;64:1920–3.
21. Panoutsakopoulos G, Pandis N, Kyriazoglou I, Gustafson P, Mertens F, Mandahl N. Recurrent t(16;17)(q22;p13) in aneurysmal bone cysts. Genes Chromosomes Cancer 1999;26:265–6.
22. Radig K, Schneider-Stock R, Mittler U, Neumann HW, Roessner A. Genetic instability in osteoblastic tumors of the skeletal system. Pathol Res Pract 1998;194:669–77.
23. Sanerkin NG, Mott MG, Roylance J. An unusual intraosseous lesion with fibroblastic, osteoclastic, osteoblastic, aneurysmal and fibromyxoid elements. "Solid" variant of aneurysmal bone cyst. Cancer 1983;51:2278–86.
24. Sciot R, Dorfman H, Brys P, et al. Cytogenetic-morphologic correlations in aneurysmal bone cyst, giant cell tumor of bone and combined lesions. A report from the CHAMP study group. Mod Pathol 2000;13:1206–10.
25. Vergel De Dios AM, Bond JR, Shives TC, McLeod RA, Unni KK. Aneurysmal bone cyst. A clinicopathologic study of 238 cases. Cancer 1992;69:2921–31.
26. Winnepenninckx V, Debiec-Rychter M, Jorissen M, Bogaerts S, Sciot R. Aneurysmal bone cyst of the nose with 17p13 involvement. Virchows Arch 2001;439:636–9.

Simple Cyst

27. Boseker EH, Bickel WH, Dahlin DC. A clinicopathologic study of simple unicameral bone cysts. Surg Gynecol Obstet 1968;127:550–60.
28. Chigira M, Maehara S, Arita S, Udagawa E. The aetiology and treatment of simple bone cysts. J Bone Joint Surg Br 1983;65:633–7.

29. Johnson LC, Vetter H, Putschar WG. Sarcomas arising in bone cysts. Virchows Arch Path Anat 1962;335:428–51.
30. Scaglietti O, Marchetti PG, Bartolozzi P. The effects of methylprednisolone acetate in the treatment of bone cysts. Results of three years follow-up. J Bone Joint Surg Br 1979;61:200–4.
31. Struhl S, Edelson C, Pritzker H, Seimon LP, Dorfman HD. Solitary (unicameral) bone cyst. The fallen fragment sign revisited. Skeletal Radiol 1989;18:261–5.

Intraosseous Ganglion

32. Schajowicz F, Clavel Sainz M, Slullitel JA. Juxta-articular bone cysts (intra-osseous ganglia): a clinicopathological study of eighty-eight cases. J Bone Joint Surg Br 1979;61:107–16.

Epidermoid Cyst

33. Roth SI. Squamous cysts involving the skull and distal phalanges. J Bone Joint Surg Am 1964;46:1442–50.

Subungual Keratoacanthoma

34. Allen CA, Stephens M, Steel WM. Subungual keratoacanthoma. Histopathology 1994;25:181–3.
35. Cramer SF. Subungual keratoacanthoma. A benign bone-eroding neoplasm of the distal phalanx. Am J Clin Pathol 1981;75:425–9.
36. Shapiro L, Baraf CS. Subungual epidermoid carcinoma and keratoacanthoma. Cancer 1970;25:141–52.

Metaphyseal Fibrous Defect

37. Arata MA, Peterson HA, Dahlin DC. Pathological fractures through non-ossifying fibromas. Review of the Mayo Clinic experience. J Bone Joint Surg Am 1981;63:980–8.
38. Caffey J. On fibrous defects in cortical walls of growing tubular bones: their radiologic appearance, structure, prevalence, natural course, and diagnostic significance. Adv Pediatr 1955;7:13–51.
39. Campanacci M, Laus M, Boriani S. Multiple non-ossifying fibromata with extraskeletal anomalies: a new syndrome? J Bone Joint Surg Br 1983;65:627–32.
40. Kyriakos M, Murphy WA. Concurrence of metaphyseal fibrous defect and osteosarcoma. Report of a case and review of the literature. Skeletal Radiol 1981;6:179–86.
41. Mirra JM, Gold RH, Rand F. Disseminated nonossifying fibromas in association with cafe-au-lait spots (Jaffe-Campanacci syndrome). Clin Orthop 1982;168:192–205.
42. Nelson M, Perry D, Ginsberg G, Sanger WG, Neff JR, Bridge JA. Translocation (1;4)(p31;q34) in nonossifying fibroma. Cancer Genet Cytogenet 2003;142:142–4.
43. Tarkkanen M, Kaipainen A, Karaharju E, et al. Cytogenetic study of 249 consecutive patients examined for a bone tumor. Cancer Genet Cytogenet 1993;68:1–21.

Periosteal Desmoid (Avulsive Cortical Irregularity)

44. Barnes GR Jr, Gwinn JL. Distal irregularities of the femur simulating malignancy. Am J Roentgenol Radium Ther Nucl Med 1974;122:180–5.
45. Bridge JA, Swarts SJ, Buresh C, et al. Trisomies 8 and 20 characterize a subgroup of benign fibrous lesions arising in both soft tissue and bone. Am J Pathol 1999;154:729–33.
46. Kimmelstiel P, Rapp I. Cortical defect due to periosteal desmoids. Bull Hosp Joint Dis 1951;12:286–97.

Fibrous Dysplasia

47. Alman BA, Greel DA, Wolfe HJ. Activating mutations of Gs protein in monostotic fibrous lesions of bone. J Orthop Res 1996;14:311–5.
48. Bianco P, Riminucci M, Majolagbe A, et al. Mutations of the GNAS1 gene, stromal cell dysfunction, and osteomalacic changes in non-McCune-Albright fibrous dysplasia of bone. J Bone Miner Res 2000;15:120–8.
49. Bridge JA, Swarts SJ, Buresh C, et al. Trisomies 8 and 20 characterize a subgroup of benign fibrous lesions arising in both soft tissue and bone. Am J Pathol 1999;154:729–33.
50. Dal Cin P, Sciot R, Brys P, et al. Recurrent chromosome aberrations in fibrous dysplasia of the bone: a report of the CHAMP study group. Chromosomes and morphology. Cancer Genet Cytogenet 2000;122:30–2.
51. Feintuch TA. Chondrosarcoma arising in a cartilaginous area of previously irradiated fibrous dysplasia. Cancer 1973;31:877–81.
52. Huvos AG, Higinbotham NL, Miller TR. Bone sarcomas arising in fibrous dysplasia. J Bone Joint Surg Am 1972;54:1047–56.
53 Jee WH, Choi KH, Choe BY, Park JM, Shinn KS. Fibrous dysplasia: MR imaging characteristics with radiopathologic correlation. AJR Am J Roentgenol 1996;167:1523–7.
54. Kaplan FS, Fallon MD, Boden SD, Schmidt R, Senior M, Haddad JG. Estrogen receptors in bone in a patient with polyostotic fibrous dysplasia (McCune-Albright syndrome). N Engl J Med 1988;319:421–5.
55. McArthur RG, Hayles AB, Lambert PW. Albright's syndrome with rickets. Mayo Clin Proc 1979;54:313-20.
56. Mikami M, Koizumi H, Ishii M, Nakajima H. The identification of monoclonality in fibrous dysplasia by methylation-specific polymerase chain reaction for the human androgen gene receptor. Virchows Arch 2004;444:56–60.

57. Nager GT, Kennedy DW, Kopstein E. Fibrous dysplasia: a review of the disease and its manifestations in the temporal bone. Ann Otol Rhinol Laryngol Suppl 1982;92:5–52.
58. Ozaki T, Lindner N, Blasius S. Dedifferentiated chondrosarcoma in Albright syndrome. A case report and review of the literature. J Bone Joint Surg Am 1997;79:1545–51.
59. Parham DM, Bridge JA, Lukacs JL, Ding Y, Tryka AF, Sawyer JR. Cytogenetic distinction among benign fibro-osseous lesions of bone in children and adolescents: value of karyotypic findings in differential diagnosis. Pediatr Dev Pathol 2004;7:148–58.
60. Pollandt K, Engels C, Kaiser E, Werner M, Delling G. Gsalpha gene mutations in monostotic fibrous dysplasia of bone and fibrous dysplasia-like low-grade central osteosarcoma. Virchows Arch 2001;439:170–5.
61. Riminucci M, Fisher LW, Shenker A, Spiegel AM, Bianco P, Gehron Robey P. Fibrous dysplasia of bone in the McCune-Albright syndrome: abnormalities in bone formation. Am J Pathol 1997;151:1587–600.
62. Ruggieri P, Sim FH, Bond JR, Unni KK. Malignancies in fibrous dysplasia. Cancer 1994;73:1411–24.
63. Sakamoto A, Oda Y, Iwamoto Y, Tsuneyoshi M. A comparative study of fibrous dysplasia and osteofibrous dysplasia with regard to Gsalpha mutation at the Arg201 codon: polymerase chain reaction-restriction fragment length polymorphism analysis of paraffin-embedded tissues. J Mol Diagn 2000;2:67–72.
64. Tanner HC, Dahlin DC, Childs DS. Sarcoma complicating fibrous dysplasia: probable role of radiation therapy. Oral Surg 1961;14:837–46.
65. Van Horn PE, Dahlin DC, Bickel WH. Fibrous dysplasia: a clinical pathologic study of orthopedic surgical cases. Proc Staff Meet Mayo Clin 1963;38:175–89.
66. Weinstein LS, Shenker A, Gejman PV, Merino MJ, Friedman E, Spiegel AM. Activating mutations of the stimulatory G protein in the McCune-Albright syndrome. N Engl J Med 1991;325:1688–95.
67. Wenig BM, Vinh TN, Smirniotopoulos JG, Fowler CB, Houston GD, Heffner DK. Aggressive psammomatoid ossifying fibromas of the sinonasal region: a clinicopathologic study of a distinct group of fibro-osseous lesions. Cancer 1995;76:1155–65.

Osteofibrous Dysplasia

68. Blackwell JB, McCarthy SW, Xipell JM, Vernon-Roberts B, Duhig RE. Osteofibrous dysplasia of the tibia and fibula. Pathology 1988;20:227–33.
69. Bridge JA, Dembinski A, DeBoer J, Travis J, Neff JR. Clonal chromosomal abnormalities in osteofibrous dysplasia. Implications for histopathogenesis and its relationship with adamantinoma. Cancer 1994;73:1746–52.
70. Bridge JA, Swarts SJ, Buresh C, et al. Trisomies 8 and 20 characterize a subgroup of benign fibrous lesions arising in both soft tissue and bone. Am J Pathol 1999;154:729–33.
71. Campanacci M. Osteofibrous dysplasia of long bones: a new clinical entity. Ital J Orthop Traumatol 1976;2:221–37.
72. Campanacci M, Laus M. Osteofibrous dysplasia of the tibia and fibula. J Bone Joint Surg Am 1981;63:367–75.
73. Hazelbag HM, Wessels JW, Mollevangers P, van den Berg E, Molenar WM, Hogendoorn PC. Cytogenetic analysis of adamantinoma of long bones: further indications for a common histogenesis with osteofibrous dysplasia. Cancer Genet Cytogenet 1997;97:5–11.
74. Kanamori M, Antonescu CR, Scott M, et al. Extra copies of chromosomes 7, 8, 12, 19, and 21 are recurrent in adamantinoma. J Mol Diagn 2001;3:16–21.
75. Kempson RL. Ossifying fibroma of the long bones. A light and electron microscopic study. Arch Pathol 1966;82:218–33.
76. Maki M, Athanasou N. Osteofibrous dysplasia and adamantinoma: correlation of proto-oncogene product and matrix protein expression. Hum Pathol 2004;35:69–74.
77. Nakashima Y, Yamamuro T, Fujiwara Y, Kotoura Y, Mori E, Hamashima Y. Osteofibrous dysplasia (ossifying fibroma of long bones). A study of 12 cases. Cancer 1983;52:909–14.
78. Sweet DE, Vinh TN, Devaney K. Cortical osteofibrous dysplasia of long bone and its relationship to adamantinoma. A clinicopathologic study of 30 cases. Am J Surg Pathol 1992;16:282–90.

Congenital Fibromatosis (Myofibromatosis)

79. Inwards CY, Unni KK, Beabout JW, Shives TC. Solitary congenital fibromatosis (infantile myofibromatosis) of bone. Am J Surg Pathol 1991;15:935–41.
80. Kindblom LG, Angervall L. Congenital solitary fibromatosis of the skeleton: case report of a variant of congenital generalized fibromatosis. Cancer 1978;41:636–40.

Fibrocartilaginous Mesenchymoma

81. Bulychova IV, Unni KK, Bertoni F, Beabout JW. Fibrocartilaginous mesenchymoma of bone. Am J Surg Pathol 1993;17:830–6.
82. Dahlin DC, Bertoni F, Beabout JW, Campanacci M. Fibrocartilaginous mesenchymoma with low-grade malignancy. Skeletal Radiol 1984;12:263–9.

Heterotopic Ossification

83. Aboulafia AJ, Brooks F, Piratzky J, Weiss S. Osteosarcoma arising from heterotopic ossification after an electrical burn. A case report. J Bone Joint Surg Am 1999;81:564–70.
84. Ackerman LV. Extra-osseous localized non-neoplastic bone and cartilage formation (so-called myositis ossificans): clinical and pathological confusion with malignant neoplasms. J Bone Surg Am 1958;40:279–98.
85. Eckardt JJ, Ivins JC, Perry HO, Unni KK. Osteosarcoma arising in heterotopic ossification of dermatomyositis: case report and review of the literature. Cancer 1981;48:1256–61.
86. Ellis R, Greene AG. Ischial apophyseolysis. Radiology 1966;87:646–8.
87. Kransdorf MJ, Meis JM, Jelinek JS. Myositis ossificans: MR appearance with radiologic-pathologic correlation. AJR Am J Roentgenol 1991;157:1243–8.
88. Shannon P, Bedard Y, Bell R, Kandel R. Aneurysmal cyst of soft tissue: report of a case with serial magnetic resonance imaging and biopsy. Hum Pathol 1997;28:255–7.
89. Smith R, Russell RG, Woods CG. Myositis ossificans progressiva. Clinical features of eight patients and their response to treatment. J Bone Joint Surg Br 1976;58:48–57.

Subungual Exostosis

90. Landon GC, Johnson KA, Dahlin DC. Subungual exostoses. J Bone Joint Surg Am 1979;61: 256–9.
91. Lucas DR, Tazelaar HD, Unni KK, et al. Osteogenic melanoma. A rare variant of malignant melanoma. Am J Surg Pathol 1993;17:400–9.
92. Urmacher C. Unusual stromal patterns in truly recurrent and satellite metastatic lesions of malignant melanoma. Am J Dermatopathol 1984;6(Suppl):331–5.

Bizarre Parosteal Osteochondromatous Proliferation

93. Choi JH, Gu MJ, Kim MJ, Choi WH, Shin DS, Cho KH. Fibrosarcoma in bizarre parosteal osteochondromatous proliferation. Skeletal Radiol 2001;30:44–7.
94. Meneses MF, Unni KK, Swee RG. Bizarre parosteal osteochondromatous proliferation of bone (Nora's lesion). Am J Surg Pathol 1993;17:691–7.
95. Nilsson M, Domanski HA, Mertens F, Mandahl N. Molecular cytogenetic characterization of recurrent translocation breakpoints in bizarre parosteal osteochondromatous proliferation (Nora's lesion). Hum Pathol 2004;35:1063–9.
96. Nora FE, Dahlin DC, Beabout JW. Bizarre parosteal osteochondromatous proliferations of the hands and feet. Am J Surg Pathol 1983;7:245–50.
97. Spjut HJ, Dorfman HD. Florid reactive periostitis of the tubular bones of the hands and feet. A benign lesion which may simulate osteosarcoma. Am J Surg Pathol 1981;5:423–33.

Stress (Insufficiency) Fracture

98. Cooper KL, Beabout JW, Swee RG. Insufficiency fractures of the sacrum. Radiology 1985;156:15–20.

Giant Cell Reparative Granuloma

99. Ackerman LV, Spjut HJ. Tumors of bone and cartilage. Atlas of Tumor Pathology, 1st Series, Fascicle 4. Washington, DC: Armed Forces Institute of Pathology; 1962:282.
100. Buresh CJ, Seemayer TA, Nelson M, Neff JR, Dorfman HD, Bridge J. t(X;4)(q22;q31.3) in giant cell reparative granuloma. Cancer Genet Cytogenet 1999;115:80–1.
101. Glass TA, Mills SE, Fechner RE, Dyer R, Martin W 3rd, Armstrong P. Giant-cell reparative granuloma of the hands and feet. Radiology 1983;149:65–8.
102. Jaffe HL. Giant-cell reparative granuloma, traumatic bone cyst, and fibrous (fibro-osseous) dysplasia of the jawbones. Oral Surg Oral Med Oral Pathol 1953;6:159–75.
103. Lorenzo JC, Dorfman HD. Giant-cell reparative granuloma of short tubular bones of the hands and feet. Am J Surg Pathol 1980;4:551–63.
104. Ratner V, Dorfman HD. Giant-cell reparative granuloma of the hand and foot bones. Clin Orthop 1990;260:251–8.
105. Wold LE, Dobyns JH, Swee RG, Dahlin DC. Giant cell reaction (giant cell reparative granuloma) of the small bones of the hands and feet. Am J Surg Pathol 1986;10:491–6.

Langerhans' Cell Histiocytosis (Eosinophilic Granuloma)

106. Kilpatrick SE, Wenger DE, Gilchrist GS, Shives TC, Wollan PC, Unni KK. Langerhans' cell histiocytosis (histiocytosis X) of bone. A clinicopathologic analysis of 263 pediatric and adult cases. Cancer 1995;76:2471–84.
107. Lichtenstein L. Histiocytosis X: integration of eosinophilic granuloma of bone, "Letterer-Siwe disease," and "Schuller-Christian disease" as related manifestations of a single nosologic entity. Arch Pathol 1953;56:84–102.
108. Lieberman PH, Jones CR, Dargeon HW, Begg CF. A reappraisal of eosinophilic granuloma of bone, Hand-Schuller-Christian syndrome and Letterer-Siwe syndrome. Medicine (Baltimore) 1969;48:375–400.

109. Shabb N, Fanning CV, Carrasco CH, et al. Diagnosis of eosinophilic granuloma of bone by fine-needle aspiration with concurrent institution of therapy: a cytologic, histologic, clinical, and radiologic study of 27 cases. Diagn Cytopathol 1993;9:3–12.
110. Willman CL, Busque L, Griffith BB, et al. Langerhans'-cell histiocytosis (histiocytosis X)—a clonal proliferative disease. N Engl J Med 1994;331:154–60.
111. Yasko AW, Fanning CV, Ayala AG, Carrasco CH, Murray JA. Percutaneous techniques for the diagnosis and treatment of localized Langerhans-cell histiocytosis (eosinophilic granuloma of bone). J Bone Joint Surg Am 1998;80:219–28.
112. Yu RC, Chu C, Buluwela L, Chu AC. Clonal proliferation of Langerhans cells in Langerhans cell histiocytosis. Lancet 1994;343:767–8.

Erdheim-Chester Disease

113. Al-Quran S, Reith J, Bradley J, Rimsza L. Erdheim-Chester disease: case report, PCR-based analysis of clonality, and review of literature. Mod Pathol 2002;15:666–72.
114. Chester W. Uber Lipoidgranulomatose. Virchows Arch Pathol Anat 1930;279:561–602.
115. Chetritt J, Paradis V, Dargere D, et al. Chester-Erdheim disease: a neoplastic disorder. Hum Pathol 1999;30:1093–6.
116. Kambouchner M, Colby TV, Domenge C, Battesti JP, Soler P, Tazi A. Erdheim-Chester disease with prominent pulmonary involvement associated with eosinophilic granuloma of mandibular bone. Histopathology 1997;30:353–8.

Mast Cell Disease

117. Metcalfe DD, Akin C. Mastocytosis: molecular mechanisms and clinical disease heterogeneity. Leuk Res 2001;25:577–82.
118. Travis WD, Li CY, Bergstralh EJ, Yam LT, Swee RG. Systemic mast cell disease. Analysis of 58 cases and literature review. Medicine (Baltimore) 1988;67:345–68.

Sinus Histiocytosis with Massive Lymphadenopathy (Rosai-Dorfman Disease)

119. Foucar E, Rosai J, Dorfman R. Sinus histiocytosis with massive lymphadenopathy (Rosai-Dorfman disease): review of the entity. Semin Diagn Pathol 1990;7:19–73.
120. Lewin JR, Das SK, Blumenthal BI, D'Cruz C, Patel RB, Howell GE. Osseous pseudotumor. The sole manifestation of sinus histiocytosis with massive lymphadenopathy. Am J Clin Pathol 1985;84:547–50.
121. Nielsen GP, Bjornsson J, Rosenberg AE, Unni KK. Primary Rosai-Dorfman disease of bone: a clinicopathologic study of 13 cases. Abstract presented at USCAP meeting, March 2002, Chicago.
122. Patterson FR, Rooney MT, Damron TA, Vermont AI, Hutchison RE. Sclerotic lesion of the tibia without involvement of lymph nodes. Report of an unusual case of Rosai-Dorfman disease. J Bone Joint Surg Am 1997;79:911–6.
123. Paulli M, Bergamaschi G, Tonon L, et al. Evidence for a polyclonal nature of the cell infiltrate in sinus histiocytosis with massive lymphadenopathy (Rosai-Dorfman disease). Br J Haematol 1995;91:415–8.
124. Rosai J, Dorfman RF. Sinus histiocytosis with massive lymphadenopathy: a pseudolymphomatous benign disorder. Analysis of 34 cases. Cancer 1972;30:1174–88.
125. Walker PD, Rosai J, Dorfman RF. The osseous manifestations of sinus histiocytosis with massive lymphadenopathy. Am J Clin Pathol 1981;75:131–9.

Osteomyelitis

126. Adeyokunnu AA, Hendrickse RG. Salmonella osteomyelitis in childhood. A report of 63 cases seen in Nigerian children of whom 57 had sickle cell anaemia. Arch Dis Child 1980;55:175–84.
127. Akbarnia BA, Wirth CR, Colman N. Fibrosarcoma arising from chronic osteomyelitis. Case report and review of the literature. J Bone Joint Surg Am 1976;58:123–5.
128. Bjorksten B, Boquist L. Histopathological aspects of chronic recurrent multifocal osteomyelitis. J Bone Joint Surg Br 1980;62:376–80.
129. Cabanela ME, Sim FH, Beabout JW, Dahlin DC. Osteomyelitis appearing as neoplasms. A diagnostic problem. Arch Surg 1974;109:68–72.
130. Fitzgerald RH Jr, Brewer NS, Dahlin DC. Squamous-cell carcinoma complicating chronic osteomyelitis. J Bone Joint Surg Am 1976;58:1146–8.
131. Jurik AG, Helmig O, Ternowitz T, Moller BN. Chronic recurrent multifocal osteomyelitis: a follow-up study. J Pediatr Orthop 1988;8:49–58.
132. McGrory JE, Pritchard DJ, Unni KK, Ilstrup D, Rowland CM. Malignant lesions arising in chronic osteomyelitis. Clin Orthop 1999;362:181–9.
133. Mollan RA, Craig BF, Biggart JD. Chronic sclerosing osteomyelitis. An unusual case. J Bone Joint Surg Br 1984;66:583–5.
134. Waldvogel FA, Medoff G, Swartz MN. Osteomyelitis: a review of clinical features, therapeutic considerations and unusual aspects. N Engl J Med 1970;282:198–206.

Paget's Disease

135. Bowerman JW, Altman J, Hughes JL, Zadek RE. Pseudo-malignant lesions in Paget's disease of bone. Am J Roentgenol Radium Ther Nucl Med 1975;124:57–61.
136. Cooper C, Dennison E, Schafheutle K, Kellingray S, Guyer P, Barker D. Epidemiology of Paget's disease of bone. Bone 1999;24(5 Suppl):3–5S.
137. Davie M, Davies M, Francis R, Fraser W, Hosking D, Tansley R. Paget's disease of bone: a review of 889 patients. Bone 1999;24(5 Suppl):11–12S.
138. Frame B, Marel GM. Paget disease: a review of current knowledge. Radiology 1981;141:21–4.
139. Guyer PB, Chamberlain AT, Ackery DM, Rolfe EB. The anatomic distribution of osteitis deformans. Clin Orthop 1981;156:141–4.
140. Harvey L, Gray T, Beneton MN, Douglas DL, Kanis JA, Russell RG. Ultrastructural features of the osteoclasts from Paget's disease of bone in relation to a viral aetiology. J Clin Pathol 1982;35:771–9.
141. Hocking LJ, Lucas GJ, Daroszewska A, et al. Domain-specific mutations in sequestosome 1 (SQSTM1) cause familial and sporadic Paget's disease. Hum Mol Genet 2002;11:2735–9.
142. Hughes AE, Ralston SH, Marken J, et al. Mutations in TNFRSF11A, affecting the signal peptide of RANK, cause familial expansile osteolysis [Letter]. Nat Genet 2000;24:45–53.
143. Laurin N, Brown JP, Morissette J, Raymond V. Recurrent mutation of the gene encoding sequestosome 1 (SQSTM1/p62) in Paget disease of bone. Am J Hum Genet 2002;70:1582–8.
144. Nakatsuka K, Nishizawa Y, Ralston SH. Phenotypic characterization of early onset Paget's disease of bone caused by a 27-bp duplication in the TNFRSF11A gene. J Bone Miner Res 2003;18:1381–5.
145. Roberts MC, Kressel HY, Fallon MD, Zlatkin MB, Dalinka MK. Paget disease: MR imaging findings. Radiology 1989;173:341–5.
146. Smith R. Paget's disease of bone: past and present. Bone 1999;24(5 Suppl):1–2S.

Infarct of Bone

147. Desai P, Perino G, Present D, Steiner GC. Sarcoma in association with bone infarcts. Report of five cases. Arch Pathol Lab Med 1996;120:482–9.

Transient Osteoporosis

148. Bramlett KW, Killian JT, Nasca RJ, Daniel WW. Transient osteoporosis. Clin Orthop 1987;222: 197–202.
149. Hunder GG, Kelly PJ. Roentgenologic transient osteoporosis of the hip. A clinical syndrome? Ann Intern Med 1968;68:539–52.

Chest Wall Hamartoma

150. Inwards CY, Unni KK, McLeod RA. Chest wall hamartoma (mesenchymoma) in infancy: a clinicopathologic study of 19 cases. Presented at the Annual Meeting of the American Society of Clinical Pathology, Orlando, Florida, October 1993.
151. McCarthy EF, Dorfman HD. Vascular and cartilaginous hamartoma of the ribs in infancy with secondary aneurysmal bone cyst formation. Am J Surg Pathol 1980;4:247–53.
152. McLeod RA, Dahlin DC. Hamartoma (mesenchymoma) of the chest wall in infancy. Radiology 1979;131:657–61.
153. Odell JM, Benjamin DR. Mesenchymal hamartoma of chest wall in infancy: natural history of two cases. Pediatr Pathol 1986;5:135–46.

Neuropathic Joint

154. Guille JT, Forlin E, Bowen JR. Charcot joint disease of the shoulders in a patient who had familial sensory neuropathy with anhidrosis. A case report. J Bone Joint Surg Am 1992;74:1415–7.
155. Raju UB, Fine G, Partamian JO. Diabetic neuroarthropathy (Charcot's joint). Arch Pathol Lab Med 1982;106:349–51.

Calcifying Pseudoneoplasm

156. Bertoni F, Unni KK, Dahlin DC, Beabout JW, Onofrio BM. Calcifying pseudoneoplasms of the neural axis. J Neurosurg 1990;72:42–8.

15 SYNOVIAL TUMORS

PIGMENTED VILLONODULAR SYNOVITIS

Definition. Pigmented villonodular synovitis is a proliferation of synovial cells that leads to thickening of the synovial membrane, with hypertrophy of the villous architecture.

General Features. It is now well recognized that the common giant cell tumor of tendon sheath is histologically identical to the more diffuse involvement of the synovium in pigmented villonodular synovitis. Occasionally, a localized form of the process involves a major joint. There are three major theories of pathogenesis: 1) a disturbance of lipid metabolism; 2) inflammation; and 3) a neoplastic proliferation (3). No theory seems to explain all the features of the disease.

Clinical Features. Patients complain of pain and swelling of a joint. There is a slight female predominance, and the mean age of the patients is 40 years, although the age range is wide (8).

Sites. The knee is involved in more than 75 percent of cases. The hip is the next most common site. Unusual sites are the temporomandibular joint (10) and the vertebral column (2,7,11).

Radiographic Findings. Plain radiographs may not show any abnormality or may show an intracapsular soft tissue swelling without mineralization. If bone is involved, lucencies usually are present on either side of the involved joint (1,4,6). Bone involvement in the form of juxtacortical lucencies is more likely in tight joints, such as the hip and facet joints, than in loose joints, such as the knee. Magnetic resonance imaging (MRI) shows low signal intensity on both T_1- and T_2-weighted images because of the presence of iron pigment. This appearance in a pathologic process involving the joint is virtually diagnostic of pigmented villonodular synovitis (fig. 15-1).

Gross Findings. The synovium is diffusely thickened and dark brown and yellow (fig. 15-2). The villous architecture is appreciated best by placing the specimen in water. In the localized form, a well-demarcated mass is seen attached by a stalk to the synovium.

Microscopic Findings. The diagnostic feature of pigmented villonodular synovitis is the proliferation of subsynovial fibrohistiocytic cells, which are small cells with uniform round to oval nuclei (fig. 15-3). Mitotic figures may be prominent, but there is no cytologic atypia and nucleoli are inconspicuous. The cells tend to be arranged in clusters and to have a clefting or alveolar pattern. They are separated by matrix consisting of collagen, but occasionally, osteoid and bone. Foam cells are always present (fig. 15-4). Benign giant cells are arranged in clusters. Iron pigment is always present. The proliferation of the synovial cells gives rise to villous hyperplasia (fig. 15-5). The villi are composed of proliferating mononuclear and giant cells, and not merely a fibrous stalk. Areas of infarct-like necrosis may be found, but they are not a prominent feature.

Genetics and Other Special Techniques. Structural rearrangements of 1p11-13 are recurrent in both the localized and diffuse forms of pigmented villonodular synovitis (9). In addition, trisomies of chromosomes 5 and 7 are nonrandom in both forms, but they are more frequent in the diffuse form. Notably, these trisomies have also been detected in malignant giant cell tumor of synovium (5).

Differential Diagnosis. Villous hypertrophy may occur in various pathologic processes affecting joints, such as degenerative joint disease and rheumatoid synovitis. However, in these conditions, the villi consist of fibrous tissue and inflammatory cells, and not synovial cells. Bleeding into the joint, as with trauma, can produce the brown discoloration typical of pigmented villonodular synovitis. However, in traumatic and hemophilic synovitis, there is no proliferation of synovial cells. After arthroplasty, a foreign body reaction can simulate the appearance of pigmented villonodular synovitis. The

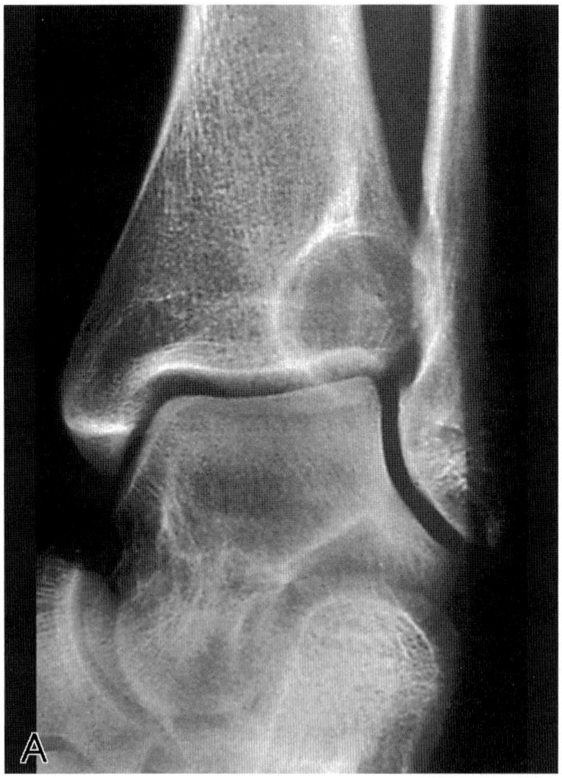

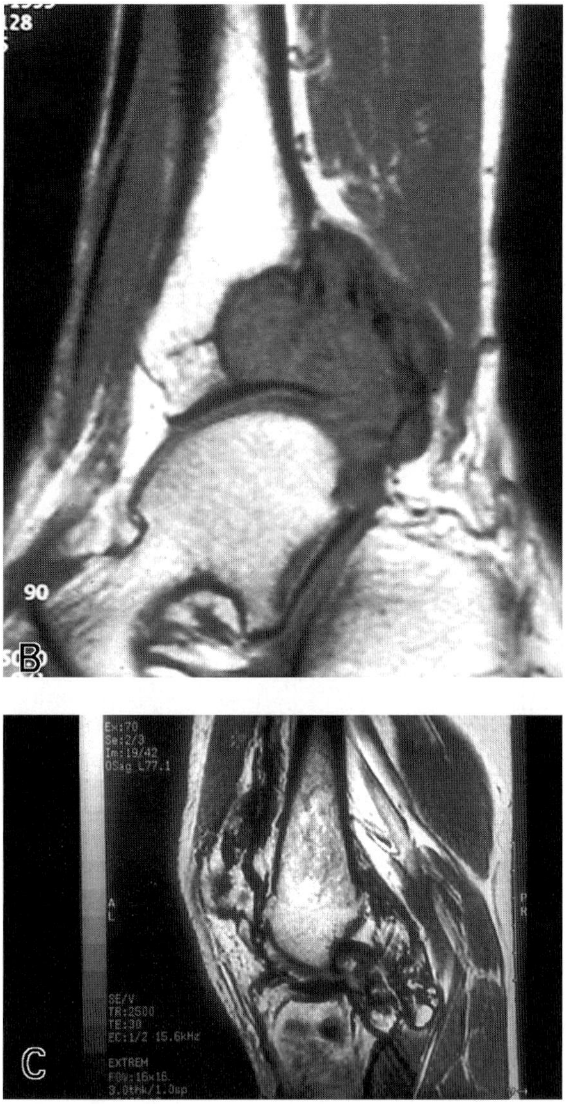

Figure 15-1

PIGMENTED VILLONODULAR SYNOVITIS

A: A lytic lesion involves the distal tibia and fibula. The lytic areas are sharply demarcated and suggest a benign process arising in the joint space.

B: T_1-weighted magnetic resonance image (MRI) shows a mass of low signal intensity involving the joint and bones.

C: T_2-weighted image of the knee shows areas of low signal intensity in the joint, corresponding to deposition of hemosiderin.

presence of crystalline material within giant cells is a clue to identifying an arthroplasty effect.

Treatment and Prognosis. Local recurrence can be a problem, and histologic features do not predict prognosis. Schwartz et al. (8) calculated that the chance of being recurrence-free at 25 years is 65 percent. Even some patients who did not have total synovectomy were free of disease. Total synovectomy is still the treatment of choice.

MALIGNANT PIGMENTED VILLONODULAR SYNOVITIS

Definition. Malignant pigmented villonodular synovitis is a sarcoma arising in association with histologically documented pigmented villonodular synovitis or arising in a joint and having histologic features similar to those of pigmented villonodular synovitis.

General Features. Malignancy in a joint is so rare that it can be considered a medical curiosity. Some studies of pigmented villonodular synovitis did not find any bona fide examples of malignancy (13,15). Weiss and Goldblum (16) suggested diagnostic criteria similar to those for diagnosing malignancy in giant cell tumor, that is, a sarcoma arising in pigmented villonodular synovitis or at the site of a previously documented pigmented villonodular synovitis. Bertoni et al. (12) modified these criteria to include sarcomas clearly centered in a synovial membrane but with cytologic features similar to

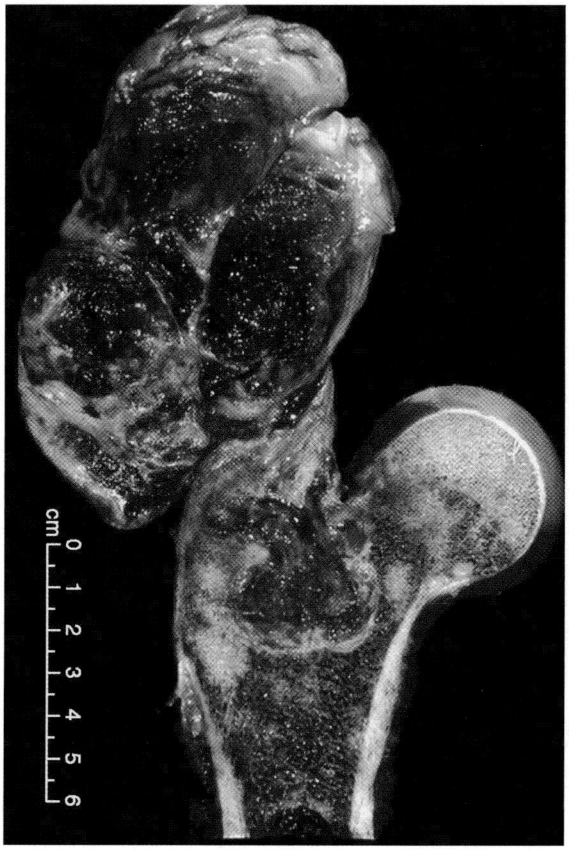

Figure 15-2

PIGMENTED VILLONODULAR SYNOVITIS

The extensive lesion of the hip joint is dark brown and yellow and invades the femur.

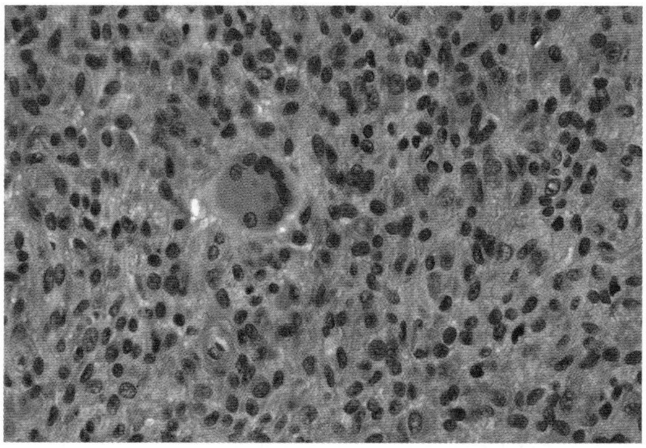

Figure 15-3

PIGMENTED VILLONODULAR SYNOVITIS

The presence of mononuclear cells with round to oval nuclei and eosinophilic cytoplasm is the diagnostic feature of pigmented villonodular synovitis. A multinucleated cell is also present.

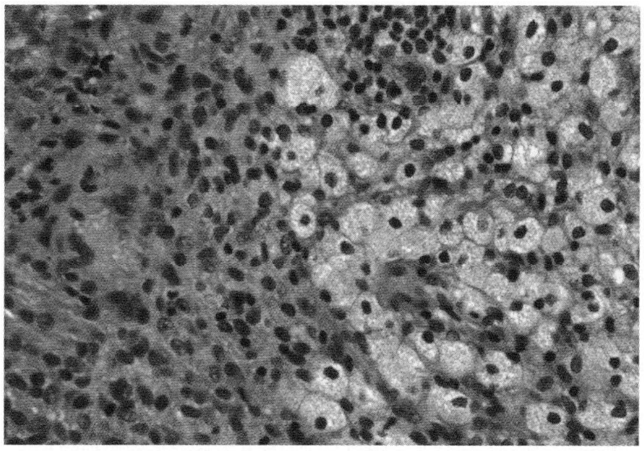

Figure 15-4

PIGMENTED VILLONODULAR SYNOVITIS

Foamy macrophages and lymphocytes are common findings.

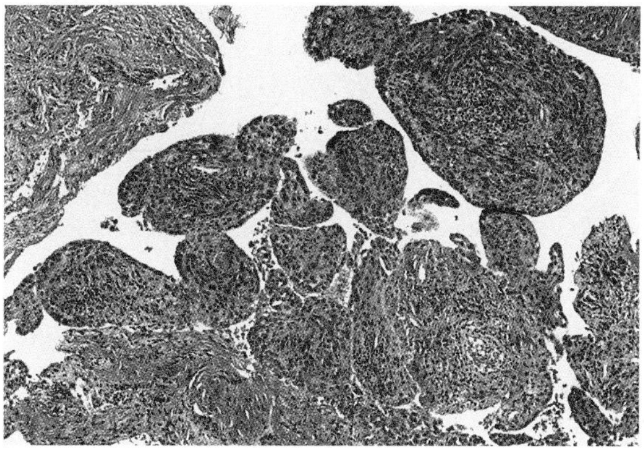

Figure 15-5

PIGMENTED VILLONODULAR SYNOVITIS

Low-power view illustrates villous hyperplasia. Hemosiderin is seen within many of the synovial nodules.

sarcomas arising in well-documented pigmented villonodular synovitis. Using these rules, Bertoni et al. reported on eight cases: three were secondary and five were primary. Layfield et al. (14) reported on two examples of malignant transformation of pigmented villonodular synovitis; both patients had received radiotherapy.

Clinical Features. There is a slight female predominance, and most patients are adults. The swelling of the joint is a consistent symptom and is sometimes associated with pain.

Sites. Many different joints have been reported to be involved, including the knee, ankle, and temporomandibular joint.

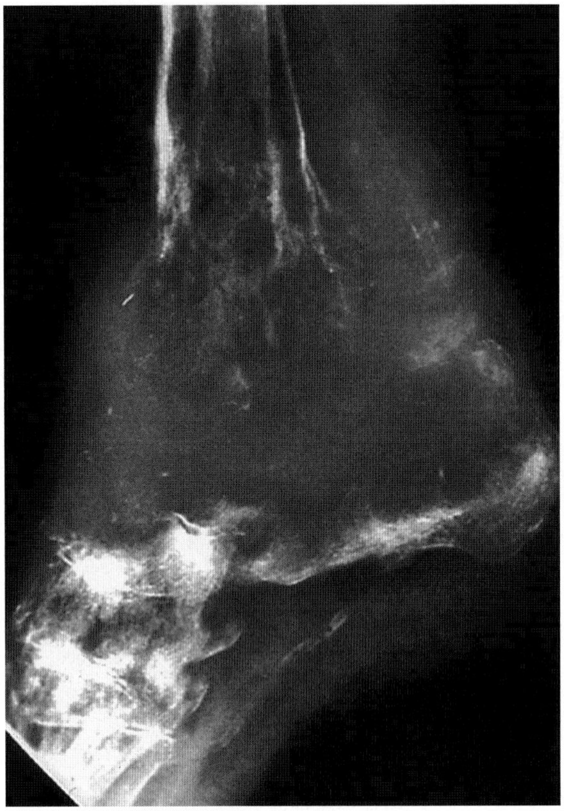

Figure 15-6

MALIGNANT PIGMENTED VILLONODULAR SYNOVITIS

An extensive destructive mass is centered in the joint.

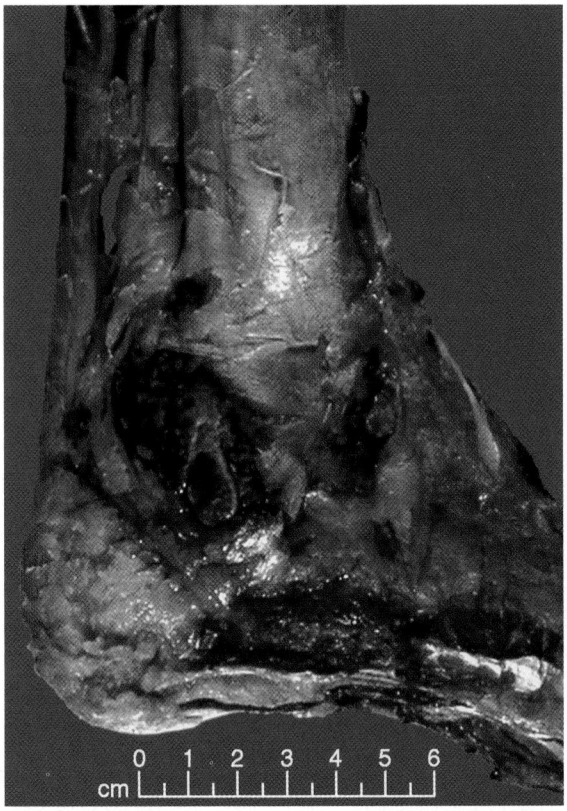

Figure 15-7

MALIGNANT PIGMENTED VILLONODULAR SYNOVITIS

An extensive lesion involves the ankle joint. The color of the lesion suggests pigmented villonodular synovitis.

Radiographic Findings. The radiographic findings are nonspecific and are essentially those of a large soft tissue mass (fig. 15-6).

Gross Findings. The tumor involves the joint cavity, but it almost always invades surrounding soft tissues or bone. The tumor consists of nodules of soft gray to yellow friable tissue (fig. 15-7).

Microscopic Findings. The tumor forms nodules that invade soft tissues. The tumor cells are uniform and have round nuclei, indistinct cell borders, and minimal pleomorphism. The cytoplasm is abundant and deep pink. Benign giant cells occur in clusters. The tumor cells are packed together tightly, and areas of infarct-like necrosis are always present (fig. 15-8).

Differential Diagnosis. Pigmented villonodular synovitis is the only diagnostic consideration. The sheet-like arrangement of uniform cells with deep eosinophilic cytoplasm is a feature of malignancy. Pigmented villonodular synovitis is polymorphic, with the proliferation containing different kinds of cells.

Treatment and Prognosis. Treatment consists of complete surgical removal of the involved joint, which may require amputation. The number of reports is not sufficient to draw conclusions about prognosis. Of the patients reported by Bertoni et al. (12), half died of pulmonary metastases.

SYNOVIAL CHONDROMATOSIS

Definition. Synovial chondromatosis is the formation of nodules of metaplastic cartilage under the surface of the synovial membrane in joints, tendons, and bursae (20).

General Features. The incidence of synovial chondromatosis is not known. Many terms have been used to describe the condition, including *synovial osteochondromatosis* and *synovial chondroma*. Moreover, the osteocartilaginous loose bodies due to conditions such as degenerative

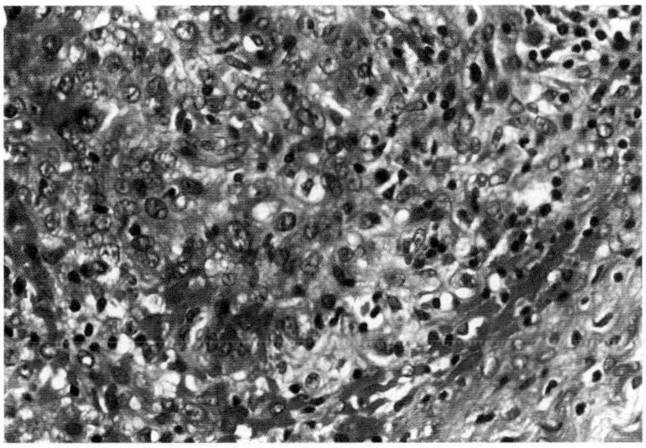

Figure 15-8

MALIGNANT PIGMENTED VILLONODULAR SYNOVITIS

There are diffuse, compact sheets of tumor cells.

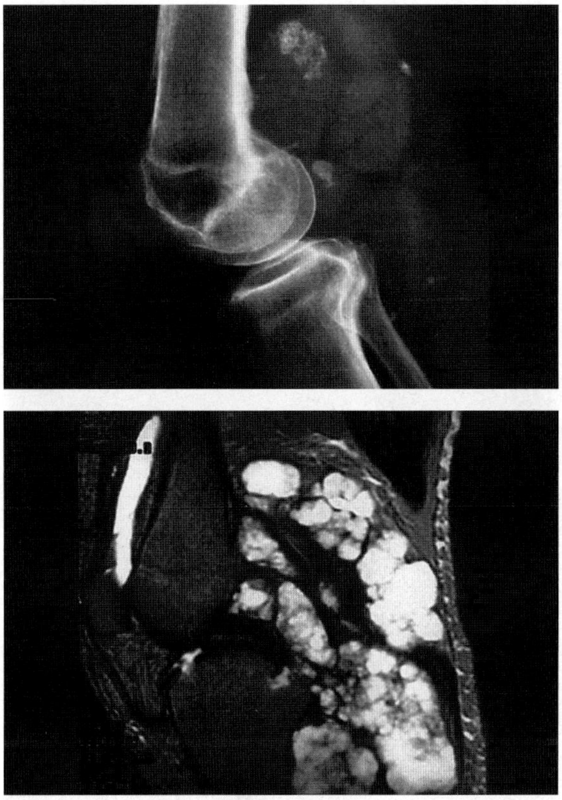

Figure 15-9

SYNOVIAL CHONDROMATOSIS

Top: Large lobulated mass in the popliteal space shows focal calcification.

Bottom: MRI shows extensive disease, with a lobulated mass that is bright on T_2-weighted images.

joint disease and osteochondritis dissecans have been included with synovial chondromatosis.

The cause is unknown. Davis et al. (18) studied the proliferative activity of the cartilage cells in synovial chondromatosis by labeling with Ki-67 and did not find labeling of the cells, which is consistent with a non-neoplastic condition. However, in 40 percent of cases of synovial chondromatosis, the cells were nondiploid, which is suggestive of a neoplastic process. The authors concluded that synovial chondromatosis lay somewhere between an enchondroma and chondrosarcoma.

Clinical Features. Pain is the most common symptom, followed by swelling. The duration of symptoms is quite variable. Patients are usually young adults, and there is a slight male predominance.

Sites. The knee is the most common site, followed by the hip. Unusual sites are the temporomandibular joint (17,21), soft tissues around joints (24), and bursae (23). The authors (KK Unni, LE Wold, CY Inwards, Mayo Clinic) have also seen rare examples in the facet joints of the vertebrae.

Radiographic Findings. Radiographs may be entirely normal or may show swelling of the soft tissue of the synovium. In typical cases, the joint contains radiopaque masses (fig. 15-9).

Gross Findings. The synovial membrane contains nodules of cartilage (fig. 15-10). These may be so numerous that the synovium is diffusely thickened and has a "cobblestone" appearance. Nodules of cartilage may break off and occur in the joint as loose bodies.

Microscopic Findings. Nodules of hyaline cartilage occur beneath a flattened synovial cell lining. The nodules contain clusters of chondrocytes and are separated by a matrix of hyaline cartilage (fig. 15-11). The chondrocytes almost always show nuclear enlargement and hyperchromasia (fig. 15-12). Double-nucleated cells are always present. Calcification in the form of powdery deposits between chondrocytes or as larger masses in the matrix is almost always present. Enchondral ossification may occur.

Genetics and Other Special Techniques. Clonal karyotypic abnormalities have been described in four cases of synovial chondromatosis; none appears specific for this entity (19,22).

Differential Diagnosis. Synovial chondromatosis has to be differentiated from osteocartilaginous loose bodies, which are secondary to degenerative joint disease. In the loose body, the

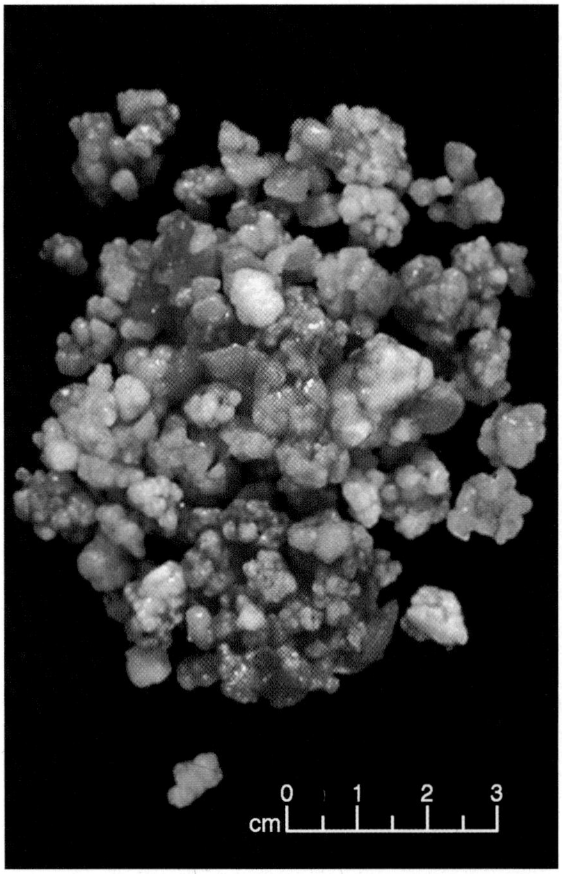

Figure 15-10

SYNOVIAL CHONDROMATOSIS

The gross specimen shows numerous light blue nodules of cartilage.

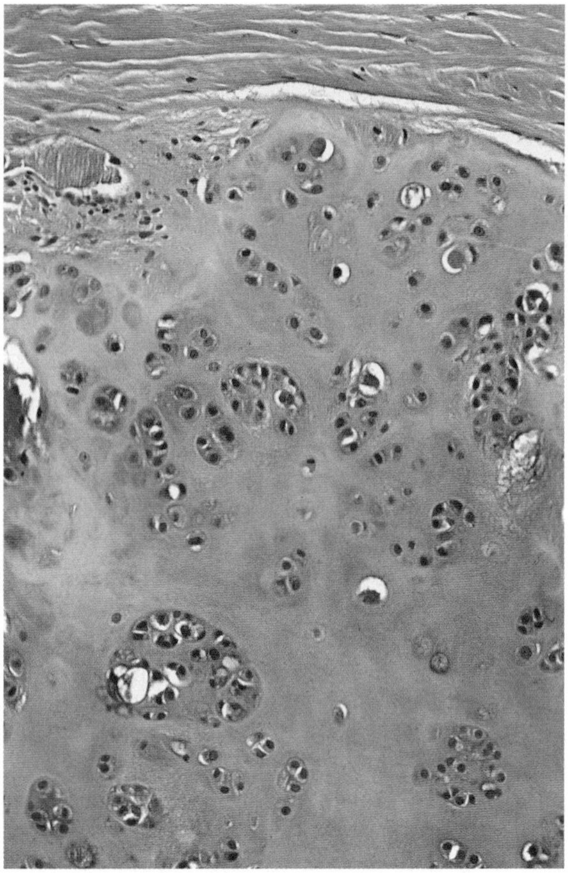

Figure 15-11

SYNOVIAL CHONDROMATOSIS

The chondrocytes are arranged in clusters separated by hyaline cartilage.

Figure 15-12

SYNOVIAL CHONDROMATOSIS

Prominent nuclear enlargement and binucleation are present. Out of context, these findings may be worrisome for malignancy. However, the chondrocytes maintain the clustering arrangement typical of synovial chondromatosis.

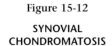

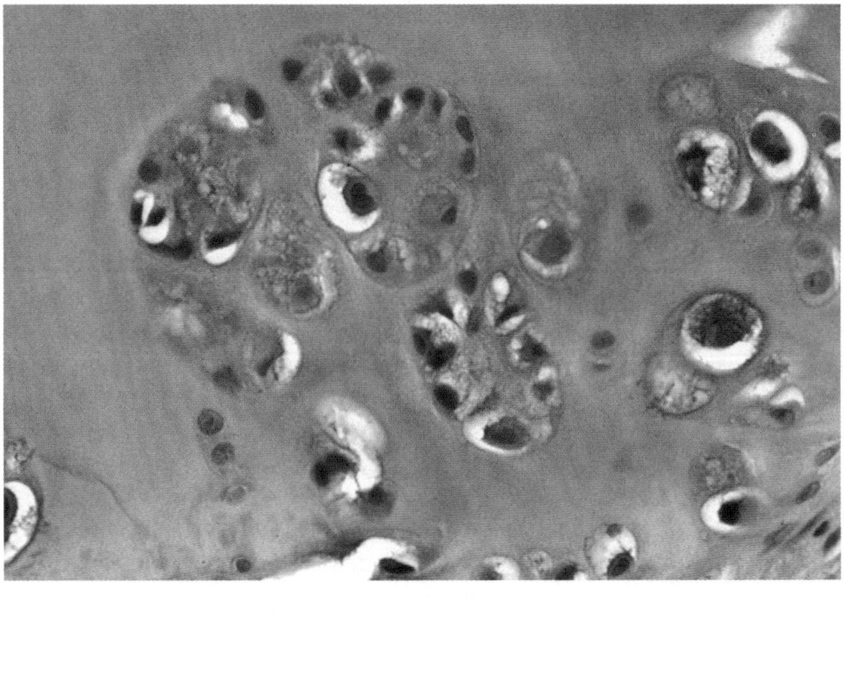

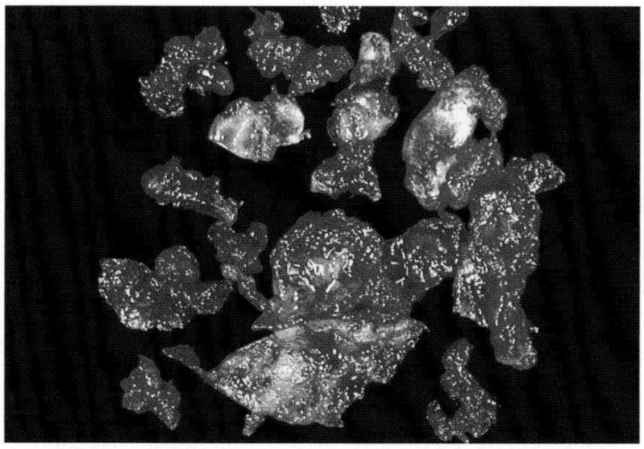

Figure 15-13

MALIGNANCY IN SYNOVIAL CHONDROMATOSIS

Although there are multiple nodules, as in synovial chondromatosis, the distinctly myxoid appearance strongly implies chondrosarcoma.

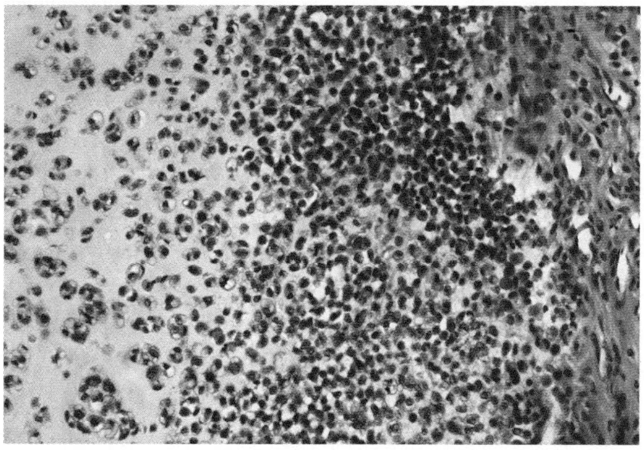

Figure 15-14

MALIGNANCY IN SYNOVIAL CHONDROMATOSIS

Dark hyperchromatic tumor cells lose the clustering arrangement to form a sheet-like pattern.

cartilage is hypocellular and has a layered effect (a central nidus of cartilage that seems to grow by the addition of concentric layers). The chondrocytes lack the neoplastic appearance of the ones seen in synovial chondromatosis.

Chondrosarcoma of bone may invade the synovium and simulate the appearance of synovial chondromatosis. Chondrosarcoma may even have the growth pattern of synovial chondromatosis. Clinical and radiographic evidence that the lesion in question is a bone tumor is the only distinguishing feature. Distinction from chondrosarcoma of the synovium is discussed with that entity, below.

Treatment and Prognosis. Complete surgical removal of the disease process is ideal; however, this may not be technically possible. The disease may recur in the joint and even erode into bone. Malignant change is uncommon (see below).

CHONDROSARCOMA OF SYNOVIUM

Definition. Chondrosarcoma of synovium is a malignancy of hyaline cartilage that arises in synovial chondromatosis or de novo in a synovial membrane.

General Features. Chondrosarcoma of synovium, either primary or secondary, is rare, and most reports are of single cases (26,27). The incidence of chondrosarcoma secondary to synovial chondromatosis is unknown.

Clinical Features. Patients complain of pain in the joint involved. There is a slight female predominance, and patients range in age from 30 to 70 years.

Sites. The knee is affected most often, followed by the hip. Other joints, including the ankle and elbow, have been reported to be involved (25).

Gross Findings. The joint cavity contains nodules of hyaline cartilage of various sizes. The nodules may have a distinctly mucoid or glistening appearance (fig. 15-13).

Microscopic Findings. Cartilaginous nodules are present within the synovium. Unlike the clustering arrangement typical of synovial chondromatosis, the chondrocytes have a sheet-like arrangement (fig. 15-14). The matrix may show marked myxoid change. Cytologic atypia is moderate to marked, and spindle cells may be present in the periphery of the chondroid lobules. When bone is involved, there is permeation of marrow spaces with entrapment of bony trabeculae. Foci of necrosis are frequent.

Differential Diagnosis. Synovial chondromatosis is frequently overdiagnosed as chondrosarcoma. The most important features favoring chondrosarcoma are: 1) marked myxoid change of the matrix; 2) sheet-like arrangement of the chondrocytes; 3) spindle cell proliferation; 4) permeation of bone; and 5) foci of necrosis.

Treatment and Prognosis. The involved joint needs to be removed, which may require amputation. The prognosis is poor: half of the patients reported by Bertoni et al. (25) died of metastatic disease.

HEMANGIOMA

Definition. Hemangioma is a benign vascular tumor of the synovium.

General Features. Tumors of the synovium are uncommon. During a 20-year period, 4,000 arthrotomies of the knee were performed at Mayo Clinic (28), of which only 95 yielded tumors. The majority of the tumors were pigmented villonodular synovitis or synovial chondromatosis. Only 11 hemangiomas were identified.

Clinical Features. Patients complain of pain, usually of long duration.

Sites. The knee is the site affected most commonly, although other joints, such as the shoulder and ankle, may be affected.

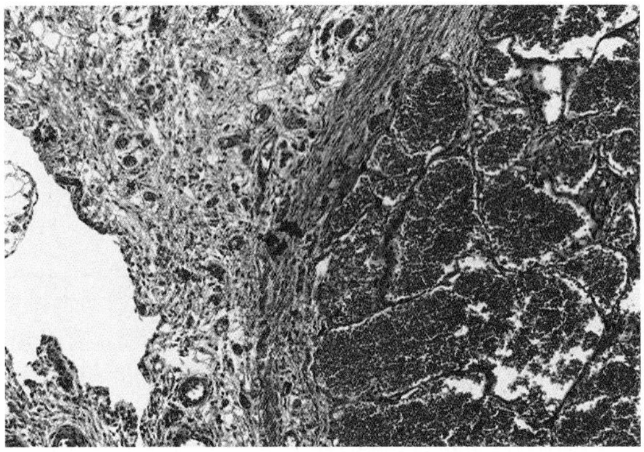

Figure 15-15

HEMANGIOMA

A tumefactive vascular proliferation involves the synovial membrane.

Radiographic Findings. Radiographs do not show specific features.

Gross Findings. The synovium appears boggy and rust colored.

Microscopic Findings. There is a proliferation of vessels, either capillary or cavernous, in the synovium (fig. 15-15).

Treatment and Prognosis. Complete surgical removal of the involved area of synovium is indicated.

LIPOMA

Definition. Lipoma is a benign neoplasm of mature adipose tissue involving the synovium.

General Features. Lipomas of the synovium are rare. Only eight lipomas of the knee were reported in a series of 4,000 arthrotomies reported from Mayo Clinic (29).

Clinical Features. Patients complain of swelling of the joint.

Sites. The knee is affected most often.

Radiographic Findings. Plain radiographs show diffuse swelling. MRI shows signal changes similar to those of subcutaneous fat.

Gross Findings. The synovium is thickened, boggy, and yellow and has excrescences on its surface (lipoma arborescens).

Microscopic Findings. The synovial membrane is filled with mature adipose tissue (fig. 15-16).

Treatment and Prognosis. Complete removal of the synovium involved by the tumor is necessary. The prognosis is excellent, and recurrence is unusual.

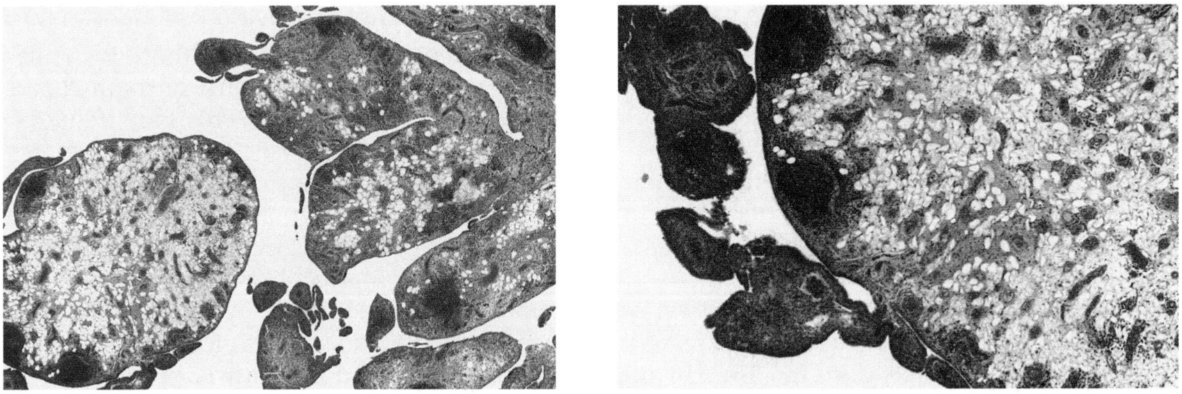

Figure 15-16

LIPOMA

Synovial hyperplasia with expansion of the synovial tissue by abundant mature adipose tissue.

REFERENCES

Pigmented Villonodular Synovitis

1. Dorwart RH, Genant HK, Johnston WH, Morris JM. Pigmented villonodular synovitis of synovial joints: clinical, pathologic, and radiologic features. AJR Am J Roentgenol 1984;143:877–85.
2. Giannini C, Scheithauer BW, Wenger DE, Unni KK. Pigmented villonodular synovitis of the spine: a clinical, radiological, and morphological study of 12 cases. J Neurosurg 1996;84:592–7.
3. Granowitz SP, D'Antonio J, Mankin HL. The pathogenesis and long-term end results of pigmented villonodular synovitis. Clin Orthop 1976;114:335–51.
4. Kindblom LG, Gunterberg B. Pigmented villonodular synovitis involving bone. A case report. J Bone Joint Surg Am 1978;60:830–2.
5. Layfield LJ, Meloni-Ehrig A, Liu K, Shepard R, Harrelson JM. Malignant giant cell tumor of synovium (malignant pigmented villonodular synovitis). Arch Pathol Lab Med 2000;124:1636–41.
6. Pantazopoulos T, Stavrou Z, Stamos C, Kehayas G, Hartofilakidis-Garofalidis G. Bone lesions in pigmented villonodular synovitis. Acta Orthop Scand 1975;46:579–92.
7. Pulitzer DR, Reed RJ. Localized pigmented villonodular synovitis of the vertebral column. Arch Pathol Lab Med 1984;108:228–30.
8. Schwartz HS, Unni KK, Pritchard DJ. Pigmented villonodular synovitis. A retrospective review of affected large joints. Clin Orthop 1989;247:243–55.
9. Sciot R, Rosai J, Dal Cin P, et al. Analysis of 35 cases of localized and diffuse tenosynovial giant cell tumor: a report from the Chromosomes and Morphology (CHAMP) study group. Mod Pathol 1999;12:576–9.
10. Tanaka K, Suzuki M, Nameki H, Sugiyama H. Pigmented villonodular synovitis of the temporomandibular joint. Arch Otolaryngol Head Neck Surg 1997;123:536–9.
11. Weidner N, Challa VR, Bonsib SM, Davis CH Jr, Carrol TJ Jr. Giant cell tumors of synovium (pigmented villonodular synovitis) involving the vertebral column. Cancer 1986;57:2030–6.

Malignant Pigmented Villonodular Synovitis

12. Bertoni F, Unni KK, Beabout JW, Sim FH. Malignant giant cell tumor of the tendon sheaths and joints (malignant pigmented villonodular synovitis). Am J Surg Pathol 1997;21:153–63.
13. Granowitz SP, D'Antonio J, Mankin HL. The pathogenesis and long-term end results of pigmented villonodular synovitis. Clin Orthop 1976;114:335–51.
14. Layfield LJ, Meloni-Ehrig A, Liu K, Shepard R, Harrelson JM. Malignant giant cell tumor of synovium (malignant pigmented villonodular synovitis). Arch Pathol Lab Med 2000;124:1636–41.
15. Schwartz HS, Unni KK, Pritchard DJ. Pigmented villonodular synovitis. A retrospective review of affected large joints. Clin Orthop 1989;247:243–55.
16. Weiss SW, Goldblum JR. Benign tumors and tumor-like lesions of synovial tissue. In: Weiss SW, Goldblum JR, eds. Enzinger and Weiss's soft tissue tumors, 4th ed. St. Louis: Mosby; 2001:1054–6.

Synovial Chondromatosis

17. Blankestijn J, Panders AK, Vermey A, Scherpbier AJ. Synovial chondromatosis of the temporomandibular joint. Report of three cases and a review of the literature. Cancer 1985;55:479–85.
18. Davis RI, Foster H, Arthur K, Trewin S, Hamilton PW, Biggart DJ. Cell proliferation studies in primary synovial chondromatosis. J Pathol 1998;184:18–23.
19. Mertens F, Jonsson K, Willen H, et al. Chromosome rearrangements in synovial chondromatous lesions. Br J Cancer 1996;74:251-4.
20. Murphy FP, Dahlin DC, Sullivan CR. Articular synovial chondromatosis. J Bone Joint Surg Am 1962;44:77–86.
21. Ronald JB, Keller EE, Weiland LH. Synovial chondromatosis of the temporomandibular joint. J Oral Surg 1978;36:13–9.
22. Sciot R, Dal Cin P, Bellemans J, Samson I, Van den Berghe H, Van Damme B. Synovial chondromatosis: clonal chromosome changes provide further evidence for a neoplastic disorder. Virchows Arch 1998;433:189–91.
23. Sim FH, Dahlin DC, Ivins JC. Extra-articular synovial chondromatosis. J Bone Joint Surg Am 1977;59:492–5.
24. Sviland L, Malcolm AJ. Synovial chondromatosis presenting as painless soft tissue mass—a report of 19 cases. Histopathology 1995;27:275–9.

Chondrosarcoma of Synovium

25. Bertoni F, Unni KK, Beabout JW, Sim FH. Chondrosarcomas of the synovium. Cancer 1991;67: 155–62.
26. Hamilton A, Davis RI, Nixon JR. Synovial chondrosarcoma complicating synovial chondromatosis. Report of a case and review of the literature. J Bone Joint Surg Am 1987;69:1084–8.
27. Perry BE, McQueen DA, Lin JJ. Synovial chondromatosis with malignant degeneration to chondrosarcoma. Report of a case. J Bone Joint Surg Am 1988;70:1259–61.

Hemangioma

28. Coventry MB, Harrison EG Jr, Martin JF. Benign synovial tumors of the knee: a diagnostic problem. J Bone Joint Surg Am 1966;48:1350–8.

Lipoma

29. Coventry MB, Harrison EG Jr, Martin JF. Benign synovial tumors of the knee: a diagnostic problem. J Bone Joint Surg Am 1966;48:1350–8.

Index*

*Numbers in boldface indicate table and figure pages.

D

E

F

G

H

I

K

L

M